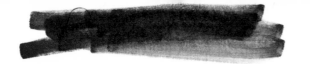

MICHAEL C. GERALD, Ph.D.

*Division of Pharmacology, College of Pharmacy,
The Ohio State University, Columbus, Ohio*

FREDA V. O'BANNON, R.N., M.S.

*Department of Nursing, California State University
at Los Angeles, Los Angeles, California*

NURSING PHARMACOLOGY AND THERAPEUTICS

Prentice-Hall, Inc., Englewood Cliffs, New Jersey 07632

Library of Congress Cataloging in Publication Data

Gerald, Michael C (date)

    Nursing pharmacology and therapeutics.

    Includes bibliographies and index.
    1. Pharmacology.   2. Chemotherapy.   3. Nursing.
I. O'Bannon, Freda V., joint author.   II. Title.
[DNLM: 1. Pharmacology—Nursing texts.   2. Drug
therapy—Nursing texts.   QV 4 G354n]
RM300.G45   615'.1   80-27022
ISBN   0-13-627505-2

Printed in the United States of America

10 9 8 7 6 5 4 3 2

Editorial production/supervision by Ellen W. Caughey
Interior design by Janet Schmid and Ellen W. Caughey
Cover design by Janet Schmid
Manufacturing buyer: John B. Hall

Prentice-Hall International, Inc., *London*

Prentice-Hall of Australia Pty. Limited, *Sydney*

Prentice-Hall of Canada, Ltd., *Toronto*

Prentice-Hall of India Private Limited, *New Delhi*

Prentice-Hall of Japan, Inc., *Tokyo*

Prentice-Hall of Southeast Asia Pte. Ltd., *Singapore*

Whitehall Books Limited, *Wellington, New Zealand*

Contents

Section III
DRUGS AFFECTING THE CENTRAL NERVOUS SYSTEM   78

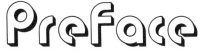

Preface

The nurse in contemporary practice is called upon to perform expertly a wide variety of drug-related activities. These include dispensing and administering medications; monitoring, recording, critically evaluating, and reporting the response of patients to drugs; providing emergency care to combat the adverse effects of drugs or poisonous chemicals; educating the patient about the safe, rational, and effective use and self-administration of prescription and nonprescription drugs; and participating in the management and rehabilitation of drug- and alcohol-dependent patients and counseling them and the members of their family.

To discharge successfully these very diverse responsibilities, the nurse must understand why a drug is being administered or being withheld, and he or she must be capable of monitoring the beneficial effects of that medication as well as anticipating, recognizing, and initiating appropriate measures to minimize drug-induced adverse effects. This text presents these therapeutic considerations and the nursing implications associated with each major class of drugs. Full appreciation of the therapeutic applications (and limitations) of the drugs currently in the clinics and those that will make their debut at some future date can only be achieved after the nurse has mastered the fundamental principles underlying drug action—namely, pharmacology. To facilitate this learning, we have presented essential background material in physiology, biochemistry, pathophysiology, and disease.

We have endeavored to prepare an introductory text that presents contemporary concepts of pharmacology and their therapeutic applications in nursing practice. While primarily intended to complement or supplement the lectures presented in a one-quarter or one-semester course, the text may be used by nursing graduates who are reading independently to maintain their competency on drug therapy.

All major classes of therapeutic agents are included, primarily arranged according to their pharmacological classification. While at first glance the reader may be overwhelmed by the number of drugs available in a given class, closer analysis reveals that a very large proportion of these drugs possesses properties that are strikingly similar to a limited number of prototype members of that group. To avoid redundancy and trivial detail, and to satisfy our objective to prepare an introductory text that is concise, readable, and stimulating, emphasis has been placed on the actions, effects, and therapeutic uses of these prototype drugs; the unique properties of similar drugs are summarized in tabular form.

Entries for individual drugs include their common names and trade names, usual doses and routes of administration, and those properties that distinguish a drug from the prototype drug and other members of the same class. Such tables provide the nurse with a readily accessible source of reference material. Table 1-1 contains a comprehensive, comparative guide to a wide variety of disparate sources of highly detailed drug information. The nurse will commonly encounter Latin abbreviations on the medication order—called a *prescription* in an ambulatory setting and a *physician*'s *order* in the hospital. We have employed these abbreviations in our tables to designate dosage and routes of administration. The two tables, located immediately after this preface, contain these standard abbreviations and equivalent volumes and weights, respectively.

This text, divided into nine sections of varying length, has been designed to provide the instructor with considerable flexibility concerning the selection of topics and the order in which subjects are presented or assigned for reading. Chapters 1 and 2 in Section I introduce the general principles that provide an essential basic foundation for the study of pharmacology and therapeutics, while Chapter 3 examines the administration of drugs. Drugs affecting the autonomic nervous system are discussed in Section II. Because of the inherent complexity of this area, some instructors may prefer to postpone consideration of this material to a later date in the syllabus.

The pharmacology and therapeutics of a wide range of central nervous system drugs are discussed in Section III. While skeletal muscle relaxants, local anesthetics, and nonnarcotic analgesics (aspirin-like drugs) do not primarily act by altering central function, we have placed them in this section because of therapeutic considerations. The nurse must be prepared to deal effectively with the many challenging problems arising from the nontherapeutic use of drugs and mind-altering chemicals. A general overview of drug misuse and abuse is presented in Chapter 24; the specific effects and potential dangers associated with the intemperate use of alcohol and the psychotomimetics and marihuana are discussed in Chapters 14 and 23, respectively. The abuse potential of clinically employed drugs is presented in their respective chapters.

Drugs used for the treatment of cardiovascular disorders, to alter the coagulability of blood, and to promote urine formation, appear in Section IV. Section V is concerned with the use of natural and synthetic hormones and hormone antagonists for the treatment of endocrine and nonendocrine disorders, as contraceptive agents, and to terminate pregnancy. Vitamins and antianemic agents are also included in this section.

Chemotherapeutic agents—drugs used for the management and cure of diseases caused by bacteria, fungi, viruses, protozoa, worms, and malignant cells—and chemicals employed to destroy microbes on skin surfaces and inanimate objects are discussed in Section VI. Drug treatment of allergic disorders and asthma and the management of peptic ulcer disease, constipation, and diarrhea appear in Sections VII and VIII, respectively. The final section examines the problem of acute chemical poisoning and its emergency treatment.

Sections II to IX are largely self-contained and, therefore, may be presented in any order. Moreover, the sequence of assignment of chapters within Sections II to VI may be altered. We strongly recommend, however, that students be first exposed to the material contained in section introductions, found in Chapters 4, 9, 25, 33, and 41. These chapters provide sufficient physiological and pharmacological background and terminology to permit the reader to comprehend more readily the succeeding chapters in that section. Some instructors might find it desirable to summarize the general principles of neuropharmacology (Chapter 4) and then proceed directly to Sections III and/or IV immediately after Section I.

Every effort has been made to check the accuracy of the contents of this book, in particular, the dosage schedules appearing in the tables. Not infrequently, however, changes are made in the recommended schedules. Hence, we strongly urge the nurse to consult the latest drug product package insert prior to administering any drug.

Many students and professional colleagues have generously provided helpful comments on and criticisms of earlier drafts of this book. The authors wish to express particular thanks to Dr. Ralf G. Rahwan who served as a frequent sounding board on many aspects and problems arising during the preparation of this text and whose critical eye scrutinized the entire manuscript. Our warm thanks are also extended to Mr. Fred Henry and Ms. Ellen Caughey and the staff of Prentice-Hall for their assistance and kind support throughout all stages of the evolution of this book.

This book is dedicated with love to Gloria, Marc, and Melissa Gerald and to the O'Bannon daughters—Kathie Davidson, Kim Garver, and Kolleen Squires.

MICHAEL C. GERALD
FREDA V. O'BANNON

Commonly Used Abbreviations

aa	of each	O.S.	left eye
a.c.	before meals	os	mouth
ad lib.	freely, as desired	O.U.	both eyes
b.i.d.	two times a day	oz.	ounce
c̄	with	p.c.	after meals
cap.	capsule	PO	by mouth
d or da.	day	PR	by rectum
dr	dram	PRN	when required
elix. or el.	elixir	q.	every
ext.	extract	q.d.	every day
g	gram	q.h.	every hour
gr	grain	q.i.d.	four times daily
gtt	a drop	q.o.d.	every other day
h	hour	q.s.	as much as required
h.s.	hour of sleep, bedtime	s.	without
IM or i.m.	intramuscular	SC or s.c.	subcutaneous
IV or i.v.	intravenous	s.o.s.	one dose if necessary
m.	minim	sp.	spirits
ml	milliliter	ss	one-half
o.d.	every day	stat.	immediately
O.D.	right eye	tab.	tablet
o.h.	every hour	t.i.d.	three times a day
o.n.	every night	tr.	tinct., tincture
		ung.	ointment

Commonly Used Approximate Equivalents

Volume

Metric	Apothecary	Household
1 ml (1 cc)	15 minims	20 drops
4 ml	1 dram	
5 ml		1 teaspoon (tsp)
15 ml		1 tablespoon (tbsp)
30 ml	1 fluid ounce (fl oz)	2 tablespoons
60 ml	2 fl oz	1 wineglass
250 ml	8 fl oz	1 measuring cup = 1 glass
500 ml	1 pint = 16 fl oz	
1000 ml = 1 liter (ℓ)	1 quart = 32 fl oz	
4000 ml	1 gallon = 4 quarts	

Weight

Metric	Apothecary
1000 μg = 1 mg	$\frac{1}{60}$ gr (gr)
60 mg	1 gr
1 g	15.4 gr
4 g	60 gr (1 dram)
30 g	1 ounce (oz)
454 g	1 pound (lb)
1000 g = 1 kg	2.2 lb

Temperature

To convert Centigrade to Fahrenheit:

$$F = \frac{9 \times C}{5} + 32$$

To convert Fahrenheit to Centigrade:

$$C = (F - 32) \times \tfrac{5}{9}$$

Section 1

GENERAL PRINCIPLES OF PHARMACOLOGY

Chapter 1

INTRODUCTION TO DRUGS

Information about drugs is of interest to all members of society regardless of their academic major, profession, or vocation. Rarely does a week pass without media reports of adverse drug reactions, medication complications arising from the use of oral contraceptives, antidiabetic or antianxiety drugs, the potential toxicity associated with food additives, marihuana or pesticides, and the experimental use of hallucinogens by governmental agencies.

Regardless of where a nurse practices, drug information is not only of general interest but is essential. Functioning autonomously—although most often in cooperation and collaboration with physicians and phar-

macists—the nurse may at times be professionally engaged in one or more of the following drug-related activities.

—Dispensing and administering medications to the patient in a hospital or an outpatient medical facility.

—Monitoring, recording, evaluating, and reporting the patient's response to drugs. When necessary, the nurse should be prepared to withhold medication or recommend to the physician a change in dosage or choice of drugs to prevent or reduce the severity of an adverse drug reaction or to maximize the benefits of the medication administered. The nurse neither administers digitalis when the

patient has a slow pulse rate nor injects insulin to the diabetic experiencing a hypoglycemic reaction. The nurse recommends that the physician reduce the dosage of a barbiturate used to produce nighttime sedation when a previously active patient is lethargic all day. Upon evaluating the results of laboratory tests, the nurse may suggest that a potassium supplement be initiated or that an alternative antibiotic be utilized when the culture reveals pathogen resistance to the drug employed.

—*Providing emergency treatment* to an individual with respiratory depression and coma caused by taking an overdose of heroin or other central nervous system depressant, or calming the patient experiencing a marihuana-induced panic reaction.

—*Educating the patient* about the possible dangers associated with indiscriminate self-medication during pregnancy; the benefits versus the risks of nonprescription drugs, including vitamins, laxatives, and antacids; the inadvisability of taking certain drugs or foods in conjunction with the prescribed medications, such as alcoholic beverages with barbiturates or antihistamines; the potential temporary impairment of mental and physical function after initiating therapy with antipsychotic drugs; the practical ways of minimizing undesirable minor but highly distressful drug-induced side effects such as dry mouth or nausea; the side effects signaling the onset of a severe adverse drug reaction that should be brought to the physician's attention; the proper storage of drugs to prevent loss of potency or accidental ingestion by children.

—*Counseling individuals* enrolled in a methadone maintenance program or providing support to an alcoholic or to the family of an alcoholic.

In this chapter we shall examine the meaning of the terms *pharmacology*, *therapeutics*, and *toxicology*; we shall also consider the general effects produced by drugs, the mechanisms responsible for these effects, and how drugs are used for the treatment of disease.

WHAT IS PHARMACOLOGY?

Pharmacology is the study of drugs. While for the most part we shall consider the term *drug* to be synonymous with medication or a chemical used for the treatment of disease, the limited boundaries imposed by this definition would soon be outgrown. The nonmedical use of heroin, alcohol, and marihuana, the treatment of accidental poisoning by insecticides, and the use of oral contraceptives to prevent pregnancy (not generally perceived to be a disease) all represent areas of interest and importance to the nurse. Let us then expand our definition and consider a drug to be any chemical, excluding food, that interacts with living organisms to produce a response. As you can observe, this definition does not distinguish between a desirable interaction that is of benefit to the patient and an undesirable or adverse interaction that harms the patient.

Therapeutics is a general term describing the *use of drugs in the treatment of disease.* This term can be modified to describe the use of drugs for specific types of diseases; for example, psychotherapeutic and chemotherapeutic agents refer to drugs used for the management of behavioral disorders and infectious diseases, respectively.

One of the most fundamental principles of pharmacology states that *all drugs are potential poisons* when taken in sufficiently high doses. Some of these toxic effects represent an intensification of the normal therapeutic effects of the drug, while other adverse effects may be unrelated to it. For example, therapeutic doses of barbiturates produce sedation and sleep, while toxic doses intensify depression of the central nervous system, producing coma. By contrast, skin rash and other allergic responses are unrelated to the therapeutic effects of barbiturates. *Toxicology* is the study of poisons and the treatment of poisoning; the boundaries circumscribing this science and those of pharmacology are often indistinct.

The rational use of drugs for the management of disease—therapeutics—is predicated upon an understanding of *pharmacodynamics*. This experimental science seeks to determine where a drug acts in the body (on what system, organ, tissue) and how it acts, that is, the physiological or biochemical mechanism responsible for the observed drug effects. Pharmacodynamics also deals with the absorption, distribution, metabolism, and eventual elimination of drugs.

unique medical problem and the therapeutic objectives sought by the physician.

The biological effects produced by a drug are the consequence of an interaction between that drug and some part of the living organism. These interactions may be highly specific and selective or, in other cases, relatively nonspecific. These general mechanisms are responsible for the therapeutic and toxicologic effects that you will observe in your patients.

Drug-Receptor Interactions

Some drugs that are highly potent—that is, produce their effects at very low doses—are

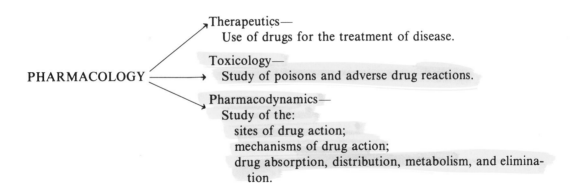

MECHANISMS
OF DRUG ACTION

One of the most fundamental principles of pharmacology is that *no drug produces one and only one effect*. Since drugs are not completely specific in their effects, it is useful for us to differentiate between the primary and secondary effects of drugs. The *primary effect* of a drug is the desired therapeutic effect; it is the effect that the physician seeks to achieve when prescribing the medication. *Secondary effects* are all other effects produced by the drug; these may be considered to be desirable or undesirable depending upon each patient's

thought to act by specifically combining with chemical groups on the surface of the cell or within the cell. These chemical groups or molecules with which the drug interacts to produce an effect are called the *pharmacological receptors*.

Classically, drug-receptor interactions have been described as being analogous to a lock and key. Just as few keys fit a given lock, so too do few drugs interact with a given receptor. Selected keys fit the lock and turn the tumblers, while others fit the keyhole but are incapable of opening the lock. In a similar manner, some drugs interact with the receptor to produce a pharmacological response; such

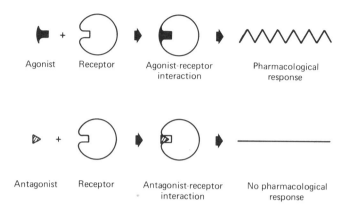

Figure 1-1. Drug-Receptor Interactions. The agonist is theorized to be capable of neatly fitting and interacting with the receptor site to produce a pharmacological response. On the other hand, the antagonist only partially fits the receptor site; its structure is such that it is unable to cause an effect. By preventing the agonist from combining with the receptor, it prevents the agonist-induced effects.

drugs are called *agonists*. By contrast, when an *antagonist* interacts with the receptor, no response is produced; moreover, in the presence of the antagonist drug, the response normally produced by the agonist is reduced or totally prevented (Figure 1-1).

The terms *affinity* and *intrinsic activity* are sometimes used to describe the nature of the drug-receptor interaction. *Affinity* refers to the tendency of a drug to combine with its receptor. *Intrinsic activity* or *efficacy* relates to the capacity of a drug to produce a pharmacological response after it has interacted with the receptor. An *agonist* is a drug that has both affinity and intrinsic activity, while an *antagonist* has affinity but lacks intrinsic activity. Two agonists interacting with a common receptor may produce an equivalent pharmacological effect at markedly different doses. While many reasonable explanations of this difference are possible, the more potent drug (that is, the drug producing its effects at the lower dose) may have greater intrinsic activity for the receptor.

(The clinical significance [or lack thereof] of differences in drug potency will be discussed later.)

Atropine and *d*-tubocurarine are antagonists of acetylcholine, and their therapeutic uses as an antiulcer and as a preoperative muscle relaxant, respectively, are predicated upon antagonism of this naturally occurring agonist. Many authorities believe that the antipsychotic effects of chlorpromazine are the result of this drug's ability to block dopamine receptor sites located in the brain. Antihistamines, drugs used for the management of allergic disorders, antagonize the actions of histamine by blocking its receptors.

Drug-Enzyme Interactions

Many drugs have been shown to produce their effects by modifying the function of enzymes, the indispensable biological catalysts. Inhibitors of the enzyme acetylcholinesterase prevent the breakdown and inactivation of acetylcholine and are used for the treatment of glaucoma; other chemicals acting by this same mechanism are employed as insecticides and as potential chemical warfare agents. Inhibitors of the enzymes monoamine oxidase and carbonic anhydrase are used for the treatment of depression and as diuretics for the removal of excessive body water, respectively.

Antimetabolites

By a series of specific biochemical reactions, living organisms are capable of converting simple starting materials into end products (metabolites) that are essential for their survival. *Antimetabolites* are drugs that resemble natural chemicals required for the biosynthesis of the essential metabolites. These drugs compete with the natural chemical and, when incorporated into the biosynthetic pathway in preference to the natural product, result in the formation of an end product that the living organism is incapable of utilizing to sustain life. Examples of commonly employed antimetabolites include the anticancer drug methotrexate and the sulfonamides ("sulfa drugs") used to combat bacterial infections.

Chelating Agents

The term *chelate*, derived from a Greek word meaning *crab's claw*, aptly describes the manner by which chelating agents grasp toxic metals present in the body to form drug-metal complexes that are nontoxic and readily eliminated. Chelating agents are used as specific antidotes for the treatment of poisoning by such heavy metals as arsenic, lead, mercury, and iron.

Drug Actions on Cell Membranes

The membrane surrounding cells selectively permits the passage of ions, nutrients, and other essential chemicals into the cell, while simultaneously excluding other substances.

The juvenile diabetic patient lacks insulin, a hormone required for glucose to go from the blood into most cells. Certain antiepileptic drugs, such as phenytoin (Dilantin), reduce the intracellular sodium and calcium content of the motor areas of the cerebral cortex. This action reduces the excitability of these nerves, which is thought to be responsible for the observed reduction in seizures. In some instances, drugs interact with receptors located on the membrane, and it is this drug-receptor interaction that is responsible for the change in membrane permeability.

Nonspecific Drug Actions

The pharmacological effects of some drugs may result from their relatively nonspecific chemical or physical properties. Iodine tincture is used to kill microbes on the surface of the skin, but as the result of its lack of specificity, healthy cells are also destroyed. Antiseptics such as iodine tincture are called *protoplasmic poisons* and act by precipitation and inactivation of protoplasmic proteins. The main ingredient of one class of nonprescription appetite suppressants is a nondigestible gum. When such products are taken with a glass of water, the gum swells in the stomach and creates a feeling of fullness, thus diminishing the desire to eat.

CATEGORIZATION OF DRUG ACTIONS

Let us now turn our attention from the mechanisms responsible for the actions of drugs to the general types of actions that drugs may have on organs, tissues, or cells. All drugs act by stimulating or depressing the functions of specific organs, replacing a deficiency of an essential chemical, killing or weakening invading foreign organisms or rapidly proliferating cells, or causing irritation. This simple categorization is not as definitive as it appears; you will find numerous examples of drugs throughout this text that fit into more than one category. Note that these actions are *not* therapeutic uses of drugs, which represent the ultimate applications of these actions for the treatment of disease.

Stimulation and Depression

Drugs may stimulate (increase) or depress (decrease) the physiological function of specific organs. Amphetamine and caffeine are stimulants of the brain, while phenobarbital and alcohol are depressants. The beneficial therapeutic effects of digitalis in the treatment of congestive heart failure have been attributed to the ability of this drug to stimulate the force of contraction of the heart while depressing the heart rate.

Replacement

Drugs may serve to replace essential body compounds that are either absent or present in less than ideal concentrations. Treatment of many endocrine disorders, such as administration of insulin to the diabetic or estrogen to the menopausal female, is predicated upon replacement therapy. In geographic areas where seafood containing iodine does not represent a regular component of the diet, hypothyroid conditions are often observed. Addition of small amounts of iodine to table salt is used to prevent such thyroid disorders.

Killing Foreign Organisms

Chemotherapeutic agents act by killing or preventing the multiplication of such disease-causing organisms as bacteria, worms, protozoa, viruses, and fungi. The effectiveness of antibiotics in the treatment of bacterial diseases cannot be attributed exclusively to the ability of these drugs to kill or inactivate bacteria; for these drugs to be maximally ef-fective, the body's immune defense mechanisms must be functioning. Antineoplastic (anticancer) agents kill or inhibit rapidly reproducing cells.

Irritation

A diverse group of drugs acts relatively non-specifically by producing irritation. Methyl salicylate (oil of wintergreen) is found in most liniments used to relieve the local pain associated with aching muscles. This compound stimulates local blood flow and produces relief of pain by causing irritation at the site of application on the skin.

TIME-RESPONSE AND DOSE-RESPONSE CONSIDERATIONS

Time-Response Relationships

Some drugs produce the desired therapeutic effects within minutes after they are administered, while others must be administered for days before their beneficial effects become evident. Three basic parameters are used to evaluate time-response relationships. The *latency* or *onset of drug action* denotes the time it takes for a drug to produce an observable effect after its administration. The *peak time* is the time required for a drug to produce its greatest effects, and the *duration of action* is the period of time a drug continues to produce its effects after it has been administered.

The nurse will observe that not all insulin preparations are equivalent. The major distinguishing characteristic of these products is based upon their time-response relationships. While regular insulin has an onset of action of less than one hour after injection and produces effects which persist for 5 to 8 hours, protamine zinc insulin exhibits its initial effects after 4 to 6 hours and continues to lower blood sugar levels for 24 to 36 hours after a single dose.

Some of the time-response factors under the direct control of the clinician include how the drug is administered (intravenous injection versus oral preparations) and what dosage form is employed (tablet versus liquid), both of which influence the rate at which the drug enters the bloodstream. Time-response parameters influenced by the unique pathophysiological state of the patient include distribution of the drug to its site of action and the rate at which the drug is chemically inactivated (metabolized) and ultimately removed (excreted) from the body. In the next two chapters, these factors will be discussed in detail.

Dose-Response Relationships

One of the most fundamental principles of pharmacology is that *the magnitude or intensity of a drug effect is dependent upon the dose administered.* Dose-response relationships may be graded to quantal.

Graded dose-response relationships   In general, as the dose administered to an individual increases, the magnitude of the effect produced by that drug will increase in a gradual and smooth fashion; this is called a *graded* or *quantitative* dose-response relationship (Figure 1-2a). A *threshold dose* refers to the lowest dose that must be administered to produce a response. The *maximum effect* or *efficacy* is the greatest response that a drug is capable of producing in an individual regardless of the dose administered.

Potency refers to the amount of a drug (that is, the dose) required to produce a given pharmacological effect. Advertisements in nursing journals will often claim that drug A is ten times more potent than drug B. Apart from indicating that the patient will require smaller tablets of drug A, this claim should *not* be thought to mean that (1) A is clinically superior to B; (2) A is less toxic or causes fewer side effects than B; or (3) A has greater efficacy than B. If, on the other hand, A *has* greater efficacy than B, this might represent a distinct clinical advantage.

Quantal dose-response relationships   Quantal dose-response relationships describe the frequency with which a given dose of a drug produces a given pharmaco-

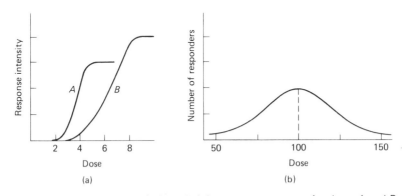

Figure 1-2.   (a) Hypothetical *graded* dose-response curves for drugs A and B. Drug A is more potent than B but B has greater efficacy. (b) A normal distribution curve depicting the *quantal* response to a theoretical drug. The median effective dose (ED50) is 100 units. Note that some subjects respond to very low doses (hyperreactive), while others respond only at very high doses (hyporeactive).

logical effect in a group of subjects. When evaluating such a drug-induced response, the investigator merely determines whether it is present or absent in the test subject at the dose tested; thus the quantal response is often referred to as an *all-or-none response.*

The quantal dose-response curve generally assumes the shape of a normal distribution (Gaussian or bell-shaped) curve (Figure 1-2b). From such a curve, the dose required to produce a specified response in 50 percent of the subjects can be determined; this is referred to as the *median effective dose*, which is commonly abbreviated ED50.

Pharmacokinetics

In summary, the concentration of a drug at its site of action determines the intensity of the drug-induced effect, and both change (increase and then decrease) with time. The drug concentration at a given instant of time is determined by the size of the dose administered and the rate and degree to which absorption

and distribution have occurred. The duration of drug action is influenced by the dose administered and the efficiency of those processes that remove a drug from its site of action, namely, redistribution, metabolism (biotransformation), and elimination. *Pharmacokinetics* is concerned with the interrelationships of dose, time, and biological response (Figure 1-3).

THERAPEUTIC USES OF DRUGS

The sites at which drugs act and the mechanisms responsible for the resulting drug effects include those aspects of pharmacology called *pharmacodynamics.* The most relevant application of this knowledge is for the development of safe and effective drugs for the treatment of disease, that is, *therapeutics.* The four therapeutic uses of drugs are for the diagnosis, prevention, cure, and symptomatic alleviation of disease. Drugs are also used to

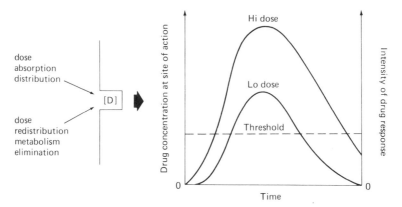

Figure 1-3. Pharmacokinetics: The Interrelationship of Dose, Time, and Biological Response. The magnitude of a drug-induced effect is proportional to the concentration of drug [D] at its site of action; [D] must be greater than a minimal (threshold) level to produce a measurable response. [D] is determined by the size of the dose administered and the rate and extent to which absorption and distribution occur. The duration of a drug-induced effect is influenced by the dose administered and by redistribution, metabolism, and elimination, processes that remove the drug from its site of action.

prevent and terminate pregnancy (contraception and abortion, respectively).

Diagnosis of Disease

Disease may be the consequence of an impairment in the normal function of the tissues or organs of the body, and drugs may be employed to detect such abnormalities. Barium sulfate is used to diagnose abnormalities of the upper gastrointestinal tract, and organic iodine compounds are employed as contrast agents to visualize the gall bladder and the presence of stones. Other commonly used chemical diagnostic agents include radioactive sodium iodide (I-131) for the identification of thyroid cancer and for assessing the functional state of the thyroid gland, sulfobromophthalein for liver function tests, and the glucose tolerance test for diagnosis of diabetes mellitus.

Prevention of Disease

The ultimate goal of medicine is to prevent disease, and drugs have played a significant role in the attainment of this objective. Vitamin deficiency diseases are relatively rare in the United States, and a marked reduction in the incidence of caries has been observed in children living in communities having fluoridated drinking water. The most dramatic examples of the prevention of disease by drugs have been the direct result of mass immunization programs employing vaccines that prevent smallpox, diphtheria, whooping cough, measles, and poliomyelitis. These vaccines have proved to be so effective that the nurse rarely, if ever, is called upon to care for patients with these formerly common diseases.

Cure of Disease

With the notable exception of the chemotherapeutic agents, most classes of drugs only re-lieve the symptoms of disease rather than produce a cure or totally eradicate the disease. Chemotherapeutic agents such as penicillin, chloramphenicol (Chloromycetin), piperazine (Antepar), and chloroquine (Aralen) have proved to be highly effective for the cure of pneumococcal pneumonia, typhoid fever, roundworm and pinworm infestations, and malaria, respectively. At present there exists an obvious and pressing need for the development of nontoxic effective chemotherapeutic agents for the cure of cancers, deep fungal infections, and diseases caused by viruses.

Alleviation of Disease Symptoms

Most of the drugs the nurse commonly administers are only capable of relieving the symptoms of disease and are incapable of directly curing the patient or altering the underlying cause of the disease. Drugs are most frequently used to establish more favorable conditions for the body to make physiological, biochemical, or psychological adjustments to eliminate or control disease.

Drugs used for the treatment of stomach ulcers prevent the secretion of gastric acid or neutralize excess acid, thus permitting stomach tissue repair to occur. Antipsychotic drugs calm violent and excessively active schizophrenic patients and reduce their aberrations in thinking, thus permitting such patients to derive maximum benefit from psychotherapy sessions. Morphine relieves the severe pain associated with terminal cancer or an acute bone fracture without modifying the metastatic process or speeding the repair of the bone.

Contraception and Abortion

Therapeutic uses of drugs are generally restricted to the aforementioned four general categories. Drugs used to prevent pregnancy,

Table 1-1   Sources of Drug Information

Handbook	Purpose and scope	Arrangement of entries	Indexed by[a]	References	Publication frequency (most recent edition)	Remarks
AMA Drug Evaluations	Objectively evaluates drugs and their therapeutic effectiveness. Emphasis on commonly prescribed, single-ingredient products.	Therapeutic classification	G, T, A, Th	No	Periodically (4th ed., 1980)	Good introduction to general properties of therapeutic class; unique characteristics, doses, dosage forms, adverse effects of individual drugs. Extensive table of drug-laboratory test interactions.
American Drug Index	Very extensive dictionarylike listing of single- and multiple-ingredient prescription and nonprescription drug products; useful for identifying drug synonyms.	Alphabetical (generic trade, chemical names)	—	No	Annually	Extensive cross-referencing monograph, lists names of drug, ingredients, uses, available dosage forms, addresses of drug manufacturers.
American Hospital Formulary Service	Provides comprehensive monographs suitable for establishing standards for hospital formulary; primarily prescription drugs.	Therapeutic classification	G, T	No	Continuing supplements to basic volume	Two-volume looseleaf binders containing both new and old single-ingredient and combination products.
Clinical Toxicology of Commercial Products	Identification, relative toxicity, first aid and emergency treatment of poisoning caused by commercial products.	Alphabetical	C, G, T	Yes	Irregularly (4th ed., 1976)	Most comprehensive handbook for the identification and treatment of acute poisoning.
Compendium of Pharmaceuticals and Specialties	Monographs of single and multiple ingredient prescription and nonprescription drugs available in Canada.	Alphabetical	G, T, C Th, M	No	Annually	Monographs based upon information provided by manufacturer. Extensive cross-indexing. Tables of abbreviations, conversions, Canadian poison control centers. Product identification color photos.
Drug Interactions (P. D. Hansten)	Monographs containing drug-drug, drug-laboratory test interactions.	Therapeutic classification	G, T, Th	Yes	Periodically (4th ed., 1979)	Each monograph provides mechanism of interaction, clinical significance (major, moderate, minor) based upon available evidence, and recommended management.

10

Title	Description	Arrangement	Information Type	Critical Evaluation	Frequency of Revision	Comments
Drugs of Choice	Contributors critically evaluate drugs and recommend their preferred treatment of disease; primarily prescription drugs.	Therapeutic classification	G, T, Th	Yes	Biennially	Recommended treatments may change with new contributors to updated editions.
Facts and Comparisons	Comprehensive and very current listing of single- and multiple-ingredient drugs; primarily prescription drugs. Tables of comparisons.	Therapeutic classification	G, T	No	Continuing supplements to basic volume	Therapeutic indications, side effects, doses, dosage forms, cost comparisons. Extensive use of tables for ready comparisons.
Handbook of Nonprescription Drugs	Comprehensive list of wide range of home remedies and nonprescription drug products and their ingredients, when known.	Therapeutic classification	G, T	Yes	Periodically (6th ed., 1979)	Review of physiology, discussion of drugs. extensive tables.
Martindale. The Extra Pharmacopoeia	Concise information of single- and multiple-ingredient prescription and nonprescription drug products. Emphasis on drugs used in United Kingdom as well as others used throughout the world (including North America).	Alphabetical	G, T, C, Th	Yes	Every 5 years (27th ed., 1977)	Contains chemical and physical properties and preparations. Excellent handbook on drugs used internationally, including their trade names. Comments on therapeutic indications and effectiveness.
Medical Letter	Objective evaluation of new drugs, therapeutic devices, and treatments; primarily prescription drugs.	Selected topics in each issue.	G, T	Yes	Semi-monthly	Highly critical and well-respected publication. Comparisons of effectiveness (and often cost) of new versus established drugs.
Merck Index	Index of chemical and physical properties of organic chemicals, a high proportion of which are of medicinal significance.	Alphabetical	G, T, C	Yes	Periodically (9th ed., 1976)	Very extensive cross-indexing of drug synonyms, including investigational numbers. Tables: radio-isotopes, weights and measures, logarithms, etc.
Modern Drug Encyclopedia and Therapeutic Index	Ready reference to prescription and nonprescription drugs containing one or more ingredients and biological products.	Alphabetical	G, T, Th, M	No	Periodically with continuing supplements to basic volume (15th ed., 1979)	Extensive cross-indexing. Simple to use. Monographs contain generic, trade and chemical names, ingredients in combination products, therapeutic indications, adverse effects, usual doses, dosage forms available.
Pediatric Drug Handbook (H.C. Shirkey)	A guide for the determination of average or generally recognized doses for children and infants.	Therapeutic classification	G, T, Th	Not specific	(1977)	Discussion of concepts of pediatric dosage followed by monographs, tables of doses, precautions, contraindications, adverse effects.

Table 1-1 (Continued)

Handbook	Purpose and Scope	Arrangement of entries	Indexed by[a]	References	Publication frequency (most recent edition)	Remarks
Physicians' Desk Reference	Detailed information provided by manufacturer and approved by Food and Drug Administration; primarily U. S. prescription drugs, containing single- and multiple-ingredients. Contains biologicals and diagnostic agents.	Alphabetical according to manufacturer, then product	G, T, C, Th, M	No	Annually with supplements	Compilation of "package inserts" selectively provided by manufacturer. Extensive cross-indexing. Product identification color photos. Names, addresses, telephone numbers of U. S. poison control centers.
Remington's Pharmaceutical Sciences	Encyclopedic volume dealing with all aspects of the theory and practice of pharmaceutical sciences. Drugs are arranged by chemical and pharmacological classifications; prescription and nonprescription drugs and biologicals including drugs with limited contemporary use.	Topical classification; information on specific drugs arranged by pharmacological classification	G, T, C, Cs, Th, M	Yes	Every 5 years (15th ed., 1975)	The most comprehensive single volume on drugs; chemistry, therapeutic monographs; dosage forms, radioisotopes, calculations. Most recent drugs not included.
The United States Dispensatory	Comprehensive information on drugs and chemicals in common use; prescription and non-prescription single-ingredient products. Older drugs included.	Alphabetical classification based on generic name, pharmacological classification.	G, T, C, Cs, Th	Yes	Periodically (27th ed., 1973)	Critical discussions of natural medicinal products, drugs and selected drug classes (with references). Monographs include drug synonyms, physical and chemical properties of drug, pharmacological actions, therapeutic uses and relative effectiveness, drug interactions, drug interactions, doses, and dosage forms. Recent drugs not included.

[a] Abbreviations: A = adverse drug reactions; C = chemical name; Cs = common synonym; G = generic name; M = manufacturer; T = trade name; Th = therapeutic indication.

oral contraceptives, and others that terminate pregnancy by inducing abortion have added new dimensions to our definition of a drug.

SOURCES
OF DRUG INFORMATION

The handbooks listed and compared in Table 1-1 are potentially useful sources of specific drug information for the nurse. A variety of health science journals represent additional invaluable sources of drug information for the nurse seeking to remain current. Nursing journals include *American Journal of Nursing*, *Nursing '81*, and *RN*. Medical and pharmacy journals include *American Journal of Hospital Pharmacy*, *Drugs*, *Journal of the American Medical Association*, and *New England Journal of Medicine*.

FACTORS MODIFYING THE THERAPEUTIC RESPONSE TO DRUGS
Chapter 2

The intensity and duration of the pharmacological effects of a drug are determined by the amount of drug reaching its site of action (tissue or drug receptor) at any given time and the length of time that the drug remains at this site in effective concentrations. You should not assume that 100 percent of the total dose administered to the patient reaches this site; indeed, only a small fraction of the dose may hit its intended biological target.

After oral administration, the drug must first be absorbed from the gastrointestinal tract into the blood, wherein it is carried or distributed to the tissues of the body; one or more of these tissues represents the desired target site. The duration of the drug's pharmacological action is determined by the extent to which the drug is bound to plasma proteins, and, more importantly, to the speed at which the drug is chemically and biologically inactivated or metabolized by enzymes and ultimately eliminated from the body. Often a rather large fraction of the total dose administered is metabolized and eliminated directly and never reaches its biological site of action (Figure 2-1).

The concentration of the drug in the body is primarily determined by the *dose*

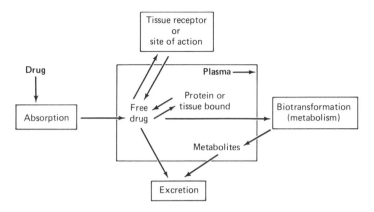

Figure 2-1.   Fate of a Drug After Absorption.

administered to the patient. Assuming that the patient has taken or has been given the medication at the correct dose and at the intended time—assumptions that are sometimes invalid—considerable variation in the intensity and duration of the therapeutic response among different patients can still be observed. In many instances we can ascribe this variation to differences in the speed and extent to which individual patients absorb, distribute, metabolize, or eliminate drugs. A better understanding of these pharmacokinetic parameters and their influence on the patient's response to drugs will enable us to individualize drug dosage to best fit the unique requirements of each patient, that is, to obtain an optimal beneficial therapeutic response with minimal adverse effects.

DRUG TRANSPORT ACROSS CELL MEMBRANES

The extent to which a drug is absorbed into the blood from the site at which it is administered, distributed to tissues and fluids throughout the body, chemically altered by drug-metabolizing enzymes in the liver, and eliminated from the body in the urine, all depend upon the ability of the drug to cross *cell membranes*. A cell membrane consists of a bimolecular layer of fat-like molecules coated with a protein layer on each surface. The relative ability of a drug to cross the barrier imposed by the membrane is dependent upon the chemical and physical properties of the drug molecule.

Drugs cross cell membranes primarily by three different processes: filtration, diffusion, and active transport (Figure 2-2). Small drug molecules are able to pass through pores in the membrane by *filtration*. Most drugs of larger size cross cell membranes by the process of *diffusion;* the relative ability of such drugs to diffuse across the membrane is directly related to their lipid (fat) solubility and their ability to dissolve in the lipid membrane. More specifically, drugs that are highly lipid soluble diffuse across the membrane rapidly, while drugs that are relatively lipid insoluble diffuse more slowly. By selectively altering the chemistry of certain drugs, we can modify their lipid solubility, and, consequently, their ability to cross cell membranes. Scopolamine is a highly effective drug for the treatment of

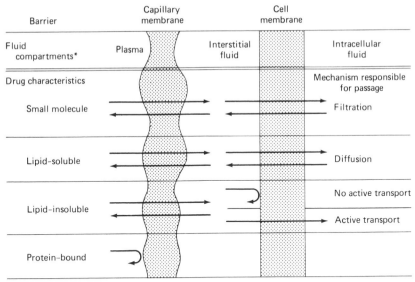

*The average 70 kg (154 lb) man is made up of 40 liters (40 quarts) of water, or about 57% of his total weight. Of these 40 liters, 25 liters are within the 100 trillion cells of the body (intracellular fluid): the remaining 15 liters of water, termed extra cellular water, are subdivided into several compartments. Two of these are the plasma (noncellular part of the blood—3 liters) and the interstitial fluid (water lying in the spaces between the cells—12 liters).

Figure 2-2.   Passage of Drugs across Membrane Barriers. Drug transfer is influenced by the size of the molecule, lipid solubility, presence of an active transport system, and protein binding. With the exception of protein-bound drugs, almost all commonly used drugs are able to cross readily the walls of the capillary membranes. This affects the transfer of these compounds from the plasma to the interstitial fluid. Small molecules enter the cell by filtration across the cell membrane; lipid-soluble drugs pass through the membrane by diffusion. Lipid-insoluble drugs of larger dimensions require an active transport carrier mechanism to cross the cell membrane. Protein-bound drugs do not leave the plasma in the bound state.

spasmodic disorders of the gastrointestinal tract; however, in high doses it produces undesirable behavioral effects. By chemically converting this drug to methscopolamine (Pamine), a much less lipid-soluble molecule, we have a drug that retains the beneficial effects of scopolamine on the gastrointestinal tract. Methscopolamine, however, is incapable of crossing cell membranes to gain access to the brain and is devoid of adverse behavioral effects; the nature of the "blood-brain barrier" will be discussed later.

Some large lipid-insoluble drugs pass across cell membranes by an *active transport* process requiring the expenditure of energy by

cells. Unlike filtration and diffusion, drugs that are active transported can be carried against a concentration gradient, that is, from areas of low drug concentration to those areas of higher concentration. Normally, after uric acid in the plasma is filtered across the glomerulus of the kidney, it is reabsorbed across the cell membranes of the proximal tubules by an active transport process and reenters the plasma. When plasma levels of uric acid become excessive, insoluble urate crystals are deposited in the joints resulting in gout. The antigout drug probenecid (Benemid) blocks the active transport system responsible for the reabsorption of urates and thereby promotes their excretion in the urine. Some diuretic agents promote urinary excretion and removal of excessive body water by inhibiting the active transport system responsible for the reabsorption of sodium.

ABSORPTION

Drugs may act at the site of their administration but more commonly act at some far removed part of the body. Antiseptics, anti-acne creams, and powders for athlete's foot all exert their beneficial therapeutic effects at the site on the skin where they are applied. Similarly, antacids neutralize gastric acid in the stomach without entering the blood. In most instances, however, the target site of the drug—for example, the brain, heart, or kidney—is inaccessible to the direct application of the drug. *Absorption* is the transfer of a drug from its site of administration to the blood, the transport vehicle. If a drug is administered directly into the blood by intravenous or intra-arterial injection, the absorption step is bypassed, and the drug is immediately available for distribution throughout the body.

The speed of drug absorption and the extent to which absorption occurs directly influences the onset of drug action after its administration, as well as the intensity of the drug-induced effects. Absorption may be modified by many factors, including the route of drug administration, the physical and chemical properties of the drug, and the surface area available for absorption.

The physical and chemical properties of the drug, the intended site of drug action, and the desired onset of drug action very often influence the *route of drug administration* selected. The protein insulin would be rapidly broken down and inactivated by enzymes located in the gastrointestinal tract if given by

mouth. Isoproterenol (Isuprel) is slowly and unreliably absorbed when taken orally and should be administered by inhalation via an aerosol to terminate an acute asthmatic attack. This drug and the anesthetic gases (halothane, nitrous oxide, and ether) are all rapidly absorbed into the blood (via an extensive network of capillaries) across the large surface area of the alveoli of the lungs. In some situations, it is desirable to prevent absorption of the drug into the blood to preclude the possibility of potential systemic toxicity. The insoluble and unabsorbable antibiotic neomycin is administered orally to reduce the bacterial population of the intestinal tract prior to abdominal surgery.

The *oral* route of drug administration is the most commonly employed because it is the easiest, safest, and least expensive method available. Drugs are more rapidly absorbed when in solution than as solids (tablets or capsules).* The entire gastrointestinal tract is capable of absorbing drugs, although the primary site of absorption is the small intestines. Since the presence of food delays the emptying time of the stomach to the small intestines, drugs are more rapidly absorbed between meals. Moreover, drug molecules may bind to food. Dairy products and certain antacids have been shown to inhibit the absorption of the tetracycline antibiotics from the gastrointestinal tract and significantly reduce their plasma levels. Some drugs have been observed to bind and reduce the absorption of other drugs or nutrients; for example, the laxative mineral oil reduces the absorption of the fat-soluble vitamins A, D, and K. A more detailed discussion of routes of administration will be presented in Chapter 3.

---

*Drugs administered as solids must first go into solution in the gastrointestinal tract. The rate of *dissolution* determines the extent and speed to which absorption will occur. Drugs administered orally in solution bypass this dissolution step.

DISTRIBUTION

The transport of a drug from the blood to the tissue sites at which the drug exerts its pharmacological effects is called *distribution*. The relative extent to which a drug is distributed to the tissues of the body, particularly to its intended site of action, determines the magnitude or intensity of the drug's pharmacological effects. This, in turn, influences the therapeutic effects produced by the medication. If less than minimum effective drug concentrations are achieved at the site of action, the patient may fail to obtain beneficial effects from the drug. Conversely, if blood (and hence, tissue) levels exceed a certain optimal concentration, it may be anticipated that the patient will experience undesirable adverse drug effects. It has been observed, for example, that the antiepileptic drug phenytoin (Dilantin) fails to control seizures when plasma levels are less than 1 milligram/deciliter (1 mg/dl) and produces toxic effects when plasma concentrations exceed 2 mg/dl. Thus seizures are effectively controlled with minimum toxic effects to the patient when drug plasma concentrations are between 1-2 mg/dl.

Once a drug has entered the blood, the rate and extent of its distribution throughout the body are determined by the physical and chemical properties of the drug and by cardiovascular considerations, namely, cardiac output (the volume of blood pumped by the heart each minute) and regional blood flow (the amount of blood supplied to a given tissue or organ). While lipid-soluble drugs readily cross cell membranes and readily gain access to most tissue and fluid compartments of the body, most lipid-insoluble drugs enter the brain and anterior chamber of the eye to only a limited extent. Because of differences in regional blood flow, drugs are rapidly distributed to the heart, liver, and kidney, but less rapidly to the muscles and skin.

Protein Binding

The extent to which drugs are able to distribute throughout the body is often influenced by their binding to plasma proteins, in particular to albumin. Unlike most molecules, the protein albumin is too large to pass through the walls of blood vessels, particularly the capillaries. Hence, when drugs are bound to albumin, they are, in effect, trapped in the plasma until they are slowly released from this binding.

For the nurse, there are many important therapeutic implications arising from the plasma-protein binding of drugs. When trapped in the blood, the drug is pharmacologically inactive because it cannot gain access to or interact at its tissue target sites. In addition, the drug cannot be inactivated by the drug-metabolizing enzymes of the liver nor excreted by the kidney (Figure 2-3). Hence, protein binding represents a storage depot for drugs.

The physical-chemical properties of a given drug determine whether and to what extent it will be bound to plasma albumin and how strong the bond will be. Drugs with properties that enable them to have a stronger attachment for plasma-protein binding sites are able to displace drugs with a weaker affinity. Rapid displacement of highly potent drugs from albumin may abruptly elevate the concentration of unbound (free) biologically active drug molecules in the plasma, resulting in an increased pharmacological effect with potentially toxic effects to the patient. The anticoagulant warfarin (Coumadin, Panwarfin) is bound to plasma proteins to the extent of 97 percent, with only 3 percent of the administered dose responsible at any given time for maintaining the optimal prothrombin (clotting) time. The anti-inflammatory drug phenylbutazone (Butazolidin) possesses greater affinity for albumin binding sites than does warfarin and is capable of displacing

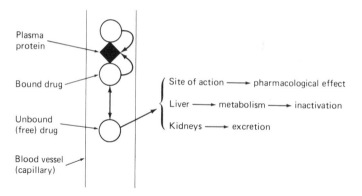

Figure 2-3. **Effects of Plasma Protein Binding of Drugs on Pharmacological Effects, Metabolism, and Excretion.**

warfarin. If phenylbutazone were to displace only 3 percent of the bound warfarin, the plasma levels of free pharmacologically active warfarin would be doubled, and the patient might experience internal bleeding with a potentially fatal outcome. The nurse should be aware of possible drug-drug interactions resulting in drug displacement from protein-binding sites and should be very cautious when coadministering such drugs.

Distribution to the Central Nervous System

While lipid-soluble drugs pass from the blood into the brain and cerebrospinal fluid with relative ease, lipid-insoluble drugs pass with great difficulty. The so-called blood-brain barrier, which is more relative than absolute, is located at the region where capillaries and the glial cells of the central nervous system meet. Under normal conditions, even after massive intravenous doses, penicillin fails to enter the central nervous system in significant amounts. However, when the meninges (membranes covering the brain and spinal cord) are acutely inflamed, penicillin more readily crosses the blood-brain barrier and can be used for the treatment of certain bacterial infections such as meningitis.

Distribution from Mother to Fetus

Since the tragic thalidomide episode of the early 1960s, nurses and other health care professionals have been concerned about the distribution of drugs from the maternal circulation to that of her fetus. Although lipid-soluble compounds preferentially cross the placenta, it is also permeable to a large number of other commonly used lipid-insoluble drugs. Drugs may have similar pharmacological effects in both mother and fetus, or they may have unique effects on the development of the fetus.

Opiates, such as heroin and methadone, readily cross the placental barrier. The clinical literature provides ample proof that many opiate-dependent mothers give birth to babies who are physically dependent upon these drugs.

The absence of drug-induced toxicity to the mother does not assure us of the drug's relative safety to her developing fetus. Suicide attempts by adults taking twenty to forty times the normal sleep-producing dose of thalidomide have proven to be unsuccessful, thus attesting to the relative safety of this compound. By contrast, when taken during the first trimester of pregnancy, as little as a single dose of this compound has been demonstrated to produce severe physical deformities (*teratogenic effects*) in the human fetus. A wide range of therapeutic agents have been reported to produce fetal malformations and abnormalities during different stages of pregnancy: anti-inflammatory cortisone-related steroids and some anticancer drugs may produce cleft palates; antithyroid drugs cause goiter and mental retardation; sex hormones (including the oral contraceptives) may produce masculinization of the female fetus, enlargement of the clitoris, and cardiac or limb anomalies. This very short and incomplete list should alert the nurse to discourage pregnant women from taking any drugs except when they are deemed to be essential by her physician.

METABOLISM

Throughout our lifetimes, we are exposed to a countless number of foreign substances. To prevent the buildup of such substances, animals have evolved a mechanism for chemically inactivating such substances and converting them to products that can be readily eliminated from the body. These chemical reactions are catalyzed by enzymes, some of which are located in the plasma and gastrointestinal tract. By far, the most important site for the *biotransformation* or *metabolism* of drugs is the *liver*, and these chemical reactions are catalyzed by the *microsomal drug metabolizing enzymes*. The microsomes are associated with the endoplasmic reticulum, a subcellular component of the liver.

In former years, biotransformation reactions involving drugs were perceived to be detoxification reactions, implying that the products (metabolites) were less toxic or biologically active than the parent drug molecule. While this is usually the case, there are noteworthy exceptions. Phenacetin is a less active analgesic (pain-relieving drug) than its metabolite acetaminophen (Tylenol, Datril). The pharmacological effects of heroin have been attributed to its metabolism to morphine.

In almost all cases, we observe that the ultimate end product of drug metabolism is less lipid-soluble and more water-soluble than the parent drug administered to the patient. For the nurse to fully appreciate the essential significance of this fact, the kidney and the types of compounds excreted by this, the most important organ of the body for the elimination of drugs (Figure 2-4), must be considered. Kidney tubules have lipid cell membranes. Hence, lipid-soluble drugs readily diffuse across the walls of the tubules and are returned to the plasma. By contrast, water-soluble drugs are not reabsorbed across the tubules and are eliminated into the urine. Thus, because the products of drug metabolism are more water-soluble, they are more readily excreted in the urine.

An understanding of drug metabolism is of particular importance to the nurse because it provides a partial explanation about why some patients are extremely sensitive to some drugs, while other patients require higher than normal doses to obtain the desired therapeutic response. In some instances, one observes that hypersensitive patients metabolize drugs more slowly than normal, resulting in drug effects that are more intense and of longer duration. Conversely, persons who are resistant to medication may metabolize and inactivate such compounds at a faster than normal rate. With repeated doses, some drugs—such as phenobarbital—are capable

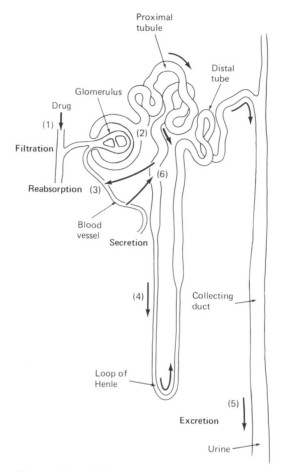

Figure 2-4. Urinary Excretion of Drugs by the Kidneys. Small blood vessels (1) carry plasma-containing drugs to the glomerulus of the kidney for filtration (2). Lipid-soluble drugs are capable of diffusing across the cell membranes of the proximal tubules (3) and thereby escape excretion. This is termed tubular reabsorption. Water-soluble compounds do not diffuse across the kidney tubules (4), are not reabsorbed, and are eventually excreted in the urine (5). Some drugs and metabolites are secreted from the plasma (6) and are thereafter eliminated from the body in the urine (5).

of enhancing their rate of metabolism or that of other drugs with which they are concurrently administered; this may potentially reduce their intensity or duration of action.

EXCRETION

Drugs and their pharmacologically active or inactive metabolites are primarily excreted (eliminated) from the body through the kidneys, alimentary tract, and lungs, with the saliva, sweat, and milk of nursing mothers of considerably lesser importance.

Volatile drugs, including the general anesthetic gases, alcohol, and the sleep-producing drug paraldehyde, are excreted in the air exhaled through the lungs. The alimentary tract is a major route for drug removal, second only to the kidney. Drugs not absorbed from the stomach or intestines are eliminated in the feces. Many drugs are carried by the blood to the liver and are excreted from this organ into the bile, which is secreted into the duodenum. While some drugs are eliminated in the feces, more often the drug and bile salts are reabsorbed from the intestines back to the liver, which has been called the *enterohepatic cycle*. Such drugs remain in this cycle until they are eventually excreted in the urine.

Kidney Excretion

The most important route of elimination of nonvolatile, water-soluble metabolites is in the urine, and for many drugs this represents the exclusive route by which drugs are removed from the body. The glomeruli of the kidneys are capable of filtering about 120 ml (4 oz) of plasma water per minute. Free unbound drugs are filtered, whereas protein-bound compounds are not. After filtration, lipid-soluble compounds are readily reabsorbed across the lipid membranes of the kidney tubules and consequently are not eliminated in the urine (Figure 2-4). Among the factors influencing the extent to which drugs are eliminated via the kidneys are kidney disease and the pH of the urine; reductions in kidney function in infants and the elderly will be considered later.

Kidney disease The dosage of drugs to be administered to patients with impaired kidney function is frequently reduced to prevent drug toxicity or further injury to the kidneys. This general rule is particularly applicable for drugs that are eliminated primarily by urinary excretion. In such cases, the initial dose administered is not generally modified. Suitable reductions must be made in the amount and frequency of subsequent doses to prevent the accumulation of toxic levels of the drug.

Urinary pH Most drugs are weak organic acids or bases, and, therefore, exist as a mixture of non-ionized (uncharged) and ionized (charged) molecules in the fluids of the body. Organic acids (such as barbiturates and aspirin) are predominately non-ionized in acidic fluids, such as the urine; however, they become ionized in the slightly alkaline environment of the plasma. The converse is true for weak organic bases (such as amphetamine and the narcotics); that is, they are ionized mainly in acidic fluids.

In general, we observe that drugs are more lipid-soluble and, therefore, more readily cross cell membranes when they are non-ionized, while ionized drugs are less lipid-soluble, have difficulty in crossing such membranes as the kidney tubules, and are relatively easily excreted in the urine.

Alkalinization of the urine with sodium bicarbonate or tromethamine (Tham-E) is sometimes employed for hastening the excretion of such acidic drugs as aspirin or barbiturates when overdoses of these drugs are taken. High doses of vitamin C can acidify the urine and modify the excretion of some basic drugs. Amphetamine is excreted 20 times more rapidly in acidic urine (pH 5) than it is in more alkaline urine (pH 8). The pH of the urine has also been observed to influence the relative effectiveness of some antibacterial agents in the treatment of urinary tract infections.

THE PATIENT
AND DRUG RESPONSE

While we speak of the average or normal response to drugs, the nurse frequently cares for patients who respond to drugs in an atypical manner. Among the major factors that may be responsible for the patient's quantitatively or qualitatively different response to medications include the age and body weight of the patient, genetic factors, route and time of drug administration, pre-existing disease, and the patient's drug history. Most of these factors have been shown to modify the normal drug response by altering such pharmacokinetic factors as drug absorption, distribution, metabolism, and elimination (Table 2-1).

Age

In general, young infants and elderly individuals are more sensitive to the effects of drugs than are young and middle-aged adults. The "average," "usual," or "normal" dose is generally based upon an individual between 20 to 60 years of age who is in good health.

When viewed pharmacologically, we cannot consider the infant to be a miniature adult. Drug metabolizing enzyme systems in the liver are poorly developed in the infant, so drugs may produce more intense effects for longer periods of time in very young patients. To compound the infants' reduced capacity to metabolize drugs, their kidneys are functionally immature, thus impairing the elimination of drugs in the urine. The nurse should inform parents of the potential dangers associated with administering drugs to their young children. A very reasonable dose of a nonprescription drug for a 3-year-old child may represent a real hazard for a 1-month-old sibling.

Elderly patients often manifest an altered response to drugs as the result of disease and the normal reduction in physiological function that is an inevitable consequence of the aging process. Drugs administered orally may not be efficiently absorbed because of reduced intestinal blood flow, thus potentially reducing the therapeutic effect obtained. More important, however, is the increased sensitivity of the elderly to drugs resulting from impaired metabolism by the liver and the decreased ability of the drug or its metabolites to be excreted by the kidneys as the result of a reduction in their normal physiological functioning.

Genetic Factors

In recent years it has become increasingly apparent that members of our species—even

Table 2-1   Selected Factors Modifying Drug Absorption, Distribution, Metabolism, and Elimination

Absorption	Distribution
Route of drug administration	Route of drug administration
Time of drug administration (meals)	Body mass
Disease	Drug history
Drug history	
Metabolism	**Elimination**
Route of drug administration	Age
Age	Disease
Genetic factors	Drug history
Disease	
Drug history	

members of relatively homogeneous populations in our society—do not possess the ability to metabolize drugs to the same degree. Among the most important emerging areas of pharmacological interest is *pharmacogenetics*, the study of the influence of genetic factors in the response to drugs.

One of the most commonly employed preoperative short-acting skeletal muscle relaxants is succinylcholine (Anectine), a compound rapidly inactivated by the plasma enzyme pseudocholinesterase. Normally, after an intravenous injection of this drug, the patient experiences muscle relaxation for several minutes and recovers the capacity to breath spontaneously within 5 minutes after the termination of drug administration. One person in 3,000 has a genetic defect resulting in the presence of an atypical plasma pseudocholinesterase, which does not readily metabolize succinylcholine. Another common hereditary abnormality observed primarily in American blacks or Mediterranean Greeks is a deficiency of glucose-6-phosphate dehydrogenase, an enzyme required for the stability of red blood cells. When susceptible individuals take certain antimalarial drugs, they often experience varying degrees of red cell hemolysis, potentially resulting in anemia.

Drug History

The prior administration of the same or different drugs may greatly influence the response of the patient to the medication taken. This response may be an intensification or a reduction in the effects normally observed. Tolerance, cumulative effects, and drug-drug interactions will be examined next.

Some drugs, after they are repeatedly administered for days or weeks, produce progressively *diminishing* effects. As a consequence of this lack of responsiveness, successive increases in dosage are required to sustain the original drug effects. This phenomenon, called *tolerance*, is often observed to develop with drugs that act primarily on the central nervous system. Tolerance is acquired to the appetite suppressing effects of amphetamine, the sedation produced by barbiturates, and to the analgesic effects of morphine. Moreover, cross-tolerance to the effects of pharmacologically related compounds, such as methadone and heroin, may develop. Tolerance may result from decreased drug absorption, increased metabolism or elimination, or as a consequence of physiological (cellular) adaptation to the drug's effects at its site of action.

By contrast, some drugs produce progressively *greater* effects with each successive dose. This is often the case when the doses administered exceed the rate at which the drug is being metabolically inactivated or eliminated. Because more drug enters the body than is being removed, a net accumulation of drug occurs, resulting in the cumulative effects observed. In the treatment of congestive heart failure, an initial dose of about 2 mg of digoxin is often administered. Thereafter, daily maintenance doses of 0.25 mg are given to replace the amount of drug excreted and thereby maintain optimal blood levels of drug. Higher maintenance doses could cause toxicity from drug cumulation. Cumulative effects are often of toxicological importance, as observed in chronic lead poisoning. Children who ingest paint chips over long periods of time accumulate lead, a metal that is very slowly eliminated from the body. Whereas ingestion of small amounts of this metal on a single occasion produce no severe adverse effects, its chronic ingestion may result in irreversible nerve and brain damage.

The effects of one drug can be increased or reduced by the prior or concurrent administration of another drug. Ingestion of alcoholic beverages with central nervous system depressants (for example, antihistamines and drugs used for the treatment of anxiety and psychosis) may produce profound depression, coma, and even death. Many accidental and intentional suicides have been attributed to this type of *drug-drug interaction.* The mechanisms underlying common drug-drug interactions are summarized in Table 2-2. Selected clinically relevant drug-drug interactions appear in summary tables in each chapter and will be pointed out throughout the text.

Thus far, biological drug-drug interactions occurring within the body have been considered; however, one cannot exclude the possibility that two drugs will be incompatible when mixed prior to being administered to the patient. Such an incompatibility can be the consequence of a chemical interaction between the drugs (such as an acidic drug neutralizing a medication that is basic) or can be based upon physical properties of a drug (such as limited solubility resulting in precipitation). Such a precipitate, when injected intravenously, can become the center of blood clots or may produce damage to the body organs. The nurse should immediately terminate an intravenous infusion if the drug added to the infusion fluid precipitates or forms crystals.

Emotional Factors

An understanding of the pharmacodynamic factors discussed thus far will enable you to predict and appreciate why patients respond differently to drugs. The patient, however, is far more than a collection of membranes, receptor sites, and enzymes. It is now well accepted that the patient's attitude about the medication taken and rapport with members of the health care team are factors of sufficient importance in that they often have a decisive influence on whether a given drug treatment will be a therapeutic success or failure.

By ordering a medication, the physician has at least tacitly implied to the patient that beneficial therapeutic effects are anticipated. Studies have revealed that patients are more likely to improve if their physicians manifest great confidence in the prescribed medication and are less likely to improve when the prescriber lacks such confidence.

The placebo   A *placebo* is a medication that produces a biological effect in the absence of any specific pharmacodynamic properties; this term is derived from the Latin "I shall please." Numerous studies have demonstrated the ability of the placebo to produce beneficial therapeutic effects, as well as adverse effects. The basis for such effects is the power of suggestion.

The placebo is traditionally thought to be a lactose or sucrose tablet or capsule or an injection of normal saline solution. It should be noted, however, that placebos are often pharmacologically active substances admin-

Table 2-2   Mechanisms Underlying Common Drug Interactions

Underlying basis of interaction	Potential consequences	Examples of drug interactions
1. *Modification of Drug Absorption*		
a. Drug binding in gastrointestinal (G-I) tract	Drug binding reduces rate or extent of intestinal drug absorption.	Antacids inhibit tetracycline absorption. Mineral oil inhibits absorption of fat-soluable vitamins.
b. Changes in rate of intestinal motility and gastric emptying time.	Increase in rate of gut motility speeds passage of drug through G-I tract can reduce drug absorption.	Laxatives (cathartics) may reduce digitalis absorption.

Table 2-2   Continued

Underlying basis of interaction	Potential consequences	Examples of drug interactions
	Decrease in gastric emptying time can reduce rate of intestinal absorption; metabolism and inactivation may occur while drug is in stomach.	Coadministration of anticholinergic (atropine-like) drugs and levodopa.
c. Inhibition of gastrointestinal enzymes	Inhibition of enzymes involved in G-I absorption of essential nutrients and vitamins can result in nutritional disorders.	Folic acid deficiency anemias in patients receiving phenytoin.
2. *Drug Displacement from Plasma Protein Binding*	Increase in plasma concentration of unbound (free) drug can result in an increased pharmacological effect or toxicity.	Displacement of warfarin (anticoagulant) or tolbutamide (oral antidiabetic agent) by phenylbutazone.
3. *Site of Action* a. Additive effects	Use of two drugs with similar actions at the same or different sites of action can result in an increased pharmacological effect or toxicity.	Coadministration of alcohol and a central nervous system depressant (barbiturate).
b. Antagonistic effects	Use of two drugs with opposing actions at the same or different sites of action can result in a reduction in the therapeutic effect. An antagonist may be used as an antidote in drug poisoning.	Naloxone is a specific antagonist of narcotics (morphine, heroin).
4. *Modification of Drug Metabolism* a. Stimulation of metabolism	Chronic administration of some drugs can stimulate the rate at which a second drug is metabolized (enzyme induction), resulting in a reduction in the intensity and/or duration of the therapeutic effect.	Chronic use of certain barbiturates (phenobarbital), an enzyme inducer, stimulates the rate of metabolism of warfarin, phenytoin, prednisone, griseofulvin.
b. Inhibition of metabolism	Administration of selected drugs inhibits the metabolism of coadministered drugs, increasing the intensity and duration of their pharmacological effects and increasing the potential risk of toxicity.	Monoamine oxidase inhibitors (tranylcypromine) inhibit the metabolism of barbiturates and meperidine.
5. *Modification of Drug Elimination* a. pH of urine	Acidification of the urine (vitamin C) increases the urinary elimination of basic drugs. Alkalinization of the urine (sodium bicarbonate, tromethamine) increases the urinary elimination of acidic drugs.	Acidic drugs as salicylates (aspirin), barbiturates. Basic drugs as amphetamine, narcotic analgesics, antihistamines.
b. Transport mechanisms	Competition between two drugs for a common transport mechanism responsible for their secretion into the urine from the plasma. This can result in a reduction in urinary elimination and an increase in drug plasma levels, increasing the intensity and duration of drug effects.	Probenecid, penicillins, salicylates, and phenylbutazone complete for common transport mechanism.

istered in subthreshold doses or a drug administered for the treatment of a disease for which it is of little, if any, proven value (for example, vitamin B_{12} injections for the treatment of weakness and fatigue in the absence of pernicious anemia).

ADVERSE RESPONSES TO DRUGS

While drugs have played a major role in the control of disease, one should not overlook drugs as the cause of many health problems. One source estimates that up to 3.5 percent of all admissions to general medical wards are primarily for the treatment of an adverse response to drugs. Since the average patient receives an average of nine different drugs during a normal period of hospitalization, it is not surprising that the walls of a hospital fail to provide the patient with protection against many adverse drug reactions. As Section III shows, many hundreds of thousands of Americans are dependent upon stimulants, depressants, and narcotics, while ten million are alcoholics.

Undoubtedly the most fundamental principle that underlies the therapeutic use of drugs involves comparing *benefits-to-risks*. When a physician prescribes a drug, an implicit decision has been made that the benefits the patient will derive from taking the drug will outweigh the real or potential risks or dangers associated with the medication. The *therapeutic index* provides a quantitative measure of the relative safety of a given drug. It is the ratio of the dose that produces toxic effects to the dose required to produce the desired therapeutic effects. Ideally, the therapeutic index must be greater than one if the drug is to have any clinical utility. The greater this ratio, the safer the drug. The therapeutic indexes of digitalis, aspirin, and

penicillin are 1.5–2, 30–50, and greater than 100, respectively. For the treatment of a life-threatening malignant disease, the antineoplastic drug selected may have an uncomfortably small ratio. In such situations, the physician's only option may be the use of such a drug, appreciating full well that the patient may suffer from severe toxicity.

Predictable and Unpredictable Adverse Reactions

Some adverse drug responses are predictable and result from excessive doses of the drug. These adverse effects are observed in all patients, although the dosage required to produce such toxic effects vary according to the susceptibility of the individual. The therapeutic class of the drug and the general pharmacological properties of that drug class usually provide a rational basis for predicting these effects; for example, an overdose of a barbiturate sedative may produce coma. The appearance of such undesirable side effects imposes a ceiling upon the highest dose that can be safely administered to the patient.

Other adverse drug reactions are unpredictable, are not dose-related (occurring with normal or even very small doses), and are exhibited only by susceptible individuals. *Idiosyncrasies* are genetically determined unusual drug responses that may quantitatively or qualitatively differ from normal. For example, as has been previously observed, succinylcholine can produce markedly prolonged muscle relaxation in some patients, a quantitatively different response; patients exhibiting excitation rather than depression after receiving barbiturates are experiencing a qualitatively unusual reaction.

Hypersensitivity reactions, sometimes called *drug allergies*, are immediate or delayed adverse responses that occur after the patient has been reexposed to a given medication or a chemically related drug and are the consequence of antigen (drug)-antibody reactions. Penicillin and aspirin have been observed to produce immediate and life-threatening anaphylactic reactions in patients severely allergic to these drugs. Common symptoms include marked bronchoconstriction, a precipitous drop in blood pressure, shock, and death in the absence of appropriate emergency treatment.

In summary, after a typical "therapeutic dose" of a given drug is administered to different patients, some may obtain the anticipated beneficial therapeutic response, others may experience severe toxicity, while not major drug effects may be observed in still other individuals.

SUPPLEMENTARY READINGS

Benet, L. Z., ed., *The Effects of Disease States on Drug Pharmacokinetics*. Washington, D.C.: American Pharmaceutical Association, 1976.

DiPalma, J. R., ed., "Part 1. Modern Approaches to Pharmacology," in *Drill's Pharmacology in Medicine* (4th ed.), ed. J. R. DiPalma, pp. 10–124. New York: McGraw-Hill Book Company, 1971.

Goldstein, A., L. Aronow, and S. M. Kalman, *Principles of Drug Action: The Basis of Pharmacology* (2nd ed.). New York: John Wiley & Sons, Inc., 1974.

Gotz, B. E., and V. P. Gotz, "Drugs in the Elderly," *American Journal of Nursing* **78**: 1347–1351 (1978).

Hanstein, P. D., *Drug Interactions* (4th ed.). Philadelphia: Lea & Febiger, 1979.

Hartshorn, E. A., *Handbook of Drug Interactions* (3rd ed.). Hamilton, Ill.: Drug Intelligence Public., 1976.

Kayne, R. C., ed., *Drugs and the Elderly*, revised. Los Angeles: University of Southern California Press, 1978.

Koch-Weser, J., "Serum Concentrations as Therapeutic Guides," *New England Journal of Medicine* **287**: 227–231 (1972).

Levine, R. R., *Pharmacology: Drug Actions and Reactions* (2nd ed.). Boston: Little, Brown & Company, 1978.

Melmon, K. L., and H. F. Morrelli, "Drug Reactions," in *Clinical Pharmacology* (2nd ed.), ed. K. L. Melmon and H. F. Morrelli, Chapter 20, pp. 951–981. New York: Macmillan, Inc., 1978.

Reidenberg, M. M., *Renal Function and Drug Action*. Philadelphia: W. B. Saunders Company, 1971.

Schwarz, R. H., and S. J. Yaffe, eds., *Drug and Chemical Risks to the Fetus and Newborn*. New York: Alan R. Liss, Inc., 1980.

Yaffe, S. J., ed., "Symposium on Pediatric Pharmacology," *Pediatric Clinics of North America* **19**(1): 1–259 (1972).

ADMINISTRATION OF DRUGS

Chapter 3

The nurse is expected to possess a thorough knowledge of the pharmacology, therapeutic applications, and potential side effects of drugs. Administration of drugs accurately, in the correct dose, and by the appropriate route of administration represents an extremely important aspect of professional nursing.

In this chapter, we shall examine the responsibilities of the nurse in handling the medication order, common routes of administration, rules for the determination of pediatric doses, and safety measures associated with the handling of drugs.

NURSING RESPONSIBILITIES AND MEDICATION ORDERS

The nurse administers drugs on the order of a licensed physician. In addition to being bound by the order, the nurse is legally and morally responsible for the safety of the patient. Any nurse who administers a drug upon an erroneous order can be held *legally responsible* for any harm resulting to the patient. Therefore a nurse cannot carry out an order automatically as written on a chart. The nurse must first consider the condition of the patient, the pharmacological effect of the drug, and the accuracy of the physician's order. The physician should be questioned about an order if any portion of the order is unclear; if the drug would seem harmful to the patient; if the dosage or frequency of successive doses is outside the usual range; or if the route of administration is not correct.

Each medication order must include the name of the drug (correctly spelled), the route of administration, the dose, and the dosage schedule to be followed. If the name of the drug is misspelled, the nurse must check with the physician or pharmacist to be sure that the correct medication has been dispensed. To read orders accurately, the nurse must know the correct interpretations of abbreviations commonly used in writing prescriptions and the hospital's usual time schedule for drug administration. The tables preceding Chapter 1 should be consulted for commonly used abbreviations and for approximate metric and apothecary equivalents.

Most hospitals have a system of discontinuing certain medications after a specified time interval as a reminder to the physician to reevaluate the need for continued therapy.

For example, an order for a narcotic will usually be discontinued in 3 days and an antibiotic may be discontinued after 5 to 7 days. The physician must rewrite the order to continue the medication beyond the specified time period. Preoperative orders are considered to be cancelled automatically after the patient has had surgery.

Routine or PRN (when needed) orders for medications that are commonly given to patients with a particular diagnosis or condition may be written in advance by a physician. The nurse may enter these on a chart to be signed later by the physician. An example of such a routine order might be for a bisacodyl (Dulcolax) suppository given daily for a patient on a bowel training program. Nurses with additional training in special care areas, such as intensive care units, coronary care units, or emergency rooms may encounter many PRN orders with specific protocols for each drug. Lidocaine (Xylocaine) may be ordered by intravenous infusion when a patient has had more than six premature ventricular contractions a minute, as determined by observing the cardiac monitor. The nurse is responsible for assessing the patient's total condition prior to administering these PRN drugs and may have to consult the physician frequently for more individualized orders.

Nurse-Patient Interactions

When a nurse enters a room to administer a medication, the patient may exhibit a variety of responses. The medication may be unquestioningly accepted because the patient identifies the nurse and physician as authority figures; or the patient may question the nurse about the purpose of the medication or may simply refuse to accept the medication. The nurse's approach to the patient and manner of speaking can greatly influence the patient's acceptance of treatment and the therapeutic effect of the medication. (The beneficial effects associated with placebo administration were discussed in Chapter 2). A suitable explanation of the therapeutic purpose of the medication combined with an expectation of favorable results may enhance the patient's response. For example, nursing studies on the variables affecting relief of pain have demonstrated a positive relationship between the nurse's approach to the patient and the amount of pain relief achieved. Permitting the patient a few minutes to ask questions and to express any fears or anxieties may make the difference between relief of pain or continued discomfort following medication.

ROUTES OF DRUG ADMINISTRATION

The route of administration of a drug is determined by its physical and chemical properties, the site of desired action, and the time course of the response desired. Drugs are administered primarily for either their local or systemic effects. Most drugs applied *topically* to the skin or mucous membrane exert their effect at the site of application, but some—such as nitroglycerin ointment—are absorbed by this route and may be given for their systemic effects. Drugs given for a *systemic* effect (orally, rectally, by inhalation, or parenterally) must be absorbed into the blood and distributed in the body to a location distant from the site of administration.

Topical Administration

Application to the skin   Most drugs applied to the intact skin exert only local effects because there is very little absorption through the outermost dead layer of epidermis. However, local application to skin that is damaged or denuded over a large area can result in systemic absorption of the medication, resulting potentially in an adverse response.

The method used for direct application of drugs will depend upon the consistency of the preparation and the purpose for which it is being administered. Ointments may be applied with a tongue depressor, a finger, or a gauze pad. Lotion or liniments should be applied with gauze using firm, gentle pressure. Rubbing or massaging the skin enhances absorption of the medication because the warmth created by friction dilates surface capillaries and increases local blood flow in tissues, enabling the medication to penetrate deeper into the tissue. Powders may be applied to dry skin to prevent caking.

Application to the mucous membranes

Mouth   Some medications are readily absorbed through the mucous membranes. Lozenges or troches are, however, used for their local effect on the mouth and throat. For optimal effectiveness, they should be allowed to dissolve gradually in the mouth and should not be chewed or swallowed whole.

Sublingual mucous membranes are capable of absorbing limited types of drugs such as nitroglycerin and proteolytic enzymes. When a patient receives a sublingual medication intended for its systemic effects, the patient should be instructed to place the tablet under the tongue until it has completely dissolved and has been absorbed by the capillaries present in the mucous membrane. The therapeutic effect of sublingual nitroglycerin on the coronary arteries of a patient with anginal pains is usually experienced in 1 to 3 minutes.

In *buccal administration*, the tablet is placed between the teeth and the mucous membrane of the cheek for local absorption. Some hormone and enzyme preparations are administered by this route.

Nose: nasal administration   Medications administered in the nose include drops and sprays containing the drug in an aqueous solution and powders which are sniffed (insufflated). When administering nose drops to a patient, the nurse should position the patient so that the drug is instilled directly into the nares without inadvertently entering the eye.

Medication may also be delivered to mucous membranes of the nose by an atomizer or nasal spray. Special care should be taken to avoid exerting too much force on the spray to prevent the drug or nasal bacteria from entering the sinuses or the eustachian tubes. Special instructions for patients using nose drops or nasal sprays may include warnings about the harmful effects of using these drugs over an extended period of time; an example of such an effect is the rebound congestion associated with the use of short-acting nasal decongestants at frequent intervals. Moreover, the systemic absorption of the drugs contained in some nasal medications can have adverse effects on the cardiovascular and central nervous systems, particularly if the spray is administered as a stream to the recumbent patient.

Eyes: ophthalmic administration Drugs may be administered in the eye for their local effect on the conjunctiva or for their effect on the structures within the anterior chamber. Aseptic technique must be used, and medication used in the eye must be specifically intended for ophthalmic use.

Ophthalmic drops and ointments are applied in a similar manner except that the ointment is squeezed from the tip of the tube onto the inverted lower eyelid. The heat of the body melts the ointment and the medication is distributed over the eye surface by the patient's eyeball movements.

Ears: otic administration   Otic drops may be instilled into the auditory canal to treat local infections or inflammatory reactions such as external otitis.

Systemic Administration

Oral administration   Administration of drugs by the oral route is the most convenient and acceptable method for the patient. The primary disadvantages of this method are variability in response and potential drug-induced gastric upset. The medication must be in solution before it can be absorbed, that is, dissolution of solid dosage forms must first occur; therefore, a liquid medication usually has a more rapid onset of action than a medication taken in a solid form. Thirty to 45 minutes is usually required before an oral medication is absorbed in sufficient amounts to have a therapeutic effect.

Oral administration of drugs is contraindicated when the patient is nauseated, vomiting, having nasogastric suction, or when the gag or swallowing reflexes are diminished or absent.

Special preparations of drugs with an *enteric coating* may be used when the drug is irritating to the mucous membrane of the stomach. While the enteric coating allows the tablet to remain intact in the acid medium of the stomach, it will disintegrate in the more alkaline medium of the small intestine. These tablets should not be crushed before administration; the patient should be instructed not to chew the tablets before swallowing them nor to swallow them with hot liquids that might dissolve their enteric coatings.

Some oral liquid medications have an extremely bitter or unpleasant taste. Methods to make the medication more palatable may vary with the patient's condition and preferences. Directions on the package insert may suggest using fruit juice as a vehicle or serving the medication with ice. The medication may be followed with water, mouth wash, or a piece of hard candy.

Rectal administration   Absorption from the rectal mucosa is slower and less predictable than absorption after oral administration. However, after rectal administration, the drug does not pass through the liver prior to entering the systemic circulation and, therefore, is not metabolized as rapidly. Drugs may be administered rectally for their local or systemic effects.

A rectal suppository may be a preferred route for an infant or a comatose or confused adult, or if oral medication is contraindicated because of nausea or vomiting.

Inhalation administration   Gases or volatile liquids may be effectively administered by inhalation to produce general anesthesia. The administration of anesthetic agents will be discussed in detail in Chapter 10. Many drugs, such as bronchodilators, mucolytics, and antibiotics, are used in conjunction with intermittent positive pressure breathing to produce primarily local effects and some systemic effects.

Parenteral administration   Literally, *parenteral* means administration of a substance by any route other than the gastrointestinal tract. In common medical usage (and in this text) parenteral routes refer to the administration of solutions or suspensions of drugs by injection and include the intradermal, subcutaneous, intramuscular, and intravenous routes.

Parenteral administration of drugs has the advantage of rapid action, which also makes it the most potentially dangerous route of administration. In addition to a thorough knowledge of drugs, parenteral administration requires specific knowledge of anatomy and aseptic technique. The effects of overdosage, resulting from an error in calculation or the double administration of a medication, is usually more critical when the drug has been injected than when it has been given orally. Once the drug has been injected, it is difficult to remove it from the body or to administer an exact antagonist to prevent its harmful effects. Preparation for administering all parenteral medications requires aseptic technique to prevent infection from contamination. While it is not possible to sterilize the skin, cleansing the site with an antiseptic solution using a circular motion outward from the injection site is recommended.

Intradermal injection   Intradermal or intracutaneous injections are given just below the surface of the skin. Tuberculin testing and allergic sensitization tests utilize this method. Local anesthetics are sometimes injected intradermally; additional, deeper injections can be subsequently given through the anesthetized superficial tissue. Areas of the body where the skin is thin, such as the inner surface of the forearm and the middle of the back, are usually used for intradermal injections.

Subcutaneous injection   A subcutaneous or hypodermic injection is given beneath the skin into the fatty connective tissue lying immediately below the dermis. This method is used for administration of drugs that are highly soluble, nonirritating, and of small volume (0.5 to 2.0 ml). An irritating solution given subcutaneously may cause a sterile abscess. Absorption will be impaired if the subcutaneous route is used for an individual with inadequate peripheral circulation, or if the injection is given in an area with scar tissue resulting from repeated injections.

Any subcutaneous tissue may be used, but the most common sites for injection are the upper lateral portion of the arms and the anterior thigh; other sites are the abdomen and buttocks. If repeated injections are required, a written plan should be used for rotating sites. Although 2 ml is usually the maximum quantity to be injected subcutaneously, large volumes of solution (500 to 1000 ml in adults) may be administered very slowly by *hypodermoclysis*. This method is used to administer nonirritating fluids to infants or adults when it is not possible to employ the intravenous route. The injection site, either the anterior thighs or the suprascapular region of the back, is first infiltrated with the enzyme hyaluronidase (Alidase, Hyazyme, Wydase). This drug facilitates absorption of fluid by decreasing the viscosity of the connective tissue.

Intramuscular injection   An intramuscular injection is used when quick or prolonged action is required. Aqueous solutions of drugs are absorbed promptly since muscle is highly vascular. When slow or gradual absorption is desirable, the medication is placed in suspension, often in an oily vehicle, and given to form a depot of drug in the tissue. The maximum volume of fluid that may be injected into one muscle is usually 5 ml. Two sites should be used to reduce pain and tissue trauma if a greater volume must be injected.

Selection of the site for intramuscular injection requires knowledge of visible anatomical landmarks and location of major nerves and blood vessels in the underlying tissue. The usual sites for intramuscular injections include the deltoid muscle in the upper arm, the dorsogluteal muscles, the ventrogluteal area, and the vastus lateralis muscle in the anterolateral portion of the thigh.

Intravenous injection   The careful administration of an entire drug dose directly into the bloodstream bypasses the need for prior absorption, and is, therefore, very useful in emergency situations when an immediate drug action is required. It is also useful for the administration of large volumes of liquid (by infusion) and for giving drugs that are too irritating to be injected into other tissues without causing undue pain and tissue damage; the irritating drug is rapidly diluted by the blood and the wall of the vein is relatively less sensitive to damage by the drug.

The rapid onset of drug action after intravenous injection also makes it among the most dangerous methods of administering a drug. Because of this, state laws and hospital policies specify who may administer drugs by this route. Once the drug enters the blood, it cannot be readily removed, nor can its distribution throughout the body be impeded. Hence it is often advisable to make such injections slowly, over a period of at least one minute. If an adverse or unanticipated reaction—such as loss of consciousness within 10 to 15 seconds—occurs, further drug administration can be discontinued.

An order for intravenous fluids must include the name and concentration of the solution, the volume of the solution, and the time span or rate at which the solution is to be infused. Each intravenous fluid bottle must be labeled prior to administration and include the name of the patient, room number, date, time started, time to be completed, medication, nurse's signature, and rate of flow.

Some of the veins commonly used for venipuncture are the basilic and cephalic veins in the forearm and antecubital fossa and the metacarpal veins on the back of the hand. The saphenous and marginal veins in the lower leg and foot may also be used.

CALCULATION OF PEDIATRIC DOSES

Administration of potent drugs to infants and children requires precise calculation of dosage since small mistakes in calculating the amount of medication to be administered results in a proportionally greater error. A variety of methods have been introduced over the years for calculating children's doses based on body weight or body surface area. These methods are *approximations* and should not be employed when established doses are available in pediatric textbooks, package inserts, or the published literature. The following are commonly used formulas.

Clark's rule for children 2 years or older:

$$\frac{\text{Weight (lb)}}{150} \times \text{adult dose}$$

$$= \text{approximate child's dose}$$

Young's rule for children 2 years and older:

$$\frac{\text{Age (yr)}}{\text{Age (yr)} + 12} \times \text{adult dose}$$

$$= \text{approximate child's dose}$$

Fried's rule for infants and children up to 2 years old:

$$\frac{\text{Age (months)}}{150} \times \text{adult dose}$$

$$= \text{approximate infant's dose}$$

Some pediatric doses are based on the body surface area of the child. The average body surface area for an adult is 1.73 square meters (m^2). Figure 3-1 contains a nomogram for estimation of a child's body surface area based upon height and weight.

$$\frac{\text{Body surface area of child } (m^2)}{1.73 \ (m^2)} \times \text{adult dose}$$

$$= \text{approximate child's dose}$$

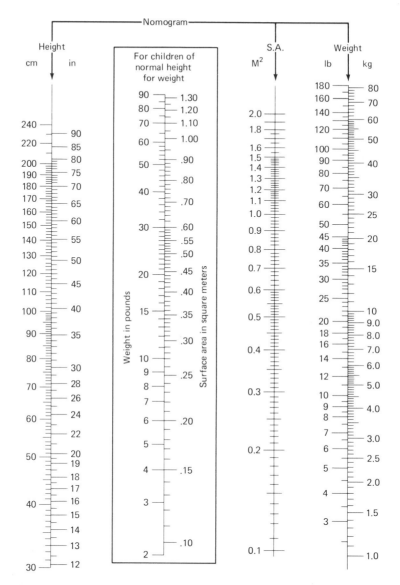

Figure 3-1   West nomogram (for estimation of surface areas). The surface area is indicated where a straight line connecting the height and weight intersects the surface area (S.A.) column or, if the patient is roughly of normal proportion, from the weight alone (enclosed area). (Nomogram modified from data of E. Boyd by C. D. West; from *Nelson Textbook of Pediatrics*, 10th ed., edited by V. C. Vaughan, III and R. J. McKay, Philadelphia: W. B. Saunders Co., 1975).

SAFETY MEASURES IN DRUG ADMINISTRATION

Each hospital has a standard procedure for drug administration that must be learned and followed. A tray with medication cards may be used to obtain drugs from a stock supply. A medication cart, with separate drawers for each patient's drugs, may be transported to each room prior to administering the medication. In unit dose dispensing, the pharmacist will prepare and label each dose of medication and place it in the patient's drawer in the medication cart.

Appropriate precautionary measures will help avoid errors and accidents in preparation and administration of drugs. Constant attention and repeated checking for accuracy is essential. The nurse who prepares a medication is legally liable if there is an error; therefore the nurse who prepares a medication must also administer it.

The patient's identification must be checked each time a medication is given, even though the nurse has cared for that particular patient all morning or for several days. The problem of identification presents an even greater hazard to the nurse who is responsible for the medications of a group of patients or perhaps an entire unit. Patients have been known to answer to names other than their own but are not likely to give the wrong name when asked to identify themselves. The nurse should check the patient's identification bracelet, ask the patient to state his or her name, and compare the medicine card information.

It is not safe to leave medications at the patient's bedside for many reasons. Drugs may accumulate, and if the patient has intentions of self-inflicting harm, there may be sufficient medication to do so. A patient may not understand the purpose of the medication and may be afraid to take it. A patient may dislike the taste or effect produced by the medication and may dispose of the medication rather than take it. Unused medication, particularly drugs subject to abuse, should be carefully accounted for to preclude their diversion to illicit sources.

Followup is an essential part of giving medication. The nurse must assess the patient to determine whether the desired action has been accomplished or if any adverse reaction has occurred.

SUPPLEMENTARY READINGS

Daniels, L., "How Can You Improve Patient Compliance," *Nursing '78* **8**(5): 40–47 (1978).

Geolot, D. H., and N. P. McKinney, "Administering Parenteral Drugs," *American Journal of Nursing* **75**: 788–793 (1975).

Hoover, J. E., "Medication Orders," in *Dispensing of Medication.* ed. J. E. Hoover, Chapter 1, pp. 1–38. Easton, Pa.: Mack Publishing Co., 1976.

Newton, M., and D. W. Newton, "Guidelines for Handling Drug Errors," *Nursing '77* 7(9): 62–68 (1977).

Shirkey, H. C., ed., *Pediatric Therapy* (5th ed.) St. Louis: The C. V. Mosby Company, 1975.

Turco, S., and R. E. King, *Sterile Dosage Forms: Their Preparation and Clinical Application.* Philadelphia: Lea & Febiger, 1974.

Ungvarski, P. J., "Parenteral Therapy," *American Journal of Nursing* **76**: 1974–77 (1976).

Section II
DRUGS AFFECTING THE AUTONOMIC NERVOUS SYSTEM

Chapter 4
INTRODUCTION TO THE AUTONOMIC NERVOUS SYSTEM

The nervous system receives stimuli, transmits this information concerning changes in the environment to higher centers, and initiates responses that generally promote the well-being of the organism. The *central nervous system* (CNS), consisting of the brain and spinal cord, receives, integrates, and interprets nerve impulses generated by these stimuli. The *peripheral nervous system*, which includes all nervous tissue outside the brain and spinal cord, serves to connect all parts of the body with the CNS. *Sensory* or *afferent nerves* detect peripheral stimuli and transmit these messages to the CNS; in turn, *motor* or *efferent nerves* from the CNS modulate the functional activity of peripheral effector cells, which include smooth and skeletal muscles, exocrine and endocrine glands, and the heart (Figure 4-1).

The *peripheral nervous system* is subdivided into the somatic and autonomic nervous systems. The *somatic motor division* innervates tissues such as skeletal muscles under voluntary or conscious influence and controls such functions as inhalation, locomotion, and posture. Neuromuscular blocking agents such as succinylcholine and tubocurarine are employed preoperatively as muscle relaxants and act by interfering with the ability of motor neurons to activate skeletal muscles.

The *autonomic nervous system* inner-

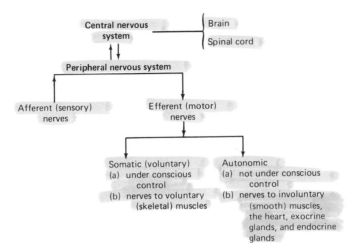

Figure 4-1   Divisions and Interrelationships of the Nervous System.

vates cells that usually are not consciously controlled. As we shall observe in subsequent chapters, many drugs employed for a diverse group of medical problems (for example, asthma, hypertension, myasthenia gravis, gastric ulcers, and nasal congestion) act by enhancing or reducing the activity of the autonomic nervous system. A fundamental knowledge of the physiology of this system is essential to the nurse for an understanding of both the therapeutic uses of these autonomic drugs and their adverse side effects. This chapter is intended to review the physiology of the autonomic nervous system and introduce you to drugs which have actions that modify the activity of this system.

AUTONOMIC NERVOUS SYSTEM

The autonomic nervous system is essentially a system that conducts information from the CNS to effector cells, with functional activity that is not consciously controlled. Autonomic nerves innervate the heart, smooth muscles in the thoracic and abdominal areas, and the endocrine and exocrine glands. This system controls blood pressure, gastrointestinal motility, glandular secretions, urinary output, and body temperature; many other bodily activities are regulated in part or entirely by the autonomic nervous system.

Information is carried by two nerve fibers that synapse at a ganglion (group of nerve cell bodies). The nerve fiber that carries nerve impulses from the CNS to the ganglion located in the periphery is called the *preganglionic neuron*. The nerve impulse is then transmitted from the ganglion to an effector cell via a *postganglionic neuron*. The preganglionic and postganglionic neurons are not contiguous, and the gap between them is called a *synapse* or *synaptic cleft*. Similarly, there is a gap between the postganglionic neuron and its effector cell, and this is referred to as the *neuroeffector junction*. The significance of these gaps will prove to be of great importance when we discuss the concept of chemical transmission of nerve impulses, which, in turn, is fundamental to our understanding of the mechanisms responsible for the actions of autonomic drugs.

Sympathetic and Parasympathetic Nervous Systems

Anatomically and physiologically, the autonomic nervous system consists of two major subdivisions, the sympathetic and parasympathetic systems. The major organs and tissues innervated by each of these systems are shown in Figure 4-2, and a comparison of the major differences between these systems is given in Table 4-1. The physiological consequences of activation of each system are noted on Table 4-2. Activation of the *sympathetic system* prepares the body to respond better to

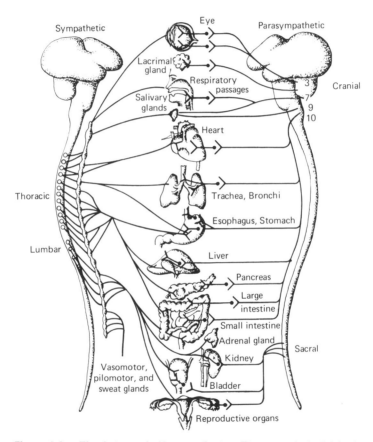

Figure 4-2   The Autonomic Nervous System. The sympathetic division is shown on the left and the parasympathetic division on the right. Note that (1) sympathetic preganglionic fibers arise from the thoracic and lumbar regions of the spinal cord; parasympathetic fibers originate from cranial and sacral areas; (2) sympathetic preganglionic fibers are short and postganglionic fibers are long; for the parasympathetic system the opposite relationship exists; (3) many postganglionic fibers arise from each sympathetic preganglionic fiber, whereas one or two postganglionic parasympathetic fibers arise from each preganglionic fiber; (4) most organs are innervated by both divisions of the autonomic nervous system.

Table 4-1   Comparison of the Sympathetic and Parasympathetic Nervous Systems

Characteristics	Sympathetic nervous system	Parasympathetic nervous system
Origin of preganglionic fibers	Thoracic & lumbar segments of spinal cord (thoracolumbar)	Cranial nerves of brain stem & sacral segments of spinal cord (craniosacral)
Relative length of fibers:		
Preganglionic fibers	Short	Long
Postganglionic fibers	Long	Short
Location of autonomic ganglia	Close to CNS	Near or on effector cell
Ratio of preganglionic to postganglionic fibers	1:10—1:20	1:1—1:2
General physiological functions	Emergency & stress responses, energy expenditure	Conservation restoration of energy, digestive processes
Neurotransmitters:		
Preganglionic	Acetylcholine	Acetylcholine
Postganglionic	Norepinephrine from nerve endings and epinephrine and norepinephrine from adrenal medulla	Acetylcholine

stress and to emergency situations ("fight or flight"), as evidenced by increases in the force and rate of cardiac contraction, dilation (widening) of the pupils and bronchioles, and breakdown of glycogen to blood glucose (sugar) to provide energy. By contrast, the *parasympathetic system* is concerned with normal vegetative functions; for example, digestion and absorption of food is promoted by increased glandular secretions and motility of the smooth muscles of the stomach and intestines.

In many instances we observe that the responses resulting from activation of each division of the autonomic nervous system are qualitatively opposite (as noted in Table 4-2). Where both autonomic divisions innervate a given effector system to produce such opposite responses, it should not be assumed that one division is "on" while the other is "off." Rather, both divisions act simultaneously to achieve a finer level of control to modulate the functional activity of the effector system. Some tissues receive innervation from both autonomic subdivisions, activation of either of which results in a similar response, while other effectors receive innervation from only one subdivision.

NEUROHUMORAL TRANSMISSION

How do autonomic nerves send their messages to the tissues of the effector system? Conduction, that is, the movement of a nerve impulse down nerve fibers, is an electrical phenomenon. The passage of this message across synapses, referred to as *transmission*, is accomplished by chemical substances that are released from nerve endings. These chemical mediators of transmission are collectively called *neurotransmitters*.

Neurotransmitters are chemicals synthesized within the neuron from simple precursor compounds provided by the diet; the biochemical reactions responsible for the formation of the neurotransmitters are catalyzed by specific enzymes. Once formed, the neurotransmitter is stored in synaptic vesicles located in the nerve endings. In response to a nerve impulse, the neurotransmitter is re-

Table 4-2   Comparison of the Responses of Effector Systems to Autonomic Nerve Impulses

Effector system	Sympathetic (adrenergic) nerve impulses	Parasympathetic (cholinergic) nerve impulses
Cardiovascular System		
Heart		
Rate of contraction	Increase	Decrease
Force of contraction	Increase	Decrease
Blood pressure	Increase	Decrease
Blood vessels		
Skin and mucous membranes	Constriction	Dilatation
Skeletal muscle	Dilatation	Dilatation
Coronary	Dilatation; constriction	——
Renal	Constriction	——
Smooth Muscles		
Stomach & intestines (motility & tone)	Decrease	Increase
Eye		
Radial muscle—iris	Dilation (mydriasis—pupil)	——
Sphincter muscle—iris	——	Contraction (constriction—pupil)
Ciliary muscle	Relaxation (focus lens for far vision)	Contraction (focus lens for near vision)
Urinary bladder sphincter	Contraction	Relaxation
Bronchial	Relaxation (dilatation)	Contraction (constriction)
Uterus	Pregnant: contraction Nonpregnant: relaxation	
Adrenal Medulla	——	Secretion of epinephrine and norepinephrine
Glands		
Sweat (cholinergic)	Generalized secretion	Localized secretion
Salivary	Slight, thick secretion	Profuse, watery secretion
Lacrimal	——	Increase in secretion
Gastrointestinal	——	Increase in secretion
Bronchial	——	Increase in secretion
Miscellaneous Responses		
Basal metabolic rate	Increase	——
Liver glycogen breakdown to blood sugar	Increase	——
Male sex organs	Ejaculation	Erection
Pancreas (islets)	Inhibit insulin secretion	——

leased from the nerve, crosses the synaptic or junctional gap, and interacts with specific receptors located on the membrane of the postganglionic neuron or the effector cell. Neurotransmitter-receptor interactions produce alterations in the permeability of the membrane to ions (sodium, potassium, chloride), resulting in an excitatory or inhibitory change in the functional activity of the innervated tissue. The released neurotransmitter is then chemically inactivated or its actions are terminated by other mechanisms.

Adrenergic and cholinergic systems

The nature of the released neurotransmitter is physiologically and pharmacologically of greater importance to the nurse studying drugs than is the anatomical differentiation of whether a given nerve is part of the sympathetic or parasympathetic nervous system. Hence it is more useful for us to classify autonomic and somatic motor neurons on the basis of the neurotransmitter substance released at their endings. All neurons that release the neurotransmitter *acetylcholine* are called *cholinergic* neurons or fibers, while those that release *norepinephrine* (noradrenaline) are called *adrenergic* neurons.

Preganglionic neurons of both the sympathetic and parasympathetic divisions of the autonomic nervous system, as well as postganglionic parasympathetic neurons, all release acetylcholine and are, therefore, cholinergic fibers. Norepinephrine is released from most postganglionic sympathetic neurons, and these are adrenergic neurons. The adrenal medulla, anatomically and functionally part of the sympathetic division, primarily secretes epinephrine (adrenaline) as well as a lesser amount of norepinephrine. Neurons innervating the sweat glands and certain blood vessels release acetylcholine; these fibers are classified as cholinergic neurons. The somatic motor neurons innervating voluntary skeletal muscle are all cholinergic. The central nervous system contains both adrenergic and cholinergic neurons. Table 4-3 summarizes the location of adrenergic and cholinergic neurons.

Adrenergic Transmission and Receptors

The primary adrenergic transmitter in the periphery and in certain areas of the brain is *norepinephrine*. The other adrenergic transmitters are *epinephrine*, released from the adrenal medulla, and *dopamine*, present in discrete regions of the brain. On the basis of their chemistry, these three compounds are referred to as *catecholamines*.

Norepinephrine is synthesized and stored in nerve ending vesicles. After its release is triggered by a nerve impulse, norepinephrine crosses the synapse and interacts with an adrenergic receptor located on neuroeffector sites such as smooth muscle, the heart muscle, or gland cells to initiate a response. Its action is terminated, primarily by reuptake into the nerve ending. Of lesser importance is its inactivation by the enzymes catechol-O-methyltransferase (COMT) and monoamine oxidase (MAO), enzymes present outside and within the adrenergic neuron, respectively.

Adrenergic receptors are classified as *alpha* (α) and *beta* (β); beta receptors are of two types: *beta*$_1$ (β_1) and *beta*$_2$ (β_2). Norepinephrine primarily activates α-receptors, isoproterenol (a synthetic catecholamine) primarily activates both β-receptor types, while epinephrine activates both α- and β-receptors (although its effects on the β-receptors predominate).

Activation of the α-adrenergic receptors produces constriction of blood vessels, dilation of the pupils (mydriasis), and relaxation of the smooth muscles of the gastrointestinal tract. Beta$_1$ activation results in an increase in the rate and force of contraction of the heart and increases in free fatty acids (lipolysis). Beta$_2$ activation causes relaxation of the smooth muscles of the bronchioles (bronchodilation), gastrointestinal tract and uterus, vasodilation of the blood vessels in skeletal muscle, and an increase in skeletal muscle contractility (muscle tremors). Beta receptor activation also results in increased blood glucose levels resulting from a breakdown of liver glycogen

Table 4-3 Cholinergic and Adrenergic Neurons

Nerve (chemical mediator)	Sites of innervation	Schematic representation
A. Cholinergic (acetylcholine; ACh)	1. All postganglionic parasympathetic fibers (neuroeffector junction) 2. All autonomic (sympathetic and parasympathetic) preganglionic fibers (autonomic ganglia) 3. Preganglionic (splanchnic nerve) fibers to the adrenal medulla 4. Postganglionic sympathetic fibers to sweat glands and certain blood vessels 5. Somatic motor nerves to skeletal or voluntary muscles (neuromuscular junction) 6. Parts of the central nervous system	*Autonomic neurons* *Sympathetic (adrenergic)* Preganglionic fiber — Ganglion (A·2) — Postganglionic fiber (B·1) — Neuroeffector junction — Receptor *Parasympathetic (cholinergic)* Ganglion (A·2) — (A·1) — Neuroeffector junction — Receptor
B. Adrenergic (norepinephrine; NE)	1. All postganglionic sympathetic fibers (except A4 above) 2. Parts of the central nervous system (norepinephrine and dopamine)	*Motor nerve* (A·5) — Neuromuscular junction — Skeletal muscle

(glycogenolysis). Adrenergic receptor antagonists are available that specifically block α- or β-receptors.

Cholinergic Transmission and Receptors

In the periphery, *acetylcholine* is the chemical mediator of nerve impulses at all autonomic ganglia (sympathetic and parasympathetic), at the postganglionic parasympathetic neuroeffector junction, and at the neuromuscular junction. After its release from nerve endings, acetylcholine interacts with cholinergic receptors to initiate a response, with the precise nature of this response dependent upon the tissue innervated. Thereafter, acetylcholine is very rapidly inactivated by the enzyme *acetylcholinesterase*.

While the cholinergic receptors at all three sites are responsive to acetylcholine-induced activation, drugs capable of mimicking the effects of acetylcholine are not equally active at each of them. Similarly, drugs that block cholinergic transmission at one site may have little or no blocking effectiveness at the other two cholinergic receptors. Based upon the differential agonistic effects of muscarine and nicotine and the antagonistic properties of atropine, tubocurarine, and hexamethonium, we commonly distinguish cholinergic receptors into one of two categories: *muscarinic receptors* at the neuroeffector (postganglionic parasympathetic) junction, and *nicotinic receptors* at the autonomic ganglion and neuromuscular junction (Figure 4-3). Muscarinic and nicotinic cholinergic receptors can also be found in the CNS.

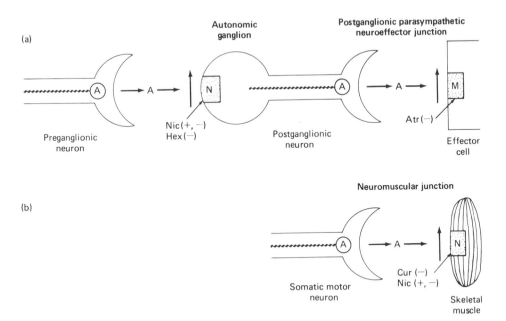

Figure 4-3   Muscarinic and Nicotinic Cholinergic Receptor Sites. Muscarinic receptor sites (M), located on effector cells, are activated by acetylcholine (A) which is released from nerve endings by nerve impulses (〜〜〜〜); these sites are blocked by atropine (Atr). Nicotinic receptor sites (N), located at the autonomic ganglion and neuromuscular junction, are blocked specifically by hexamethonium (Hex) and tubocurarine (Cur), respectively. Nicotine (Nic) has both stimulatory and inhibitory effects at these two sites.

General Overview of Autonomic Drugs

Drugs are capable of increasing or decreasing the functional activity of the autonomic nervous system by a variety of mechanisms (Table 4-4). Increasing the release of the neurotransmitter from vesicles in the nerve endings or inhibiting processes that result in termination of the neurotransmitter's actions result in an increase in the functional activity of that subdivision of the autonomic nervous system; other drugs directly activate the receptor site. Conversely, many drugs decrease the functional activity of the autonomic nervous system by inhibiting the synthesis, storage, or release of the neurotransmitter or by blocking the receptor site and thereby preventing the interaction between the neurotransmitter and its respective receptor. As we saw in Chapter 2, the neurotransmitter is an *agonist* and the receptor blocker is an *antagonist*.

Drugs that mimic effects observed when norepinephrine is released from adrenergic nerves are called *adrenergic* or *sympathomimetic* agents (Chapter 5). Specific receptor antagonists are classified as *alpha-* and *beta-adrenergic* (β_1, β_2) *blocking agents* (Chapter 6). Compounds that mimic the muscarinic effects of acetylcholine at the postganglionic parasympathetic neuroeffector junction are called *cholinergic, parasympathomimetic*, or *muscarinic* agents (Chapter 7); antagonists at these sites are called *cholinergic blocking agents* or *antimuscarinic drugs* (Chapter 8). Since both preganglionic sympathetic and parasympathetic nerves release acetylcholine, drugs that mimic or block acetylcholine at these sites are called *ganglionic stimulants* or *ganglionic blocking agents*, respectively. Drugs preventing the activation of skeletal muscle after the release of acetylcholine from somatic motor nerves are called *neuromuscular blocking agents* (Chapter 11).

Table 4-4   Drugs Modifying the Function of the Autonomic Nervous System

Mechanism of drug action	Neurotransmitter	
	Acetylcholine[a] (cholinergic)	Norepinephrine (adrenergic)
Inhibits neurotransmitter synthesis	Hemicholinium[b]	α-methyltyrosine[b]
Inhibits neurotransmitter storage in nerve ending vesicles	——	Reserpine
Increases neurotransmitter release	Carbachol	Amphetamine
Inhibits neurotransmitter release	Botulinum toxin[b]	Guanethidine
Activates receptor directly (mimics neurotransmitter)	A. Nicotine[b] B. Pilocarpine, muscarine[b] C. Nicotine[b]	α-receptor: phenylephrine β_1 and β_2-receptor: isoproterenol β_2-receptor: metaproterenol
Blocks receptor site (inhibitory effects)	A. Hexamethonium B. Atropine C. Tubocurarine	α-receptor: phentolamine β_1 and β_2-receptor: propranolol β_1-receptor: practolol
Inhibits termination of action of neurotransmitter (enhances effects of neurotransmitter)	Neostigmine Isoflurophate	Amphetamine Cocaine Imipramine

[a] Cholinergic sites of action: A. Autonomic ganglia; B. Neuroeffector junction; C. Neuromuscular junction.
[b] Pharmacological tool—not employed therapeutically.

SUPPLEMENTARY READINGS

Appenzeller, O., *The Autonomic Nervous System: An Introduction to Basic and Clinical Concepts* (2nd ed.). Amsterdam: North-Holland Publishing Company, 1976.

Blaschko, H. and E. Muscholl, ed., "Catecholamines." *Handbook of Experimental Pharmacology*, Vol. 33. Berlin: Springer-Verlag, 1972.

Burn, J. H., *The Autonomic Nervous System for Students of Physiology and Pharmacology* (5th ed.). Oxford: Blackwell Scientific Publications Ltd, 1975.

Cooper, J. R., F. E. Bloom, and R. H. Roth, *The Biochemical Basis of Neuropharmacology* (3rd ed.). New York: Oxford University Press, Inc., 1978.

Johnson, R. H., and J. M. K. Spaulding, *Disorders of the Autonomic Nervous System*. Philadelphia: F. A. Davis Company, 1974.

Mayer, S. E., "Neurohumoral Transmission and the Autonomic Nervous System," in *Goodman and Gilman's The Pharmacological Basis of Therapeutics* (5th ed.), ed. A. G. Gilman, L. S. Goodman, and A. Gilman, Chapter 4, pp. 56–90. New York: Macmillan, Inc., 1980.

McLennan, H., *Synaptic Transmission* (2nd ed.). Philadelphia: W. B. Saunders Company, 1970.

Rang, H. P., ed., *Drug Receptors*. Baltimore: University Park Press, 1973.

Turner, P., *Clinical Aspects of Autonomic Pharmacology*. Philadelphia: J. B Lippincott Company, 1970.

Volle, R. L., "Introduction to the Autonomic Nervous System," in *Drill's Pharmacology in Medicine* (4th ed.), ed. J. R. DiPalma, Chapter 30, pp. 559–83. New York: McGraw-Hill Book Company, 1971.

Chapter 5

SYMPATHOMIMETIC (ADRENERGIC) DRUGS

Sympathomimetic or *adrenergic agents* are drugs that produce pharmacological effects similar to those observed when adrenergic (postganglionic sympathetic) nerves or the adrenal medulla are stimulated. The primary therapeutic uses of these drugs are predicated upon their pronounced effects on the heart, blood vessels, and certain smooth muscles such as the bronchi.

In your nursing practice, you shall encounter numerous sympathomimetic agents. The pharmacological effects of these drugs are very similar to the prototype drugs epinephrine, norepinephrine, and isoproterenol, differing primarily in their relative selectivities and time courses of action.

ADRENERGIC RECEPTORS

Adrenergic receptors, as previously discussed (Chapter 4), are classified as alpha, beta$_1$, or beta$_2$. The nature of the pharmacological response produced by a given sympathomimetic drug is dependent upon its relative ability to activate one or more of these receptor types and on the relative distribution of these receptors in a given tissue (Table 5-1). Norepinephrine and phenylephrine preferentially activate α-receptors, isoproterenol activates β_1- and β_2-receptors, metaproterenol activates β_2-receptors, while epinephrine acts on all three adrenergic receptor types.

When a sympathomimetic agent such as norepinephrine activates α-receptors, you would anticipate observing vasoconstriction of splanchnic and subcutaneous blood vessels (with a resulting reduction in blood flow and an increase in systemic blood pressure) and pupilary dilation. Isoproterenol-induced activation of β_1-receptors increase the rate and force of contraction of cardiac muscle and elevates blood levels of free fatty acids; β_2-receptor activation causes vasodilation of

Table 5-1 Responses of Effector Organs to Sympathetic Activation by Catecholamines or Sympathomimetic Drugs[a]

Effector organ	Adrenergic receptor	Predominant physiological or pharmacological effects	Predominant response observed
Eye			
Iris, radial muscle	α	Contraction	Mydriasis[b]
Ciliary muscle	β	Relaxation	Accommodation
Heart			
Sinoatrial node	β_1	↑ Rate	↑ Heart rate[b]
Conduction tissues	β_1	↑ Conduction velocity	↑ Heart rate
Myocardium	β_1	↑ Contraction	↑ Force of contraction
Arteries and arterioles			
Renal; abdominal viscera	α	Vasoconstriction	↓ Local blood flow[b] ↑ Systemic blood pressure[b]
Subcutaneous	α	Vasoconstriction	↓ Local blood flow[b]
Skeletal muscle	β_2	Vasodilation	↑ Local blood flow[b] ↓ Systemic blood pressure[b]
Veins	α	Vasoconstriction	↑ Venous return ↑ Cardiac output
Kidney	β_2	↑ Renin secretion	↑ Sodium reabsorption ↑ Blood pressure
Lungs			
Bronchial smooth muscle	β_2	Relaxation	Bronchodilation[b]
Gastrointestinal tract			
Intestinal smooth muscle	α, β_1	Relaxation	↓ Motility
Uterus			
Pregnant	α	Contraction	↑ Motility
	β_2	Relaxation	↓ Motility
Liver	β	↑ Glycogen breakdown	↑ Blood glucose[b]
Pancreas	α	↓ Insulin secretion	↑ Blood glucose[b]
Adipose (fat) tissue	β_1	↑ Fat breakdown	↑ Blood free fatty acids[b]

[a]Abbreviations: ↑ = increase; ↓ = decrease.
[b]Most significant reponses after administration of therapeutic doses of sympathomimetic agents.

blood vessels in skeletal muscles, relaxation of bronchial, gastrointestinal, and genitourinary smooth muscle, and increases in blood glucose levels.

Mechanism of Action

Some sympathomimetic agents interact *directly* with adrenergic receptors located on effector cells to initiate a pharmacological response, while others act *indirectly* by stimulating the release of norepinephrine from nerve endings. Examples of direct-acting drugs include epinephrine, norepinephrine (levarterenol), isoproterenol, and phenylephrine; amphetamine and ephedrine, by contrast, are indirect-acting drugs.

The distinction between these mechanisms of action assumes great therapeutic significance when these drugs are employed as pressor agents, that is, to elevate blood pressure. Unlike direct-acting drugs, continuous infusions or frequent repeated injections of indirect-acting sympathomimetic agents progressively diminish the ability of these latter drugs to elevate blood pressure. This diminished response, occurring over a period of hours, is called *tachyphylaxis* and results from the depletion of norepinephrine from nerve endings more rapidly than it can be replenished by biosynthetic processes.

PHARMACOLOGY

Based upon similarities in chemical structure, epinephrine, norepinephrine (levarterenol) and the synthetic sympathomimetic drug isoproterenol are collectively referred to as *catecholamines*. The pharmacological properties and therapeutic applications of epinephrine, the prototype sympathomimetic agent, will be considered in greatest detail, followed by discussions of the other two catecholamines, with emphasis placed on their differences and similarities to epinephrine. Clinically employed sympathomimetic agents are summarized in Table 5-2. The pharmacology of amphetamine, a central nervous system stimulant, will be discussed in Chapter 22.

Epinephrine (Adrenaline)

Epinephrine, commonly called *adrenaline*, is a hormone that is discharged from the adrenal medulla when an individual is subjected to emotional stress, pain, trauma, and emergency situations. The pharmacological actions of epinephrine, most prominently observed on the heart, blood vessels, and bronchial smooth muscle, may be attributed to its ability to activate α-, β_1-, and β_2-adrenergic receptors when this compound is administered in a clinical situation.

Table 5-2   Commonly Used Sympathomimetic Drugs

Generic name	Selected trade names	Usual adult dose	Remarks
A. *Levarterenol-like vasopressor agents (α-adrenergic effects)*			
Levarterenol (norepinephrine)	Levophed	IV infusion: 2–4 μg/min diluted in 5% dextrose sol.	Extremely potent; short duration of action (1–2 min); avoid extravasation; patient not to be left unattended; see text.
Ephedrine		SC: 15–50 mg; IV: 20 mg	Less potent, longer duration of action than levarterenol; tachyphylaxis with repeated injections.
Metaraminol	Aramine	IV infusion: 15–100 mg	Pressor effects last 90 min; avoid subcutaneous administration.
Methoxamine	Vasoxyl	IM: 5–20 mg; IV: 3–10 mg	Alpha activation only; no cardiac arrhythmias with general anesthetics.

Table 5-2   (Continued)

Generic name	Selected trade names	Usual adult dose	Remarks
Phenylephrine	Neo-Synephrine	SC or IM: 1-10 mg; IV: 0.25-1 mg	Same as methoxamine; suitable for IV, IM and SC injection; longer duration of action.
Dopamine	Intropin	IV infusion: 2.5-20 μg/kg/min	Useful in treatment of shock; increase in cardiac output and blood pressure without increasing heart rate; enhances blood flow to kidneys and splanchnic areas by activating dopaminergic receptors.

B. Epinephrine-like cardiac stimulants (β_1-adrenergic effects)

Epinephrine (adrenaline)	Adrenalin	SC: 0.1-0.5 mg	Danger of ventricular fibrillation, anginal pain, and cerebral hemorrhaging. Solutions should not be used if brown in color or containing a precipitate.
Isoproterenol	Isuprel	IM or SC: 0.01-0.20 mg	No danger of ventricular fibrillation. Avoid using any dosage form of isoproterenol that is brown in color.
Dobutamine	Dobutrex	IV infusion: 2.5-10 μg/kg/min	Inotropic activity with little chronotropic, hypertensive, arrhythmogenic and vasodilatory effects. Used for short-term treatment of congestive heart failure. (See Chapter 26.)

C. Isoproterenol-like bronchodilators (β_2-adrenergic effects)[a]

Isoproterenol	Isuprel; Norisodrine	Inhalation: 0.5 ml of 0.5% sol.	Used by aerosol and injection to abort acute bronchial asthmatic attacks; adverse cardiovascular effects.

D. Nasal Decongestants (α-adrenergic effects)

Ephedrine	———	PO: 25 mg 3-4 times daily	Orally active; adverse cardiovascular and central stimulating effects.
Pseudoephedrine	Sudafed	PO: 30-60 mg 3-4 times daily	Orally active; fewer adverse cardiovascular effects than ephedrine.
Phenylpropanolamine	Propadrine	PO: 25-50 mg 3-4 times daily	Orally active; less central stimulation than ephedrine.
Phenylephrine	Neo-Synephrine	2 gtts of 0.25% sol.	Nasal solution; effective decongestant.
Naphazoline	Privine	2 gtts of 0.05% sol.	Nasal solution; effective but rebound congestion; vasopression and reduction in heart rate reported.
Tetrahydrozoline	Tyzine	2 gtts of 0.05-0.1% sol.	Nasal solution; cardiac slowing observed in an infant.
Oxymetazoline	Afrin, Duration	2-4 gtts of 0.05% sol.	Nasal solution for adults and children over 6 yr; long duration of action (8-12 h)
Xylometazoline	Otrivin	2-3 gtts of 0.1% sol.	Nasal solutions for adults and children; long duration of action (8-10 h).
Propylhexedrine	Benzedrex	1-2 inhalations	Nasal inhaler; some stimulatory effects on the heart, but not on the central nervous system.

[a]See Table 54-1.

Cardiovascular System

Blood pressure The effects of epinephrine on the cardiovascular system depend primarily upon its dose and speed of administration. The increase in pulse pressure observed after the slow intravenous infusion of low doses (10 μg/minute) result from an increase in systolic pressure and a fall in diastolic pressure; mean arterial pressure is not generally changed. Epinephrine possesses both vasoconstrictor (α-mediated) and vasodilator (β_2-mediated) effects; blood vessels in the skin and splanchnic (viseral) areas are constricted (α), while those in skeletal muscle are dilated (β_2). At low doses vasodilation predominates and a decrease in total peripheral resistance is observed. By contrast, after rapid intravenous injection of epinephrine, a rapid and pronounced increase in mean arterial blood pressure results; blood pressure then falls below normal prior to returning to pre-drug levels. This latter hypertensive response is the consequence of marked vasoconstriction and may cause a cerebral hemorrhage if the blood pressure is permitted to rise to dangerously high levels.

Heart Epinephrine is a potent stimulant of the heart, increasing both the rate and force of contractions. These β_1-mediated effects serve as the basis for the use of epinephrine for emergency treatment of cardiac arrest. Cardiac arrhythmias may occur after high doses of epinephrine; this drug reduces the refractory period of atrial and ventricular muscles and increases ventricular automaticity.

Epinephrine greatly increases oxygen consumption by the heart muscle and is, therefore, contraindicated in angina pectoris; extreme chest pain occurs in this coronary artery disease when the oxygen requirements of the heart muscle exceed the oxygen supply (Chapter 29).

Blood vessels The *vasoconstrictor* effects of administered epinephrine on superficial blood vessels can be readily detected by blanching and a reduction in skin temperature. Clinical uses of epinephrine based upon vasoconstriction include the arrest of hemorrhaging from small blood vessels and the prevention of the diffusion of local anesthetic agents from their site of injection. While epinephrine is an effective vasoconstrictor of the mucous membranes of the nasal passages after topical application, its clinical utility as a nasal decongestant is limited by rebound vasodilation resulting in "after congestion."

Smooth muscle The effects of epinephrine on the smooth muscle of blood vessels have been described above. Epinephrine relaxes smooth muscle of the gastrointestinal tract, the urinary bladder, and the uterus and dilates the pupils by causing contraction of the radial muscle of the eye.

A prominent action of epinephrine is on smooth muscle of the *bronchioles*, where activation of β_2-adrenergic receptors causes relaxation of these muscles, resulting in *bronchodilation*. This effect, occurring in conjunction with constriction of swollen mucous membranes of the respiratory tract and inhibition of excessive bronchial secretions, is of life-saving significance to the asthmatic patient experiencing severe respiratory impairment resulting from bronchoconstriction and congestion.

During the last month of pregnancy, epinephrine inhibits *uterine contractions* but short duration of action and adverse cardiovascular effects preclude its use for this purpose. By contrast, selective β_2 agonists such as metaproterenol have been employed clinically to delay premature labor.

Metabolic effects Epinephrine enhances the breakdown of liver glycogen, thereby increasing *blood glucose* levels, and also promotes the release of free fatty acids from adipose tissues. The increase in available glucose and free fatty acids represents important sources of energy.

Plasma *potassium* concentrations rise temporarily after epinephrine injection, followed by a prolonged fall in the plasma levels of this cation; hypokalemia results from the movement of plasma potassium into cells.

Therapeutic uses   The actions of epinephrine on blood vessels, the heart, and bronchial muscle serve as the basis for the clinical uses of this drug. It is employed as a vasoconstrictor agent to arrest bleeding from superficial capillaries and to prolong the duration of action of local anesthetics. The stimulating properties of this drug on cardiac muscle are of value for the emergency treatment of cardiac arrest. Epinephrine is also used for the treatment of bronchial asthma and to achieve rapid relief from the hypotensive symptoms of allergic reactions to drugs and other allergens. The therapeutic applications of epinephrine and other sympathomimetic agents will be considered in greater detail later in this chapter.

Adverse effects and nursing precautions   Administration of normal therapeutic doses of epinephrine may cause anxiety, fear, headache, and palpitations. These effects are greatly disquieting to the patient, yet are not generally dangerous. Prior to administering this drug, the nurse should advise the patient that such effects may occur. Remaining with the patient after epinephrine injection can help in allaying the fear and anxiety. Far more significant, however, are *cerebral hemorrhage* and *cardiac arrhythmias* (in particular, ventricular fibrillation) produced by epinephrine overdosage. Elderly patients and those with a history of heart dis-

ease, hypertension, and hyperthyroidism are particularly susceptible to the adverse effects of this drug. Great caution should be exercised when epinephrine is administered to a patient receiving digitalis therapy for the treatment of congestive heart failure; both these drugs can precipitate cardiac arrhythmias and can potentiate each other's adverse effects on the heart. Epinephrine may also induce anginal pain in patients with a history of angina pectoris. Additional nursing implications are given at the end of this chapter.

Levarterenol (Norepinephrine)

Norepinephrine, the neurotransmitter substance released from peripheral sympathetic postganglionic (adrenergic) nerves, acts to maintain the normal function of tissues innervated by the sympathetic division of the autonomic nervous system. There is strong evidence supporting the concept that norepinephrine is also a neurotransmitter in selected areas of the brain. The discussion in this text will be limited to the cardiovascular effects of levarterenol (norepinephrine) because only these effects are therapeutically significant in humans.

Cardiovascular effects   Levarterenol is predominantly an α-adrenergic stimulant. Hence it should be anticipated that the effects of this drug on blood vessels will be almost exclusively *vasoconstrictor* in nature.

Therapeutic doses of levarterenol administered by slow intravenous infusion elevate both systolic and diastolic pressures. These effects can be attributed to vasoconstriction of blood vessels with a resulting increase in total peripheral resistance. The vasoconstrictor actions of this drug also reduce blood flow to the kidney, splanchnic areas, placenta, and skeletal muscle.

The nurse will generally observe brady-cardia after levarterenol administration, although this drug has direct stimulating effects on cardiac muscle. Drug-induced vasoconstriction increases blood pressure causing a reflex increase in vagal activity and a reduction in heart rate.

The therapeutic use of levarterenol for the treatment of shock will be considered later in this chapter.

Adverse effects and nursing precautions The adverse effects associated with levarterenol at therepautic doses are similar to those caused by epinephrine, but occur less frequently. Overdose of this drug can cause severe hypertension, possibly resulting in cerebral hemorrhaging, chest pain, sweating, and vomiting. Levarterenol should not be administered to patients with mesenteric thrombosis, because of the danger of increasing ischemia and extending the area of the infarction.

Extreme care must be exercised when administering this drug intravenously to prevent its leakage into tissues surrounding the vein. Contact of this potent vasoconstrictor drug with subcutaneous tissues can result in ischemia, necrosis, and tissue sloughing. If tissue infiltration, denoted by blanching of the skin, is detected, the infusion should be immediately terminated and started in another vein. The area of tissue infiltration should be promptly treated with the α-adrenergic blocking agent phentolamine (Regitine) in normal saline solution. Other nursing implications are summarized at the end of the chapter.

Isoproterenol

Isoproterenol (Isuprel) is a synthetic catecholamine which has pharmacological effects that can be attributed almost exclusively to activation of β_1- and β_2-receptors. The major effects of this drug are on the cardiovascular system and on bronchial smooth muscle.

Cardiovascular effects Intravenous infusion of isoproterenol increases the force and rate of cardiac contractions (β_1-effects) and reduces total peripheral resistance as a consequence of its general vasodilatory effects (β_2-effects). Small doses of this drug cause modest reductions in mean arterial pressure, while high doses produce a dramatic fall in mean blood pressure.

Dobutamine (Dobutrex), a recently developed isoproterenol-like drug, increases the force of cardiac contractions with relatively weak effects on heart rate or blood pressure. The properties of this drug and its use for the treatment of congestive heart failure will be discussed in Chapter 26.

Smooth muscle Isoproterenol relaxes almost all smooth muscle, with its actions on bronchial muscle most prominent and of greatest therapeutic significance. Injection or inhalation of this drug produces pronounced *bronchodilation*. The use of isoproterenol for the treatment of cardiac arrest will be discussed in a later section of this chapter; its use in the management of bronchial asthma will be discussed in Chapter 54.

Administration of Catecholamines

Neither epinephrine nor levarterenol are effective after oral administration, since both drugs are readily destroyed by enzymes in the gastrointestinal tract. Epinephrine is administered by intravenous, subcutaneous, or intramuscular injection, applied topically on the skin or mucous membranes, or used as an inhalant aerosol. Levarterenol is safely administered only by intravenous injection; severe ischemia and necrosis, resulting from arteriolar vasoconstriction, occur at the site of subcutaneous injections. Isoproterenol is most effective when inhaled via an aerosol or injected intravenously; absorption of oral and sublingual tablets are undependable.

THERAPEUTIC USES OF SYMPATHOMIMETIC DRUGS

Dozens of sympathomimetic agents are employed as therapeutic agents; some of the most important of these are listed in Table 5-2. This section discusses the clinical uses of the catecholamines and other representative sympathomimetic drugs the nurse is likely to encounter in professional practice. Clinically

significant drug interactions involving this drug class appear in Table 5-3.

Control of Bleeding

Topical application of epinephrine in a dilution of 1:20,000 to 1:1,000 is employed to control superficial bleeding from capillaries and arterioles resulting from nose bleeds, tooth extractions, and surgical procedures. This drug should not be used to attempt to stop hemorrhaging from large blood vessels.

Use With Local Anesthetics

Epinephrine, at low concentrations (1:100,000 to 1:200,000), is often added to solutions containing local anesthetic agents. The vaso-

Table 5-3   Selected Clinically Significant Drug Interactions Involving Sympathomimetic Agents

Sympathomimetic agent	Interacting drug class	Potential consequences
Epinephrine	Anesthetics, general Cyclopropane Halothane (Fluothane)	Sensitization of heart muscle to arrhythmias.
Amphetamine Ephedrine Phenylpropanolamine Phenylephrine Pseudoephedrine	Antidepressants, monoamine oxidase inhibitors (MAOI) Isocarboxazid (Marplan) Phenylzine (Nardil) Tranylcypromine (Parnate)	Inhibition of metabolism of sympathomimetic agents resulting in their buildup potentially causing acute hypertensive crisis and cerebral hemorrhaging. The hazards associated with the ephedrine-MAOI interaction are well documented.
Epinephrine	Antidepressants, tricyclic Amitriptyline (Elavil) Imipramine (Tofranil) Protriptyline (Vivactil)	The antidepressants markedly enhance the pressor response to epinephrine and may cause cardiac arrhythmias.
Amphetamine Ephedrine	Antihypertensives Guanethidine (Ismelin) Methyldopa (Aldomet) Reserpine (Serpasil)	Antagonism of antihypertensive effect, with loss of control of blood pressure.
Epinephrine	Digitalis-cardiac glycosides Digoxin (Lanoxin) Digitoxin (many brands)	Epinephrine-induced reduction in plasma potassium levels may increase risk of digitalis toxicity. Epinephrine and digitalis glycosides should be used concurrently with great caution since each drug is capable of causing cardiac arrhythmias; this risk is greatly increased when these drugs are used in combination.

constriction produced by this catecholamine greatly reduces the diffusion of the local anesthetic from its site of administration, thereby prolonging the duration of its action and decreasing the risk of systemic toxicity (Chapter 12).

Hypotension

Sympathomimetic drugs are extensively employed as *vasopressor agents*, that is, to elevate blood pressure in certain cases of severe hypotension.

A marked drop in blood pressure may be observed during spinal anesthesia; normal blood pressure can be usually restored in the absence of drugs by simply tilting the operating table to raise the patient's legs, thereby facilitating the venous return of blood to the heart. Should this procedure fail, long-acting α-adrenergic vasopressor agents such as methoxamine, phenylephrine, or ephedrine may be administered intramuscularly.

Sympathomimetic vasopressor agents should be used with extreme caution for the management of hypotension produced by such general anesthetic agents as cyclopropane and halothane (Fluothane). These drugs sensitize the heart to the arrhythmic actions of endogenously circulating and exogenously administered epinephrine. The ideal vasopressor agent selected should possess minimal excitatory effects on the heart. Methoxamine (Vasoxyl), the drug of choice in such situations, is a very potent vasopressor agent that reportedly inhibits cardiac arrhythmias produced by cyclopropane.

Shock   *Shock* is a state of cardiovascular insufficiency characterized, in part, by severe hypotension, low cardiac output, and generalized vasoconstriction. As a consequence, vital organs such as the brain, the heart, and the kidneys fail to receive an adequate supply of blood, with irreversible tissue damage and death the inevitable consequence if effective treatment is delayed. Causes of shock include trauma, hemorrhage, myocardial infarction, and septicemia. Shock resulting from an inadequate circulating blood volume should first be treated with fluids and electrolytes or plasma expanders, such as dextran. While no general agreement exists among clinicians as to the best method of treating shock, the general objective is to increase blood flow to vital organs and not merely to increase blood pressure.

Alpha-adrenergic stimulants, such as levarterenol, methoxamine, and phenylephrine (Table 5-2A), all constrict the smooth muscles of the arterioles, which increases total peripheral resistance, thereby elevating and maintaining blood pressure. Unfortunately, these effects are accomplished at the expense of further reducing regional blood flow to tissues and reflexly reducing cardiac output.

The major potential hazard attendant with the use of levarterenol is an excessive elevation in blood pressure, potentially resulting in a stroke or a fatal cardiac arrhythmia. When the intravenous infusion is first started, the nurse should check the rise in blood pressure every two minutes. After the desired blood pressure—usually a systolic blood pressure of 90 to 100 mg Hg is attained, it should be monitored no less frequently than at 5-minute intervals. When methoxamine and phenylephrine are employed as vasopressor agents, blood pressure can be monitored at less frequent intervals after it has stabilized.

Some physicians prefer to treat shock by using drugs, such as isoproterenol, which increase cardiac output while improving blood flow to vital organs by producing vasodilation. Caution must be exercised when using such drugs to prevent an excessive increase in heart rate or cardiac arrhythmias.

Dopamine (Intropin), a naturally occurring catecholamine, has been shown to possess unique pharmacological properties on the cardiovascular system, which make it a useful drug for the treatment of certain cases of shock. This drug enhances cardiac output without significantly increasing heart rate. While dopamine elevates blood pressure by constricting blood vessels in the skin and skeletal muscles, it also increases blood flow to the kidneys and splanchnic regions by a vasodilatory action. The major cardiovascular effects of this drug have been attributed to its effects on α- and β-receptors, as well as on dopaminergic receptors on splanchnic and renal blood vessels.

Nasal decongestion Nasal decongestants represent one of the most widely used classes of drugs. These drugs are employed alone (Table 5-2D) or as one of a conglomeration of ingredients in cough and cold products.

One of the least pleasant symptoms of the common cold results from vasodilation of the mucous membranes of the nasal passage leading to obstruction or a "stuffed nose." Sympathomimetic vasoconstrictor agents such as phenylephrine (Neo-Synephrine) and naphazoline (Privine) activate α-receptors and thus produce decongestion.

Decongestants are either locally administered as drops, sprays, or inhalants or are orally ingested in tablets, capsules, or liquids. *Locally administered* nasal decongestants generally provide immediate and either temporary or prolonged symptomatic relief, depending upon the preparation used. Oxymetazoline (Afrin, Duration) and xylometazoline (Otrivin) produce a decongestant action lasting 6 to 12 hours, whereas most other drugs provide more temporary relief. Among the potentially undesirable consequences of

excessive use of decongestants includes impairment of the normal protective activities of the nasal cilia, damage to the nasal mucosa, and chronic nasal congestion; this latter effect, called *rebound congestion* or *after congestion*, results from compensatory vasodilation and is frequently encountered with short-acting preparations. In the absence of proper health care counseling, the patient often attempts to combat this rebound congestion by administering more drug, thus perpetuating this vicious cycle. Indiscriminate use of topically administered nasal decongestants is a very common example of drug misuse.

After *oral administration* of these drugs, the vasoconstrictor reaches the α-adrenergic receptors via the blood stream. This route of administration is effective regardless of the amount of mucus present in the nasal passages and is longer acting than topical drug administration but has a greater potential risk of side effects, particularly in patients with cardiovascular diseases.

The dangers associated with the use of these decongestants include hazards beyond the confines of the nose. Among the side effects observed include nervousness, insomnia, cardiac palpitations, and depression of the central nervous system and coma, the latter observed most commonly in children following drug overdosage. Nurses should never administer nasal sprays to patients who are in a recumbent position; the resulting stream of drug solution may cause severe toxicity.

Cardiac uses Prior to administering drugs for the treatment of cardiac arrest, physical means should be employed to maintain respiration (artificial ventilation) and restore the heart beat (an electrical pacemaker, if available, or a sharp blow on the chest). Should these procedures prove unsuccessful, epinephrine may be injected intravenously or directly into the heart to stimulate ventricular contractions. In recent years, isoproterenol has gained favor for the treatment of cardiac arrest and Stokes-Adams syndrome, a condition in which the heart slows to very low rates or temporarily stops. Unlike epinephrine, there is less risk of inducing ventricular fibrillation, a potentially life-threatening emergency, using isoproterenol.

Asthma   Bronchial asthma results from a spasmodic contraction of the smooth muscle of the bronchi, causing an impairment in the ability of the patient to exhale air from the lungs. Isoproterenol and epinephrine, administered by inhalation or by injection, have proved to be highly effective for the termination of acute asthmatic attacks. These drugs relax bronchial smooth muscle, producing bronchodilation by activating β_2-receptors. The treatment of bronchial asthma will be considered in detail in Chapter 54.

Allergic disorders   For many decades epinephrine has been the drug of choice for the treatment of acute hypersensitivity reactions caused by allergens and serum sickness. A subcutaneous injection of epinephrine provides rapid relief from itching, hives, swelling of the tongue, lips, and eyelids, and swelling of the glottis, which might otherwise result in suffocation. The management of allergic disorders will be considered in Chapter 53.

Ophthalmic uses   Topical administration of adrenergic agents (ephedrine, hydroxyamphetamine, and phenylephrine) dilate the pupil and are used for diagnostic examinations of the fundus of the eye. Epinephrine and phenylephrine are also used for the treatment of open-angle glaucoma. These drugs, when locally applied, decrease the production of aqueous humor by virtue of their vasoconstrictor activity, resulting in a decrease in intraocular pressure (Chapter 7).

Central nervous system uses   Amphetamine and related drugs are used for the treatment of narcolepsy, appetite suppression, and hyperkinetic disorders in children. These therapeutic uses will be discussed in Chapter 22.

Sympathomimetic Drugs:
nursing implications

Epinephrine [adrenaline] (Adrenalin)

1. Observe patient constantly when giving drug IV. Blood pressure (BP) should be checked repeatedly during the first 5 min, then every 3 to 5 min until stabilized. The drug may cause life-threatening ventricular fibrillation.

2. Epinephrine solutions should be clear and colorless. Discard solutions that are discolored, contain sedimented materials, or are past expiration date.

3. Check the type of solution prescribed, concentration, dosage, and route of administration. Carefully aspirate before subcutaneous (SC) injection. The IV injection of usual SC or IM doses can result in sudden hypertension.

Levarterenol (Levophed)

1. Observe patient constantly when administering this drug. Take BP and pulse prior to drug administration, every 2 min thereafter until desired BP is obtained, and then every 5 min. In normotensive patients, the flow rate should be adjusted to maintain BP at low-normal levels, usually 80 to 100 mm Hg systolic. In previously hypertensive patients, the systolic BP is generally maintained no more than 40 mm Hg below preexisting level.
2. Discard colored solutions or those past expiration date.
3. A double-bottle setup should be used to maintain the IV infusion even if drug administration must be discontinued.
4. The recommended infusion site is the large antecubital vein. If blanching of the skin results from drug infiltration, stop the infusion immediately and start in another vein. Phentolamine (Regitine) should be available for local infiltration in the event of ischemia.
5. Emergency drugs should be available in the event of cardiac abnormalities: atropine for bradycardia; propranolol (Inderal) for cardiac arrhythmias.

Isoproterenol (Isuprel, Norisodrine)

1. Here IV administration is regulated by continuous EKG monitoring and frequent evaluation of BP, pulse, and precordial distress.
2. Oral Inhalation:
   a. Carefully instruct patient in the proper use of the nebulizer and to take the lowest effective dose to obtain relief from an asthmatic attack.
   b. Advise patient to rinse mouth immediately after inhalation therapy to help prevent dryness and irritation of the throat. Explain to patient that saliva and sputum may appear pink.
   c. If respiratory condition worsens after therapy or if parotid gland swelling occurs, drug administration should be discontinued.

Ephedrine

1. This is a commonly abused drug. Advise patients of side effects and dangers and caution to take medication only as directed.
2. Instruct older male patients to report any difficulty in urinating, which may result from drug-induced urinary retention.
3. Reduced clinical effectiveness with rebound congestion may occur if drug is frequently administered or used over prolonged periods of time. Drug withdrawal for several days may restore effectiveness.

SUPPLEMENTARY READINGS

Aviado, D. M. *Sympathomimetic Drugs*. Springfield, Illinois: Charles C Thomas, Publisher, 1970.

Blashko, H. and E. Muscholl, ed. "Catecholamines," *Handbook of Experimental Pharmacology*, Vol. 33, Berlin: Springer-Verlag, 1972.

Eckstein, J. W. and F. M. Abboud, "Circulatory Effects of Sympathomimetic Amines," *American Heart Journal* **63**: 119–35 (1972).

Euler, U. S. von, "Adrenergic Neurotransmitter Functions," *Science* **173**: 202–206 (1971).

Goldberg, L. I., "Cardiovascular and Renal Actions of Dopamine: Potential Clinical Applications," *Pharmacological Reviews* **24**: 1–29 (1972).

Levy, B. and R. P. Ahlquist, "Adrenergic Drugs," in Drill's *Pharmacology in Medicine*, (4th ed.), ed. J. R. DiPalma, Chapter 33, pp. 627–674, New York: Mc-Graw-Hill Book Company, 1971.

Moyer, J. H. and L. C. Mills, "Vasopressor Agents in Shock," *American Journal of Nursing* **75**: 620–625 (1975).

Weiner, N., "Norepinephrine, Epinephrine and the Sympathomimetic Amines," in *Goodman and Gilman's The Pharmacological Basis of Therapeutics* (6th ed.), ed. A. G. Gilman, L. S. Goodman, and A. Gilman, Chapter 8, pp. 138–175. New York: Macmillan, Inc., 1980.

Whelan, R. F., "The Effects of Adrenergic Drugs on the Systemic Circulation," in *Physiological Pharmacology*. ed. W. S. Root and F. G. Hofmann, Vol. 4, pp. 29–95, New York: Academic Press, Inc., 1967.

ADRENERGIC BLOCKING AGENTS

Chapter 6

Adrenergic blocking agents are drugs that inhibit the actions of endogenously released catecholamines (epinephrine and norepinephrine) or sympathomimetic drugs at their effector cell receptor sites. In this class are drugs that selectively block either α-, β_1-, or β_2-adrenergic receptors, and each will be considered separately. You should not confuse this drug class with adrenergic neuron blocking agents such as guanethidine (Ismelin) that act by preventing the release of norepinephrine from postganglionic sympathetic neurons. Adrenergic neuron blocking agents will be considered in Chapter 28, when antihypertensive agents are discussed.

ALPHA-ADRENERGIC BLOCKING AGENTS

Alpha-adrenergic blocking agents are more effective in their ability to antagonize the actions of circulating catecholamines than in their capacity to block the actions of norepinephrine released by stimulation of adrenergic nerves. Most blood vessels contain both α- and β-adrenergic receptors (Chapter 5). Activation of α-receptors produces vasoconstriction, while stimulation of β_2-receptors causes vasodilation. Since α-adrenergic blockers antagonize the vasoconstrictor effects of endogenous catecholamines on the arterioles, vasodilation results after their administration, causing a reduction in arterial blood pressure and an increase in blood flow.

Alpha-adrenergic blocking agents are employed clinically for the diagnosis and treatment of pheochromocytoma and for the management of certain peripheral vascular disorders (Table 6–1). These drugs were formerly used for the treatment of hypertension, but they have been replaced by equally effective drugs that have fewer undesirable side effects (Chapter 28).

Pheochromocytoma

In relatively rare instances, hypertension may be caused by tumors of the chromaffin tissues of the adrenal medulla, and these tumors secrete extremely large amounts of epinephrine and norepinephrine. The tumor responsible for this hypertensive condition is called *pheochromocytoma*. In the absence of this disorder, intravenous administration of the α-blocker *phentolamine* (Regitine) causes only a small reduction in blood pressure; by contrast, patients with pheochromocytoma exhibit a fall of 35 mm Hg systolic and 25 mm Hg diastolic pressures within 2 minutes. This diagnosis is often confirmed by measuring urinary catecholamine metabolites; in cases of pheochromocytoma, the concentration of VMA (3-methoxy-4-hydroxymandelic acid), the principal metabolite of norepinephrine and epinephrine in the urine, may be 10 to 50 times higher than normal lev-

Table 6-1   Adrenergic Blocking Agents

Generic name	Trade name(s)	Adverse effects	Therapeutic uses (Usual daily oral dose)
A. Alpha-adrenergic blocking agents			
Phenoxybenzamine	Dibenzyline	Orthostatic hypotension; tachycardia; nasal congestion	Pheochromocytoma; Raynaud's disease (20-60 mg)
Tolazoline	Priscoline	Gooseflesh; less commonly, flushing and tachycardia	Peripheral vascular diseases (100-300 mg)
Phentolamine	Regitine	Like phenoxbenzamine	Diagnosis and preoperative treatment of pheochromocytoma (5 mg, IM or IV, 1-2 h preoperative)
B. Beta-adrenergic blocking agents			
1. Approved drugs			
Propranolol Nadolol	Inderal Corgard	Bradycardia; gastrointestinal disorders; hypoglycemia; bronchoconstriction (asthmatics)	Cardiac arrhythmias, angina pectoris, hypertension, pheochromocytoma, thyrotoxicosis (30-240 mg)
2. Other drugs[a]		*Distinguishing Characteristics*	
Practolol Alprenolol Metoprolol[b] Oxprenolol Tolamolol	Eraldin Aptin Lopressor Trasicor Coptin	More selective blockade of cardiac β_1 receptors than on bronchial smooth muscle; less bronchoconstriction.	

[a]More selective β_1-blocking agents approved for use in Europe, but not in the United States.
[b]Approved for use in the United States.

els. *Phenoxybenzamine* (Dibenzyline), a long-acting α-blocker, is used to manage pheochromocytoma preoperatively and also in patients who are poor risks for the surgical removal of this tumor. The combined use of phenoxybenzamine and the β-blocker, propranolol, for the treatment of this condition is discussed later. Nursing implications associated with the use of phenoxybenzamine are summarized at the end of the chapter.

Metyrosine *Metyrosine* (Demser), recently approved for use in pheochromocytoma, inhibits the enzyme tyrosine hydroxylase resulting in a reduction in catecholamine synthesis by 35 to 80 percent. This drug is useful for preoperative treatment prior to surgery, the management of patients for whom surgery is contraindicated, and the chronic treatment of patients with malignant pheochromocytoma. This drug may be administered alone or in combination with an α-adrenergic blocking agent.

Almost all patients treated with metyrosine experience moderate-to-severe sedation and should, therefore, be warned about the potential dangers associated with the concurrent use of other central nervous system depressants. Other adverse effects are observed in behavior (confusion, disorientation, depression, hallucinations), extrapyramidal function (drooling, speech difficulties, tremors), and gastrointestinal function (diarrhea). To minimize the risk of crystalluria and urolithiasis, particularly when daily doses exceed 2 g, fluid intake should be increased to permit patients to maintain daily urinary output of at least 2000 ml. The usual maintenance oral dose of metyrosine is 250 to 500 mg four times daily.

Peripheral Vascular Disorders

Alpha-blockers are employed for the treatment of *Raynaud's disease* and related peripheral vascular disorders caused by vasoconstriction that reduce blood flow to the extremities. The vasodilatory effects of *tolazoline* (Priscoline) and related drugs have been attributed to blockade of α-receptors on the smooth muscle of the arterioles as well as direct relaxation of this muscle. The most disturbing side effects associated with tolazoline involve the heart (tachycardia, anginal pains, and cardiac arrhythmias) and gastrointestinal tract (abdominal pain, nausea, vomiting, diarrhea and exacerbation of peptic ulcer).

Nylidrin (Arlidin), a stimulant of β2-receptors, increases blood flow to skeletal muscles by causing direct dilation of arteries and arterioles. It is used for the treatment of peripheral vascular disease. The clinical value of this drug has not been established.

BETA-ADRENERGIC BLOCKING AGENTS

Activation of β1-adrenergic receptors causes an increase in the heart rate and force of cardiac contraction, while β2-activation produces vasodilation and relaxation of bronchial smooth muscle. Recent years have witnessed the development of drugs that are relatively specific β-receptor blocking agents, drugs that many experts believe will have a significant impact on the treatment of a variety of cardiovascular diseases, including angina pectoris and cardiac arrhythmias.

Propanolol (Inderal) is the prototype systemic β-blocking agent so the pharmacological properties and therapeutic uses of this drug will be emphasized. This compound and Nadolol (Corgard) block both β1- and β2-receptors. Metoprolol (Lopressor) is a more selective β2-blocker that primarily inhibits stimulation of the heart; similar drugs, currently in the investigational stage and not clinically available in the United States, are listed on Table 6–1. The use of timolol maleate (Timoptic) for the treatment of glaucoma will be considered in Chapter 7.

Pharmacological Effects

Propranolol exerts its most important actions on the cardiovascular system, in particular, on the heart. Its effects on bronchial smooth muscle, the central nervous system, and on blood sugar result in its undesirable effects.

Cardiovascular system Propranolol inhibits the excitatory effects of sympathetic innervation of the heart resulting in a decrease in heart rate and a reduction in the force of cardiac contractions. While these effects are observed when the patient is at rest, they are most pronounced during periods of exercise. Generation of impulses at the sinoatrial node (the pacemaker) is reduced, as is atrioventricular conduction, and the refractory period during diastole is prolonged. In addition to these effects, all of which can be attributed to blockade of cardiac β_1-receptors, propranolol also possesses direct antiarrhythmic actions similar to quinidine (Chapter 27), producing a suppression of ectopic (abnormal) ventricular pacemakers and the reduction of abnormal ventricular rhythms.

This drug also inhibits the release of renin from the kidney, an effect that may contribute to its beneficial antihypertensive effects (Chapter 28).

Bronchial smooth muscles Propranolol blocks β_2-receptors in bronchial smooth muscle, which may result in pronounced bronchoconstriction in patients with bronchial asthma or other obstructive respiratory disorders. Metoprolol, by contrast, possesses relatively selective β_1-blocking effects on the heart while having much less effect on the bronchial β_2-receptors.

Therapeutic Uses

At present, propranolol is approved for use in the United States for the treatment of angina pectoris, cardiac arrhythmias, pheochromocytoma, hypertrophic subaortic stenosis, hypertension, and thyrotoxicosis.

Angina pectoris The pain of angina results from an inadequate supply of oxygen to the cardiac muscle. Propranolol may reduce the oxygen consumption of the heart muscle by blocking catecholamine-induced increases in heart rate, systolic blood pressure, and the speed and force of cardiac contractions. The treatment of angina pectoris will be discussed in greater detail in Chapter 29.

Cardiac arrhythmias Propranolol has been demonstrated to be effective for the treatment of digitalis-induced arrhythmias (Chapter 26) and ventricular arrhythmias arising from other causes. The antiarrhythmic properties of this drug have been ascribed to its β_1-blocking activity and to its quinidine-like ability to suppress ectopic pacemakers in the ventricles; these effects will be discussed in Chapter 27.

Pheochromocytoma The use of α-blocking agents (such as phenoxybenzamine) for the treatment of pheochromocytoma prior to surgical removal of the tumor has been discussed earlier in this chapter. Propranolol can be used in combination with an α-blocker to control tachycardia, which may be present. Should propranolol therapy be initiated, an α-blocker must also be administered to prevent a marked elevation in blood pressure.

Hypertrophic subaortic stenosis In this disorder, hypertrophy of the septal wall causes an obstruction of inflow or outflow in the ventricles, producing such symptoms as respiratory difficulty, fatigue, cardiac pain, and fainting after exercise. Propranolol reduces the systolic pressure gradient and the

Table 6-2   Potential Drug Interactions Involving Propranolol

Interacting drug/class	Potential consequences
Antidepressants, monoamine oxidase inhibitors	Combined administration with propranolol contraindicated; potential hypertensive reaction.

Antidiabetic agents
    Insulin
    Oral hypoglycemics
	Propranolol reduces blood sugar; combined use with antidiabetic agents may produce hypoglycemic crisis. Well-documented interaction.

Digitalis-cardiac glycosides	Digitalis-induced bradycardia may be potentiated by propranolol.
Epinephrine	Administration of epinephrine may result in an enhanced pressor response and a reflex reduction in heart rate.
Isoproterenol (Isuprel)	Propranolol can inhibit the β-adrenergic stimulatory effects of isoproterenol.
Skeletal muscle relaxants Tubocurarine	Propranolol may intensify the magnitude and prolong the duration of muscle relaxation produced by tubocurarine.

force of ventricular contraction, thus relieving the obstruction.

Hypertension The precise mechanism underlying the antihypertensive effects of propranolol have not been determined, yet it has been observed that its ability to reduce elevated blood pressure is greatly enhanced when used in combination with other drugs (Chapter 28). Propranolol may act, in part, by reducing cardiac output, as well as by inhibiting the secretion of renin by the kidney.

Thyrotoxicosis Excessive secretion of thyroid hormones can lead to a state of toxic hyperthyroidism referred to as *thyrotoxicosis*. Some of the symptoms associated with this disorder include an increase in heart rate, palpitations, and extreme anxiety. Propranolol does not modify the hyperactivity of the thyroid gland, but it has been found to be a useful drug in controlling these symptoms prior to the onset of action of more specific antithyroid agents (Chapter 35).

Precautions and Drug Interaction

Propranolol is contraindicated in patients with asthma or other obstructive respiratory diseases, atrioventricular heart block, hypotension, and congestive heart failure.

In diabetic patients or individuals predisposed to diabetes, propranolol has been observed to modify carbohydrate metabolism via multiple and complex mechanisms, causing a reduction in blood sugar. Hence the patient should be advised that reductions in the dosage of insulin or oral hypoglycemic agents (Chapter 36) may be necessary to prevent severe hypoglycemic episodes. Table 6–2 lists other potential drug interactions, the clinical significance of which have not been fully documented to date. A summary of nursing implications associated with the use of propranolol appears on page 62.

Adrenergic Blocking Agents:
nursing implications

Phenoxybenzamine (Dibenzyline)

1. Administer with food or milk to reduce gastric irritation.
2. During periods of dosage adjustments, monitor BP every 4 h while patient is in supine and erect positions.
3. Instruct patient to make changes in position slowly, especially from recumbent to upright position, and to dangle legs for several minutes before standing.
4. Inform patient that postural hypotension and palpitations usually disappear with continued therapy but may reappear with situations that promote vasodilation, such as after alcohol ingestion or exercise.
5. Treat overdose by maintaining the patient in a flat position for 24 h with pressure bandages on the legs and use of an abdominal binder. If severe hypotension occurs, levarterenol may be administered.

Propranolol (Inderal)

1. Preferably give orally before meals and at bedtime, since food in the stomach delays absorption.
2. Do not give to patients with a history of respiratory allergies, asthma, or other obstructive pulmonary disorders because drug may cause bronchiolar constriction even in normal patients.
3. Carefully monitor EKG, BP, and central venous pressure during IV administration. Emergency drugs should be available: atropine for excessive bradycardia; vasopressors for excessive hypotension; isoproterenol (Isuprel) or aminophylline for bronchospasm.
4. Observe diabetics; drug may mask symptoms of hypoglycemia (nervousness, tremor, sweating, hunger, increased pulse rate) and may prolong drug-induced hypoglycemia. Reduced doses of insulin or oral hypoglycemic agents may be necessary.
5. Gradually reduce dosage when propranolol administration is to be discontinued. Abrupt withdrawal in patients with angina pectoris may cause myocardial infarction or serious arrhythmias.
6. Advise patient to avoid excessive use of alcohol, coffee, and food and not to smoke, if possible; smoking may increase BP in some patients.

SUPPLEMENTARY READINGS

Dollery, C. T., J. W. Paterson, and M. E. Conolly, "Clinical Pharmacology of Beta-Receptor Blocking Agents," *Clinical Pharmacology and Therapeutics* 10: 765–799 (1969).

Epstein, S. E. and E. Braunwald, "Beta-Receptor Blocking Agents: Mechanisms of Action and Clinical Applications," *New England Journal of Medicine* 275: 1106–1112, 1175–1183 (1966).

Morrelli, H. F., "Propranolol," *Annals of Internal Medicine* 78: 913–917 (1973).

Petrie, J. C., D. B. Galloway, T. A. Jeffers, and J. Webster, "Adverse Reactions to Beta-Blocking Drugs: A Review," *Postgraduate Medical Journal* **52** (Suppl 4): 63–69 (1976).

Weiner, N., "Drugs That Inhibit Adrenergic Nerves and Block Adrenergic Receptors," in *Goodman and Gilman's The Pharmacological Basis of Therapeutics* (6th ed.), ed. A. G. Gilman, L. S. Goodman, and A. Gilman, Chapter 9, pp. 176–210. New York: Macmillan, Inc., 1980.

CHOLINERGIC AGENTS

Chapter

7

Cholinergic or *parasympathomimetic agents* are those drugs that are capable of imitating *acetylcholine* or intensifying the effects of endogenously released acetylcholine at its effector sites. In either case, we observe effects that—to a great extent—are qualitatively similar to those observed after activation of cholinergic nerves.

Drugs in this class are employed for the treatment of glaucoma, as postoperative agents for the treatment of urinary retention and abdominal distention, and for the management of myasthenia gravis. Moreover, we are concerned with the acute toxicity of some of these compounds because of their use as insecticides.

CHOLINERGIC TRANSMISSION

Acetylcholine is the chemical mediator of nerve impulses at the postganglionic parasympathetic neuroeffector junction (muscarinic receptor), at all (sympathetic and parasympathetic) autonomic ganglia, and at the neuromuscular junction (nicotinic receptors) discussed in Chapter 4.

The synthesis of acetylcholine is controlled by the enzyme choline acetyltransferase, which mediates the transfer of an acetyl group from acetyl coenzyme A to choline, the latter being a normal constituent of the diet. After its release from storage vesicles present in cholinergic nerve endings, acetylcholine interacts with the cholinergic receptor to initiate a response. The neurotransmitter is then very rapidly hydrolyzed and inactivated by the enzyme *acetylcholinesterase.*

Effects of Cholinergic Stimulation

Notwithstanding the paramount role acetylcholine plays in physiology, this compound is only rarely used as a therapeutic agent for two important reasons. Acetylcholine is very rapidly inactivated by acetylcholinesterase and produces widely diverse effects on many tissues throughout the body. The cholinergic agents employed clinically are useful because of longer duration and greater specificity of action.

What major effects might be seen after the subcutaneous injection of a moderate dose of acetylcholine? Among the earliest effects observed are flushing of the face and a rise in skin temperature, both the result of peripheral vasodilation. Acetylcholine stimulates secretions from several exocrine glands, causing profuse sweating, salivation, and tearing. Breathing becomes difficult as the result of bronchoconstriction, the heart rate is markedly reduced, and the pupils are constricted. Stimulation of gastrointestinal smooth muscle increases peristalsis, which may result in defecation, while its effects on the urinary bladder can cause urination. Exogenously administered acetylcholine is rapidly destroyed; within 5 minutes, this alarming reaction is terminated.

Classification of Cholinergic Agents

Cholinergic agents are generally divided into two major categories based upon their mechanism of action: direct-acting cholinergic agents and cholinesterase inhibitors. The *direct-acting* drugs activate those receptor sites innervated by cholinergic nerves. *Cholinesterase inhibitors* or *anticholinesterase agents* do not directly interact with the cholinergic receptor, but rather act indirectly by preventing the enzyme acetylcholinesterase from inactivating acetylcholine. Inhibition of this enzyme permits the buildup of acetylcholine at its receptor site, resulting in more intense and prolonged activation of effector cells by this transmitter agent.

DIRECT-ACTING CHOLINERGIC AGENTS

The direct-acting cholinergic agents mimic the effects of endogenously released acetylcholine at the postganglionic parasympathetic neuroeffector junction, that is, at *muscarinic* receptor sites (Chapter 4). These drugs resist hydrolysis by acetylcholinesterase, and, therefore, have a longer duration and greater specificity of action than acetylcholine. For the most part, while drugs in this class (Table 7-1) have been replaced by safer, more effective compounds, several continue to be employed therapeutically.

Bethanechol

Following abdominal surgery, gastrointestinal smooth muscle may lose its tone, resulting in distention of the intestinal walls and impairment of normal peristaltic activity. In such situations, food and other contents are not propelled down the gastrointestinal tract. Another unpleasant consequence of abdominal surgery may be a loss of the tone of the smooth muscle of the urinary bladder, causing retention and an inability to urinate. *Bethanechol* (Urecholine), possessing relatively specific effects on the smooth muscle of the gastrointestinal tract and urinary bladder, is clinically em-

Table 7-1   Direct-Acting Cholinergic Agents

Generic name	Trade name	Route of administration and usual daily dose	Therapeutic uses
Bethanechol	Urecholine Myotonachol	PO: 15–120 mg SC: 7.5–20 mg	Postoperative urinary retention; intestinal and abdominal distention; postvagotomy; gastric atony.
Carbachol	Isopto-carbachol	Conjunctival: 0.1 ml of 0.75–3% sol.	Miotic agent for the treatment of open-angle glaucoma.
Methacholine	Mecholyl	SC: 10–25 mg	Peripheral vascular diseases; atrial tachy-cardia (rarely used).
Pilocarpine		Conjunctival: 0.1 ml of 0.5–6% sol. 1–6 times daily	Counteract mydriasis produced by atropine in eye examinations; open-angle glaucoma.

ployed to restore parasympathetic tone and relieve postoperative abdominal distention and urinary retention. Nursing responsibilities for such patients include accurate maintenance of records of urinary output and checking for bowel sounds by abdominal auscultation. Other nursing implications are summarized at the end of the chapter.

Pilocarpine, after administration into the conjunctival sac of the eye, produces pupillary constriction and is employed to counteract the mydriatic effects of atropine and related drugs in ophthalmologic examinations. It is also used for the treatment of open-angle glaucoma, as discussed in a later section.

ANTICHOLINESTERASE AGENTS

Anticholinesterase agents act by chemically combining with acetylcholinesterase to prevent this enzyme from inactivating acetylcholine. Such compounds cause activation of both muscarinic and nicotinic receptors. These drugs enjoy extensive therapeutic use for the treatment of glaucoma and myasthenia gravis, are employed in agriculture

as insecticides, and are among the most effective compounds available for conducting chemical warfare.

Cholinesterase inhibitors are classified as reversible or irreversible inhibitors of acetylcholinesterase, a distinction predicated upon their duration of action. Physostigmine and neostigmine are reversible anticholinesterase agents; over a period of several hours, these inhibitors are slowly hydrolyzed and acetylcholinesterase is slowly regenerated. By contrast, the effects of *organophosphorous* anticholinesterase agents persist for days or weeks, with normal acetylcholinesterase activity restored only after the biosynthesis of new enzyme molecules. Organophosphorous anticholinesterase agents such as isoflurophate are referred to as *irreversible inhibitors*.

Reversible Anticholinesterases: Physostigmine and Neostigmine Type

Physostigmine (eserine) is an alkaloid derived from the Calabar or ordeal bean of West Africa, a plant used by some tribes to attempt to establish the guilt or innocence of an individual accused of witchcraft; drug-induced vomiting was interpreted as innocence on the part of the defendant. Formerly used for the treatment of myasthenia gravis, physostigmine has since been replaced by neostigmine and safer drugs. Physostigmine is currently employed for the treatment of glaucoma and to reverse atropine-induced mydriasis. Topical application of physostigmine into the conjunctival sac causes constriction of the pupils and a reduction in intraocular pressure. We shall discuss the use of this drug for the treatment of glaucoma in a later section of this chapter.

Neostigmine, a synthetic compound, differs from physostigmine in two major respects. While both drugs are reversible inhibitors of acetylcholinesterase, neostigmine also possesses direct actions at nicotinic receptors at the neuromuscular junction. Physostigmine readily crosses the blood-brain barrier after oral administration, producing adverse effects in the central nervous system. By contrast, neostigmine is a lipid-insoluble quaternary ammonium compound, which gains very limited access to the brain.

The therapeutic uses of neostigmine are based upon its actions at muscarinic and nicotinic receptor sites. In addition to being employed for the treatment of glaucoma, neostigmine is used postoperatively to enhance gastrointestinal smooth muscle tone and to treat urinary retention. The major therapeutic application of this drug is for the treatment of muscle fatigue associated with myasthenia gravis. The adverse effects associated with neostigmine administration will be discussed in a later section of this chapter; potential drug interactions involving cholinergic agents appear in Table 7-3.

Myasthenia gravis Myasthemia gravis is a chronic disease characterized by abnormal skeletal muscle weakness and fatigability. During the early stages, weakness is restricted to the muscles of the eye, producing ptosis (drooping of the eyelids) and diplopia (double vision). As the disease progresses, weakness spreads to the muscles of the face, causing difficulties in chewing, swallowing, and talking, and to the muscles of the legs, arms, and hands. The major danger in this disease is the development of weakness of the respiratory muscles, creating the risk of death from respiratory failure. This disorder, most commonly afflicting women between the ages of 20 and 50, is associated with spontaneous remissions and exacerbations. The incidence of myasthenia is estimated to be approximately one case in 15,000 to 20,000; it is likely that an equal number of mild cases remain undetected.

It is generally believed that the muscle weakness associated with this disorder results from an autoimmune (antibody mediated) degradation and blockade of the acetylcholine receptor on the motor end plate of skeletal muscle.

Drug therapy Reversible anticholinesterase agents represent the major class of drugs currently employed for the diagnosis and symptomatic treatment of this disease. Intravenous injection of the short-acting anticholinesterase agent *edrophonium* (Tensilon) produces a brief increase in the muscle strength of the extremities; this test is sufficiently specific to confirm a suspected diagnosis of myasthenia.

After the diagnosis has been established, oral administration of neostigmine (Prostigmin), pyridostigmine (Mestinon), or ambenonium (Mytelase) can be initiated; varying durations of action are the primary differences of clinical significance among these drugs (Table 7-2). The use of corticotropin for the treatment of myasthenia is discussed in Chapter 34. The patient should be instructed that the optimal dosage may vary on a daily basis, with emotional and physical

Table 7-2 Commonly Employed Anticholinesterase Agents

Generic name	Trade name	Route of administration and usual dose	Duration of action	Distinguishing characteristics
Drugs for myasthenia gravis				
Ambenonium	Mytelase	PO: 5–25 mg, 3–4 times daily	6–8 h	Long duration of action limits accurate control of dosage.
Edrophonium	Tensilon	IV: 2 mg	1–2 h	Diagnosis of myasthenia and differentiation of myasthenic and cholinergic crisis; treatment of tubocurarine overdosage (Chapter 12).
Neostigmine	Prostigmin	PO: 15–45 mg q.i.d.	2–4 h	Short duration of action limits usefulness for chronic treatment.
Pyridostigmine	Mestinon	PO: 120–300 mg q. 4 h	4–6 h	Most widely used drug for myasthenia; see nursing implications at the end of the chapter.
Drugs for glaucoma				
Demecarium	Humorsol	Conjunctival: 0.03–0.06 ml of 0.25% sol. twice weekly	2–4 da	Potent and long-acting; stable in aqueous solutions.
Echothiophate	Phospholine	Conjunctival: 0.1 ml of 0.06–0.125% sol. o.d.	3–7 da	Potent, long-acting, very effective; stable in solution for 1 month at room temperature.
Isoflurophate	Floropryl	Conjunctival: 0.05–0.1 ml of 0.1% sol. q. 12–72 h	1 week	Potent and long-acting; unstable in water; oily vehicle may be unpleasant; reported to occasionally elevate intraocular pressure.
Physostigmine (eserine)	———	Conjunctival: 0.1 ml of 0.25% sol. 2–4 times daily	6–12 h	Short duration of action necessitates frequent drug administration; unlike above drugs, little or no danger of cataracts; solutions decompose on exposure to light. See the nursing implications at the end of the chapter.
Timolol maleate	Timoptic	Conjunctival: 1 drop of 0.25 *or* 0.5% sol. b.i.d.	12–24 h	β-adrenergic blocker used for open-angle glaucoma and ocular hypertension. Contraindicated in bronchial asthma and certain heart diseases (Chapter 6).

stresses, infections, and menstruation usually requiring an increase in the size or frequency of drug administration.

Complications Myasthenic and cholinergic crises are major complications of myasthenia, with both characterized by respiratory failure but arising from different causes. *Myasthenic crisis* is caused by an acute exacerbation of the disease, commonly precipitated by upper respiratory infections or physical fatigue. The nurse should not overlook the possibility that the patient is failing to take the medication at the recommended doses or intervals. This disease complication is managed by increasing the daily dosage of the anticholinesterase agent. Signs of myasthenic crisis include pupillary constriction, sweating, salivation, tearing, and diarrhea. *Cholinergic crisis*, by contrast, is the result of an overdosage of medication, and is characterized by symptoms reflecting excessive muscarinic and nicotinic activation, the latter manifested by muscle twitching and paralysis. The patient should be advised by the nurse that accidental overdosage of cholinergic agents may cause muscle weakness rather than increased strength. Should overdosage be suspected, all cholinergic medication must be immediately terminated and artificial respiration initiated without delay. The edrophonium test can be used to differentiate between myasthenic and cholinergic crisis. Edrophonium-induced muscle strength is indicative of inadequate medication rather than drug overdosage.

Precautions Great caution must be exercised when administering drugs to the myasthenic patient, particularly drugs that may increase muscle weakness or produce respiratory depression. Drugs capable of producing muscle weakness include tubocurarine, polymyxin, and aminoglycoside antibiotics (streptomycin, kanamycin, neomycin, and gentamicin), quinine, quinidine, and procainamide. Myasthenic individuals are particularly sensitive to the respiratory depressant effects of sedative-hypnotics and morphine-like opiates, and these drugs should be administered judiciously and in reduced dosage to such patients. Potential drug interactions are summarized in Table 7-3.

Irreversible Anticholinesterases: Organophosphates

In the years immediately prior to the onset of World War II and during the war years, a relatively new class of compounds was examined by German scientists for potential use as insecticides and later as chemical warfare agents. Among these *organophosphates* were parathion, a very widely employed insecticide, and sarin and soman, compounds developed but never used for military use. The latter irreversible cholinesterase inhibitor nerve gases are odorless, tasteless, and provide their unfortunate recipients with no advance warning of their presence. They are highly effective in extremely low concentrations and are capable of producing death within minutes after exposure. The toxi-

Table 7-3 Selected Clinically Significant Drug Interactions Involving Cholinergic Agents

Cholinergic drug	Interacting drug/class	Potential consequences
Anticholinesterase agents: exposure to insecticides, anti-glaucoma drugs (echothiophate), anti-myasthenic drugs (edrophonium).	Succinylcholine (Quelicin, Anectine)	Inhibition of pseudocholinesterase: enzyme metabolizes succinylcholine resulting in prolonged muscle relaxation, potential respiratory failure.
Neostigmine Edrophonium	Tubocurarine	Antagonism of muscle-relaxing effects; use as antidote for tubocurarine overdosage.
Cholinergic agents, employed for treatment of glaucoma	Steroids Dexamethasone (Decadron, Gammacorten) Hydrocortisone Prednisone (Deltasone, Meticorten)	Systemic steroid administration may increase intraocular pressure in open-angle glaucoma making control of pressure more difficult.

cological effects of these compounds will be discussed later in this chapter.

Isoflurophate (DFP) was initially prepared for military applications but was subsequently investigated for the treatment of glaucoma and myasthenia gravis. While isoflurophate and chemically related organophosphates have not proved to be practical for the treatment of myasthenia, they have been found to be effective for the treatment of certain types of glaucoma. When applied to the eye, they reduce intraocular pressure for days or weeks after a single dose.

Glaucoma It is estimated that two million individuals in the United States are afflicted with glaucoma, with 10 to 20 percent of the blindness in this country attributed to this disease. Glaucoma is a major cause of blindness in persons over the age of 40. There are two major types of primary glaucoma, open-angle (wide-angle) and angle-closure (narrow-angle); the former accounts for 90 percent of all diagnosed cases of glaucoma and the latter less than 5 percent. Prior to discussing the treatment of glaucoma and the rational basis for this treatment, the nurse should be acquainted with factors responsible for this disease.

Classification Aqueous humor is a fluid formed in the posterior chamber of the eye; it passes through the pupil and into the anterior chamber. This fluid is drained from the anterior chamber and the eye by way of the trabecular meshwork through the canal of Schlemm. The rate of fluid inflow into the canal is normally equal to the outflow, with a constant pressure of 15 mm Hg created. If the fluid fails to drain normally and continues to accumulate, the intraocular pressure increases several-fold, leading to compression of the retina and optic nerve and eventually causing visual loss and blindness.

The increased intraocular pressure associated with *open-angle glaucoma*, which is slow in onset, is caused by degenerative changes in the trabecular membrane and the canal of Schlemm that interfere with fluid outflow. Drugs have proved highly useful in the treatment of this disorder. In *angle-closure glaucoma*, excessive dilation of the pupil and relaxation of the ciliary muscle cause the iris to block aqueous humor outflow. The resulting abrupt and marked increase in intraocular pressure produces severe pain and visual loss and is generally considered to be a medical emergency. While drugs are useful in controlling an acute attack, long-term management requires surgery.

Therapy Drugs employed for the treatment of glaucoma act by constricting the pupil, thereby enhancing the drainage of aqueous humor (cholinergic and sympathomimetic agents), or by reducing the formation of aqueous humor (sympathomimetics and carbonic acid inhibitors).

Cholinergic Agents. Topical application of ophthalmic solutions or ointments containing pilocarpine or anticholinesterase to the conjunctival sac constrict the pupil, cause contraction of the ciliary muscle, and— by mechanisms that are poorly understood— facilitate the outflow of aqueous humor.

Cholinergic agents (Table 7-2) are most frequently used for the treatment of primary open-angle glaucoma. While the irreversible anticholinesterase agents demecarium (Humorsol), echothiophate (Phospholine), and isoflurophate (Floropryl) require less frequent administration and control intraocular pressure overnight, the use of these drugs for periods exceeding 6 months carries a very high risk of the development of specific types of *cataracts*. Since pilocarpine and physostigmine are not associated with cataract formation, it is generally recommended that these drugs be employed as long as they continue to control pressure prior to initiating therapy with the long-acting anticholinesterase agents. Commonly encountered adverse effects with cholinergic agents include blurred vision, headache, difficulties in light accommodation, and such potential systemic effects as salivation, nausea, diarrhea, and abdominal cramps.

Sympathomimetic Agents.   By mechanisms that are not presently well understood, sympathomimetic agents with mydriatic properties (epinephrine and phenylephrine) reduce intraocular pressure by reducing the rate of aqueous humor secretion and increasing the outflow of this fluid. These drugs are employed for the treatment of open-angle glaucoma. When timolol maleate (Timoptic), a β-adrenergic blocker, is applied topically, it reduces intraocular pressure with little or no effect on pupil size or visual acuity. This new drug can be administered 1–2 times daily for the management of open-angle glaucoma and ocular hypertension.

Carbonic Anhydrase Inhibitors. When cholinergic miotic agents fail to provide adequate control, systemic administration of such carbonic anhydrase inhibitors as *acetazolamide* (Diamox), dichlorphenamide (Daranide, Oratrol), ethoxzolamide (Cardrase, Ethamide), or methazolamide (Neptazane) may be employed to reduce intraocular pressure for 4 to 10 hours in the treatment of angle-closure glaucoma. Drugs in this class reduce the formation of aqueous humor.

Precautions   Sympathomimetics, glucocorticoids (cortisone-like steroid drugs), and atropine-like anticholinergic agents have been implicated as causes of glaucoma, with the anticholinergic agents generally contraindicated in patients with this ocular disease. Based upon the available clinical evidence, many experts believe these fears to be exaggerated. The following general statements

may assist the nurse in evaluating the potential dangers of a given medication in such patients. The risk of precipitating glaucoma by administration of drugs directly into the eye is greater than when the same drug is given systemically. Since acute angle-closure is regarded as a medical emergency, drugs suspected of inducing glaucoma should be used with great caution; when this type of glaucoma has been established, suspected drugs are contraindicated. Withholding the systemic administration of compounds possessing anticholinergic activity (including antiulcer, tricyclic antidepressant, and antipsychotic drugs) for fear of inducing open-angle glaucoma appears to have little justification in many cases; each case, however, requires individual judgment.

Nursing responsibilities   The nurse should assume a major responsibility in the education of patients, teaching them about the nature of glaucoma and the proper administration of medications. The patient should be informed that medications should be taken on a regularly scheduled basis and applied only in the eye for which they have been ordered. In addition, the patient should be advised that extra lights may be required in the home and that difficulties may be encountered in night vision because the miotic agents employed prevent normal mydriasis.

Acute Anticholinesterase Toxicity

Anticholinesterase agents, in particular the organophosphates, are extremely poisonous substances even in very low concentrations. Since the organophosphates are employed as insecticides (parathion, malathion, TEPP, and systox), individuals working or living on farms are the most common victims of poisoning. Exposure may result from inhalation, absorption through the unbroken skin, and by ingestion. Aircraft sprayers of insecticides and other handlers are most frequently exposed; contamination may also result from residues remaining on work clothing or after conveyance of these compounds in the air. Other causes of organophosphate poisoning include accidents during transportation or ingestion by children.

Symptoms of poisoning involve the peripheral cholinergic system, with the intensity of the symptoms dependent upon the concentration of poison. Common symptoms include constriction of the pupils, runny nose, bronchoconstriction with respiratory impairment, profuse salivation and tearing, nausea, vomiting, diarrhea, muscle weakness and paralysis, extreme anxiety and mental confusion, convulsions, and eventual death resulting from respiratory failure.

Artificial respiration must be initiated as soon as possible. The victim's contaminated clothing should be removed and the skin thoroughly washed with soap and water. The specific muscarinic receptor blocking agent *atropine*, intravenously administered, is highly effective in antagonizing the peripheral muscarinic effects of organophosphates and other symptoms adversely affecting the central nervous system. Since atropine is ineffective in blocking the nicotinic actions of acetylcholine at the neuromuscular junction, it will not terminate muscle twitching or skeletal muscle weakness of the limbs and those involved in respiration.

Pralidoxime (Protopam) is effective in antagonizing the effects of anticholinesterase organophosphate agents on skeletal muscle after intravenous administration. This compound reactivates acetylcholinesterase by combining with the organophosphate and "pulling" it away from the enzyme. The reactivated enzyme is then available to metabolize and inactivate acetylcholine, thereby reducing organophosphate toxicity at both muscarinic and nicotinic sites in the periphery.

Cholinergic Drugs:
nursing implications

Bethanechol (Urecholine)

1. To determine minimum effective dose, an initial test dose of 5–10 mg may be given and repeated at 15- to 30-min intervals for a maximum of 4 doses until a satisfactory response or disturbing side effects occur.

2. Early signs of overdose are salivation, sweating, flushing, abdominal cramps, and nausea. A syringe (0.6 mg) containing atropine should be available if severe symptoms occur.

Pyridostigmine (Mestinon)

1. Failure to show improvement in myasthenia may result from drug overdosage or underdosage. Increasing muscular weakness, cramps, or fasciculations should be reported. The edrophonium (Tensilon) test differentiates between myasthenic and cholinergic crisis; improvement after edrophonium indicates inadequate medication.

2. Relative drug effectiveness may vary with physical and emotional stress, as well as the severity of myasthenia.

Physostigmine [eserine]

1. Teaching plan for patients with glaucoma should include proper administration of eye drops; adverse symptoms to be reported; and activities that increase intraocular pressure and that should be avoided, such as straining at defecation or heavy exertion.

2. Drops may cause lid twitch, temporary blurring of vision, and difficulty in seeing in dim light; advise the patient of appropriate safety precautions.

3. Emphasize to the patient the need to take medication under close medical supervision. Untreated glaucoma can cause blindness.

4. Long-acting anticholinesterase agents increase the risk of development of specific types of cataracts.

SUPPLEMENTARY READINGS

Drachman, D. B., "Myasthenia Gravis," *New England Journal of Medicine* **298:** 136–142, 186–193 (1978).

Grob, D., ed., "Myasthenia Gravis," *Annals of the New York Academy of Sciences* **214:** 1–682 (1976).

Havener, W. H., *Ocular Pharmacology* (4th ed.). St. Louis: The C. V. Mosby Company, 1978.

Kosterlitz, W. H., "Effects of Choline Esters of Smooth Muscle and Secretions," in *Physiological Pharmacology*, Vol. 3, *The Nervous System*, Part C: *Autonomic Nervous System Drugs*, ed. W. S. Root and F. G. Hofmann, pp. 97–161. New York: Academic Press, Inc., 1967.

Rand, M. J. and A. Stafford, "Cardiovascular Effects of Choline Esters," in *Physiological Pharmacology*, Vol. 3, *The Nervous System*, Part C: *Autonomic Nervous System Drugs*, ed. W. S. Root and F. G. Hofmann, pp. 1–95. New York: Academic Press, Inc., 1967.

Taylor, P., "Anticholinesterase Agents," in *Goodman and Gilman's The Pharmacological Basis of Therapeutics* (6th ed.), ed. A. G. Gilman, L. S. Goodman, and A. Gilman, Chapter 6, pp. 110–119. New York: Macmillan, Inc., 1980.

Watson, P. G., ed., "Glaucoma," *British Journal of Ophthalmology* **56:** 145–318 (1972).

Volle, R. L., "Cholinomimetic Drugs," in *Drill's Pharmacology in Medicine* (4th ed.), Chapter 31, pp. 584–607, ed. by J. R. DiPalma. New York: McGraw-Hill Book Company, 1971.

ATROPINE AND RELATED ANTIMUSCARINIC AGENTS

Chapter 8

Atropine and related drugs antagonize the *muscarinic* effects of acetylcholine at effector cells innervated by postganglionic parasympathetic nerves and are, therefore, commonly referred to as *antimuscarinic agents*. Less precise designations of this drug class include *anticholinergic agents*, *cholinergic blocking agents*, and *parasympatholytic agents*.

The extensive clinical uses of antimuscarinic agents are based upon their actions on the gastrointestinal tract, the eye, exocrine glands, and the central nervous system. Dozens of antimuscarinic agents are employed in therapeutics; almost all of these agents differ only quantitatively from atropine, the prototype of this drug class.

ATROPINE AND THE BELLADONNA ALKALOIDS

The *Solanaceae* family of plants has been used for centuries for its pharmacological and toxicological effects and for cosmetic purposes. The leaves and roots of *Atropa belladonna* are the natural sources of the alkaloids atropine and scopolamine (hyoscine).

During the sixteenth century, Italian women squeezed the berries of this plant into their eyes to widen and brighten their pupils; hence the name belladonna or beautiful lady. Medieval poisoners used *Atropa belladonna* as a common tool of their nefarious profession, thus accounting for the common name of this plant, the "deadly nightshade." Hyoscyamine is another belladonna alkaloid obtained from the Jimson or Jamestown weed (*Datura stramonium*), a plant well known to Indian tribes of the United States and Mexico for its mind-altering effects. Inhalation of fumes from burning stramonium powder has been employed for many years for the treatment of asthma.

Pharmacological Effects

Atropine is a potent antagonist of the muscarinic actions of acetylcholine. The major effects of this drug are on the exocrine glands, smooth muscle of the gastrointestinal and urinary tract, the eye, the cardiovascular system, and the central nervous system.

Exocrine glands   Secretions from exocrine glands are inhibited by atropine. *Salivation is blocked* at therapeutic doses, resulting in dryness of the mouth; this is the most common adverse effect associated with antimuscarinic agents. Inhibition of secretions from the sweat glands accounts for the extreme hyperthermia observed after the ingestion of toxic doses of these drugs by young children. Relatively high doses of atropine are required to inhibit the secretion of gastric acid.

Smooth muscles   The normal tension (tone) and spontaneous movements (motility) of the smooth muscles of the gastrointestinal tract are reduced; these are referred to as the *antispasmodic effects* of atropine. This drug produces similar effects on the smooth muscle of the urinary bladder and also contracts the sphincter. These effects result in *urinary retention*, which is primarily observed in elderly men. The bronchodilatory effects of atropine are less pronounced than epinephrine and isoproterenol (Isuprel).

Eye   Antimuscarinic agents produce marked dilation of the pupils (*mydriasis*) and paralysis of the ciliary muscles of accommodation (*cycloplegia*). The pupil of an eye treated with atropine fails to respond to light. While drug-induced cycloplegia interferes with the capacity of the eye to focus upon near objects, causing *blurred vision*, the patient retains the ability to see distant objects clearly. Local application of atropine produces mydriasis and cycloplegia that persists for more than 1 week. While systemic administration of atropine in normal therapeutic doses (0.5 mg) does not modify ocular parameters, high doses will produce such effects which persist for several hours.

Systemic administration of antimuscarinic agents has no effect on the intraocular pressure of a normal eye and rarely elevates intraocular pressure in patients with wide-angle glaucoma. By contrast, atropine-like drugs may precipitate attacks of previously undiagnosed narrow-angle glaucoma (Chapter 7).

Cardiovascular system   Ordinary therapeutic doses of atropine temporarily and slightly reduce heart rate, while moderate to high doses increase heart rate by blocking the inhibitory influences of the cholinergic vagus nerve on the cardiac pacemaker (sinoatrial node). Atropine has little or no effect on blood pressure at therapeutic doses, but may induce vasodilation and flushing of the face and neck.

Central nervous system   Clinical doses of atropine do not produce marked changes in behavior. Toxic doses, by contrast, cause excitation manifested by euphoria, restlessness, irritability, hallucinations, delirium, and coma; at lethal doses, the respiratory centers in the medulla become depressed and death results from respiratory failure.

Scopolamine, a compound closely resembling atropine both chemically and pharmacologically, usually produces drowsiness, amnesia, and dreamless sleep at normal doses. Nonprescription products designed to induce sleep formerly contained scopolamine.

Therapeutic Uses

The diverse pharmacological effects of atropine and related antimuscarinic drugs in the periphery and central nervous system serve as the basis for the extensive clinical applications of this class of drugs. Conversely, these same wide-ranging effects result in a relative lack of specificity and an equally diverse array of side effects, as discussed later. Attempts to obtain greater therapeutic benefit by increasing their dosage is often thwarted by a concurrent increase in the spectrum and intensity of undesirable effects. Prior to the administration of antimuscarinic agents, the nurse should ascertain whether the patient has a history of or symptoms suggestive of narrow-angle glaucoma; patients over 40 years of age may have this disease without being aware of its existence. A summary of nursing implications associated with atropine administration appears at the end of this chapter.

Preoperative uses Atropine or scopolamine is frequently administered prior to surgery to inhibit salivary and bronchial secretions stimulated by certain general anesthetic agents. During induction of anesthesia with cyclopropane or halothane (Fluothane), the vagal (cholinergic) influence on the heart may be increased, causing reflex bradycardia; administration of these belladonna alkaloids prior to anesthesia prevents this problem. Since the postoperative patient often experiences a very dry mouth—particularly after the use of these drugs—the nurse should administer cold drinks if oral fluids are permitted; hard candy and gum are also helpful in treating dry mouth.

Uses in ophthalmology Local administration of antimuscarinic agents to the eye produces mydriasis and cycloplegia. Mydriasis is often desirable for diagnostic examinations of the retina and optic disc and for the treatment of inflammatory conditions of the iris and uveal tract. Cycloplegia is induced prior to diagnostic examinations of the eye for the purpose of fitting corrective lenses. While atropine is a powerful mydriatic and cycloplegic agent, its long duration of action (7 to 12 days) represents the major deterrent to its use. Short-acting antimuscarinic drugs intended for these ophthalmic effects are available (Table 8-1); eucatropine (Euphthalmine) produces only mydriasis, in the absence of cycloplegia, and, therefore, does not impair vision of near objects.

Gastrointestinal disorders Antimuscarinic agents reduce gastric acid secretion, decrease smooth muscle motility, and delay gastric emptying time. Although their therapeutic benefit in the treatment of *peptic ulcer disease* has not been clearly established, they are widely used for the management of duodenal ulcers. Synthetic derivatives of atropine have been developed that have marked antispasmodic activity and are employed for the treatment of a wide variety of intestinal spastic and hypermotility disorders. The uses of atropine-like drugs in the treatment of intestinal diseases, in particular peptic ulcers, will be discussed in Chapter 55, with representative antimuscarinic agents listed in Table 55-3.

Common cold The belladonna alkaloids have been used as ingredients of nonprescription products promoted for treatment of the common cold. These drugs inhibit secretion from the nasopharynx and lower respiratory tract and thereby provide symptomatic relief of acute inflammation of the mucous membranes of the nose (rhinitis); the patient may feel better as a result, but the normal duration of the common cold is not shortened. These drugs may be harmful to patients with chronic respiratory disorders. Drug-induced inhibition in the secretion of respiratory tract fluids may produce a thickening of these fluids, obstructing respiratory passages and further increasing the distress encountered by the patient.

Table 8-1 Antimuscarinic Mydriatic-Cycloplegic Agents

Generic name	Trade name	Duration of action	Unique properties
Atropine	——	7–12 days	Long duration (disadvantage).
Cyclopentolate	Cyclogyl	12–24 h	—
Eucatropine	Euphthalmine	6–12 h	No cycloplegia.
Homatropine hydrobromide	——	1–3 days	—
Tropicamide	Mydriacyl	15–20 min	Very short duration of action.

Motion sickness For trips of short duration that are characterized by vigorous motion, scopolamine is probably the most effective drug available for preventing the nausea and vomiting of motion sickness. This drug has not been observed to prevent nausea and vomiting arising from other causes. Scopolamine is most effective when taken *prior* to the onset of these symptoms, and therefore, should be employed on a prophylactic basis. The use of antihistamines for the prevention of motion sickness will be considered in Chapter 53.

Parkinson's disease Prior to the introduction of levodopa in the late 1960s, selected tertiary antimuscarinic agents were the most widely used drugs for the reduction of tremors and rigidity associated with Parkinson's disease. The use of these drugs and levodopa for the treatment of this neurological disorder will be discussed in Chapter 19. Antimuscarinic drugs continue to be used for the relief of parkinsonism-like symptoms produced by phenothiazine and butyrophenone antipsychotic agents (Chapter 15).

Administration and Fate

The belladonna alkaloids are rapidly absorbed after oral administration (the most common route); the average adult dose of atropine sulfate is 0.5 mg four times daily. Atropine may also be administered by injection (subcutaneously or intravenously) and in an ophthalmic solution (1 percent).

Atropine is distributed throughout the entire body. It is primarily eliminated in the urine, both unchanged and as a metabolite; traces of atropine are found in various secretions, including nursing milk.

Side Effects and Acute Toxicity

Therapeutic doses of antimuscarinic agents commonly produce dry mouth, blurred vision, photophobia, urinary retention (in older men), and constipation.

Apart from infants and young children, who are highly susceptible to the toxic effects of the belladonna alkaloids, these drugs have a very wide margin of safety in adults; for example, while doses of 10 mg or less may prove lethal for children, fatal doses of atropine in adults are approximately 100 mg. Potential drug interactions involving antimuscarinic agents are listed in Table 8-2.

Symptoms of overdosage give rise to distinctive signs, including a rapid but weak pulse, mydriasis, dry, flushed skin, extreme thirst, restlessness, excitability, confusion, and delirium. In children, body temperatures

Table 8-2 Potential Drug Interactions Involving Antimuscarinic Agents

Drug/class	Potential consequences
Antidepressants, tricyclics Antihistamines Antipsychotic phenothiazines Meperidine (Demerol)	These drugs possess antimuscarinic properties and may, therefore, enhance the side effects produced by the belladonna alkaloids and synthetic antimuscarinic agents.
Levodopa (Bendopar, Dopar, Larodopa, Levopar)	Antimuscarinic agents delay gastric emptying, which prolongs the stay of levodopa in stomach. Levodopa is inactivated in stomach; less active drug is absorbed into blood, which may reduce its antiparkinson effects.
Amantadine (Symmetrel)	Amantadine may potentiate antimuscarinic side effects when these drugs are given at high doses.
Methotrimeprazine (Levoprome)	Extrapyramidal (parkinsonism) side effects have been reported in patients receiving scopolamine and methotrimeprazine.

of 107°F (41.7°C) or more have been reported. In severe cases of poisoning, circulatory collapse develops, causing a drop in blood pressure. After a period of coma, death may result from respiratory failure.

Gastric lavage is of value to reduce intestinal absorption of antimuscarinic agents after their oral administration. Slow intravenous administration of physostigmine (but not neostigmine) reverses atropine-induced delirium and coma. Low doses of diazepam (Valium) may prove beneficial in calming the excited poison victim or in controlling convulsions. Artificial respiration with oxygen may be required. Ice bags and alcohol sponge baths assist in the reduction of fever.

Antimuscarinic Agents: nursing implications

Atropine

1. Oral atropine is usually given 30 min before meals.
2. Postural hypotension may result if patient ambulates too soon after parenteral administration; slowing of the heart for 1–2 min may occur.
3. Older patients should be observed for tachycardia, increased intraocular pressure, and urinary retention.
4. Advise patients to avoid hazardous activities if blurred vision, dizziness, or drowsiness occurs.
5. Advise parents of infants and children that atropine flush results from vasodilation and not from a fever.
6. Be alert for symptoms of atropine poisoning, especially in infants and children: hot, dry, flushed skin; fever; tachycardia; increased respiratory rate; behavioral confusion; muscle weakness and incoordination; respiratory depression; and death.
7. Discomfort resulting from dry mouth can be minimized by sucking hard candy, chewing gum, or rinsing the mouth with water.

SUPPLEMENTARY READINGS

Collumbine, H., "Cholinergic Blocking Drugs," in *Drill's Pharmacology in Medicine* (4th ed.), ed. J. R. DiPalma. Chapter 32, pp. 608–626. New York: McGraw-Hill Book Company, 1971.

Greenblatt, D. J. and R. I. Shader, "Anticholinergics," *New England Journal of Medicine* **288**: 1215–1219 (1973).

Weiner, N., "Atropine Scopolamine, and Related Antimuscarinic Drugs," in *Goodman and Gilman's The Pharmacological Basis of Therapeutics* (6th ed.), ed. A. G. Gilman, L. S. Goodman, and A. Gilman, Chapter 7, pp. 120–137. New York: Macmillan, Inc., 1980.

Section III

DRUGS AFFECTING THE CENTRAL NERVOUS SYSTEM

Chapter 9

INTRODUCTION TO THE CENTRAL NERVOUS SYSTEM

The central nervous system is responsible for the coordination and direction of all the organ systems of the body. Such control enables us to adapt by maintaining a relatively constant internal environment (*homeostasis*) in an ever-changing external environment.

Sensory information is transmitted along peripheral nerve fibers to the spinal cord and brain. The brain filters this information, and, via motor nerves, activates effector organs or tissues to make an appropriate response. A large number of drugs are able to modify the actions of the central nervous system by increasing or decreasing the functional activity of one or more component areas. Drugs are capable of reducing our perception of pain, increasing our level of mental and physical activity, and controlling seizures and abnormal behavior. By contrast, other drugs produce behavioral and neurological dysfunctions.

In this chapter we shall review the primary physiological functions of the major areas of the central nervous system. Although we shall consider each of these regions separately, you should bear in mind that there are extensive neural connections that permit communication, feedback, and interactions among these regions.

PHYSIOLOGICAL FUNCTIONS OF THE CENTRAL NERVOUS SYSTEM

The brain is commonly separated into two primary divisions, namely, the forebrain and the hindbrain or brain stem (Figure 9-1).

Forebrain

The forebrain may be subdivided into the *telencephalon* or *cerebral hemispheres* (consisting of the cerebral cortex and basal ganglia) and the *diencephalon* (including the thalamus and hypothalamus). The limbic system includes regions from both the telencephalon and diencephalon.

The *cerebral cortex* receives sensory information from the external and internal environment, processes this information, and then transmits messages to the appropriate parts of the body. The sensory, motor, and association areas of the cortex participate in these activities. The sensory areas are concerned with the reception of information from the five senses. Motor areas are responsible for the direction of all voluntary and associated* motor movement. The most highly sophisticated regions of the cerebral cortex, the association areas, collect, interpret, and integrate information from all parts of the central nervous system. These areas direct our highest mental activities, namely, memory, learning, reasoning, and judgment. Directly or indirectly, a variety of drugs affect the function of the cerebral cortex, including the stimulants amphetamine and caffeine and the depressants alcohol and barbiturates.

---

*The movement of arm swinging is "associated" with the primary motor act of walking; facial expressions and hand gestures are "associated" with talking.

The *basal ganglia*, consisting of several anatomically distinct but functionally interconnected structures, direct motor functions that are not under conscious control. Deficiencies in the neurotransmitter substance dopamine have been associated with Parkinson's disease, resulting in altered muscle tone and abnormal movements. This neurological disease is characterized by tremors occurring at rest, rigidity, and difficulties in initiating movement. Antipsychotic agents, such as haloperidol (Haldol) and trifluoperazine (Stelazine), produce a parkinsonian syndrome by blocking the actions of dopamine in the basal ganglia.

The *thalamus* serves as a relay station for the transmission of sensory information from the peripheral nervous system to the cerebral cortex. Crude sensations such as pain and emotions can be appreciated by the thalamus. It has been suggested that morphine reduces the perception of pain by depressing thalamic neurons.

The *hypothalamus* is primarily responsible for the central control of both the sympathetic and parasympathetic divisions of the autonomic nervous system; it also influences regulation of the cardiovascular system, maintenance of body temperature, body water content, and feeding behavior. Aspirin reduces the elevated body temperature by its actions on the thermoregulatory centers in the hypothalamus, while amphetamines are thought to suppress appetite by inhibiting the activity of the feeding center located in this area of the brain. The hypothalamus modulates the activity of the pituitary gland, which in turn controls the activity of endocrine glands.

The *limbic system* has been implicated in modulating emotional behavior. Among the many neuronally interconnected structures that comprise the limbic system are the hypothalamus, septal areas, amygdala, and

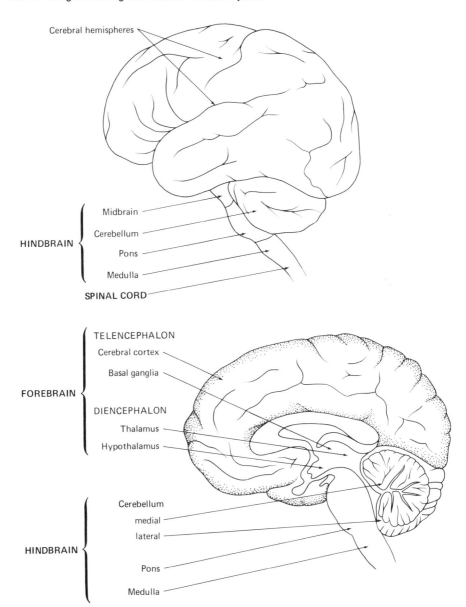

Figure 9-1 The Human Brain. Top: lateral view; bottom: sagittal section through midline of the brain.

hippocampus. There is experimental evidence suggesting that the antipsychotic agents (for example, chlorpromazine) and anti-anxiety agents (for example, diazepam) may exert their beneficial therapeutic effects by acting in the limbic system.

Hindbrain (Brain stem)

The cerebellum, medulla, pons, and midbrain are the four structures making up the hindbrain or brain stem. We shall consider only the first two of these brain parts.

The *cerebellum* coordinates the fine movements of voluntary muscles throughout the body, permitting us to carry out smooth and accurate body movements. It modulates neural impulses arising from the motor areas of the cerebral cortex, basal ganglia, and spinal cord that are concerned with voluntary movements. The cerebellum, in conjunction with the vestibular system of the inner ear, maintains posture and equilibrium. Drugs that interfere with the function of the cerebellum cause a loss of balance, dizziness, and uncoordinated jerky movements.

Many of the body's most vital functions are controlled by the *medulla oblongata.* Centers controlling respiration and cardiovascular function are located in the medulla; the vasomotor and cardiac centers control blood pressure and heart rate, respectively. Toxic doses of alcohol, barbiturates, general anesthetics, and narcotics are capable of causing death by depressing these centers, particularly those controlling respiratory function. The cough and vomiting centers are also found in this part of the brain. Codeine and dextromethorphan are widely used cough suppressants that act by inhibiting the medullary cough center.

Reticular Formation

The *reticular formation* is a diffuse network of neurons that travel from the upper portion of the spinal cord and brain stem through the midbrain and into the forebrain (Figure 9-2). It serves both excitatory and inhibitory functions. The ascending reticular activating system of the reticular formation receives sensory messages from all parts of the body; these are transmitted to the cerebral cortex, which arouses the cortex and maintains a state of consciousness. It is believed that stimulants increase alertness and depressants cause drowsiness and loss of consciousness by virtue of their opposite effects on the reticular

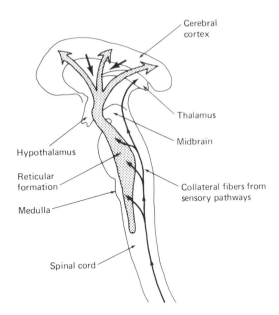

Figure 9-2   Arousal of Cerebral Cortex by the Reticular Formation (RF). Neural pathways from the RF are responsible for activating the cortex. In turn the cortex sends messages back to the RF.

formation. The inhibitory functions of the reticular formation are manifested by a reduction in voluntary movements and sleep.

Spinal Cord

The *spinal cord* serves as a conduit for the transmission of information between the peripheral nervous system and the brain. Ascending nerves transmit sensory impulses up the spinal cord to higher levels of the central nervous system, whereas descending nerve tracts send instructions to effector cells via motor nerve fibers. Convulsions induced by strychnine have been attributed to the effects of this drug on motor neurons in the spinal cord. Local anesthetics may be injected into the spinal cord (spinal anesthesia) to prevent pain and yet permit the maintenance of consciousness during operations and in childbirth.

CHEMICAL TRANSMISSION IN THE CENTRAL NERVOUS SYSTEM

It is generally accepted that transmission of nerve impulses across synapses located in the central nervous system is accomplished by chemicals, or *neurotransmitters*, as in the periphery. A better understanding of the functional role of such chemicals in the brain might provide us with a rational basis for the treatment of psychoses, disorders of mood, and other neuropsychiatric diseases.

At present there are varying degrees of evidence to suggest that the catecholamines (norepinephrine, dopamine), serotonin, acetylcholine, and gamma-aminobutyric acid (GABA) are neurotransmitters in the central nervous system. It is theorized that abnormalities in the functional activity of norepinephrine, and possibly of serotonin, underlie affective disorders (mania and depression). There is strong evidence to suggest that Par-kinson's disease is associated with a deficiency of dopamine, while an excess in the functional activity of this compound has been implicated in schizophrenia. The behavioral aberrations associated with lysergic acid diethylamide (LSD) and some related compounds are thought to result from an interaction of these psychotomimetic (hallucinogenic) substances with serotonin.

SUPPLEMENTARY READINGS

Carpenter, M. B., *Human Neuroanatomy* (7th ed.). Baltimore: Williams & Wilkins Company, 1976.

Cooper, J. R., F. E. Bloom, and R. H. Roth, *The Biochemical Basis of Neuropharmacology* (3rd ed.). New York: Oxford University Press, Inc., 1978.

Eccles, J. C., *The Understanding of the Brain.* New York: McGraw-Hill Book Company, 1973.

Krnjević, K., "Chemical Nature of Synaptic Transmission in Vertebrates," *Physiological Reviews* **54:** 418–540 (1974).

Mountcastle, V. B., ed., *Medical Physiology* (15th ed.), Vol. 1. St. Louis: The C. V. Mosby Company, 1974.

"The Brain," *Scientific American* **241**(3): 44–232 (1979).

GENERAL ANESTHETICS

Prior to the 1840s many patients preferred to suffer the agonies of disease rather than submit to the surgeon's scalpel. The reputation of the surgeon of this period was largely predicated upon speed, with the duration of operations measured in minutes. Notwithstanding the technical perfection of the operation, the apprehension and extreme pain experienced by the patient often resulted in surgical shock and death.

The discovery of the general anesthetic agent ether in 1846 transformed this torture chamber filled with the agonizing screams of the patient into an operating room, and it enabled the surgeon to operate deliberately on an unconscious patient free of pain. Surgery could then become an art and science. In the opinion of many, the discovery of general anesthetics represents one of the major, if not *the* major, contribution of the medical sciences to humanity.

General anesthetics are drugs that produce a loss of sensation throughout the body and a loss of consciousness. This chapter considers the clinical objectives of general anesthesia, the administration of inhalation anesthetics (including factors modifying the uptake, distribution, and elimination of these drugs and the general methods employed for their administration), and the signs and stages of anesthesia. The specific pharmacological characteristics of representative general anesthetic agents will then be discussed.

OBJECTIVES OF GENERAL ANESTHESIA

General anesthesia has four major objectives, namely, to produce narcosis, analgesia, muscle relaxation, and hyporeflexia.

Narcosis

Narcosis is a general term referring to a state of continuing and progressive central nervous system depression leading to unconsciousness. The general anesthetics and other central nervous system depressants (sedative-hypnotics, alcohol, opiate narcotics) are all capable of producing various levels of narcosis depending upon the dosage administered. In most operative procedures, it is desirable to induce a state of anesthesia in which the patient is totally unconscious and lacks the perception of sensation.

Since the turn of the century, numerous theories have been proposed to explain the mechanism by which these drugs produce anesthesia. Considerable experimental evidence suggests that these drugs act by depressing the ascending reticular activating system and thereby inhibit the transmission of nerve impulses from the periphery to the cortex. The precise mechanism by which general anesthetics depress these multisynaptic pathways has not been clearly established.

Analgesia and Muscle Relaxation

Analgesia, the loss of the sensation of pain, is independent of narcosis and is produced by some general anesthetics (ether, nitrous oxide) but not others (halothane, thiopental sodium). *Skeletal muscle relaxation* is desirable and at times essential in many operative procedures, such as abdominal surgery. Varying degrees of reduction in muscle tone may be achieved, but the reduction should not be so great that the function of those muscles required to maintain respiratory function is compromised. Ether and methoxyflurane possess excellent muscle-relaxing properties, while nitrous oxide is devoid of such effects.

Hyporeflexia

Hyporeflexia refers to a reduction in reflex actions that compromise the patient's ability to carry out normal respiratory and cardiovascular responses. Ether, for example, is irritating to the respiratory tract and reflexly stimulates secretions that may obstruct normal breathing; thiopental sodium produces hyperactivity of laryngeal reflexes, provoking laryngospasms. While no currently available general anesthetic effectively blocks these reflexes, both reflex responses may be inhibited by pretreatment with atropine.

Preoperative Medication and Balanced Anesthesia

The *ideal* general anesthetic agent should be nonflammable and nonirritating; should rapidly and pleasantly induce anesthesia and readily and safely maintain the desired level of anesthesia; should produce effective analgesia and muscle relaxation and suppress undesirable reflex responses; should be nontoxic to the heart, liver, and kidneys; and should permit a rapid recovery devoid of postoperative nausea and vomiting.

Tables 10-1 and 10-2 (pp. 85–86) reveal that no currently available general anesthetic possesses all these desirable attributes. Hence, to accomplish these objectives, the nurse will commonly observe that a combination of drugs are employed preoperatively and during the operative procedure; this has been called *balanced anesthesia*. Preanesthetic agents often employed include (1) a short-acting barbiturate (secobarbital, pentobarbital) on the evening prior to surgery to reduce apprehension and provide the patient with a restful night's sleep; (2) a narcotic analgesic (morphine, meperidine) 45 to 60 minutes prior to surgery to produce sedation, reduce anxiety and tension, and provide relief of pain; and (3) an anticholinergic agent (atropine, scopolamine) 45 to 60 minutes preoperatively to inhibit respiratory secretions, laryngospasms, and vagal-mediated bradycardia. Induction of anesthesia may be rapidly and pleasantly produced with nitrous oxide or by intravenous administration of thiopental sodium or another ultrashort-acting barbiturate. A curare-like drug (tubocurarine) may be used to promote skeletal muscle relaxation. If ether is employed as the general anesthetic, a muscle relaxant may not be required.

Preoperative preparation of the patient for anesthesia by the nurse can facilitate smooth induction of anesthesia and can re-

Table 10-1 Comparative Properties of Volatile Liquid Inhalation

Generic name (trade name)	Ether [diethyl ether]	Chloroform	Vinyl ether (Vinethane)	Halothane (Fluothane)	Methoxyflurane (Penthrane)	Enflurane (Enthrane)
Flammable and explosive	Yes.	No.	Yes.	No.	No.	No.
Complete/incomplete anesthesia	Complete.	Complete.	Complete.	Complete.	Complete.	Complete.
Induction						
Onset	10–20 min	2–5 min	1–2 min	10 min	10–20 min	7–10 min
Pleasant	No.	Yes.	Yes.	Yes.	Yes.	Yes.
Recovery	Slow.	Rapid.	Rapid.	More rapid than ether.	Slow.	Rapid.
Respiratory effects						
Irritating to mucosa	Yes.	No.	Yes.	No.	No.	No.
Alteration of respiration	Initial stimulation, later depression.	Progressive depression.	Same as ether.	Progressive depression.	Depression.	Same as halothane.
Cardiovascular effects						
Blood pressure	Stage III, plane 3, decrease.	Decrease.	Same as ether.	Decrease.	Slight decrease.	Some decrease.
Heart rate	Stage III, plane 3, decrease.	Decrease.	Same as ether.	Decrease.	Slight decrease.	No change.
Sensitization of myocardium to catecholamines	No.	Yes.	At high concentrations.	Yes.	Less than halothane.	Yes.
Skeletal muscle relaxation	Excellent.	Good.	Less than ether.	Modest.	Excellent.	Good.
Analgesia	Yes.	Yes.	Yes.	Poor.	Yes.	Yes.
Miscellaneous properties	Postoperative nausea and vomiting; slow onset and recovery; wide range of safety.	Narrow range of safety.	Rapid induction and recovery; liver and kidney toxicity.	Possible liver toxicity.	Most potent agent; similar to halothane; long recovery period.	Similar to halothane, no liver toxicity, good muscle relaxation. Convulsions at high doses.
Major therapeutic uses	Major operations of long duration; childbirth.	Rarely used: explosive, cardiac arrhythmias; liver toxicity.	Operations of short duration.	Most widely used agent; often employed with nitrous oxide.	Childbirth.	Abdominal surgery.

Table 10-2   Comparative Properties of Inhalation Gases and Intravenous General Anesthetics

Generic name (trade name)	Nitrous oxide	Cyclopropane	Thiopental sodium (Pentothal sodium)	Droperidol-Fentanyl (Innovar)	Ketamine (Ketaject, Ketalar)
Physical state	Gas.	Gas.	Liquid.	Liquid.	Liquid.
Route of Administration	Inhalation.	Inhalation.	Intravenous.	Intravenous.	Intravenous.
Flammable & explosive	No.	Yes.	No.	No.	No.
Complete/Incomplete anesthesia	Incomplete.	Complete.	Complete.	Incomplete.	Incomplete.
Induction					
Onset	1–2 min	2–3 min	1 min	3–5 min	1 min
Pleasant	Yes.	Yes.	Yes.	Yes.	Yes.
Recovery	Rapid.	Rapid.	Rapid, at low doses.	Rapid.	Rapid.
Respiratory effects					
Irritating to mucosa	No.	No.	No.	No.	No.
Alteration of respiration	No change.	Depression at high concentrations.	Pronounced depression.	Depression.	No change.
Cardiovascular effects					
Blood pressure	No change.	No change.	Decrease.	Decrease.	Increase.
Heart rate	No change.	Slight changes.	Decrease.	Decrease.	Increase.
Sensitization of myocardium to catecholamines	No.	Yes.	No.	No.	Rarely.
Skeletal muscle relaxation	Poor.	Good.	Poor.	Muscle rigidity.	No.
Analgesia	Yes.	Yes.	No.	Yes, continuing to postoperative period.	Yes.
Miscellaneous properties	Extremely safe; low potency; anoxia at high concentrations.	Wide margin of safety; little postop nausea and vomiting.	Rapid and pleasant induction and recovery; cannot terminate effect rapidly; laryngospasm.	Neuroleptic analgesia; Postoperative respiratory depression.	Dissociative anesthesia. Postoperative disturbing dreams and hallucinations.
Major therapeutic uses	Used extensively in minor operations and for induction in balanced anesthesia.	Uncommonly used; explosive; cardiac arrhythmias; myocardial sensitization.	Operations of short duration; induction in major operations.	Diagnostic procedures; burn dressings.	Procedures of short duration; head and neck surgery; burn treatment; useful in children.

duce complications during the postoperative period. Preanesthetic medications must be administered at the correct or appropriate time to allow sequential development of balanced anesthesia. A narcotic agent given too close to the administration of the general anesthetic may cause severe respiratory depression. Preoperative education of the patient facilitates cooperation postoperatively. The importance of turning, coughing, and deep breathing should be explained to, demonstrated to, and practiced by the patient, with emphasis placed on specific techniques to suit the patient's individual needs. The principle of splinting an abdominal incision with a pillow is more readily understood prior to surgery than postoperatively, when attention is focused primarily on incisional pain. If the patient exhibits a high level of anxiety or expresses fear of death, this should be reported to the physician. Severe anxiety or fear can adversely affect the autonomic and central nervous systems, necessitating high levels of anesthetic, with potential adverse effects.

ADMINISTRATION OF INHALATION ANESTHETICS

General anesthetic gases (nitrous oxide) and volatile liquids vaporized prior to their use (ether, halothane) are administered by inhalation. This section examines the uptake, distribution, and elimination of these drugs and then considers the general methods employed for their administration.

Uptake, Distribution, and Elimination

The anesthetic agent is delivered into the alveoli of the lungs from the inspired air by an appropriate delivery apparatus, as discussed shortly. The drug diffuses across the alveolar membrane into the arterial blood flowing through the lungs and is subsequently distributed to many tissues of the body, in particular to those such as the brain receiving a rich blood supply (Figure 10-1).

During the induction stage of anesthesia, the concentration (or more correctly, the partial pressure) of the anesthetic gas is lower in the tissues than in the arterial blood, and this gradient is responsible for the movement of the anesthetic from the arterial blood to the tissues. After continued anesthetic administration, this gradient no longer exists; when equilibrium is established, the rate at which the drug leaves the tissues in the venous blood is equal to the rate at which the drug is supplied to the tissues by the arterial blood. After the administration of the anesthetic agent is terminated, the net flow of gas is from the tissues to the venous blood to the expired alveolar air. The concentration of anesthetic in tissues that have a rich blood supply (brain) declines more rapidly than in those tissues that are poorly perfused (fat).

Most anesthetic agents are eliminated from the body in the exhaled air without chemical modification. Halothane is metabolized to a limited extent, and it has been suggested that a metabolite of this drug may be responsible for its liver toxicity. The nurse will observe a direct relationship between the rate of induction and the rate of recovery; for example, rapid induction and recovery periods are associated with cyclopropane and nitrous oxide, while a delayed onset and a prolonged recovery period are noted with ether, halothane, and methoxyflurane (Table 10-1).

Anesthetic Delivery Systems

An anesthetic delivery system intended for the administration of a gas or volatile liquid

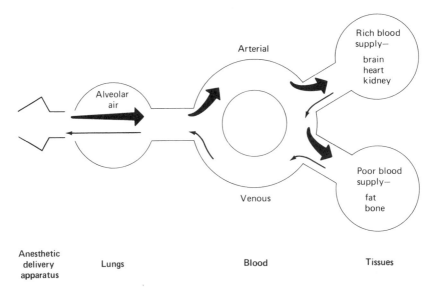

Anesthetic
delivery   Lungs   Blood   Tissues
apparatus

Figure 10-1 Arrows depict the transfer of an inhalation anesthetic during induction from the inspired alveolar air of the lungs to the arterial blood to the tissues. After the termination of anesthetic administration, the net flow of the anesthetic is in the opposite direction, in effect, from the tissues to the venous blood to the expired air.

by inhalation must provide sources of oxygen and anesthetic, as well as provide for the maintenance of respiration and the removal of carbon dioxide. Three such basic systems include the *open*, *semiclosed*, and *closed* methods.

Open method   A volatile liquid is dropped on a cotton or gauze mask placed over the patient's nose. Oxygen and carbon dioxide exchange with the air and there is no mechanical support of respiration. While this method is simple, its use is limited to operations of short duration.

Semiclosed method   In this procedure, the patient inhales a mixture of oxygen and the anesthetic gas or vapor through a mask, which is equipped with a valve to permit expiration outside the system.

Closed method   The patient continuously rebreathes the contents of a reservoir bag containing a mixture of the anesthetic

agent and oxygen, in which the rate of flow of each can be carefully regulated. The exhaled air is directed to flow through and be trapped by a carbon dioxide absorber. Since the anesthetic is rebreathed and contained in a closed system, this method is economical and also reduces the hazards of fire or explosion associated with flammable anesthetics. This is the method most commonly used in hospitals.

STAGES OF ANESTHESIA

The depth of anesthesia can be assessed by monitoring characteristic signs associated with each of four stages. These signs were originally described for ether and will differ somewhat when preanesthetic medication is used prior to ether or when anesthetic agents other than ether are employed.

Stage I. Analgesia

The onset of administration of the anesthetic and the loss of consciousness mark the beginning and end, respectively, of this first stage. In addition to not responding to painful stimuli, the patient may experience feelings of drifting, giddiness, and choking, as well as dreams or hallucinations.

Stage II. Excitement

The patient, while unconscious during this stage, exhibits signs of excitement and involuntary movements including laughing, shouting, and thrashing about. Pupils are dilated and reflexes become overactive, causing salivation, swallowing, coughing, and vomiting. Respiration is rapid and irregular, with alternating periods of breath holding and deep breathing often encountered; blood pressure and heart rate are both increased. The anesthetist generally attempts to pass the patient through this phase as rapidly as possible. When anesthesia is induced with rapidly acting, intravenously administered barbiturates—as is often the case—this stage may not be observed.

Stage III. Surgical Anesthesia

In this stage the patient is unconscious and reflexes are depressed. This stage is divided into four planes.

Plane 1 This plane begins with the loss of eyelid reflex and ends with a cessation of ocular movements, with the eyes looking directly ahead; the pupils are no longer dilated as in stage II and appear normal. Excessive reflex activity disappears and muscle relaxation of the limbs is noted.

Plane 2 Respiration is regular and deep. Sufficient muscle relaxation is produced to permit most surgical procedures to be performed at this plane.

Plane 3 This plane begins with the first signs of intercostal muscle paralysis and ends with complete paralysis of these muscles, which are involved in respiration. The pupils are once again dilated and reflex constriction of the pupils to light is lost. This is the deepest intended level of anesthesia for major surgery.

Plane 4 Respiration is rapid and shallow resulting from paralysis of the intercostal muscles and diaphragm.

Stage IV. Medullary Paralysis

This toxic stage begins with central (medullary) paralysis and progresses to vasomotor collapse, cardiac failure, and death unless the administration of the anesthetic is terminated and respiration reestablished. During emergence from anesthesia, the signs of the various stages occur in the reverse order until normal reflex activity and consciousness are present.

The depth of anesthesia produced by general anesthetics differs. In the absence of preanesthetic medication, ether, cyclopropane, and halothane can take the patient to stage III, plane 4, a level of anesthesia sufficient for all major operations; such drugs are referred to as *complete* or 100 percent anesthetics. By contrast, nitrous oxide possesses considerably less efficacy than ether and, when used in safe anesthetic concentrations, can carry the patient only to stage III, plane 1, a level insufficiently deep for major surgical procedures; nitrous oxide is referred to as an *incomplete* or 25 percent anesthetic.

CHARACTERISTICS OF SPECIFIC GENERAL ANESTHETICS

Anesthetic agents fall into three major categories, namely, gases, volatile liquids—both of which are administered by inhalation— and fixed or intravenous agents (Tables 10-1 and 10-2). Representative drugs of each of these classes will be discussed in this section.

Inhalation Agents

Ether Ether is a clear, colorless liquid, possessing a characteristic odor. The vapors of this compound are highly flammable.

Ether produces progressive depression of the central nervous system. The induction period is slow (10 to 20 minutes) and often unpleasant. The vapors of ether are highly irritating to the mucosa of the respiratory tract, initially resulting in a reflex stimulation of respiration. In addition, these irritating effects increase bronchial secretions, which may impair free breathing; pretreatment with an anticholinergic agent, such as atropine or scopolamine, inhibits these secretions. Cardiovascular functions are well maintained until stage III, plane 3, at which time blood pressure and heart rate decrease.

Ether causes excellent skeletal muscle relaxation even in the absence of d-tubocurarine or other similar drugs. Muscle relaxation has been attributed to the ability of ether to inhibit the transmission of nerve impulses along the corticospinal tract as well as by producing blockade at the neuromuscular junction by an action similar to that of curare-like drugs (Chapter 11).

This drug is a relatively safe anesthetic and can be safely employed for surgical procedures of long duration; a wide margin of safety exists between anesthetic and toxic doses. Few anesthetics are capable of rivaling its excellent muscle-relaxing properties. The major disadvantages associated with ether, which have caused it to fall into disfavor in recent years, include its potential explosiveness, its long onset of action and slow recovery, and the high incidence of postoperative nausea and vomiting. Drug interactions with ether are summarized in Table 10-3.

Halothane Halothane (Fluothane) is a nonexplosive volatile liquid that is among the most commonly used contemporary general anesthetics. This complete anesthetic pleasantly produces induction in approximately 10 minutes, with emergence more rapid than with ether. The pharmacological properties of halothane differ from those of ether.

Unlike ether, halothane is not irritating to the respiratory mucosa, and, therefore, it neither increases respiratory secretions nor stimulates respiration. With increasingly deeper levels of anesthesia, progressive depression of the cardiovascular system is observed. This compound produces myocardial depression and arterial hypotension, the latter often utilized as a measure of the depth of anesthesia. Halothane, like chemically similar halogenated hydrocarbons (chloroform, methoxyflurane, enflurane), may sensitize the heart muscle to arrhythmias induced by circulating and endogenous catecholamines, in particular, to epinephrine.

Major advantages associated with the use of halothane include its lack of explosiveness, ease of administration, smooth and pleasant induction period, and the absence of postoperative nausea and vomiting. Since halothane has a long onset of action, nitrous oxide or an intravenously administered barbiturate is often employed to induce anesthesia.

Disadvantages include the expense of this drug, its poor muscle-relaxing and analgesic activities, its depressing effects on the cardiovascular system, and its tendency to sensitize the myocardium to arrhythmias. *Liver toxicity* has been associated with the use of halothane, and this risk may be increased when the patient is reexposed to this drug. Drug interactions with halothane are summarized in Table 10-3.

Table 10-3   Potential Drug Interactions Involving General Anesthetics

General anesthetic	Interacting drug/class	Possible consequences	Mechanism(s) underlying interactions
Halothane (Fluothane) Methoxyflurane (Penthrane)	Epinephrine (Adrenalin) Levarterenol (Levophed) Isoproterenol (Isuprel)	Ventricular arrhythmias.	Increased sensitization of myocardium to circulating epinephrine.
Ether Halothane (Fluothane) Methoxyflurane (Penthrane)	Aminoglycoside antibiotics streptomycin kanamycin (Kantrex) gentamicin (Garamycin) viomycin (Viocin) tobramycin (Nebcin) Polypeptide antibiotics polymyxin B (Aerosporin) colistin (Coly-Mycin)	Prolonged neuromuscular blockade, with possible respiratory depression and arrest.	Additive neuromuscular blockade.
Methoxyflurane (Penthrane)	Aminoglycoside antibiotics Tetracycline antibiotics tetracycline (Achromycin, Tetracyn, Tetrex, and others) demeclocycline (Declomycin) methacycline (Rondomycin) doxycycline (Vibramycin) minocycline (Minocin, Vectrin)	Kidney toxicity.	Additive nephrotoxicity.

Miscellaneous volatile liquid anesthetics   *Chloroform* is a highly potent, complete anesthetic with an onset of action of 2 to 5 minutes. This compound is rarely employed because of the high incidence of cardiac arrhythmias and liver toxicity associated with its use.

Methoxyflurane (Penthrane) is a highly potent, nonflammable, complete anesthetic with a long onset of action and slow recovery period. The outstanding features associated with this drug include its ability to produce excellent muscle relaxation and analgesia. Liver and kidney damage may occur after the use of methoxyflurane. The primary use of this drug is an obstetrical anesthetic agent.

Nitrous oxide   Nitrous oxide, the oldest and safest of all general anesthetics, is the only anesthetic gas in common usage. This nonexplosive agent, commonly called *laughing gas*, produces a very pleasant and rapid induction of anesthesia (1 to 2 minutes) and rapid recovery. Nitrous oxide is very commonly used as a component of balanced anesthesia to produce anesthesia and good analgesia. Apart from the danger of hypoxia when used in concentrations of more than 70 percent, nitrous oxide produces no significant adverse effects on the liver or cardiovascular and respiratory systems.

If nitrous oxide were a complete anesthetic with muscle-relaxing properties, it would possess all the characteristics of an ideal agent. It is commonly employed alone in dental procedures and obstetrics and for induction prior to the use of other anesthetics in major surgical procedures.

Cyclopropane Cyclopropane is a complete anesthetic gas with a very pleasant and rapid onset of action and recovery period. This compound possesses a wide margin of safety, good muscle relaxing properties, and causes no severe depression of respiration or blood pressure. Cyclopropane is rarely used because it is extremely explosive, induces cardiac arrhythmias, and produces postoperative nausea and vomiting.

Intravenous Anesthesia

In addition to the inhalation anesthetics previously considered, selected central nervous system depressants may be administered intravenously to induce a state of general anesthesia. Intravenous anesthetics, such as the ultrashort-acting barbiturates, pleasantly induce anesthesia within seconds after their administration. Such drugs are devoid of fire or explosion hazards, are simple to administer in trained hands, do not produce respiratory irritation, and permit rapid recovery in the absence of nausea and vomiting. Unlike the inhalation anesthetics, once injected, the depressant effects of these drugs cannot be readily terminated.

Thiopental sodium Thiopental sodium (Pentothal Sodium) is the most commonly employed intravenously administered ultrashort-acting barbiturate. As noted, this drug induces pleasant and smooth general anesthesia and, when administered in low doses, recovery is rapid. The high lipid solubility of thiopental is responsible for the rapid uptake of this drug into the brain, resulting in its rapid onset of action. After intravenous administration is discontinued, this drug rapidly redistributes to muscle and fat; this redistribution is primarily responsible for the termination of its anesthetic effects. When high doses of thiopental are employed, the recovery period is often protracted.

Extreme care must be exercised when administering thiopental; therapeutic doses are capable of producing severe respiratory and circulatory depression. Since thiopental has a tendency to cause laryngospasm, bronchospasm, and cough, this drug should be used cautiously in patients with chronic respiratory diseases such as asthma or emphysema. Thiopental lacks analgesic activity, and skeletal muscle relaxation occurs only at very deep levels of anesthesia.

Thiopental is clinically employed as the sole anesthetic for operations of short duration and to induce anesthesia prior to the administration of inhalation agents. *Methohexital sodium* (Brevital Sodium) and *thiamylal sodium* (Surital Sodium) are other ultrashort-acting barbiturates possessing pharmacological effects similar to those of thiopental. Since emergence from methohexital anesthesia is very rapid, this drug is very popular for operations of short duration, such as dental procedures.

Innovar: Neuroleptanalgesia *Neuroleptanalgesia* is a state characterized by quiescence, emotional indifference to the environment, and analgesia, in which the patient retains consciousness. This state is valuable when it is desirable to have the patient conscious and capable of cooperating in such diagnostic procedures as x-ray studies, bronchoscopy or cystoscopy, and during neurosurgery.

Innovar is a product containing both the neuroleptic agent droperidol and the narcotic analgesic fentanyl. Droperidol (Inapsine) is a butyrophenone derivative related in haloperidol (Chapter 15). This drug produces calmness, emotional detachment, and drowsiness and reduces the incidence of postoperative nausea and vomiting associated with the use of narcotic agents. Fentanyl (Sublimaze) is a highly potent meperidine derivative (Chapter 20) with a rapid onset (5 to 15 minutes) and a duration of analgesic action of 1 to 2 hours.

Peak anesthesic effects are observed within 3 to 5 minutes after the intravenous administration of Innovar, and emergence is rapid. This product is also employed 45 to 60 minutes preoperatively as a preanesthetic medication prior to nitrous oxide. The primary disadvantages associated with Innovar include pronounced respiratory depression and droperidol-induced extrapyramidal movements such as tremors; the latter effect is observed in approximately 1 percent of the patients 6 to 12 hours postoperatively.

Ketamine: Dissociative anesthesia

Dissociative anesthesia refers to a state in which the patient is awake but not responsive to the environment. During this state, the patient's eyes are open; the patient feels no pain during the procedure and experiences amnesia postoperatively.

Ketamine (Ketaject, Ketalar), the principal drug used to induce dissociative anesthesia, is a rapid-acting drug that has little effect on respiration and that elevates arterial blood pressure, cardiac output, and heart rate; skeletal muscle relaxation is poor.

During the recovery period, approximately 15 percent of the patients experience disagreeable dreams and hallucinations, the latter sometimes reoccurring at unpredictable intervals days or even weeks postoperatively. Nurses in the recovery room can reduce the incidence or severity of such adverse psychic effects by protecting the patient against visual, tactile, or auditory stimuli during the recovery period. Ketamine rarely produces hallucinations in children. *Phencyclidine*, a veterinary anesthetic chemically related to ketamine, is a commonly used "street drug" that produces marked adverse behavioral effects (Chapter 23).

Ketamine is employed in head and neck operations, providing the surgeon with a clear operative field unobstructed by anesthetic masks and ventilation equipment. The drug is also used for the debridement of burns and in painful diagnostic procedures.

General Anesthetics:
nursing implications

1. Preanesthetic medications should be administered at the time ordered to permit sequential development of balanced anesthesia.
2. If the patient exhibits a high level of anxiety or fear preoperatively, this should be reported; such symptoms can affect the autonomic and central nervous systems, necessitating greater anesthetic requirements and potentially resulting in adverse effects.
3. Preoperative patient teaching should include:
   (a) Explanation of preoperative activities (scrubs, shaves, enemas, and so on), and operation (loss of consciousness, recovery), including what will be expected of the patient.
   (b) Activities required during the postoperative recovery period: turning, coughing, deep breathing, splinting incisions.
   (c) Explanations of medications to be administered: IV fluids, parenteral or oral analgesics, or other drugs.
   (d) Practice nondrug pain-reducing procedures or techniques.

SUPPLEMENTARY READINGS

Adriani, J., *The Pharmacology of Anesthetic Drugs: A Syllabus for Students and Clinicians* (5th ed.). Springfield, Ill.: Charles C Thomas, Publisher, 1970.

Cullen, S. C., and C. P. Larson, Jr., *Essentials of Anesthetic Practice.* Chicago: Year Book Medical Publishers, Inc., 1974.

DiPalma, J. R., ed. *Drill's Pharmacology in Medicine* (4th ed.), Chapters 7–10 and 12, pp. 127–89, 211–24. New York: McGraw-Hill Book Company, 1971.

Dripps, R. D., J. E. Echenhoff, and L. D. Vandam, *Introduction to Anesthesia. The Principles of Safe Practice* (5th ed.). Philadelphia: W. B. Saunders Co., 1977.

Goodman, L. S. and A. Gilman, ed., *The Pharmacological Basis of Therapeutics* (5th ed.), Chapters 2–8, pp. 53–101. New York: Macmillan, Inc., 1975.

Ngai, S. H., L. C. Mark, and E. M. Papper, "Pharmacologic and Physiologic Aspects of Anesthesiology," *New England Journal of Medicine,* **282:** 479–491, 541–556 (1970).

Smith, R. M., *Anesthesia for Infants and Children* (4th ed.). St. Louis: The C. V. Mosby Company, 1978.

SKELETAL MUSCLE RELAXANTS

Chapter 11

Three separate and distinct classes of drugs are available clinically to produce skeletal (voluntary) muscle relaxation. These classes—the neuromuscular blocking agents, the centrally acting muscle relaxants, and the direct-acting muscle relaxants—differ with respect to their chemistry, sites and mechanisms of action, therapeutic uses, and side effects, and will, therefore, be considered individually. Prior to examining the pharmacological and therapeutic properties of each of these drug classes, the physiological basis for skeletal muscle contraction will be briefly considered.

PHYSIOLOGY OF SKELETAL MUSCLE CONTRACTION

Skeletal muscles are innervated by motor nerves that originate in the anterior horn cells of the gray matter of the spinal cord (Figure 11-1). As a single motor nerve approaches the muscle, it divides and sends branches to multiple muscle fibers. A *motor unit* consists of a motor neuron and the muscle fibers it innervates. When a motor nerve is stimulated, all the muscle fibers within the muscle unit contract. The termi-

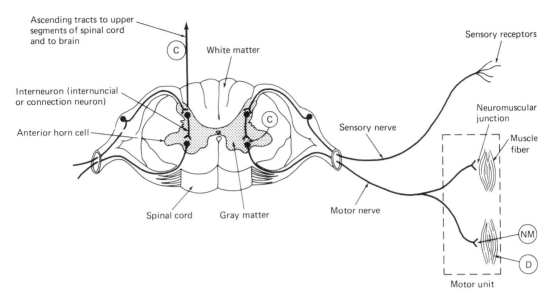

Figure 11-1   Innervation of Skeletal Muscle by Motor Nerves and Sites of Action of Skeletal Muscle Relaxants. The motor nerve originates in the anterior horn cell of the gray matter of the spinal cord. Upon reaching the muscle, the nerve sends branches to individual muscle fibers. The motor nerve and muscle fibers innervated by it constitute the motor unit. Sites of action of skeletal muscle relaxants include: NM = neuromuscular junction; D = direct-acting drugs whose effects are on the skeletal muscle; and C = centrally acting drugs that act in the brain and at motor synapses within the spinal cord, such as at interneurons.

nation of the motor nerve ending lies in close association with the motor end-plate of the muscle fiber; the space or synapse between the nerve ending and the muscle is called the *neuromuscular* or *myoneural junction*.

The nerve ending contains packets of the neurotransmitter substance *acetylcholine*. As a nerve impulse reaches the nerve ending, it triggers the release of acetylcholine across the neuromuscular junction to stimulate cholinergic nicotinic receptor sites. This acetylcholine-receptor interaction induces changes in the muscle membrane initiating a spread of depolarization from the motor end-plate along the muscle fiber and resulting in contraction of the muscle. After its interaction with the cholinergic receptor, acetylcholine is very rapidly inactivated by the enzyme acetylcholinesterase.

NEUROMUSCULAR BLOCKING AGENTS

Neuromuscular blocking agents produce skeletal muscle relaxation by altering the ability of acetylcholine to activate the postsynaptic cholinergic receptor on the motor end-plate of the muscle fiber. Based upon the mechanism of action and the characteristics associated with the neuromuscular blockade produced by these drugs, the neuromuscular blocking agents are divided into two groups: *competitive* (antidepolarizing, *nondepolarizing*, or *stabilizing*) agents such as tubocurarine and the *depolarizing* (*noncompetitive*) blocking agents, the most important of which is succinylcholine. The nurse should understand the mechanisms by which these two groups of drugs produce neuromuscular blockade to appreciate the rationale underlying factors that modify the response to these drugs and the treatment of their overdosage.

These drugs are employed primarily to produce muscle relaxation during general anesthesia as well as to facilitate endotracheal intubation. As will be evident in later discussions, the neuromuscular blocking agents are highly potent and, if employed without adequate precautions or by inadequately trained personnel, are readily capable of producing respiratory paralysis and death.

Competitive Neuromuscular Blocking Agents: Tubocurarine

For many centuries, South American Indians living along the banks of the Amazon and Orinoco Rivers used plant extracts containing *curare* as an arrowhead poison to kill wild animals for food; the cause of death in these animals was paralysis of the skeletal muscles required for respiration. The active constituent in curare, *d-tubocurarine* (Tubarine, Tubadil), is a useful skeletal muscle relaxant, and its pharmacological properties are typical of other competitive neuromuscular blocking agents.

Tubocurarine combines with cholinergic nicotinic receptor sites at the motor endplate of the muscle membrane and prevents acetylcholine from interacting with these receptors; acetylcholine fails to produce depolarization and contraction of the muscle. Tubocurarine blockade of muscle contractions can be overcome (in cases of overdosage) by increasing the amount of acetylcholine in the area of the neuromuscular junction with a cholinesterase inhibitor.

Pharmacological effects   Neither competitive nor depolarizing neuromuscular blocking agents are effectively absorbed into the blood stream after oral administration and are generally given by intravenous or intramuscular injection. Within 3 to 5 minutes after an intravenous injection of tubocurarine, muscles are relaxed in the following order: muscles of the eyes, face, neck, and pharynx, followed by muscles of the abdomen and limbs; the muscles of respiration—the diaphragm, in particular—are the last to be affected. It should be noted, however, that in surgical procedures requiring relaxation of the abdominal muscles, the normal ability of the diaphragm to contract will be impaired. Hence, in almost all instances in which tubocurarine is employed, the patient will require artificial respiratory assistance. Muscle strength returns within 30 to 60 minutes, with the muscles of the diaphragm recovering first and those of the eyes last.

In addition to its neuromuscular blocking effects, tubocurarine can also impair transmission at the autonomic ganglion and stimulate the release of histamine. These effects are responsible for the hypotension and bronchospasm, respectively, that are sometimes observed when this drug is administered. The neuromuscular blocking agents do not cross the blood-brain barrier. Table 11-1 compares the pharmacological properties of the various competitive neuromuscular blocking agents. The therapeutic uses of these drugs will be discussed below.

Overdosage   and   its   treatment
When an excessive dosage is administered, tubocurarine and related drugs severely depress contraction of the diaphragm muscle, causing respiratory paralysis, hypoxia, and death. Treatment includes establishing an open airway with an endotracheal tube and initiating positive pressure artificial respiration with oxygen. Antagonism of tubocurarine-induced blockage of respiratory muscles may be accomplished by intravenous

Table 11-1   Commonly Employed Neuromuscular Blocking Agents

Class	Generic name (Synonym)	Trade name(s)	Peak onset of action	Duration of action	Unique properties
Competitive	Tubocurarine (d-tubocurarine)	Tubadil, Tubarine	3-5 min	30-60 min	Ganglionic blockade (hypotension), histamine release (bronchospasm).
	Dimethyl tubocurarine iodide (metocurine iodide)	Metubine	3-5 min	15-90 min	Three times as potent as tubocurarine; avoid use in patients sensitive to iodides.
	Gallamine triethiodide	Flaxedil	3 min	15-35 min	No ganglionic blockade or histamine release; produces tachycardia.
	Pancuronium bromide	Pavulon	2-3 min	35-40 min	No ganglionic blockade or histamine release; five times as potent as tubocurarine.
Depolarizing	Succinylcholine chloride (Suxamethonium)	Anectine, Quelicin Sucostrin Sux-Cert	1 min	5 min	Excellent for short procedures; bradycardia, hypotension.
	Hexafluorenium bromide	Mylaxen	———	———	Used only as an adjunct to succinylcholine to prolong its duration of action and reduce muscle twitches.
	Decamethonium bromide	Syncurine	4-8 min	20 min	Rarely used, unpredictable at times.

administration of a cholinesterase inhibitor such as neostigmine or edrophonium; these drugs, while highly effective in reversing muscle paralysis, may worsen the hypotension or bronchospasm produced by tubocurarine.

The danger of tubocurarine-induced respiratory depression may be increased by elevated body temperature and electrolyte imbalances, in particular, hypokalemia; patients with a history of myasthenia gravis are at greater risk. Selected general anesthetic agents and antibiotics, which when employed alone are capable of producing neuromuscular blockade, have been clinically observed to potentiate the respiratory depression caused by competitive neuromuscular blocking agents. These and other drug interactions are listed in Table 11-2.

Depolarizing Neuromuscular Blocking Agents: Succinylcholine

The depolarizing agents succinylcholine and decamethonium resemble acetylcholine both chemically and pharmacologically. The mechanism responsible for the neuromuscular blockade produced by these drugs is highly complex and only partially understood at present. Drugs in this class produce initial muscle stimulation followed by a prolonged period of depolarization blockade. The initial stimulation is characterized by fascicula-

Table 11-2   Potential Drug Interactions Involving Neuromuscular Blocking Agents

Neuromuscular blocker	Interacting drug/class	Mechanism underlying interaction and possible consequences

Competitive and depolarizing	Aminoglycoside antibiotics
	   Gentamicin (Garamycin)
	   Kanamycin (Kantrex)
	   Neomycin (Mycifradin)
	   Streptomycin
	Polypeptide antibiotics
	   Colistin (Coly-Mycin)
	   Polymyxin B
	Magnesium salts
	Phenothiazines
		Many of these antibiotics have been shown to possess neuromuscular blocking activity in high doses. Combination may produce additive muscle relaxation increasing its intensity or duration with greater risk of respiratory failure.

	Procainamide (Pronestyl) Propranolol (Inderal) Quinidine	May potentiate neuromuscular blockade potentially resulting in respiratory failure.
	Narcotic analgesics Methotrimeprazine (Levoprome)	Produce respiratory depression and may potentiate similar effects by blockers.

Competitive	General anesthetics
	   Cyclopropane
	   Ether
	   Fluoroxene (Fluomar)
	   Halothane (Fluothane)
	   Methoxyflurane (Penthrane)
		These inhalation anesthetics possess muscle relaxing properties. Can be used in combination with blockers if dose of blocker is reduced.

	Diuretics, potassium depleting
	   Chlorthalidone (Hygroton)
	   Ethacrynic acid (Edecrin)
	   Furosemide (Lasix)
	   Thiazides
	Amphotericin B (Fungizone)
		May produce hypokalemia, which potentiates blockade by competitive agents.

Depolarizing	Antidepressants, monoamine oxidase inhibitors Cyclophosphamide (Cytoxan) Echothiophate iodide (Phospholine) Edrophonium (Tensilon) Thiotepa Neostigmine (Prostigmin)	Inhibition of plasma pseudocholinesterase, retards blocker metabolism and inactivation, thus potentiating action of blocker.
Succinylcholine	Lidocaine (Xylocaine)	Displaces succinylcholine from plasma protein binding sites, thus increasing its blocking activity.
	Digitalis glycosides	Increased risk of cardiac arrhythmias.

tions or twitches of muscle fibers of the neck or back. The subsequent depolarization blockade renders the muscle unresponsive to motor nerve activation and results in flaccid paralysis.

Succinylcholine (Anectine, Quelicin) is considered by many to be the ideal drug when muscle relaxation of short duration is sought. It produces maximum effects in 2 minutes, with recovery observed within 5 minutes. The short duration of action has been attributed to rapid inactivation by the enzyme pseudocholinesterase. In occasional patients, apnea is observed after succinylcholine administration, with muscle paralysis persisting for 1 or more hours. In some cases, this intensified drug response has been associated with a genetically determined defect in the pseudocholinesterase enzyme.

No specific antagonists are available to counteract the respiratory depressing effects of the depolarizing neuromuscular blockers; neostigmine and edrophonium *intensify* the muscle-relaxing properties of these drugs, and are, therefore, contraindicated. Moreover, echothiophate (Phospholine) and other long-acting cholinesterase inhibitors used for the treatment of glaucoma enhance the effects of succinylcholine and should be discontinued 2 to 4 weeks prior to surgery if this muscle relaxant is to be employed. Drug interactions involving the depolarizing blockers are given in Table 11-2.

Therapeutic Uses of Neuromuscular Blocking Agents

The primary use of this drug class is to produce a state of skeletal muscle relaxation in *surgical anesthesia*. In the absence of adequate muscle relaxation, it may be extremely difficult for the surgeon to operate. While some general anesthetic agents are capable of producing muscle relaxation when employed alone, the anesthetic concentration required is often uncomfortably close to that capable of causing irreversible respiratory failure. Neuromuscular blocking agents abolish muscle tone, permitting the use of lighter levels of the anesthetic agents.

These drugs are also used to facilitate *endotracheal intubations* and in *orthopedic procedures* involving the correction of dis-

locations or the alignment of fractures. When electroconvulsive or chemoconvulsive therapy is used for the treatment of psychiatric disorders, the seizure produced may be sufficiently severe to cause dislocations or fractures. To preclude this problem, succinylcholine is routinely used in these convulsive therapies. A summary of nursing implications associated with tubocurarine and succinylcholine appears at the end of the chapter.

CENTRALLY ACTING SKELETAL MUSCLE RELAXANTS

The skeletal muscle relaxation produced by the neuromuscular blocking agents discussed in the previous section is not clinically useful for the relief of muscle spasticity and rigidity associated with neurological disorders, local injury, or inflammatory conditions, including cerebral palsy, hemiplegia, sprains, strains of the ligaments, myositis, arthritis, and bursitis. The treatment objective in these disorders is to relieve the often painful muscle spasms without causing the loss of voluntary muscle function or impairing cerebral function. It is the impression of many clinicians that the beneficial effects derived from the centrally acting muscle relaxants may be largely attributed to their antianxiety properties rather than their abilities to produce actual muscle relaxation.

The mechanism of action of these drugs has not been clearly defined at this time. These drugs may act on interneuronal spinal neurons to depress polysynaptic pathways controlling spinal reflexes, as well as possibly depressing selected areas of the brain that control skeletal muscle function.

Central skeletal muscle relaxants may be of value for the relief of spasms resulting from injury or inflammation; however, most are ineffective for the treatment of spasms arising as the result of neurological disorders.

Table 11-3   Representative Centrally-Acting Muscle Relaxants

Generic name	Trade name	Usual oral daily doses	Remarks
Mephenesin carbamate	Tolseram	3–9 g	Oldest drug in this class; very short duration of action (3 h); limited effectiveness.
Methocarbamol	Robaxin	2.25–4.5 g	Longer duration of action than mephenesin.
Chlorphenesin carbamate	Maolate	0.8–3.2 g	Related to mephenesin.
Meprobamate	Equanil, Miltown	1.2–1.6 g	Purported muscle-relaxing properties may be attributed to antianxiety effects; abuse potential demonstrated.
Carisoprodol	Rela, Soma	1.4 g	Related to meprobamate, somewhat more effective.
Chlorzoxazone	Paraflex	0.75–3 g	Jaundice has been associated with this drug.
Metaxalone	Skelaxin	2.4–3.2 g	Liver toxicity and gastrointestinal upset.
Diazepam	Valium	4–40 mg	Widely used to relieve spasticity associated with back strains; effective in cerebral palsy.
Cyclobenzaprine	Flexeril	20–40 mg	New drug used for relief of muscle spasm associated with acute, painful musculoskeletal disorders. Short-term use (2–3 wk) only. Common side effects: drowsiness, dizziness, dry mouth.
Baclofen	Lioresal	40–80 mg	Uses similar to cyclobenzaprine. Abrupt withdrawal may result in hallucinations. Common side effects: drowsiness, dizziness, weakness, fatigue.

Representative drugs in this class are listed in Table 11-3. Common adverse effects associated with this drug class include drowsiness, dizziness, lethargy, and gastrointestinal upset. It is generally recommended that these drugs not be administered for more than 3 weeks.

DIRECT-ACTING SKELETAL MUSCLE RELAXANT: DANTROLENE

In contrast to the previously discussed classes of muscle relaxants, dantrolene (Dantrium) relieves spasticity by a direct action on skeletal muscle. This drug is thought to act on the contractile mechanism of the muscle, perhaps by reducing the availability of calcium. This drug has no effect on the conduction of nerve impulses in the motor nerve, nor does it interfere with neuromuscular transmission.

Dantrolene has been used successfully for the relief of spastic disorders resulting from stroke, cerebral palsy, multiple sclerosis, and spinal cord injury. It is not recommended for the treatment of spasticity associated with rheumatoid arthritis. Dantrolene has been recently approved for intravenous use for the treatment of *malignant hyperthermia*, a rare, genetically determined condition caused by drugs used in general anesthesia. No specific treatment was previously available for this condition which was associated with a 50 to 70 percent mortality rate.

In adults, the initial oral dose is 25 mg once or twice daily; this dose is increased in general increments up to 100 mg (and rarely to 200 mg) four times daily. Each dosage level increment should be maintained for 4 to 7 days to assess the patient's response and the incidence of acceptable side effects.

The primary adverse effect associated with the use of this drug is skeletal muscle weakness, which undoubtedly represents an extension of its primary effects on muscle.

Dizziness, drowsiness, and fatigue are often observed during the early phases of drug treatment. Impairment of liver function may occur when this drug is used for over 60 days.

Skeletal Muscle Relaxants: nursing implications

Tubocurarine

1. Administered primarily by anesthesiologist.
2. Determine serum electrolytes prior to drug administration. Electrolyte imbalances, especially potassium and magnesium, can potentiate drug effects.
3. Monitor vital signs and airway until complete recovery. Drug side effects include hypotension, increased salivation, and bronchospasm.
4. Muscle paralysis in specific order, recovery in opposite order: respiratory muscles (diaphragm) last paralyzed, first to recover. Muscle function usually restored within 90 min.

Succinylcholine (Anectine, Quelicin)

1. Administered primarily by anesthesiologist.
2. Electrolyte imbalance can potentiate drug effects.
3. Transient apnea common at time of maximum drug effect, usually within 1–2 min. Spontaneous respiration should return within seconds or at most 3–4 min.
4. Monitor vital signs and maintain clear airway. Observe for and report residual muscle weakness. Postprocedural muscle stiffness and pain caused by initial fasciculations after injection.

Methocarbamol (Robaxin) and Related Central Muscle Relaxants

1. The patient should remain recumbent for 15 min after IV to reduce postural hypotension. Changes in position should be made slowly, especially from recumbent to upright position.
2. Mild and transient symptoms of drowsiness or dizziness may occur after oral therapy. Activities requiring mental alertness and physical coordination should be avoided until response to drug is well established.

SUPPLEMENTARY READINGS

Argov, Z., and L. Mastaglia, "Disorders of Neuromuscular Transmission Caused by Drugs," *New England Journal of Medicine* **301**: 409–413 (1979).

Carlson, F. D., and D. R. Wilkie, *Muscle Physiology.* Englewood Cliffs, New Jersey: Prentice-Hall Publishing Co., Inc., 1974.

Cheymol, J., ed., "Neuromuscular Blocking and Stimulating Agents," Vol. 1. *International Encyclopedia of Pharmacology and Therapeutics*, Sec. 14. Oxford: Pergamon Press, Inc., 1972.

Feldman, S. A., *Muscle Relaxants*. Philadelphia: W. B. Saunders Company, 1973.

Foldes, F. F., ed., *Muscle Relaxants*. Philadelphia: F. A. Davis, 1966.

Grob, D., "Neuromuscular Blocking Drugs," in *Physiological Pharmacology*, Vol. 3, *The Nervous System—Part C: Autonomic Nervous System Drugs*, ed. W. S. Root and F. G. Hofmann, pp. 389–460. New York: Academic Press, Inc., 1967.

Mayer, N., S. A. Mecomber, and R. Herman, "Treatment of Spasticity with Dantrolene Sodium," *American Journal of Physical Medicine*, **52:** 18–29 (1973).

Smith, C. M., "Relaxants of Skeletal Muscle," in *Physiological Pharmacology*, Vol. 2, *The Nervous System—Part B: Central Nervous System Drugs*, ed. W. S. Root and F. G. Hofmann, pp. 2–96. New York: Academic Press, Inc., 1965.

Symposium, "Spasticity—Its Etiology, Physiology and the Pharmacology of a New Agent," *Archives of Physical Medicine and Rehabilitation*, **55:** 331–392 (1974).

Waud, D. R., and B. E. Waud, "Agents Acting on the Neuromuscular Junction and Centrally Acting Muscle Relaxants," in *Drill's Pharmacology in Medicine*, ed. J. R. DiPalma, 4th ed., Chapter 36, pp. 735–769. New York: McGraw-Hill Book Company, 1971.

Zaimis, E., ed., "Neuromuscular Junction," *Handbook of Experimental Pharmacology*, Vol. **42:** Berlin: Springer-Verlag, 1976.

Chapter 12

LOCAL ANESTHETICS

Local anesthetics are drugs used to temporarily and reversibly block the perception of pain in a restricted region of the body. Such drugs enjoy widespread usage for minor operative procedures of the eye, nose, and throat, for the removal of small tissue growths, suturing lacerations, dental procedures, and for labor and delivery. We shall first discuss the desired and adverse pharmacological effects produced by these drugs.

PHARMACOLOGICAL EFFECTS

The major pharmacological effects of local anesthetics are on nerves and their ability to transmit nerve impulses signaling pain. These drugs are potentially dangerous when used in high doses and are capable of producing central nervous system and cardiovascular toxicity.

Effects on Nerves

Local anesthetics can act on all parts of the nervous system and on all types of nerve fibers; however, we observe that some types of nerve fibers are more susceptible to the effects of therapeutic doses of these drugs than others. After the administration of a local anesthetic agent, the nurse will observe that loss of function occurs in the following order: pain, temperature sensitivity to cold and warmth, touch, proprioception (sensations arising from within the body), and skeletal (voluntary) muscle tone.

These drugs are thought to prevent the conduction of nerve impulses by interfering with the movement of ions across the cell membrane of nerve fibers. As a consequence, depolarization fails to occur, thus preventing transmission of nerve impulses and abolishing all sensations.

The duration of action of local anesthetics is directly proportional to the time the drug is in contact with the nerve fibers. While it is possible to increase the duration of action by increasing the dose administered locally, the use of higher doses increases the likelihood of drug diffusion from the site of administration and potential systemic toxic effects. Local anesthetic agents are frequently coadministered with vasoconstrictors (Chapter 5), such as epinephrine (1:100,000), which both prolong the action of the local anesthetic and reduce the risk of systemic toxicity.

Adverse Effects

Toxic effects associated with local anesthetic administration are usually attributable to the inadvertent injection of the drug into a blood vessel or the diffusion of the drug into the systemic circulation. The latter problem is usually the consequence of the use of highly concentrated drug solutions or the administration of large volumes of diluted solutions.

To preclude this problem, local anesthetics should be administered at the lowest effective concentration, in the smallest effective volume, or with a vasoconstrictor such as epinephrine.

The use of excessive doses produces cardiovascular and central nervous system toxicity in virtually all patients. In addition, some patients experience allergic reactions to certain local anesthetics.

Cardiovascular effects The cardiovascular system is depressed by toxic doses of the local anesthetics. Hypertension and tachycardia may be observed initially, followed by hypotension and bradycardia; this leads to a reduction in cardiac output with a potentially fatal outcome. This hypotensive state can be treated with a vasopressor such as phenylephrine (Neo-Synephrine) or methoxamine (Vasoxyl).

Central nervous system effects Overdosage of local anesthetics may result in central nervous system stimulation followed by depression. The stimulatory phase is associated with anxiety, excitability, irritability, tremors, and convulsions. Postconvulsive depression, characterized by respiratory paralysis, cardiovascular failure, and death, may ensue.

Allergic reactions Hypersensitivity reactions to local anesthetics have been documented but are not common. The nature of this allergic response may vary from allergic dermatitis to an asthmatic attack or a fatal anaphylactic reaction. These reactions occur with local anesthetics of the ester type (for example, procaine) but not with the amides (for example lidocaine; see Table 12-2). The patient's previous experiences with and responses to local anesthetics, such as during dental procedures, should be recorded as part of the drug history.

Table 12-1   Comparison of Methods of Local Anesthetic Administration

Method of anesthesia	Site of drug administration	Representative drugs employed	Therapeutic uses	Comments
Topical or surface	Application of solution, ointment, cream, or powder to the skin, a mucous membrane surface (oral cavity, pharnyx, tracheobronchial tree, genitourinary tract) or cornea.	Lidocaine Tetracaine Proparacaine Cyclomethycaine	Bronchoscopy Conjunctival exam. Local pain, itch. Corneal anesthesia.	Limit dose to prevent rapid systemic drug absorption.
Infiltration	Injection into tissue area surrounding nerve endings.	Lidocaine Procaine Mepivacaine	Minor operations. Dental procedures. Suture lacerations.	Often intradermal followed by subcutaneous drug administration.
Nerve block	Injection as close as possible to main nerve trunk innervating area.	Lidocaine Procaine	Limb operations. Dental procedures.	Various techniques employed.
Spinal (subarachnoid block)	Injection into subarachnoid space which contains cerebrospinal fluid. Level of anesthesia controlled by position of patient and specific gravity of drug solution.	Tetracaine Lidocaine Mepivacaine	Perineal area surgery. Abdominal operations. Obstetrics.	Various techniques employed. Advantages: complete analgesia, muscle relaxation; no loss of consciousness. Disadvantages: levels of anesthesia unpredictable; headache; sudden hypotension; possible respiratory failure.

METHODS OF LOCAL ANESTHETIC ADMINISTRATION

Local anesthetics may be administered by topical application, by infiltration into the tissues surrounding the nerve fibers, by injection into areas directly adjacent to a nerve (nerve block), or by injection into the subarachnoid space (Figure 12-1). The major characteristics, therapeutic applications, and some local anesthetics employed by each method are summarized in Table 12-1.

SPECIFIC LOCAL ANESTHETICS

Cocaine

Cocaine, the first of the local anesthetic agents, is the active constituent of *Erythroxylon coca*. The leaves of this plant were chewed for their central nervous system stimulating properties by Peruvian Indians centuries prior to the arrival of the Spanish conquistadors in the 1530s. Cocaine was first employed as a local anesthetic agent in ophthalmology in 1884 and, within several years, was used in dentistry and general surgery.

While cocaine produces excellent topical anesthesia when applied to the mucous membranes of the nose and throat, it is too toxic to be injected into tissues and produces corneal ulcerations when applied to the eyes. The introduction of newer synthetic local anesthetic agents that are less toxic and devoid of abuse potential have markedly limited the contemporary medical use of cocaine. The central stimulating properties of cocaine and its abuse are discussed in Chapter 22.

Several dozen local anesthetic agents are currently available for use; examples are given in Table 12-2. By convention, the names of local anesthetics end in *caine*. We shall now discuss the pharmacology and therapeutic applications of the representative local anesthetics procaine, lidocaine, benzocaine, and cyclomethycaine.

Procaine Procaine (Novocain), the oldest synthetic local anesthetic (1905) continues to be very widely used because of its

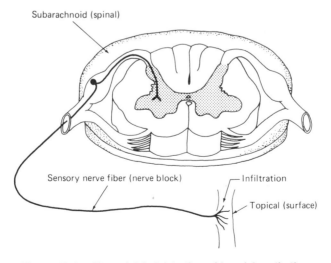

Figure 12-1   Sites of Administration of Local Anesthetics

Table 12-2 Commonly Employed Local Anesthetics

Generic name (synonym)	Trade name(s)	Ester or amide	Concentration	Onset of action	Duration of action	Remarks
Cocaine	——	Ester	5–10% nose and throat	1 min	1 h	Too toxic for injection. High abuse liability. Corneal irritation and mydriasis.
Procaine	Novocain	Ester	0.75–2%	2–5 min	1 h	Not employed topically. Relatively low toxicity. Potential for allergic reaction.
Tetracaine (Anethaine)	Anacel Pontocaine	Ester	0.5–2% topically 0.25% injection	5–10 min	2 h	Very slow onset of action.
Lidocaine (Lignocaine)	Xylocaine	Amide	1–2%	1 min	1–2 h	Widely used, versatile anesthetic. Toxic doses associated with sedation and cardiovascular dysfunctions.
Mepivacaine	Carbocaine	Amide	1–2%	1 min	2 h	Similar to lidocaine.
Proparacaine	Ophthaine Ophthetic	Ester	0.5%	0.5 min	15 min	Used for corneal anesthesia. Little or no irritation after administration; no corneal irritation or mydriasis. No cross-sensitization with procaine
Benzocaine (Ethylamino-benzoate)	Americaine	Ester	5–20%	Immediate	As long as in contact with skin.	Surface anesthesia only on skin or mucous membranes.
Cyclomethycaine	Surfacaine	Ester	0.25–1%	Immediate	As long as in contact with skin or mucous membranes.	Similar to benzocaine. Used for skin irritation, minor burns, insect bites, hemorrhoids, prior to urologic examination. Little effect on tracheobronchial tree, eyes, and nose.

high degree of effectiveness and relatively low toxicity. While it is poorly absorbed from mucous membranes, which renders it unsuitable for topical anesthesia, it is a valuable drug for infiltration, nerve block, and spinal anesthesia. The relatively short duration of action of this drug (1 hour) can be prolonged by coadministering it with the vasoconstrictor agent ephinephrine.

The incidence of cardiovascular and central nervous system toxicity is relatively low with procaine. By contrast, allergic reactions such as allergic dermatitis with this ester-type local anesthetic are not uncommon. One of the major metabolites of procaine is para-aminobenzoic acid, and this metabolite interferes with the antibacterial activity of sulfonamides. Therefore procaine should not be employed as a local anesthetic when patients are being treated with sulfonamides.

Lidocaine Lidocaine (Xylocaine) is among the most widely used local anesthetic agents and possesses several distinct advantages when compared with procaine. It is extensively used for infiltration, nerve block, and spinal anesthesia and is also effective when applied topically to the mucous membranes of the mouth, throat, and tracheobronchial tree. Lidocaine has a shorter onset of action than procaine, a longer duration of action, and—since it is an amide-type drug—can be safely employed in patients that are sensitive to procaine.

In contrast to most other local anesthetics that produce central stimulation in toxic doses, lidocaine causes *depression* (dizziness and drowsiness); dysfunctions of the heart, including cardiac arrest, may be observed with high doses of this drug. The use of lidocaine for the treatment of cardiac arrhythmias will be discussed in Chapter 27.

Surface anesthetics Benzocaine (Americaine) and cyclomethycaine (Surfacaine) are drugs that are very slightly soluble in water (and, therefore, cannot be administered by injection) and are slowly absorbed into the blood when applied to the skin and mucous membranes. Such drugs, used exclusively as surface or topical anesthetics, are applied to wounds and ulcerated surfaces as ointments or dusting powders. They produce immediate anesthesia which lasts as long as the drug retains contact with the skin.

Cyclomethycaine is applied to intact or abraded mucous membranes of the rectum and genitourinary tract and is employed to relieve itching and pain associated with skin irritations, minor burns, insect bites, and hemorrhoids, as well as in urethral instillation prior to urologic examinations.

Local Anesthetics: nursing implications

1. These should be administered in the lowest effective concentrations and in the smallest volume.
2. The patient's pulse rate and blood pressure should be checked and recorded prior to the administration of local anesthetics to provide a baseline for recognizing drug-induced changes in cardiovascular parameters.

3. Injections should be made slowly and cautiously. If blood is aspirated when syringe plunger is pulled back, a new injection site should be selected.

4. Oxygen, diazepam (Valium), or ultrashort-acting barbiturates such as thiopental sodium (Pentothal) and vasopressor agents should be readily available when local anesthetics are administered.

5. Solutions containing preservatives should not be used for spinal or epidural blocks.

6. Oral topical anesthetics may interfere with swallowing, gag, and cough reflexes. Foods or liquids should not be taken for at least 60 minutes after their administration, especially in pediatric, geriatric, or debilitated patients.

SUPPLEMENTARY READINGS

Adriani, J. "The Clinical Pharmacology of Local Anesthetics," *Clinical Pharmacology and Therapeutics* **1**: 645–673 (1960).

Covino, B. G., and H. G. Vassallo, *Local Anesthetics—Mechanisms of Action and Clinical Use*. New York: Grune & Stratton, Inc., 1976.

de Jong, K. H., *Physiology and Pharmacology of Local Anesthesia*. Springfield, Ill.: Charles C Thomas, Publisher, 1970.

Greene, N. N. *Physiology of Spinal Anesthesia* (2nd ed.). Baltimore: The Williams & Wilkins Company, 1970.

Lechat, P., ed., *Local Anesthetics, Vol. 1. International Encyclopedia of Pharmacology and Therapeutics*, Section 8. Oxford: Pergamon Press, Inc., 1971.

Scott, D. B., ed., "Proceedings of a Symposium on Local Anesthesia," *British Journal of Anaesthesia* **47** (Supplement): 163–333 (1975).

SEDATIVES AND HYPNOTICS

Chapter 13

Although its physiological role is obscure, there is a definite biological need for sleep. While most individuals require between 7 and 8 hours of sleep each night, some need as little as 5 hours. The most common sleep disturbance is *insomnia*, which is highly variable in nature and includes the inability to fall asleep as readily as desired, the inability to stay asleep during the night, or sleep that does not prove to be refreshing. It has been suggested that 25 million Americans are the victims of some degree of insomnia.

Insomnia is often a symptom of an underlying physical or emotional disorder. The hospitalized patient may be unable to sleep because of the anxiety or physical discomfort associated with a medical problem, the foreign surroundings of a hospital, an uncomfortable bed, or a stuffy room.

One of the most common methods of treating insomnia is with drugs. Indeed, such drugs are among the most widely prescribed. *Hypnotics* are drugs that are intended to induce a state that resembles normal sleep; these drugs are sometimes referred to as *soporifics* or *somnifacients*. In smaller doses, many of these same drugs are employed as *sedatives*, compounds used to calm the patient and relieve anxiety. Drugs used specifically for their antianxiety properties will be discussed in Chapter 16.

THE IDEAL HYPNOTIC

What characteristics might a nurse look for in an ideal hypnotic agent? This drug should rapidly induce sleep and have a sufficiently long duration of action to maintain sleep throughout the night and enable the patient to awaken refreshed in the morning without residual drowsiness or feelings of a hangover. The state of sleep produced by the drug should be identical to natural sleep without disrupting normal sleep patterns. Tolerance should not develop to its hypnotic effects, nor should psychological or physical dependence develop after repeated doses. The drug should possess a very wide margin of safety to preclude it from becoming an accidental or intentional instrument for poisoning or suicide. Unfortunately, no available drug satisfies all these criteria. Moreover, since sleep disturbances are of different types (for example, difficulty in falling asleep, in staying asleep, or in early morning awakening), no single hypnotic agent is best for all patients.

Most of the available drugs hasten the onset of sleep, reduce the periods of involuntary awakening during the night, and increase the total sleep time. With repeated usage, their hypnotic effectiveness is reduced and changes in normal sleep patterns occur.

Sleep

Two major normal patterns of sleep have been identified: a state characterized by rapid eye movements (REM) that is associated with dreaming, and four stages of nonrapid eye movement (NREM) sleep, which range from a period of drowsiness to one of deep sleep. Dreaming sleep appears essential; periods of REM deprivation have been shown to produce irritability, anxiety, and other more severe behavioral aberrations. Regular use of hypnotic agents at normal therapeutic doses reduces REM sleep and certain stages of NREM sleep. Upon termination of hypnotic drug therapy, the body attempts to make up for lost REM sleep, and this "REM rebound" often results in restlessness, vivid nightmares, and more intense insomnia. To suppress these adverse effects, the patient may again seek the use of these drugs, which in time, leads to drug tolerance, psychological dependence, and potential physical dependence. To preclude this problem hypnotics should only be used for short periods. To reduce the discomfort and medical hazards associated with abrupt drug withdrawal, the dose of these drugs should be gradually reduced.

Sedative-hypnotics may be classified on the basis of their chemistry into three major categories: the barbiturates, nonbarbiturates-nonbenzodiazepines; and the benzodiazepines. There are many pharmacological properties common to these classes and, with the possible exception of the benzodiazepine derivative flurazepam, few therapeutically significant differences.

BARBITURATES

Medical interest in the barbiturates began in 1903, the year barbital (Veronal) was synthesized and found to possess excellent hypnotic properties. More than 2,500 barbiturates have been prepared in laboratories over the years, and about one dozen of these are currently employed as sedative-hypnotics, anesthetics, and antiepileptic agents. By convention, the American names of all barbiturates end in "al," while the British names end in "one."

Pharmacological Actions

Sedative-Hypnotic At normal therapeutic doses, barbiturate-induced depression of the central nervous system is the major effect the nurse will observe. This results from the extreme sensitivity of the neurons of the brain to the actions of these drugs. The magnitude of the central nervous system depression seen for a given barbiturate is dose-dependent and will range from mild sedation to hypnosis to anesthesia to coma and even death.

Many theories have been postulated to explain the mechanism by which barbiturates produce sedation and hypnosis. The multisynaptic pathways of the ascending reticular formation are readily inhibited by low doses of these drugs. Depression of the reticular formation prevents activation of the cerebral cortex, making the cortex less responsive to the external stimuli of the environment, thus promoting sedation and sleep.

Anticonvulsant When administered at anesthetic doses, all barbiturates are capable of arresting convulsion resulting from strychnine poisoning or tetanus. However, some barbiturates (such as phenobarbital) possess specific anticonvulsant activity at doses that do not produce general depression; such drugs are employed for the treatment of epilepsy.

Analgesia At therapeutic doses, the barbiturates lack analgesic activity, that is, they do not relieve pain. Moreover, barbiturates may cause patients to exhibit an increased sensitivity to pain; this is called *hyperalgesia*. Patients experiencing severe pain may become excited and agitated when administered hypnotic doses of barbiturates.

Respiration Barbiturates cause dose-dependent depression of respiration. While normal hypnotic doses depress respiration only slightly, breathing becomes slow and shallow after toxic amounts are taken, and death results from depression of the respiratory center in the medulla.

Therapeutic Uses

Barbiturates are widely used in contemporary therapeutics, although somewhat less than in the last decade (Table 13-1). The long-acting barbiturates, in low doses, are employed as *sedatives* to calm the anxious patient suffering from neurotic disorders or for the hypertensive individual whose mild hypertension may be partly attributed to nervousness. At somewhat higher doses, the short- or intermediate-acting barbiturates are used as *hypnotics* to induce or maintain sleep; after regular administration for several weeks, barbiturates lose their hypnotic effectiveness. Short-acting barbiturates are often employed as *preanesthetic agents*, administered on the preoperative night to permit the patient to enjoy a restful sleep and also given on the morning of the operation. Ultrashort-acting agents are utilized as *surgical anesthetics* because of the ease and rapidity with which they induce anesthesia (Chapter 10).

Some barbiturates are used as *anticonvulsant agents* to control or prevent seizures associated with tetanus or caused by strychnine or nicotine poisoning. Selected barbiturates, most notably phenobarbital, are valuable drugs for the treatment of epileptic seizures (Chapter 18).

Amobarbital and pentobarbital, intravenously administered at doses that produce deep sedation, are used in psychiatry. Inhibitions are suppressed, and the patient becomes more relaxed and more receptive to communicating with the clinician, thereby facilitating psychotherapy.

Table 13-1   Classification of Barbiturate Hypnotics According to Onset and Duration of Action

Classification based upon duration of action	Onset	Duration (half-life)	Generic name	Trade name	Usual adult oral hypnotic dose (mg)
Ultrashort (intravenous anesthetics)	Seconds	Minutes (3-8 h)	Hexobarbital Methohexital Thiamylal Thiopental[a]	Evipal Brevital Surital Pentothal	
Short	10-15 min	3-4 h (14-42 h)	Pentobarbital[a] Secobarbital[a]	Nembutal Seconal	100 100-200
Intermediate	40-60 min	4-6 h (14-42 h)	Amobarbital[a] Butabarbital	Amytal Butisol	100-200 50-100
Long	1-2 h	6-12 h (24-96 h)	Barbital Mephobarbital Phenobarbital[a]	Veronal Mebaral Eskabarb Luminal	300-600 100-200 100

[a] Most widely used drugs.

Administration and Fate

The barbiturates are rapidly absorbed into the blood stream after oral administration, and this route is most commonly employed. The sodium salts of barbiturates are used for preparations intended for injection. Table 13-1 summarizes the approximate onset and duration of action of some of the frequently used drugs in this class. These time-response parameters should be viewed not in absolute terms, but merely as a guide; moreover, some authors view this classical time-response classification to be unsound.

With the exception of barbital, which is excreted in the urine unmetabolized, virtually all other barbiturates in common use are metabolically inactivated in the liver prior to their elimination by the kidney. Barbiturates should be administered with caution to patients with liver disease. Moreover, when kidney function is impaired, normal therapeutic doses of these drugs may produce severe central nervous system depression.

Side Effects and Toxicity

The most common side effects associated with the barbiturates are most often observed on the morning after their use and are collectively referred to as *hangover symptoms*. These are characterized by listlessness, emotional disturbances, nausea, and vomiting. Certain individuals, especially older patients, may experience such idiosyncratic reactions as hyperexcitability, bad dreams, delirium, and hallucinations. Skin rashes spread widely over the trunk and limbs, urticaria, and swelling of the face are common symptoms of *allergic responses* to barbiturates. Patients found to be allergic to one barbiturate will probably be allergic to all others; nonbarbiturate sedative-hypnotics are indicated in such individuals.

Barbiturate poisoning Whether the result of accidental or intentional overdosage, acute barbiturate poisoning represents one of the leading causes of drug-induced toxicity.* Severe acute toxicity may result from the ingestion of five to ten times a hypnotic dose while lethality may occur after ten to fifteen times the normal sleep-producing dose. Alcohol and other central nervous system depressants act additively with barbiturates and enhance their toxicity. Table 13-3 lists potential drug interactions involving barbiturates and other sedative-hypnotic agents.

Symptoms of acute barbiturate poisoning include confusion and excitement prior to the onset of deep sleep and coma; at this time, respiration becomes slow and shallow, reflexes are reduced or absent, body temperature is below normal, blood pressure drops, and the pupils are constricted and may not respond to light. Death is generally attributed to depression of the respiratory centers in the medulla.

At this time, no specific pharmacological antagonists are available for the treatment of barbiturate overdosage. Treatment objectives include attempts to remove any unabsorbed drug from the stomach (by gastric lavage or by inducing emesis with syrup of ipecac) and the maintenance of respiration and circulation. In addition, efforts may be initiated to facilitate the removal of the drug by administering alkaline osmotic diuretics (mannitol) or by employing hemodialysis. In previous years, analeptic agents (stimulants of the respiratory center in the medulla) were extensively used to stimulate barbiturate-depressed respiration. Since such drugs may induce convulsions and are less effective than

*While barbiturate-related deaths have been declining in recent years, during the first quarter of 1976 they were implicated in 14.5 percent of all drug-related deaths; barbiturates and nonbarbiturate hypnotics accounted for over 15 percent of the drugs listed in emergency room episodes involving drug abuse.

mechanical methods of supporting respiration, analeptic agents are rarely employed.

Drug Dependence

Chronic medical or nonmedical use of the barbiturates and other sedative-hypnotics may result in a drug-dependent state. Some individuals who have habitually used these drugs for years to relieve anxiety or combat insomnia find it very difficult to give up this habit. Nursing responsibilities include counseling the patient about ways to improve sleep without using medications. Increasing the level of physical activity during the daytime and employing relaxation techniques at bedtime can often improve sleep. Sometimes the patient may simply need reassurance that the amount of sleep he or she is getting is adequate for good health.

The number of persons using sedative-hypnotic agents for nonmedical purposes is generally believed to exceed those abusing opiates. High doses of these drugs produce effects similar to those observed after alcohol intoxication. The user first experiences a euphoric feeling, followed by mental and physical sluggishness. Thoughts, speech, and comprehension are achieved with difficulty, and memory, judgment, attention span, emotional stability, and motor coordination are all impaired.

Significant tolerance develops to the hypnotic and behavioral effects of these depressants, enabling the individual to ingest ten to fifteen times the hypnotic dose. However, like alcohol (but unlike opiates) the lethal dose of the barbiturate and nonbarbiturate sedative-hypnotics is not much greater for the chronic user than for the nonuser.

While psychological dependence to the sedative-hypnotics may appear in individuals who are taking normal hypnotic doses for extended periods of time, physical dependence does not develop. Physical dependence

generally develops to barbiturates after four to six times the hypnotic dose has been taken on a daily basis for several months. Upon abrupt drug withdrawal, the user may experience a withdrawal syndrome characterized by nausea, vomiting, a drop in blood pressure, extreme weakness, delirium, and grand mal convulsions, which can be fatal. *Barbiturate withdrawal is potentially far more hazardous and life-threatening to the user than is opiate withdrawal.*

In view of these dangers, barbiturate withdrawal should be carried out in a hospital where the patient can be carefully monitored. Pentobarbital (Nembutal) is generally administered in a dose sufficient to stabilize the patient; the dose of this drug is very *gradually* reduced by 100 mg a day until complete withdrawal is accomplished.

NONBARBITURATE-NONBENZODIAZEPINE SEDATIVE-HYPNOTICS

Prior to the discovery of the barbiturates in the early years of this century, nonbarbiturate agents such as sodium bromide, paraldehyde, and chloral hydrate were the major sedative-hypnotic agents available. In recent years attempts have been made to develop newer nonbarbiturate sedative-hypnotics that are as effective as the barbiturates, but that are devoid of an abuse potential, are safer when taken in overdosage, and produce a more natural sleep without altering normal sleep patterns. Notwithstanding the introduction of many such drugs purported to possess such advantages, clinical experience has failed to support these claims.

The therapeutic uses, toxic effects, and abuse potential of the nonbarbiturate-nonbenzodiazepines are quite similar to the barbiturates. Among the many nonbarbiturates available (Table 13-2), we shall now

Table 13-2 Selected Nonbarbiturate Sedative-Hypnotic Agents

Generic name	Trade name(s)	Usual adult oral hypnotic dose	Duration of action	Comments[a]
Bromide salts		2-5 g	Long	Slow acting; chronic use causes depression, confusion, lethargy. Little justification for continued use; neither safe nor effective.
Chloral hydrate	Noctec, Somnos	500-1000 mg	Short	Effective drug with low abuse potential; gastric irritation.
Triclofos	Triclos	1500 mg	Short	Derivative of chloral hydrate produces less gastric irritation.
Ethchlorvynol	Placidyl	500-1000 mg	Short	Effective drug; P-D; problem with acute toxicity; no advantages.
Flurazepam	Dalmane	15-30 mg	Intermediate	Effective hypnotic; little disturbance of sleep patterns; low abuse potential; wide margin of safety; slow tolerance development; not enzyme inducer.
Glutethimide	Doriden Rolathimide	500 mg	Intermediate	Acute overdosage difficult to treat; P-D; no advantages.
Methaqualone	Quaalude, Sopor, Mequin, Parest	150-300 mg	Short	High-abuse liability; P-D; no advantages.
Methyprylon	Noludar	200-400 mg	Short	P-D; no advantages.
Paraldehyde		4-8 ml	Short	Effective drug; offensive odor and taste; used for institutionalized patients.
Pyrilamine	Cope, Compoz, Nervine, Quiet World, Sleep-Eze, Sominex	50 mg		Questionably effective primary ingredient in nonprescription sleep-aid products.

[a] P-D is physical dependence with barbiturate-like syndrome demonstrated.

consider the distinguishing properties of several drugs that are more widely used.

Chloral Hydrate

Chloral hydrate (Noctec, Somnos) is the oldest hypnotic agent that continues to be widely used in modern therapeutics. After oral doses of 1 to 2 g of this drug, sleep generally occurs within 30 minutes and lasts for 4 to 8 hours. A refreshing sleep is produced with only modest disturbances of normal sleep patterns.

Normal therapeutic doses do not depress respiration or blood pressure. Overdosage has been observed to depress the cardiac muscle, especially in patients with a history of heart disease. The major disadvantage associated with this drug is the relatively high incidence of gastric irritation. To minimize this problem, chloral hydrate capsules or syrup should be taken with water or milk. The chloral derivative, triclofos (Triclos) is reported to produce less gastric irritation than chloral hydrate.

Methaqualone and Glutethimide

Methaqualone (Quaalude) and glutethimide (Doriden), short- and intermediate-acting sedative-hypnotics, respectively, possess no clearly demonstrable advantages over the barbiturates, yet are noteworthy because of their acute toxicity and abuse potential. Unique aspects of severe glutethimide overdosage include laryngospasms and convulsions and sudden death after restoration of consciousness. The abuse potential of both drugs has been clearly demonstrated, and, at periodic intervals over the years, has been very extensive. Withdrawal after chronic use of high doses may result in marked behavioral changes and convulsions, which are symptoms of the abstinence syndrome associated with physical dependence to these drugs.

BENZODIAZEPINE SEDATIVE-HYPNOTIC

Flurazepam

Flurazepam (Dalmane) is a benzodiazepine derivative chemically related to the antianxiety agents chlordiazepoxide (Librium) and diazepam (Valium). The widespread acceptance of this drug as a hypnotic agent* may be attributed to several advantages it possesses when compared with the barbiturates and other nonbarbiturate sedative-hypnotics.

Unlike these drugs, flurazepam does not suppress REM sleep patterns immediately; REM deprivation is only observed after this drug has been administered on a daily basis for several weeks. Withdrawal of most hypnotic drugs after their administration for several days or weeks results in immediate rebound REM sleep patterns that have been associated with insomnia, nightmares, and other sleep disturbances. Discontinuation of

---

*In 1976, approximately one-half of all prescriptions for hypnotic agents filled in American retail pharmacies were for flurazepam.

flurazepam causes very slight rebound REM with a continued pattern of improved sleep for several days after the last dose. This "carry-over" effect permits "drug holidays"— five days on the drug and two days off—which reduce the tendency for the development of psychic dependence and tolerance to its hypnotic effects. Unlike other hypnotics, flurazepam possesses a very high therapeutic index (lethal dose to hypnotic dose); massive doses of this drug, when ingested alone, have not been observed to produce fatalities. Nevertheless, patients should be cautioned to avoid the concurrent use of alcohol with this drug as well as with other sedative-hypnotics. Moreover, tolerance to the hypnotic effects develops much more slowly than to barbiturates, nor does flurazepam interfere with the metabolism of coadministered drugs (that is, it is not an enzyme inducer; see below).

Numerous minor side effects have been reported after flurazepam administration. Excessive drowsiness, dizziness, and falling are not infrequently observed in elderly patients.

DRUG INTERACTIONS INVOLVING SEDATIVE-HYPNOTICS

Drug interactions involving the sedative-hypnotic agents are of two major types and have been well documented in the clinical literature. Barbiturates and nonbarbiturate sedative-hypnotics should be cautiously administered with alcohol and other central nervous system depressants (Table 13-3). These latter drugs may enhance the depressant effects of the sedative-hypnotics, resulting in sluggishness, drowsiness, impaired motor activity, coma, and even death. To reduce this undesirable depression, the dose of the sedative-hypnotic should be reduced.

Barbiturates and some nonbarbiturate

Table 13-3   Potential Drug Interactions Involving Sedative-Hypnotics

Sedative-hypnotics	Interacting drug/class	Possible consequences
Barbiturates Nonbarbiturates	Alcohol, acute Analgesics, narcotic Antihistamines Antidepressants Antipsychotics	Combined use of sedative-hypnotics with other CNS depressants may impair mental and physical performance (for example, motor vehicle operation) and result in lethargy, respiratory depression, coma, or death.
	Antidepressants, monoamine oxidase inhibitors Sulfonylurea oral hypoglycemic agents	These drugs may enhance the sedative effects of barbiturates and nonbarbiturates.
Chronic barbiturates Chloral hydrate Ethchlorvynol Glutethimide Meprobamate	Anticoagulants, oral (Coumarin)	Increased rate of coumarin anticoagulant metabolism, decreasing plasma levels of coumarin and reducing its ability to prevent blood coagulation; higher dose of coumarin required. When barbiturate withdrawn and dose of coumarin not reduced, bleeding episode may occur.
Barbiturates	Corticosteroids	Increased metabolism of corticosteroids when used for treatment of asthma; worsening of asthma.
	Doxycycline (Vibramycin)	Increased metabolism of doxycycline, decreased plasma levels, possible reduction in antibacterial effects.
	Griseofulvin (Fulvicin, Grifulvin, Grisactin)	Decreased antifungal effects of griseofulvin due to increased rate of metabolism and inhibition of absorption.

sedative-hypnotics (but not flurazepam) (Table 13-3) can interact with other drugs by increasing their rate of metabolism and inactivation. Phenobarbital, when administered for 48 hours, has been shown to increase the activity of drug-metabolizing enzymes located in the liver; this is called *enzyme induction*. Coadministration of an enzyme inducer such as phenobarbital with many drugs that are metabolized in the liver can result in a lowering of the plasma levels of such drugs, reducing their therapeutic effectiveness. To overcome this interaction, it may be necessary to increase the dosage of the drugs coadmin-istered with the barbiturates to maintain their desired effectiveness. After discontinuation of the administration of the enzyme inducer, the effective dose of the coadministered drugs will be increased, since their rate of inactivation will no longer be as rapid in the absence of the inducer. Thus, to prevent toxicity, the dosage of such drugs should be reduced upon discontinuation of the barbiturate to maintain the desired plasma levels and therapeutic effect.

Nursing implications associated with the administration of sedative-hypnotics are summarized on the following page.

Sedatives and Hypnotics:
nursing implications

1. Explore pattern of insomnia and possible causes. When appropriate, utilize nursing measures, including backrub, warm drink, pleasant and quiet atmosphere instead of drugs to promote relaxation and sleep. Educate patient in ways to improve sleep habits and sleep environment.
2. Warn the patient about driving, operating machinery, or engaging in potentially hazardous activities when taking drugs.
3. Caution the patient that alcohol, barbiturates, nonbarbiturate sedative-hypnotics, and other CNS depressants have additive depressing effects and should not be taken in combination without specific instructions from the physician.
4. Chronic barbiturate administration can reduce the therapeutic effectiveness of concurrently administered drugs (Table 13-3).
5. Administering barbiturates (especially by injection) to children or elderly patients may cause excitement and confusion.
6. Drugs do not possess analgesic activity and may produce restlessness and increased sensitivity when given to patients in pain.
7. During IV barbiturate administration: monitor rate of infusion to prevent overdosage; check IV site frequently for thrombophlebitis; record vital signs at least every hour or more frequently, if indicated; maintain airway. Resuscitation and drugs should be available for immediate use.
8. Warn the patient not to leave or store hypnotics on bedside table to reduce potential risk of unintentional overdosage.
9. Because of their high abuse potential, duration of drug administration should be as short as possible.
10. When administering orally, be sure the patient is actually swallowing the medication.
11. After chronic administration, sudden drug withdrawal may cause REM rebound with increased periods of dreaming, nightmares, and insomnia.
12. Drug withdrawal after chronic administration should be achieved slowly under close medical supervision. Abrupt withdrawal can cause anxiety, insomnia, weakness, delirium, confusion, and potentially life-threatening convulsions.
13. Side effects that a patient on long-term therapy should report include fever, sore throat, malaise, easy bruising or bleeding, petechiae, jaundice, or rash.

SUPPLEMENTARY READINGS

Anders, T., and P. Weinstein, "Sleep Disorders in Children: A Review," *Pediatrics* **50**: 312–324 (1972).

Essig, C. F., "Addiction to Nonbarbiturate Sedative and Tranquilizing Drugs," *Clinical Pharmacology and Therapeutics* **5**: 334–43 (1964).

Gerald, M. C., and P. M. Schwirian, "Nonmedical Use of Methaqualone," *Archives of General Psychiatry* **28**: 627–31 (1973).

Harvey, S. C., "Hypnotics and Sedatives," in *Good-*

man and Gilman's *The Pharmacological Basis of Therapeutics*, ed. A. G. Gilman, L. S. Goodman, and A. Gilman, 6th ed., Chapter 7, pp. 339–375. New York: Macmillan, Inc., 1980.

Kales, A., and J. Kales, "Sleep Disorders: Recent Findings in the Diagnosis and Treatment of Disturbed Sleep," *Journal of the American Medical Association* **290**: 487–499 (1974).

Jinks, M., "Insomnia and its Treatment," *Journal of the*

American Pharmaceutical Association **NS16**: 613–16 (1976).

Maynert, E. W., "Sedative and Hypnotics," in *Drill's Pharmacology and Medicine*, ed. J. R. DiPalma, 4th ed., Chapters 13, 14, pp. 229–49, 250–74. New York: McGraw-Hill Book Company, 1970.

Williams, D. "Sleep and Disease," *American Journal of Nursing*, **71**: 2321–24 (1971).

ALCOHOL AND ALCOHOLISM

Chapter 14

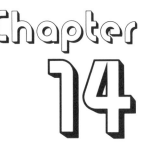

The general term *alcohol* is used in chemistry to designate a class of compounds that are hydroxy (—OH) derivatives of aliphatic hydrocarbons. Many common alcohols should be familiar to you—methyl alcohol (methanol or wood alcohol), a compound, which, when ingested, can produce impaired vision, blindness, and even death; isopropyl alcohol, a skin disinfectant; and the antifreeze diethylene glycol.

In this chapter, however, when the term *alcohol* is used without additional qualification, the alcohol referred to is *ethyl alcohol*, a liquid also known as *ethanol*, grain alcohol, or proof spirit. Our interest in alcohol is not predicated upon its use as a

medication, which is of only limited importance, but rather its toxicological significance. Moreover, the chronic abuse of this compound, *alcoholism*, currently represents the most widespread type of drug abuse in the United States. Prior to discussing alcoholism, we shall first consider some pertinent aspects of the pharmacology of alcohol.

PHARMACOLOGY OF ALCOHOL

In this section, the absorption and fate of alcohol and the local and systemic effects of this compound will be discussed.

Absorption and Fate of Alcohol

Alcohol is rapidly absorbed into the blood stream from the stomach and small intestines. On an empty stomach, peak blood alcohol levels are attained within one hour; the presence of food or milk in the stomach can delay the rate of absorption of alcoholic beverages.

Once in the blood stream, alcohol gains access to all the tissues and fluids of the body. Brain concentrations of alcohol rapidly approach those of blood due to the rich blood supply to this organ. Hence, determination of blood-alcohol concentrations provide a reasonable measure of brain alcohol levels. Alcohol also readily crosses the placental barrier. Recent evidence suggests that chronic alcoholism can lead to physical and functional deformities of the newborn, a condition known as the *fetal alcohol syndrome* discussed later.

From 90 to 98 percent of the total alcohol ingested is ultimately oxidized to carbon dioxide and water, with the generation of 7 kcal of energy per gram of alcohol or 200 kcal per ounce. Since alcohol provides energy, it is a food; it cannot be stored, however, nor does it provide vitamins. Regardless of the quantity of alcohol consumed, it is broken down at a constant rate of approximately 10 ml of alcohol (or about 20 ml of whiskey) per hour. Unmetabolized alcohol is primarily eliminated from the body in the exhaled air and urine.

Central Nervous System Effects

Although alcohol is distributed throughout the body, its effects on the brain are most evident. Contrary to popular belief, the increased activity, laughter, and voluble speech observed after the ingestion of moderate amounts of alcohol are not the consequences of drug-induced central stimulation. *Alcohol is always a central nervous system depressant.*

In small quantities alcohol depresses the association areas of the cortex controlling restraint and judgment. With increasing doses, sensory functions (vision, proprioception, pain), systematic thought processes, memory, and concentration all become impaired. Interference with motor coordination is first observed, followed by an unsteady and staggering gait, and ultimately a total inability to walk. Table 14-1 summarizes the correlation between blood-alcohol concentrations and these behavioral deficits.

The nurse should warn patients about the potential dangers associated with the combined use of alcohol with other drugs (Table 14-2). Of the 100 most frequently prescribed drugs, more than half contain at least one ingredient known to interact adversely with alcohol. Such interactions result in an estimated 2,500 deaths and 47,000 emergency-room admissions annually. The most common problems arise when alcohol is taken with central nervous system depressants such as barbiturate and non-barbiturate sedative-hypnotics, antianxiety, antipsychotic, and antidepressant drugs, antihistamines, and narcotic analgesics. Reasonable amounts of alcoholic beverages taken with normal therapeutic doses of these drugs are often capable of producing profound sedation. Many deaths, both unintentional and intentional, have been attributed to respiratory failure induced by a combination of alcohol and a central depressant.

Peripheral Effects

Alcohol also produces systemic effects on the cardiovascular system, gastrointestinal tract, and kidney. In addition, it is commonly em-

Table 14-1   Correlation of Blood-Alcohol Concentrations with Behavioral Effects[a]

Approximate intake (ml spirits[b])	Blood-alcohol levels[c]		Behavioral effects
	mg %	%	
	Up to 10	Up to 0.01	Effects doubtful.
Up to 60	10-50	0.01-0.05	Effects slight.
60	50	0.05	False sense of well-being; some impairment of vision.
60-120	60-100	0.06-0.10	Effects definite, but not pronounced.
120	100	0.10	Some impairment of reaction time; motor incoordination; legally considered to be "driving under the influence" in many states.
180	150	0.15	Clearly intoxicated; very marked impairment of reaction time; behavioral changes; legally intoxicated in all states.
Over 240	Over 200	Over 0.20	Very marked impairment to fatal outcome.
240	200	0.20	Emotional instability; physical and mental depression.
240-420	200-350	0.20-0.35	Confusion; slurred speech; staggering gait; blackout.
360-480	300-400	0.30-0.40	Stupor.
420-540	350-450	0.35-0.45	Coma.
540-	450-	0.45-	Fatal outcome.

[a]Underlined entries are major subdivisions of the table. They describe the effects that occur at blood-alcohol levels within that range. Effects not underlined refer to those observed at specific blood-alcohol levels.

[b]These approximate volumes of imbibed spirits required to produce the indicated blood levels refer to a 150-lb man. About 30 ml = 1 ounce. A "shot" of spirits containing 45 ml or 1.5 oz (40-50% alcohol), a 5-oz glass of wine (12% alcohol), and 16 oz of beer (5% alcohol) all provide 0.75 oz of alcohol.

[c]mg % = milligrams of alcohol per 100 ml blood; % = grams of alcohol per 100 ml blood. Conversion: % × 1000 = mg %.

ployed by nurses for its local effects on the skin.

Cardiovascular system   Vasodilation of the blood vessels of the skin, with feelings of warmth, are readily observed after the ingestion of alcohol. This drug has been shown to relieve the pain associated with attacks of angina pectoris, an effect not resulting from improved coronary blood vessel circulation. Both the peripheral vasodilatory effects and the relief of anginal pain are thought to result from alcohol's central effects. Recent studies suggest that the chronic use of small amounts of alcoholic beverages may improve cardiovascular function.

Gastrointestinal tract and kidney
Small quantities of alcohol increase the appetite; gastric acid and salivary secretions are stimulated. By contrast, concentrated alcoholic beverages inhibit gastric acid secretions and are irritating to the gastric mucosa. Chronic gastritis is commonly observed in heavy drinkers. Alcohol should be avoided by patients with peptic ulcers.

Alcohol exerts a definite diuretic effect as the result of its ability to inhibit the release of antidiuretic hormone (ADH) from the posterior pituitary gland.

Local effects   Rubbing alcohol is a useful cleansing agent and germicide when applied to the skin at a 70 percent concentration. When alcohol is used to cleanse the skin prior to an injection, friction over the surface area to be used is as important as the

Table 14-2   Potential Alcohol-Drug Interactions (1)

Interacting drug/class	Representative drugs	Mechanism underlying interaction and potential consequences
Alcohol deterrent	Disulfiram (Antabuse)	Interaction results in acetaldehyde accumulation, causing a rise in blood pressure, increase in heart rate, facial flushing, pounding headache, dizziness, rapid breathing, nausea, vomiting, weakness, fainting, potentially fatal.
Analgesics, nonnarcotic	Acetaminophen (Datril, Tylenol) Aspirin Sodium salicylate	Alcohol can intensify salicylate-induced inflammation of the gastric mucosa (gastritis) and gastrointestinal bleeding. The combination can delay clotting (by inhibiting blood clot aggregation) resulting in possible bleeding episodes. Alcohol abuse may increase susceptibility to liver damage resulting from acetaminophen overdosage.
Anesthetics, general	Ether Halothane (Fluothane)	Cross-tolerance develops between these drugs; chronic alcoholics require greater doses of anesthetics to induce sleep. After anesthesia has been induced, if alcohol is present in the body a deeper level of narcosis will be induced and the lethal concentration of anesthetic will be reduced.
Antianginal, antihypertensive agents, and peripheral vasodilators.	Guanethidine (Esimil, Ismelin) Hydralazine (Apresoline, Dralzine) Methyldopa (Aldomet) Nitroglycerin Propranolol (Inderal)	Alcohol may enhance the blood pressure lowering capacity of these drugs causing postural hypotension, fainting, and loss of consciousness. In addition, propranolol may mask the signs and symptoms (rapid heartbeat, profuse sweating) of alcohol-induced hypoglycemia.
Antianxiety agents ("minor tranquilizers")	Meprobamate (Equanil, Miltown) Benzodiazepines (Librium, Valium)	Additive central nervous system (CNS) depression impairing mental and physical performance.
Anticonvulsants	Phenytoin (Dilantin)	Alcohol increases the rate of phenytoin metabolism decreasing its anticonvulsant (antiepileptic) effects.
Antidepressants	Tricyclics Amitriptyline (Elavil) Desipramine (Norpramin, Pertofrane) Monoamine oxidase inhibitors (MAOI) Tranylcypromine (Parnate)	Depending upon their relative sedative or stimulant activity, tricyclics can antagonize or potentiate alcohol depression; desipramine (a stimulant) and amitriptyline (a depressant) antagonize and enhance alcohol-induced depression, respectively. Tricyclics increase susceptibility to convulsions and should be used cautiously during alcohol withdrawal. MAOI inhibit alcohol metabolism, increasing the degree of alcohol intoxication. Alcoholic beverages containing tyramine (Chianti wine, beer) form dangerous and even lethal effects; MAOI inhibition of tyramine metabolism leads to its build-up causing release of norepinephrine from nerve endings potentially resulting in a hypertensive crisis.
Antidiabetic/hypoglycemic agents	Acetohexamide (Dymelor) Chlorpropamide (Diabinese) Tolazamide (Tolinase)	After acute consumption of large quantities of alcohol, these drugs interact *via* multiple mechanisms causing loss of control of blood sugar and severe

121

Table 14-2   (Continued)

Interacting drug/class	Representative drugs	Mechanism underlying interaction and potential consequences
	Tolbutamide (Orinase)	hypoglycemia. Chronic high dose alcohol consumption can increase enzyme activity and the metabolism of tolbutamide and related drugs, reducing the antidiabetic effects. Use of alcohol with these drugs may result in a disulfiram-like reaction (see page 121).
Antihistamines	Chlorpheniramine (Chlor-Trimeton) Diphenhydramine (Benadryl)	Additive CNS depression impairing mental and physical performance.
Antimicrobial/anti-infective agents	Chloramphenicol (Chloromycetin) Furazolidone (Furoxone) Griseofulvin (Fulvicin, Grifulvin, Grisactin) Isoniazid (INH) Metronidazole (Flagyl) Quinacrine (Atabrine)	Interaction may result in disulfiram-like reaction, although milder and less predictable than with disulfiram.
Antipsychotic agents (neuroleptics)	Chlorpromazine (Thorazine) Thioridazine (Mellaril)	Combination may produce severe disruption of mental and physical performance, depression (potentially fatal) of the respiratory center in the medulla, and impairment of liver function. Hypotension, often produced by antipsychotic agents, can be intensified by alcohol. Phenothiazines increase seizure susceptibility and, therefore, their use to control chronic alcohol withdrawal can be hazardous.
Narcotic analgesics	Hydromorphone (Dilaudid) Meperidine (Demerol) Morphine Propoxyphene (Darvon)	Additive CNS depression, impairment in mental and physical performance, and depression (potentially fatal) of the respiratory center in the medulla.
Sedative-hypnotics	Barbiturates Phentobarbital (Nembutal) Secobarbital (Seconal) Nonbarbiturates Glutethimide (Doriden) Chloral hydrate (Noctec) Flurazepam (Dalmane) Methaqualone (Quaalude, Sopor)	Best-established and potentially most dangerous interaction. Lethal dose for barbiturates is almost 50% lower in the presence of alcohol than in absence. Symptoms of severe alcohol-barbiturate intoxication: vomiting, severe motor impairment, loss of consciousness, coma, death. Use of combination in sublethal doses can cause severe impairment of physical and mental performance. Cross-tolerance and cross-dependence develops between alcohol and barbiturates. Interaction between alcohol and chloral hydrate can result in enhanced CNS depression ("Mickey Finn," "knockout drops") and profound vasodilation, the latter resulting in an increase in heart rate, palpitations, facial flushing, and feelings of apprehension.

alcohol. This drug is not useful against spores or viruses. When alcohol is rubbed on the skin, it dries and hardens the epithelial skin layer and helps prevent bed sores. It is also employed to reduce fever because of its ability to readily evaporate and cool the skin when applied locally. However, if the skin surface is irritated or has lost its integrity, alcohol can cause increased tissue damage and, therefore, should not be used.

Acute Alcohol Intoxication

The severely intoxicated individual is stuporous or comatose, has cold skin and reduced body temperature, breathes slowly and noisily, and has a slow heart rate. If coma persists for over 8 to 10 hours, a severe risk of hypostatic pneumonia exists, with death resulting from respiratory failure.

The patient should be kept warm and respiration stimulated mechanically. Patients emerging from states of acute intoxication are often agitated. There is no uniform agreement as to the best treatment for this hyperexcitable state; among the drugs used in different clinics are the barbiturates (such as pentobarbital [Nembutal]), chloral hydrate, paraldehyde, and diazepam (Valium).

CHRONIC ALCOHOLISM

Chronic abuse of alcohol may result is psychological and physical dependence, a deterioration of the individual's physical and mental health, and destruction of the family unit, resulting in a broken home. Alcohol abuse may directly or indirectly lead to one-half of all auto fatalities and homicide victims each year. There are approximately ten million alcoholics in the United States, only 3 to 5 percent of whom are the skid row derelicts. Let us look at the characteristics of this drug-dependent state.

Characteristics of Alcohol Dependence

The chronic alcoholic has an extreme psychological dependence upon this compound. While such an individual can consume relatively large amounts of alcohol and not manifest obvious signs of intoxication, tolerance is not acquired to its lethal effects; the lethal blood-alcohol levels in the chronic alcoholic are not substantially higher than those required to kill the abstainer or social drinker.

Chronic ingestion of large volumes of alcohol produces unequivocal *physical dependence*, with the intensity of the withdrawal symptoms proportional to the degree of intoxication and its duration. *Delirium tremens*, the most serious type of alcohol withdrawal, is characterized by anxiety, tremors, terrifying visual and auditory hallucinations, fever, cardiovascular collapse, and occasionally grand mal seizures. Treatment of delirium tremens includes the use of depressant drugs (paraldehyde, barbiturates, chlordiazepoxide [Librium], or phenothiazine antipsychotic agents) to reduce agitation and the intravenous administration of fluids, electrolytes, and vitamins (thiamine, nicotinic acid, and ascorbic acid) to replace deficiencies resulting from inadequate intake or excessive loss.

Medical and Psychological Problems

The major medical problems associated with chronic alcoholism involve the nervous system, digestive system, and liver. Teratogenic effects are observed in infants born to alcoholic mothers.

Nervous system Alcoholic polyneuropathy is a neurological disease characterized by weakness, numbness, and pain, in which the patient suffers from sensory and motor impairments of the limbs. The most serious neuropsychiatric complications of chronic alcoholism are Wernicke's syndrome and Korsakoff's psychosis. The former is characterized by dizziness, paralysis of the eyes, mental confusion, and disorientation. Korsakoff's psychosis is manifested by a severe impairment of memory and learning.

Digestive system and liver   Ingestion of large amounts of alcohol have a direct irritating effect on the mucosal cells of the stomach. Gastritis and stomach ulcers are frequently observed in alcoholics.

Approximately three-fourths of all alcoholics lose some degree of liver function, with one in ten developing *cirrhosis*, a disorder characterized by widespread scarring. In advanced cases, death often results from uncontrolled bleeding, liver failure, or infections. Successful treatment necessitates total abstinence from alcohol and a nutritious, high-calorie, high-protein diet.

Psychological problems   The alcoholic often has an inadequate ego function (a poor self-image), a limited ability to restrain impulses, an unsatisfactory relationship with others (including family, friends, business associates), wide mood swings, and a low tolerance for anxiety and frustration. Whether these problems represent the cause or effect of alcoholism remains to be determined.

Teratogenic effects   Reports appearing in recent years suggest that infants born to mothers who are chronic alcoholics may exhibit multiple teratogenic effects. Babies born of mothers who are binge drinkers experience the highest incidence of adverse effects. Among the most common characteristics of the *fetal alcohol syndrome* include low birth weight and abnormalities of the head, face, heart, joints, and genital organs. Postnatally, there is a higher incidence

of mortality, as well as a reduction in the rate of increase of weight and growth and marked mental and motor retardation.

Treatment of Alcoholism

While the etiology of alcoholism is presently unknown, it appears highly unlikely that a single cause will be identified that applies to all cases. There is a growing body of recent evidence suggesting a genetic predisposition to alcoholism. Contemporary treatment is primarily empirical and attempts to provide *symptomatic relief*, with little realistic hope for an immediate and dramatic cure.

A fundamental premise underlying the successful treatment of alcoholism is the patient's realization that he or she cannot control his or her drinking, and that he or she does not merely "have a problem with alcohol," but rather that he or she is an alcoholic in need of help. While the decision to enter a treatment program must ultimately be that of the patient, the physician and nurse should be available to provide the necessary support during periods of low morale and relapse.

Two general treatment modalities are used for the treatment of alcoholism: emotional rehabilitation and deterrent drugs, with the former far more successful.

Emotional rehabilitation   Emotional rehabilitation may be conducted in many settings, including individual or group psychotherapy, counseling, family therapy, and psychodrama, among others. All have the same fundamental objective: to help the alcoholic find and adjust to a new way of life and adapt to normal pressures without seeking the escape previously found in the bottle.

The most successful approach to the treatment of this drug dependent state has been *Alcoholics Anonymous* (AA), an informal fellowship of reformed alcoholics whose goal is the rehabilitation of others. Although accurate statistics are lacking, it has been estimated that one-half of the individuals who enter this program intent upon rehabilitation have no relapses, while many others remain abstinent, notwithstanding occasional backsliding.

Deterrent drugs: Disulfiram   Disulfiram (Antabuse) does not cure alcoholism, but rather provides a chemical crutch or deterrent for the sporadic or spree drinker who is likely to impulsively relapse from an abstinent state when confronted with anxiety, frustration, or pressure. Within 5 to 10 minutes after the ingestion of alcohol, the patient treated with disulfiram experiences flushing, dizziness, palpitations of the heart, a precipitous drop in blood pressure, a severe headache, nausea, and vomiting; these effects may last for anywhere from 30 minutes up to several hours. Since the patient is warned of these consequences of drinking *prior* to initiating disulfiram therapy, the alcoholic is deterred from having even "just one drink."

What is the pharmacological basis for this intended alcohol-drug interaction? In the absence of disulfiram, alcohol is metabolize to acetaldehyde, which is very readily converted to acetate. Disulfiram retards this second reaction; as a consequence, the acetaldehyde levels rapidly accumulate in the body, producing many of the effects described earlier.

Treatment with disulfiram is justified only for those patients who are truly resolute in their desire to stop drinking. Medical and psychological treatment should be used in conjunction with this drug. Patients should be advised to refrain from the use of alcoholic beverages for 6 to 12 days after the last drug dose. Nursing implications associated with the use of disulfiram are summarized below.

Alcohol and Disulfiram:
nursing implications

1. Pregnant women should be warned that the risk of the fetal alcohol syndrome increases if they engage in binge drinking. Such women should be cautioned to limit their alcohol consumption to no more than 2 drinks per day.

2. Disulfiram is used as an adjunct to supportive and psychiatric therapy and only in patients who are motivated to fully cooperate and who are forewarned of the nature of the alcohol-disulfiram reaction.

3. The patient should carry an identification card stating that he or she is taking disulfiram, describing symptoms of reaction with alcohol and their treatment, and the name of the patient's physician. Cards may be obtained from Ayerst Laboratories, 685 Third Ave., New York, NY 10017.

4. Advise the patient to avoid alcohol in disguised form, such as in foods, cough syrups, tonics, other medicines, and shaving lotion.

5. Alcohol-disulfiram reaction occurs within 5–10 min after alcohol ingestion and may last for 30–60 min up to several hours. The intensity of the reaction varies among individuals, but is generally proportional to the amount of alcohol taken.

6. Reaction to alcohol may occur as long as 2 wk after a single dose of disulfiram.

7. During the first 2 wk of therapy, the patient may experience a metallic or garlic-like after-taste and other minor side effects, including drowsiness, headache, fatigue, and acne-form skin eruption. These dose-related symptoms usually disappear with continued therapy.

SUPPLEMENTARY READINGS

Forney, R. B., and F. W. Hughes, *Combined Effects of Alcohol and Other Drugs.* Springfield, Ill.: Charles C Thomas, Publisher, 1968.

Goodwin, D., *Is Alcoholism Hereditary?* New York: Oxford University Press, 1976.

Isler, C., "The Alcoholic Nurse," *RN* **41**(7): 48–55 (1978).

Israel, Y., and J. Mardones, eds. *Biological Basis of Alcoholism.* New York: John Wiley & Sons, Inc., 1971.

Kissin, B., and H. Begleiter, eds., *The Biology of Alcoholism.* 4 vols. New York: Plenum Publishing Corporation, 1971–1976.

Seixas, F. A., ed., "Nature and Nurture in Alcoholism," *Annals of the New York Academy of Sciences* **197**: 1–229 (1972).

Tobias, E. A., "Confronting Alcoholism—How One Medical Surgical Unit Faced the Problem," *Nursing '77* 7(5): 56–61 (1977).

Wallgren, H., and H. Barry, III, *Actions of Alcohol.* 2 vols. New York: American Elsevier Publ., 1970.

ANTIPSYCHOTIC AGENTS

Chapter 15

Psychotherapeutic or psychotropic agents, drugs that are used to treat behavior disorders, are among the most frequently prescribed classes of drugs. These include drugs employed for the treatment of psychoses (antipsychotic agents), neuroses (antianxiety agents), and alterations in mood or affective disorders (antidepressants and antimanic agents). It is of interest to note that the major prototype drugs in each of these classes was introduced between 1949 and 1960. None of these drugs is capable of curing psychiatric illnesses; rather, they favorably alter the behavior of the patient. This chapter considers the antipsychotic agents, and the next two chapters discuss drugs used for the treatment of anxiety and affective disorders, respectively. The nature of psychoses is examined first.

PSYCHOSES

The *psychotic patient* lives in a world of his or her own, possessing only a marginal appreciation of reality. Psychotic disorders are characterized by disturbances in thinking that impair the patient's ability to successfully interact with others; the patient may sometimes experience delusions and hallucinations. Such an individual often exhibits a lack of responsiveness to others and manifests changes in mood that are inappropriate to the events that are transpiring. Behavioral aberrations, including the performance of bizarre acts, are common.

Schizophrenia is the most prevalent type of the major psychoses. It has been estimated that 1 percent of the population will experience a schizophrenic illness during the course of a lifetime, and, for many, this may become an incapacitating chronic illness.

There is a mounting body of evidence to suggest that a biochemical aberration may be involved in schizophrenia. Recent evidence suggests that the functional activity of the *dopaminergic* system may be overactive in the brains of these patients, and that antipsychotic agents act by blocking the activity of dopamine. There also appears to be a genetic predisposition for schizophrenia.

DRUG TREATMENT OF PSYCHOSES

The *antipsychotic agents*, also called *neuroleptic agents* and *major tranquilizers*, belong to three major classes, namely, the phenothiazines, thioxanthenes, and butyrophenones (Table 15-1). Since these classes share many common pharmacological properties, the phenothiazines, the most extensively used class of antipsychotic agents, will be emphasized.

Phenothiazines

During the course of clinical studies designed to reduce the incidence of surgical shock, patients to whom *chlorpromazine* was administered were observed to retain consciousness, and yet were calm, relaxed, and noticeably indifferent to the normal anxieties associated with surgery. The potential therapeutic applications of chlorpromazine for the treatment of the mentally ill were rapidly appreciated; this single drug was administered to more than 50 million patients around the world between 1955 and 1965.

Overview of comparative pharmacological properties The discovery of chlorpromazine (Thorazine) led to the introduction of numerous phenothiazine antipsychotic derivatives (Table 15-1). The nurse will encounter three chemical classes of phenothiazines in practice: the *aliphatic* phenothiazines, including chlorpromazine (Thorazine); the *piperidine* phenothiazines, such as thioridazine (Mellaril); and the *piperazine* derivatives, such as trifluoperazine (Stelazine). While classes of phenothiazines are not strikingly different in their antipsychotic effectiveness nor in their general pharmacological properties, notable differences are seen in their potency (reflected by dosage) and side effects (Table 15-1).

The aliphatic agents are the least potent and cause considerable sedation and orthostatic hypotension. The piperazines are the most potent drugs and produce the highest incidence of extrapyramidal side effects, but cause little sedation and hypotension. The piperidine derivatives are of intermediate potency and are least likely to cause extrapyramidal side effects. The pharmacology of chlorpromazine as the prototype phenothiazine agent will be discussed.

Pharmacological effects Chlorpromazine produces an extremely diverse spectrum of pharmacological effects, which involve primarily the central and autonomic nervous systems and the cardiovascular and endocrine systems.

Table 15-1 Comparative Properties of Selected Antipsychotic Agents

Antipsychotic class	Generic name	Trade name(s)	Adult usual oral daily dosage (mg)	Adverse side effects[a]			
				Sedative effects	Extrapyramidal effects	Hypotensive effects	Antiemetic properties
Phenothiazines							
Aliphatic (Dimethylaminopropyl) Derivatives							
	Chlorpromazine	Thorazine	200–800	+++	++	+++	Yes.
	Triflupromazine	Vesprin	50–200	++	+++	++	Yes.
Piperazine Derivatives							
	Mesoridazine	Serentil	25–200	+++	+	++	Yes.
	Piperacetazine	Quide	20–40	++	++	+	
	Thioridazine	Mellaril	100–600	+++	+	++	
Piperazine Derivatives							
	Acetophenazine	Tindal	40–80	++	++	+	
	Butaperazine	Repoise	15–100	++	+++	+	
	Carphenazine	Proketazine	75–400	++	+++	+	
	Fluphenazine	Permitil, Prolixin	2–10	+	+++	+	
	Perphenazine	Trilafon	8–32	++	+++	+	Yes.
	Prochlorperazine	Compazine	75–150	++	+++	+	Yes.
	Trifluoperazine	Stelazine	4–15	+	+++	+	Yes.
Thioxanthenes							
	Chlorprothixene	Taractan	50–400	+++	++	+++	Yes.
	Thiothixene	Navane	6–30	+	+++	+	Yes.
Butyrophenones							
	Haloperidol	Haldol	2–6	+	+++	+	
Miscellaneous							
	Loxapine	Daxolin, Loxitane	15–40	++	+++	+	
	Molindone	Lidone, Moban	15–60	++	++	+	

[a]Key to incidence of adverse side effects: + = minimal to low; ++ = moderate; +++ = high.

Central nervous system   Chlorpromazine exerts effects on all levels of the central nervous system. These effects are responsible for this drug's antipsychotic, antimanic, and antiemetic properties, as well as its adverse effects on the extrapyramidal system.

Chlorpromazine alleviates many of the symptoms of schizophrenia. Violent, hostile, hyperactive, and panic-stricken patients become calm and quiet, with thought disturbances, hallucinations, and illusions gradually dissipating. Unlike the barbiturates, which produce general central depression, chlorpromazine does not markedly cloud consciousness in normal therapeutic doses. Apathetic and withdrawn schizophrenic patients become more alert and communicative.

Contemporary thinking suggests that schizophrenia may be associated with *excessive dopaminergic activity* in the limbic areas of the central nervous system. The phenothiazines, thioxanthenes, and butyrophenones all block dopaminergic receptor sites and increase the rate of dopamine turnover (synthesis and breakdown). These drugs are also thought to improve the filtering capabilities of the ascending reticular activating system, thereby selectively reducing the flow of sensory stimuli to the cerebral cortex.

At low doses, chlorpromazine and other selected phenothiazine derivatives (Table 15-1) inhibit the chemoreceptor trigger zone located in the medulla, thereby preventing nausea and vomiting. The antiemetic effects of the phenothiazines are of great therapeutic importance.

Autonomic nervous system   Chlorpromazine possesses anticholinergic properties that are responsible for the observed dry mouth, blurred vision, failure of accommodation for near objects, constipation, and— less commonly—urinary retention.

Orthostatic hypotension is frequently observed after administration of the aliphatic and piperidine phenothiazine derivatives. This effect results from the α-adrenergic blocking properties of these drugs, as well as depression of centrally mediated vasomotor reflexes.

Endocrine system   Chlorpromazine administration enhances the release of prolactin from the anterior pituitary gland, which may result in galactorrhea (the spontaneous flow of milk), an effect that may be observed in men and nonnursing females. Disturbances in the normal menstrual cycle (delayed menstruation or amenorrhea) and infertility in both sexes may be observed as a result of chlorpromazine-induced inhibition of the release of follicle-stimulating hormone and luteinizing hormone from the anterior pituitary gland.

Adverse effects   Although a number of severe adverse effects are associated with the use of the phenothiazines, these drugs have a high therapeutic index. Unlike the barbiturates and antianxiety agents, chronic administration of the phenothiazines does not result in drug dependence. Nursing implications and potential drug interactions involving the antipsychotic agents (Table 15-2) are both found at the end of this chapter and on page 130, respectively.

Commonly encountered side effects include atropine-like effects, orthostatic hypotension, liver and blood dyscrasias, and extrapyramidal signs.

Orthostatic hypotension, which may result in fainting, is most often observed with the aliphatic phenothiazines (chlorpromazine). Although tolerance generally develops to this hypotensive response within several weeks, it may persist to some degree as long as therapy is continued. Should orthostatic hypotension prove greatly incapacitating to

Table 15-2   Potential Interactions Involving Antipsychotic Agents

Antipsychotic agent	Interacting drug/class	Possible consequences
Phenothiazines	Antacids, oral	Antacids may inhibit absorption of orally administered phenothiazines.
Phenothiazines Aliphatic (Chlorpromazine) Piperidine (Thioridazine)	Central Depressants Ethanol Barbiturates Nonbarbiturate sedative-hypnotics Antianxiety agents Antihistamines Narcotic analgesics	Additive central nervous system depression increasing the risk of mental or physical impairment of performance.
Phenothiazines Aliphatic Piperidine	Anticholinergic agents Antiulcer Antiparkinsonism	Additive atropine-like side effects. Anticholinergics reduce gastric motility, resulting in enhanced intestinal metabolism of phenothiazines and reduced absorption.
Phenothiazines Thioxanthenes Butyrophenones	Levodopa (Bendopa, Larodopa, Levopa)	Antiparkinsonism effects of levodopa may be antagonized by antipsychotic agents.
Phenothiazines Chlorpromazine	Guanethidine (Ismelin)	Chlorpromazine antagonizes antihypertensive effects of guanethidine.
	Amphetamine-like drugs	Phenothiazines may antagonize the appetite-suppressing effects of these drugs.

the patient, a piperazine phenothiazine (fluphenazine) may be used.

Jaundice and blood dyscrasias are among the most dangerous adverse effects associated with phenothiazine therapy. *Jaundice* of the obstructive type, observed in 2 to 4 percent of patients, most commonly appears between the second and fourth week after the initiation of drug administration, with the incidence diminishing thereafter. This condition, thought to be a hypersensitivity reaction, is usually reversible after the discontinuation of therapy.

Blood dyscrasias, including leukopenia and agranulocytosis, are rare but have a high mortality rate. The nurse should be vigilant for the sudden onset of an apparent upper respiratory tract infection (sore throat, fever, weakness); a complete blood count should be initiated without delay upon the appearance of these symptoms.

Skin reactions, including urticaria or dermatitis, are seen in about 5 percent of patients taking chlorpromazine. Long-term, high-dosage administration of phenothiazines—in particular, chlorpromazine—may result in abnormal blue-gray pigmentation of the skin upon exposure to sunlight. This problem may be obviated by the nurse recommending that the patient wear protective clothing over exposed skin areas. Opacities in the cornea and lens have been noted after chlorpromazine, which, in extreme cases, may impair vision; administration of thioridazine may cause pigmentation of the retina. Patients receiving moderate to high doses of these drugs over extended periods of time should have periodic ocular examinations.

Extrapyramidal signs Among the most important adverse effects associated with the use of antipsychotic agents are neurological disorders affecting the extrapyramidal system. These problems are most frequently observed with the piperazine phenothiazines (fluphenazine, trifluoperazine) and the butyrophene agent haloperidol, while their incidence is much lower with the piperidine derivatives (thioridazine).

These extrapyramidal effects include a parkinsonian syndrome, akathisia, and acute dystonic reaction, which all appear during the early phases of drug therapy, and tardive dyskinesia, observed after chronic drug administration or upon discontinuation of the antipsychotic agent.

The *parkinsonian syndrome* mimics idiopathic parkinsonism (Chapter 19), and is characterized by akinesia, rigidity, and tremors. Patients manifesting *akathisia* are in constant movement, with the patient feeling compelled to walk about. *Acute dystonic reactions* are associated with facial grimacing and torticollis, a twisting of the neck into unnatural positions. All three of these extrapyramidal symptoms respond to a reduction in the dosage of the antipsychotic agent. The administration of an anticholinergic antiparkinsonism drug such as benztropine (Cogentin) is often highly effective in managing these disorders and may be therapeutically justified in severe cases.

Tardive dyskinesia is a neurological complication recently reported in 43 percent of psychiatric outpatients. It is typically observed after the withdrawal of chronic antipsychotic medication (in particular, the piperazine phenothiazines) or when chronic high doses are abruptly reduced; the incidence of this disorder is higher in patients chronically receiving anticholinergic antiparkinsonism drugs with their antipsychotic agents. Symptoms include involuntary movements of the lips, tongue, and jaw, and purposeless, quick darting movements of the extremities. Since there exists no effective treatment for tardive dyskinesia at present, attempts must be made to prevent its occurrence. Such preventive measures include the initiation of drug holidays, limitations imposed on the duration of antipsychotic drug therapy, and avoidance of the routine coadministration of anticholinergic antiparkinsonism drugs unless these drugs are absolutely required.

THERAPEUTIC USES

The phenothiazines are therapeutically employed for the treatment of psychoses (see below) and mania and to prevent nausea and vomiting. The antimanic properties of the phenothiazines and butyrophenones will be discussed in greater detail in Chapter 17.

Nausea and Vomiting

Chlorpromazine and several other phenothiazine derivatives (Table 15-1) are used in nonsedative doses to prevent vomiting caused by various diseases, radiation sickness, and some drugs (narcotic analgesics, anticancer agents, and general anesthetics). Among the phenothiazine derivatives devoid of antipsychotic activity that are employed for their antiemetic effects are promazine (Sparine), promethazine (Phenergan), and thiethylperazine (Torecan). Unlike chlorpromazine, the antihistamine phenothiazine agent promethazine has been found to be highly effective in preventing motion sickness.

Thioxanthenes

The chemistry and pharmacological properties of the thioxanthenes closely resemble those of the phenothiazines (Table 15-1). *Chlorprothixene* (Taractan) is the thioxanthene analog of chlorpromazine and possesses equivalent properties, including low potency, marked sedative effects, a high incidence of orthostatic hypotension, a moderate incidence of extrapyramidal effects, and effective antiemetic properties. The effects of thiothixene (Navane) are similar to the piperazine phenothiazines, namely, high potency and a low incidence of sedation and orthostatic hypotension, while causing a high incidence of extrapyramidal side effects. There is no compelling evidence to suggest these drugs have any advantages over the older phenothiazine derivatives as antipsychotic agents.

Butyrophenones

Haloperidol (Haldol) is the only butyrophenone approved for use as an antipsychotic agent in the United States at this time. The pharmacological profile of haloperidol is qualitatively similar to the piperazine phenothiazines. This drug is of high potency, possesses little anticholinergic activity, and causes minimal sedation and orthostatic hypotension.

Adverse effects associated with haloperidol include a high incidence of extrapyramidal side effects, and, not infrequently, leukopenia. The therapeutic use of haloperidol for the treatment of psychoses will be discussed in the next section of this chapter; the antimanic properties of this drug will be considered in Chapter 17.

Droperidol (Inapsine), a compound chemically and pharmacologically similar to haloperidol, is used in combination with the narcotic analgesic fentanyl and is employed in anesthesiology to produce neuroleptanalgesia (Chapter 10).

Therapeutic Aspects of Psychoses

Clinical studies have clearly demonstrated that the phenothiazine, thioxanthene, and butyrophenone drugs listed in Table 15-1 are highly effective for the treatment of acute and chronic schizophrenic patients. These drugs reduce the disordered thinking, lack of affect, social withdrawal, hostility, hyperexcitability, behavioral aberrations, and other symptoms associated with schizophrenia. Not withstanding the dramatic effects often observed after the administration of these antipsychotic agents, the nurse should bear in mind that these drugs do not cure schizophrenia, but merely provide symptomatic relief, thereby enhancing the potential benefits to be derived from psychotherapy.

Drug selection   There is no compelling evidence that there is a drug of choice among the many antipsychotic agents; all drugs in common therapeutic use are equal to chlorpromazine in the therapeutic efficacy. However, certain factors should be considered in order to make a rational drug selection. When there is reason to suspect that the outpatient will not take the medication as directed, biweekly intramuscular or subcutaneous injections of fluphenazine decanoate or ethanate may be indicated. Piperazine derivatives or haloperidol are preferred in patients with cardiovascular disease who are prone to hypotension. When a strong risk of the development of extrapyramidal symptoms exists, thioridazine is the most useful drug.

Dose and administration   The optimal dose administered is highly individualized; acutely ill schizophrenic patients may require daily doses of chlorpromazine that range from 300 to 2000 mg.

Some physicians gradually increase the dose over a period of days to weeks until an adequate therapeutic response is obtained or until troublesome side effects are manifested. By contrast, other physicians prefer to parenterally administer chlorpromazine or other antipsychotic agents to acutely agitated schizophrenics every 30 to 60 minutes until improvement is observed and then stabilize the patient with daily doses.

Once the dosage has been stabilized, a single dose at bedtime is often preferred to multiple daily doses. A single bedtime dose has advantages since there is better patient compliance, the sedative properties facilitate sleep, and many of the undesirable side effects (atropine-like effects, orthostatic hypotension) will be maximal while the patient is at sleep.

Time course of therapy Often 3 weeks of drug therapy are required to demonstrate the beneficial effects of antipsychotic agents in hospitalized schizophrenics, with maximal effects achieved within 6 weeks to 6 months. Abrupt termination of drug therapy is associated with a very high incidence of relapse and the appearance of tardive dyskinesia. Both problems are attenuated when dosage is gradually reduced and trial periods of drug-free holidays are attempted. Since these drugs are slowly removed from the body, signs of relapse may not be observed for days or weeks.

For supplementary readings, see page 145 in Chapter 17.

Antipsychotic Drugs:
nursing implications

1. Prior to initiating therapy and at periodic intervals thereafter, a general examination should include evaluation of blood pressure, liver function and the eyes, and a complete blood count.

2. Postural hypotension, dizziness, and sedation are common during the first few weeks of chlorpromazine (Thorazine) therapy. Changes in position should be made slowly, especially from the recumbent to the upright position; the patient should dangle legs prior to ambulating. IM preparations should be slowly injected; the patient should remain in recumbent position for at least 1 h after parenteral medication.

3. Avoid contact of drug with skin, eyes, and clothing. Contact dermatitis has been reported.

4. Observe the patient for extrapyramidal effects such as tremors, muscle rigidity, impairment of motor function, increased muscle tone or spasms, involuntary rhythmic movements or restlessness, or inability to sit still or sleep.

5. Observe and report to the physician early symptoms of tardive dyskinesia, including involuntary movements of the mouth, lips, or tongue.

6. Observe menstrual irregularities, breast engorgement, lactation, changes in libido (increased in women, decreased in men). Reassure the patient that such effects are drug-induced.

7. Observe and report to the physician early symptoms of cholestatic jaundice, such as high fever, upper abdominal pain, nausea, diarrhea, and rash. Withhold drug and report if signs of cholestatic jaundice appear, including yellowing of the skin, mucous membranes, or sclera of eyes.

8. Alert the patient about side effects that should be reported: fever with sore throat and weakness (suggesting blood dyscrasias), change in vision, and change in tolerance to heat or cold.

9. Abnormal pigmentation of the skin induced by chlorpromazine in the presence of sunlight may be prevented by recommending that the patient wear protective clothing over exposed areas.

10. Many weeks may be required for the beneficial effects of the medication to be clearly manifested. Teaching the patient or family the importance of continuing to take the prescribed medication as directed and remaining under close medical supervision is essential for treatment success.

11. After chronic therapy, the drug should be slowly withdrawn over a period of several weeks to minimize the risk of an exacerbation of the psychotic state or the appearance of tardive dyskinesia.

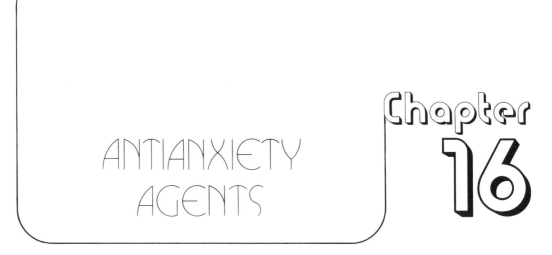

ANTIANXIETY AGENTS

Chapter 16

Neuroses are probably the most common group of disorders afflicting mankind. It has been estimated that 50 percent of patients visiting their physicians have underlying emotional disorders that are to varying degrees responsible for their physical complaints. The *antianxiety agents*, drugs employed for the treatment of neuroses, are the most extensively prescribed class of drugs—in many cases, with little medical justification.

NEUROSES

The emotions and reactions of the neurotic patient are exaggerations of those exhibited by the normal individual. Neurotic disorders are manifested by anxiety and tension, which may be exhibited during periods of stress. *Anxiety* is characterized by extreme apprehension, irritability, and emotional liability, while *tension* is manifested by such physical symptoms as a rapid heart beat, excessive perspiration, flushing, cold extremities, and headaches. While thinking and judgment may, at times, be impaired, there is minimum loss of appreciation of reality, and the patient generally realizes that he or she is ill. There does not appear to be an underlying biochemical basis for or genetic predisposition to neurotic disorders.

ANTIANXIETY AGENTS

The antianxiety agents are sometimes referred to as "minor tranquilizers," a term implying that their pharmacological properties and therapeutic uses are similar to the "major tranquilizers" or antipsychotic agents but of lesser degree. This is not the case! The antianxiety agents have sedative-hypnotic properties and abuse potential like the barbiturates and produce skeletal muscle relaxation by a central mechanism. By contrast, unlike the antipsychotic phenothiazine agents, the antianxiety agents do not cause extrapyramidal side effects or alterations in autonomic function, such as orthostatic hypotension. The use of barbiturates as antianxiety agents has previously been considered (Chapter 13).

Meprobamate and the benzodiazepine derivatives will be discussed as representative antianxiety agents. The properties of these drugs and other miscellaneous drugs in this therapeutic class are summarized in Table 16-1. A summary of nursing implications associated with the administration of antianxiety agents appears at the end of this chapter.

Meprobamate

Meprobamate (Equanil, Miltown) was originally developed as a centrally-acting skeletal muscle relaxant with a longer duration of action than mephenesin. Meprobamate produces dose-related progressive degrees of central nervous system depression, resulting in sedation, drowsiness, and ataxia.

While many, but not all, studies have demonstrated meprobamate to be superior to a placebo, it is generally accepted that this drug is no better than the barbiturates for the relief of anxiety. Meprobamate is not an hypnotic agent but, by virtue of its sedative properties, may facilitate the onset of sleep.

The major side effects associated with this drug include drowsiness with high doses and allergic reactions, including skin rash and itching.

The acute toxicity of meprobamate is considered to be relatively low, with the average adult lethal dose approximately 28 g or 70 tablets each containing 400 mg of meprobamate. Meprobamate should be used cautiously with alcohol and other central nervous system depressants because of additive effects. Physical dependence has been documented when this drug is taken at daily doses of 3,200 mg (twice the usual daily dose) for several months. Abrupt drug withdrawal may result in abstinence syndrome similar to that associated with the barbiturates and characterized by tremors and convulsions.

Benzodiazepines

The benzodiazepine derivatives, including chlordiazepoxide (Librium), diazepam (Valium), and oxazepam (Serax), are the most widely prescribed class of antianxiety agents (Table 16-1). Flurazepam (Dalmane) is a benzodiazepine used exclusively as a hypnotic agent (Chapter 13).

Pharmacological effects While the benzodiazepines normally reduce anxiety, in high doses they may—paradoxically— increase anxiety. The antianxiety effects of this drug class have been attributed to their abilities to inhibit electrical discharges and neuronal transmission in the limbic system at low doses that fail to depress other areas of the brain. Higher doses of the benzodiazepines may cause disinhibition, a state characterized by excitement and increased hostility, rage, and aggressive behavior. The benzodiazepines, diazepam in particular, produce skeletal muscle relaxation and anticonvulsant effects by central mechanisms that are not well understood at this time.

Table 16-1   Representative Nonbarbiturate Antianxiety Agents

Generic name	Trade name(s)	Usual adult oral daily dosage (mg)	Distinguishing properties
Meprobamate	Equanil, Miltown	1200–1,600	Mild sedation, muscle relaxation. Abuse potential documented.
Tybamate	Tybatran	750–1,500	Meprobamate-like properties.
Benzodiazepines			
Chlordiazepoxide	Librium	20–75	Antianxiety, muscle relaxing effects. Treatment of anxiety, chronic alcohol withdrawal, musculoskeletal disorders.
Diazepam	Valium	4–40	Most extensively used antianxiety agent; more effective for treatment of muscle spasms than chlordiazepoxide; drug of choice for status epilepticus.
Oxazepam	Serax	30–60	Antianxiety agent with sedative properties. Rapid onset, short duration of action.
Clorazepate	Tranxene, Azene	30, 26	Antianxiety agent. Long duration of action.
Lorazepam	Ativan	2–6	Antianxiety agent.
Prazepam	Verstran	20–40	Antianxiety agent.
Hydroxyzine	Atarax, Vistaril	25–100	Antianxiety agent, with antihistaminic, sedative, and antiemetic properties.
Propiomazine	Largon	20 (IM or IV)	Phenothiazine agent used preoperatively to alleviate anxiety. Enhances the depressing effects of barbiturates and narcotics.

Therapeutic uses   The benzodiazepines are employed clinically for the treatment of neuroses, chronic alcohol withdrawal, neuromuscular disorders, preoperative anxiety, and in labor and delivery. We will consider diazepam's beneficial anticonvulsant effects for the emergency treatment of status epilepticus in Chapter 18.

Neuroses   The benzodiazepines are effective drugs for the treatment of anxiety, although they are not more effective than the barbiturates. When compared to the barbiturates, these drugs possess several distinct advantages that undoubtedly account for their widespread popularity among clinicians. Relief of anxiety and tension is accomplished in the absence of sedation and ataxia. While psychological and physical dependence have been clearly documented after chronic administration of high doses, the benzo-

diazepine withdrawal syndrome, which appears up to one week after the last dose, is generally mild. Withdrawal symptoms resemble those associated with barbiturates and alcohol and include convulsions, tremors, abdominal and muscle cramps, vomiting, and sweating. The most important advantage of the benzodiazepines is their very wide margin of safety even when taken in very high doses, thus markedly reducing the risk of potential suicide.

Alcohol withdrawal   Chlordiazepoxide is the most extensively used drug for preventing the abstinence syndrome associated with the withdrawal of chronic alcohol ingestion or suppressing the syndrome (tremors, seizures, delirium) after its onset (Chapter 14). A sufficiently high dose of chlordiazepoxide is administered to stabilize the alcoholic patient and is then slowly reduced.

Table 16-2   Potential Interactions Involving Benzodiazepine Antianxiety Agents

Benzodiazepine	Interacting drug/class	Possible consequences
Benzodiazepines	Alcohol	Potential additive central depression.
Diazepam	Barbiturates	Intravenous administration of diazepam and barbiturates for the treatment of status epilepticus and nonepileptic convulsive disorders has been reported to result in respiratory depression or hypotension.

Neuromuscular disorders   Diazepam has been found to be useful in providing relief of spasticity in patients with multiple sclerosis, cerebral palsy, and traumatic spinal cord lesions. It is often prescribed for the treatment of common musculoskeletal disorders including back strain and "slipped disc" (Chapter 11).

Anesthesia   Chlordiazepoxide and diazepam are used as preanesthetic antianxiety agents, to facilitate induction prior to the administration of general anesthetics (Chapter 10). They are also employed as adjuncts to analgesic agents during labor and delivery, reducing the dosage of analgesic required; these drugs reportedly produce amnesia.

Adverse effects and toxicity   The most frequently observed adverse side effects associated with benzodiazepine administration include drowsiness, ataxia, and muscle weakness. Other undesirable effects include paradoxical excitement (disinhibition), impairment of sexual functions and desires, and menstrual irregularities. Potential drug interactions involving the benzodiazepines are summarized in Table 16-2. Recent studies suggest that the use of the benzodiazepines and meprobamate during the first trimester of pregnancy may increase the risk of birth defects.

The toxicological consequences of benzodiazepine overdosage are rarely severe. Successful treatment involves the support of respiratory and cardiovascular functions, which are depressed after very high doses.

For supplementary reading, see page 145 in Chapter 17.

Antianxiety Agents:
nursing implications

1. Elderly and debilitated patients are more prone to dizziness, drowsiness, and the hypotensive effects; therefore the usual dosage should be reduced in such patients.

2. Blood pressure should be monitored before and after medication is administered. Increased motor activity with impaired coordination requires the use of side rails.

3. Strongly advise the patient to refrain from drinking alcoholic beverages while taking antianxiety drugs because of their combined depressant effects.

4. Since these drugs impair physical and mental abilities, the patient should be warned not to drive a car, operate machinery, or engage in other potentially hazardous activities until their drug response has been fully assessed.

5. Look for symptoms of chronic intoxication suggesting that the patient is either extremely sensitive to the drug or taking doses in excess of those prescribed. Withhold dose if patient is ataxic, has slurred speech, or is otherwise excessively depressed.

6. Sudden drug withdrawal after prolonged periods of administration may exacerbate the anxiety and precipitate a withdrawal syndrome characterized by anxiety, insomnia, confusion, tremors, muscle twitching, and convulsions.

7. Observe and report symptoms of cholestatic jaundice such as high fever, abdominal pain, nausea, diarrhea, or rash. Withhold drug and report yellowing of the skin, mucous membranes, or sclera of the eyes.

8. The patient should be instructed to immediately report any symptoms of blood dyscrasias such as sore throat, fever, weakness, or easy bruising.

ANTIDEPRESSANT AND ANTIMANIC AGENTS

Chapter 17

The *affective disorders*, depression and mania, are characterized by extreme changes in mood, which differ from normal fluctuations in mood in their intensity, duration, and the nature of the symptoms manifested. This chapter discusses drug treatments of these mood disorders.

AFFECTIVE DISORDERS

Depression is characterized by extreme sadness and some, but not necessarily all, of the following symptoms: sleep disturbances, most commonly, insomnia, lack of energy, loss of interest in family, job, or other activities; feelings of guilt, helplessness, and worthlessness, agitation, or retardation; disturbances in thinking or concentration; and recurrent thoughts of suicide or death. In the absence of treatment, a depressive episode may persist for many months, followed by spontaneous remission.

Depressive illnesses are classified as reactive or endogenous, on the basis of their presumed etiology. *Reactive (exogenous) de-*

pression results from environmental or emotional stresses, frustrations, or losses. Certain drugs, including the oral contraceptives, reserpine, and high doses of the glucocorticoid steroids have been observed to cause depression in some patients. By contrast, *endogenous depressive disorders* are of unknown etiology and are thought to have a biochemical basis and a genetic predisposition.

Mania is characterized by extreme euphoria or irritability and some of the following symptoms: hyperactivity, apparent lack of fatigue, decreased sleep, and distractability, with many projects initiated but quickly abandoned. A manic episode persists an average of 3 months in the absence of treatment.

Affective disorders are often classified as *bipolar*, characterized by depression and mania, or *unipolar*, characterized only by depression. There appears to be a strong genetic predisposition for bipolar manic-depressive illnesses. The treatment of depression and mania, respectively, will be discussed next.

ANTIDEPRESSANTS

Two major classes of drugs are employed for the treatment of depression, namely, the monoamine oxidase (MAO) inhibitors and the tricyclic antidepressants (Table 17-1). Since the MAO inhibitors are less effective and more toxic and are capable of interacting with foods and beverages and many other drug classes to produce adverse reactions, these antidepressants have fallen into disfavor in recent years. In rare cases, the central nervous system stimulants dextroamphetamine (Dexedrine) and methylphenidate (Ritalin) are used to treat short-lived and mild exogenous depressive disorders. The pharmacology of these stimulants will be discussed in Chapter 22. Nursing implica-

tions associated with the use of the antidepressants appear at the end of this chapter.

While the neurochemical basis for depression has not been determined with certitude, indirect evidence suggests that deficient amounts of the biogenic amines (norepinephrine and/or serotonin) may exist. Drugs that elevate the mood are thought to act by increasing the concentrations of biogenic amines available to interact at receptor sites in critical areas of the brain associated with mood. As implied by their name, the MAO inhibitors block MAO, an enzyme that catalyzes the inactivation of serotonin, norepinephrine, and dopamine. The tricyclic antidepressants inhibit the reuptake of norepinephrine and serotonin after their endogenous release, thus making one or both of these biogenic amines available to interact with their respective receptor sites; this class of antidepressants has little effect on dopamine reuptake or dopaminergic receptor sites. Dextroamphetamine stimulates the release of norepinephrine and dopamine from their nerve endings and also inhibits the reuptake of these catecholamines.

Monoamine Oxidase Inhibitors

During the course of clinical trials conducted in 1951 designed to evaluate iproniazid (Marsilid) for the treatment of tuberculosis, it was observed that this drug produced a state of euphoria. This drug was later discovered to be an MAO inhibitor and was employed clinically as an antidepressant for a number of years.

The MAO inhibitors are of two chemical types, the hydrazides (isocarboxazid and phenelzine) and the nonhydrazides (tranylcypromine) (Table 17-1). The antidepressant properties of these drugs have been attributed to their ability to inhibit MAO, thereby increasing the brain concentrations of norepinephrine and serotonin and also producing central nervous stimulation. Since these

Table 17-1 Comparative Properties of Antidepressant Agents

Generic name	Trade name(s)	Usual adult oral daily dosage (mg)	Distinguishing properties
Monoamine Oxidase Inhibitors			
Isocarboxazid	Marplan	10-30	These two hydrazide MAO inhibitors possess questionable effectiveness. These drugs have a slow onset of action (2-4 wk), a long duration of action, and may cause postural hypotension, liver and blood disorders, and behavioral disturbances.
Phenelzine	Nardil	15-30	
Tranylcypromine	Parnate	20-30	This nonhydrazide MAO inhibitor possesses amphetamine-like stimulation. It has a faster onset of action than the hydrazides, is clinically more effective, and does not cause liver or blood disorders; postural hypotension commonly occurs.
Tricyclic Antidepressants			
Imipramine	Antipress, Imavate, Janimine, Presamine, SK-Pramine, Tofranil	50-150	Effective antidepressants, lacking stimulatory effects, with onset of action of 1-2 wk. Side effects include orthostatic hypotension and atropine-like effects (dry mouth, blurred vision, constipation, and urinary retention in men). Imipramine is useful for treatment of enuresis (bed wetting).
Desipramine	Norpramin, Pertofrane	75-150	
Amitriptyline	Elavil, Endep	50-150	Amitriptyline is a widely used and effective antidepressant with properties similar to imipramine, but more pronounced depression and lower incidence of atropine-like effects.
Nortriptyline	Aventyl	20-100	
Doxepin	Adapin, Sinequan	50-150	High incidence of sedation; antianxiety-antidepressant properties.
Protriptyline	Vivactil	10-40	Stimulant properties; useful in withdrawn and lethargic depressed patients. Should not be used in patients with anxiety. Produces more cardiovascular side effects than other tricyclics. In elderly patients, monitor cardiovascular function carefully if daily dose exceeds 20 mg.
Trimipramine	Surmontil	50-150	Indicated for treatment of mild depression; less effective in severe cases.

drugs are less effective, have a slower onset of action, and are more toxic than the tricyclic antidepressants, their contemporary usage is primarily limited to those patients who fail to respond favorably to the tricyclic agents.

Adverse effects Commonly encountered side effects associated with the MAO inhibitors include orthostatic hypotension, nervousness, insomnia, and, in high doses, tremors and convulsions. Hepatotoxicity and blood dyscrasias may occur after the use of the hydrazide derivatives.

Tranylcypromine and the other MAO inhibitors have been reported to produce severe headaches and sometimes fatal hypertensive crises in patients who have ingested

Table 17-2   Potential Interactions Involving Monamine Oxidase Inhibitors

MAO inhibitors	Interacting drug/class	Possible consequences
Isocarboxazid Phenelzine Tranylcypromine	Tricyclic antidepressants	Concurrent use has resulted in severe toxicity including excitation, fever, delirium, convulsions, and death; 10 da should elapse prior to administering tricyclics after last dose of MAO inhibitor.

	Sympathomimetic amines
	    Dextroamphetamine
	    Ephedrine
	    Metaraminol (Aramine)
	    Phenylephrine
	    Phenylpropanolamine
		MAO inhibitors block metabolism of many sympathomimetic amines resulting in marked rise in blood pressure, fever, convulsions, and death. Patients should be advised to use nonprescription cough and cold preparations containing these drugs with extreme caution.

	Meperidine (Demerol)	Potentiation of central depressing effects of meperidine (respiratory depression and hypotension), restlessness, muscle twitching, fever, and death. Combination is contraindicated.
	Barbiturates	Potentiation of barbiturate depression.
	Insulin Oral hypoglycemic agents	MAO inhibitors may potentiate the reduction in blood sugar levels when these drugs are administered to diabetic patients.
	Levodopa	Transitory elevation in blood pressure.

	Tyramine-rich foods and beverages
	    Cheeses (cheddar, Camembert,
	        Gruyére)
	    Wines (Chianti), beer
	    Chicken liver
	    Pickled herring
	    Broad beans
	    Bananas
		MAO inhibitors prevent normal metabolism of tyramine which accumulates and stimulates the release of norepinephrine. Adverse effects include severe headaches, hypertensive crises, heart palpitations, and possible death.

	Doxapram (Dopram)	Adverse cardiovascular effects of doxapram (hypertension, arrhythmias) are potentiated.

tyramine-rich foods and beverages. The nurse should warn patients taking these drugs about the hazards of such *drug-food interactions* (Table 17-2). The MAO inhibitors are also capable of inhibiting the metabolism of a wide range of drugs, thereby potentiating their toxicity (Table 17-2). Severe adverse reactions have been associated with the combined use of the MAO inhibitors and tricyclic antidepressants.

Tricyclic Antidepressants

In 1958 clinical trials designed to investigate the potential antipsychotic activity of phenothiazine-related compounds revealed that imipramine (Tofranil) was an effective anti-depressant agent. Imipramine, amitriptyline (Elavil), and chemically-related compounds (Table 17-1) have been clearly demonstrated to be effective for the relief of the symptoms of endogenous depression and, to a lesser degree, reactive depression. Some tricyclic agents (amitriptyline, nortriptyline, doxepin) also possess sedative properties that make these drugs useful for the treatment of depression accompanied by anxiety.

The tricyclic agents do not produce acute central nervous system stimulation or euphoria. Patients receiving these drugs exhibit early signs of mood elevation and increased mental alertness and physical activity within days after the initiation of therapy; therapeutic benefit is usually obtained within 1 to 2 weeks, although drug administration is often continued for several months to achieve complete reversal of the depressive episode. The patient should be advised that complete clinical improvement may be slow and should be encouraged not to prematurely discontinue use of the medication. The dosage of both the tricyclics and MAO inhibitors should be gradually reduced.

Adverse effects The anticholinergic actions of the tricyclic agents are responsible for dryness of the mouth, blurred vision, constipation, and urinary retention. Other common side effects include hypotension, tachycardia, cardiac arrhythmias, and occasional allergic reactions, such as skin rashes and photosensitivity. Drug interactions involving this drug class appear in Table 17-3.

Doses of tricyclic agents in excess of 1,200 mg can cause severe toxicity, and fatalities are often observed at doses exceeding 2,500 mg. Symptoms of overdosage include depression of respiratory and cardiac function, fever, and neuromuscular irritability. The most dangerous aspects of drug overdosage are disturbances of cardiac rhythm and conduction, resulting in *arrhythmias* and cardiac arrest. These potentially life-threatening effects are effectively treated with anticholinesterase agents, such as pyridostigmine (Mestinon) or physostigmine (eserine). Drug elimination can be enhanced by forced diuresis with mannitol.

ANTIMANIC AGENTS

Acute manic episodes are effectively controlled with phenothiazine or butyrophenone antipsychotic agents (Chapter 15) or with lithium carbonate.

Phenothiazines and Butyrophenones

The phenothiazine derivative *chlorpromazine* (Thorazine) was among the first drugs found to be effective in suppressing manic excitement and agitation. Control of a severe manic episode is achieved by initiating therapy with intramuscular drug administration followed by orally administered chlorpromazine. A return to normal behavior is generally achieved within 4 to 5 days. Although

Table 17-3   Potential Interactions Involving Tricyclic Antidepressants and Lithium Carbonate

Drug	Interacting drug/class	Possible consequences
Tricyclics	MAO inhibitors	See Table 17-2.
Amitriptyline Nortriptyline Doxepin	Alcohol, other central nervous system depressants	Additive, central depression resulting in potential physical or mental impairment.
Tricyclics, exept doxepin	Guanethidine (Ismelin) Methyldopa (Aldomet)	Antagonism of the antihypertensive effects with loss of control of blood pressure.
Imipramine	Chlorpromazine (Thorazine) Haloperidol (Haldol) Anticholinergic agents	Additive atropine-like effects.
Lithium	Vasopressin (endogenous)	Lithium may interfere with antidiuretic action of vasopressin, resulting in diabetes insipidus, which causes excessive urination.
Lithium	Diuretics	Diuretic-induced sodium depletion enhances lithium toxicity. Conversely, increased sodium intake interferes with antimanic effects of lithium.

other antipsychotic phenothiazines have been used with some success, the pronounced sedative properties of chlorpromazine make it the phenothiazine of choice.

Haloperidol (Haldol), a butyrophenone, substantially reduces behavioral and motor hyperactivity within 3 days after the initiation of therapy, and in a high percentage of cases, abolishes all manic symptoms within 4 to 5 days. Recent studies suggest that chlorpromazine and haloperidol possess approximately equivalent antimanic activity, with haloperidol superior in certain aspects.

Lithium Carbonate

In normal individuals, therapeutic doses of lithium have no behavioral effects, and, in this respect, it differs from all other psychotherapeutic agents. This drug produces a normalization of mood and motor activity, making the manic patient feel normal in the absence of a "drugged feeling."

Lithium carbonate (Eskalith, Lithonate, Lithane) has been shown to be at least as effective as chlorpromazine for the treatment of acute mania and also appears to be useful when employed chronically to prevent manic episodes and wide mood swings. Since the full antimanic effects of lithium are only manifested after 7 to 10 days of treatment, this drug is commonly administered with an antipsychotic agent to obtain more immediate beneficial effects.

Optional therapeutic effects are achieved when plasma lithium concentrations are maintained between 0.9 to 1.4 milliequivalents per liter, levels normally obtained when 1,800 mg are administered in divided daily doses. Adverse effects observed at normal therapeutic doses include fatigue, slurred speech, muscle weakness, and tremors. Toxic doses of lithium cause muscle rigidity, convulsions, and coma. Table 17-3 summarizes drug interactions involving lithium. Nursing implications appear at the end of this chapter.

Antidepressants and Lithium:
nursing implications

1. Preparation and education of the patient and family is essential to promote patient compliance. Information to be included should be the nature of depressive illnesses; that approximately 2–3 wk of drug therapy are required for clinical improvement to be manifested; that the drug must be taken precisely as prescribed; and that return appointments must be kept to evaluate the effectiveness of therapy.

2. Monitor pulse and blood pressure when therapy is initiated and at regular intervals thereafter. To avoid hypotensive reactions, instruct the patient to make changes in position slowly, avoid standing in place for long periods of time, and avoid hot baths or showers, which cause vasodilation.

3. Advise the patient to avoid the use of any other prescription or nonprescription drugs or alcoholic beverages while taking antidepressant drugs and for 2–3 wk after discontinuing them without first consulting their physician.

4. Monoamine oxidase inhibitors (MAOI) and tricyclic antidepressants should not be administered together without the expressed consent of the physician, who should be

fully apprised of the potential dangers of this combination. At least 10 days should elapse between discontinuing MAOI therapy and initiating the use of tricyclics.

5. Observe the patient closely for indications of contemplated suicide. Patients receiving these drugs are most prone to attempt suicide when the response to therapy begins and after they emerge from the depths of depression.

6. Observe diabetic patients for potential loss of control of blood sugar. MAOI potentiate the hypoglycemic effects of insulin and sulfonylurea compounds; reduced dosage may be necessary. Tricyclics may produce hypoglycemia or hyperglycemia in some patients.

Monoamine Oxidase Inhibitors

1. Maximum antidepressant effects may require 2-6 wk. If no beneficial effects occur after 3-4 wk, the MAOI is usually discontinued and another drug substituted for it.

2. Ingestion of foods containing tyramine can cause a severe hypertensive reaction. Provide the patient or a responsible family member with a list of foods and beverages to be avoided during therapy and for 2-3 wk after therapy has been discontinued (see Table 17-2). Excessive use of beverages containing caffeine (coffee, tea, cocoa, cola) may increase the risk of a hypertensive reaction.

3. Instruct the patient to immediately report any headache or palpitations, symptoms which may indicate an impending hypertensive crisis.

4. Caution the patient to avoid overexertion because these drugs may suppress anginal pain, which serves as a warning of myocardial ischemia.

5. The patient receiving prolonged therapy may develop optic damage. Changes in red-green vision may be the first indication of such damage and should be checked periodically.

6. Medication for the treatment of drug overdose should be readily available: phenothiazine antipsychotic agents for agitation; phentolamine (Regitine) for excessive pressor response.

Tricyclic Antidepressants

1. Maximum antidepressant effects generally appear within 2-3 wk. If no therapeutic response is observed after 4 to 8 wk, the drug is usually discontinued and another substituted.

2. The patient should be instructed to report fever, malaise, sore throat, or sore mouth, which are early signs of agranulocytosis. The patient should be placed in protective isolation pending results of blood evaluation.

3. Check for abdominal distention, which may result from urinary retention or constipation.

4. High doses increase the frequency of seizures in epileptic patients and may cause eliptiform seizures in normal individuals.

Lithium Carbonate (Eskalith, Lithane, Lithonate)

1. During initiation of therapy, plasma lithium levels and blood tests should be determined once or twice weekly and monthly thereafter.

2. The patient and his or her family should be alerted that tremors, diarrhea, weakness, and fatigue are early signs of drug overdosage. Lithium therapy should be immediately discontinued, and the patient should report to the physician.

3. The patient should be advised to maintain a high intake of fluids (31 daily) and a normal salt intake.

SUPPLEMENTARY READINGS

Baldessarini, R. J., "Drugs and the Treatment of Psychiatric Disorders," in *Goodman and Gilman's The Pharmacological Basis of Therapeutics* (6th ed.), ed. A. G. Gilman, L. S. Goodman, and A. Gilman, Chapter 19, pp. 391–447. New York: Macmillan, Inc., 1980.

Barchas, J. D., P. A. Berger, R. D. Ciaranello, and G. R. Elliott, eds., *Psychopharmacology—From Theory to Practice*. New York: Oxford University Press, 1977.

Clark, W. G., and J. delGiudice, eds., *Principles of Psychopharmacology*, 2nd ed. New York: Academic Press, Inc., 1978.

Cole, J. O., A. M. Freedman, and A. J. Friedhoff, eds., *Psychopathology and Psychopharmacology*. Baltimore: Johns Hopkins University Press, 1973.

DiMascio, A., and R. I. Shader, eds., *Clinical Handbook of Psychopharmacology* New York: Science House, 1970.

Frazer, A., and A. Winokur, eds., *Biological Bases of Psychiatric Disorders*. New York: Spectrum Publications, Inc., 1977.

Hollister, L. E., "Adverse Reactions to Psychotherapeutic Drugs," in *Drug Treatment of Mental Disorders*. Edited by L. L. Simpson, pp. 267–88. New York: Raven Press, 1976.

————, *Clinical Pharmacology of Psychotherapeutic Drugs*. New York: Churchill Livingstone, 1978.

Klein, D. F., and J. M. Davis, *Diagnosis and Drug Treatment of Psychiatric Disorders*. Baltimore: The Williams & Wilkins Company, 1969.

Lipton, M. A., A. DiMascio, and K. F. Killam, ed., *Psychopharmacology: A Generation of Progress*. New York: Raven Press, 1978.

Newton, M., K. L. Godbey, D. W. Newton, and A. L. Godbey, "How Can You Improve the Effectiveness of Psychotic Drug Therapy?" *Nursing '78* 3(7): 46–55 (1978).

Reading, A., and T. N. Wise, eds., "Symposium on Psychiatry in Internal Medicine," *Medical Clinics of North America*, 61(4): 701–941 (1977).

Rodman, M. J., "Controlling Acute and Chronic Schizophrenia," *RN* 41(4): 75–83 (1978).

Shader, R. I., ed., *Manual of Psychiatric Therapeutics*. Boston: Little, Brown & Company, 1975.

Shader, R. I., and A. DiMascio, *Psychotropic Drug Side Effects: Clinical and Theoretical Perspectives*. Baltimore: Williams & Wilkins Company, 1970.

Simpson, L. L., ed., *Drug Treatment of Mental Disorders*. New York: Raven Press, 1976.

Wheatley, D., *Psychopharmacology in Family Practice*. London: William Heinemann Medical Books, Ltd., 1973.

ANTIEPILEPTIC AGENTS

Reports of epilepsy appear in medical writings authored thousands of years ago. While we know that the behavioral changes associated with this disorder are the consequence of abnormalities in the functional activity of neurons in the brain, until the last century its etiology was generally ascribed to the presence of supernatural forces within the patient.

Epilepsy is among the most common neurological disorders, affecting approximately one million individuals in the United States. While the available drugs cannot cure epilepsy, antiepileptic agents are capable of effectively controlling seizures, reducing their frequency and severity in a large percentage of patients. This chapter first discusses the nature of epilepsy and then considers the most important antiepileptic agents employed in contemporary therapeutics.

EPILEPSY

Epilepsy (more accurately, "the epilepsies") is a collective term referring to neurological disorders characterized by alterations in the normal states of consciousness resulting from a sudden, excessive, and self-limiting firing of neurons within the brain. The abnormal electrical brain waves generated during an epileptic seizure can be detected utilizing the electroencephalogram (EEG); the recordings generated are employed for the differential diagnosis of the specific type of seizure and the selection of the most appropriate drug for therapy.

In view of the social stigma associated with the designation of a patient as an epileptic, as well as the restrictions in jobs and driving that often follow, the nurse should recognize that not all patients with seizures are epileptics and not all epileptics have seizures.

A number of specific factors have been identified as being responsible for precipitating epilepsy, although in most cases this condition is of unknown origin. Some of the known causes include brain tumors, head trauma, high fevers, infections (encephalitis, meningitis), metabolic disturbances, and an inadequate supply of oxygen or glucose to the brain. Seizures may also be observed following abrupt withdrawal of chronic administration of alcohol, barbiturates, and nonbarbiturate sedative-hypnotics.

Classification of the Epilepsies

Epilepsies are classified as generalized or localized seizures. *Generalized seizures* (including grand mal and petit mal) are bilaterally symmetric, do not have a local onset, and are characterized by motor disturbances or disturbed consciousness. *Partial seizures* (including focal and psychomotor seizures) begin locally and do not generally result in the loss of consciousness. Patients may experience more than one type of seizure or have mixed seizures on a given occasion.

Grand mal seizures ("generalized tonic-clonic seizures" is now the preferred designation) are most frequently encountered by the nurse; 90 percent of all epileptic patients experience this type of condition. Prior to the loss of consciousness, many patients experience an aura or unusual sensory sensation. While the patient is unconscious, rapid extension of the muscles of the back and limbs and then jerking movements of the arms and legs are seen. Breath holding, tongue biting and swallowing, and involuntary urination or defecation may occur. Within minutes after the onset of an attack, the patient regains consciousness and, thereafter, may fall into a deep sleep for several minutes to hours; upon awakening the patient often has no recollection of the events that have transpired.

In *status epilepticus*, a medical emergency, there is a series of consecutive or continuous grand mal convulsions, which may last for hours or even days with variable intervals between seizures in the absence of the restoration of consciousness. Nursing responsibilities when observing a seizure include protecting the patient from injury, maintaining an open airway, and recording a description of the seizure.

In children and adolescents, the most common type of epilepsy is *petit mal* or *absences*. These seizures result in a brief lapse of consciousness (of 1 to 30 seconds in duration), during which time the patient is motionless and exhibits a flickering of the eyelids or a gap in conversation. Teachers may mistake such seizures as a lack of attention on the part of the child. In some variants of this disorder, muscle jerking of the limbs occurs.

Focal seizures originate in one part of the body and may spread. *Focal motor* or *Jacksonian seizures* often begin with a twitching of the muscles of the fingers, which spread up the arm and down the leg on the same side of the body. If both sides of the body are involved, a grand mal seizure may result.

Psychomotor or *temporal lobe epilepsy* ("partial seizures with complex symptomatology" is the current preferred designation) is extremely variable in nature; it is characterized by a temporary clouding of consciousness, during which period the patient repetitively performs automatic grimaces, movements of the limbs, or bizarre behavorial acts.

ANTIEPILEPTIC AGENTS

No single drug is capable of controlling all types of epilepsy (Table 18-1). The mechanisms of action of drugs in this therapeutic class are highly complex. Available evidence suggests that most of the commonly employed drugs exert their effects on normal neurons that surround the epileptic focus to prevent the spread of the hyperexcitable discharge to other normal parts of the brain.

Antiepileptic agents control but do not cure epilepsy. To achieve maximum therapeutic benefits from such drugs, the patient must take them as directed, on a daily basis for years or even a lifetime. Ideally, the drug should prevent seizures without producing drowsiness or impairing the ability of the

Table 18-1 Antiepileptic Agents

Generic name	Trade name	Therapeutic uses[a]	Daily oral adult dose (mg)	Common side effects	Remarks
Phenobarbital[b]		GM, PsM	100-200	Sedation.	Highly effective. Abrupt withdrawal may precipitate seizures.
Mephobarbital	Mebaral	GM	120-600	Sedation.	See Phenobarbital. Metabolized to phenobarbital.
Metharbital	Gemonil	GM	300-800	Sedation.	Metabolized to barbital.
Primidone	Mysoline	GM, PsM	500-1,500	Sedation, dizziness.	Metabolized to phenobarbital.
Phenytoin[b] (diphenylhydantoin)	Dilantin Dihycon Ekko	GM, PsM	300-600	Ataxia, nystagmus, diplopia, gingival hypertrophy, excitement.	Highly effective, no sedation, check plasma levels.
Mephenytoin	Mesantoin	GM, PsM	200-600	Sedation, blood and liver disorders.	Less gingival hypertrophy.
Ethotoin	Peganone	GM, PsM	2,000-3,000	Skin rash, gastrointestinal upset, drowsiness.	Less toxic, but less effective than phenytoin.
Ethosuximide[b]	Zarontin	PM	500-1,000	Gastrointestinal upset, drowsiness, blood dyscrasias.	Highly effective.
Methsuximide	Celontin	PM, PsM	300-1,200	Similar to ethosuximide.	Less effective than ethosuximide. Used with other drugs for PsM.
Phensuximide	Milontin	PM	2,000-4,000	Similar to ethosuximide.	Limited effectiveness.
Trimethadione	Tridione	PM	400-1,500	Sedation, hemeralopia, decreases neutrophils.	Effective, but more toxic than ethosuximide.
Paramethadione	Paradione	PM	900-1,500	Similar to trimethadione.	Fewer adverse effects than trimethadione.
Diazepam[b]	Valium	SE	2-20 mg slow IV	Thrombosis, cardiovascular failure.	Highly effective for controlling status epilepticus.
Clonazepam[b]	Clonopin	PM, MS	1.5	Drowsiness, confusion, hallucinations.	New drug, useful substitute for ethosuximide.
Carbamazepine	Tegretol	GM, PsM	600-1,200	Gastric upset, visual problems, blood dyscrasias, cardiovascular disorders, atropine-like effects.	Effective antiepileptic and for treatment of trigeminal neuralgia. Potential for severe toxicity.

Table 18-1 (Continued)

Generic name	Trade name	Therapeutic uses[a]	Daily dose adult dose (mg)	Common side effects	Remarks
Acetazolamide	Diamox	PM	500–1,000	Drowsiness, paresthesia.	Rapid development of tolerance. Used in combination with other antiepileptic drugs.
Phenacemide	Phenurone	PsM	1,500–2,000	Adverse personality disorders, hepatitis, blood dyscrasias, skin rashes.	Effective against all epileptic types; severe toxicity limits use to PsM when all other drugs fail.
Sodium valproate Valproic acid	Depakane	PM, PsM	1,200	Gastrointestinal upset, nausea, drowsiness, atoxia; potential liver and blood disorders.	Potentially useful drug for PsM; new drug requiring more evaluation. Liver function should be assessed prior to and every 2 mo after initiation of therapy.

[a] Key to abbreviations: GM = grand mal and focal seizures; MS = myoclonic spasms and akinetic seizures; PM = petit mal (absences); PsM = psychomotor (temporal lobe) epilepsy; SE = status epilepticus.
[b] Most widely prescribed.

patient to normally carry out daily activities. Because the drug may often be employed for a protracted period of time, it should be devoid of chronic toxicity, tolerance development, or abuse potential. Among the most commonly prescribed drugs are phenobarbital, phenytoin, ethosuximide, and clonazepam. The properties of these agents and related alternative drugs are summarized in Table 18-1; drug interactions involving antiepileptic agents are summarized in Table 18-2 and nursing implications appear at the end of this chapter.

Phenobarbital

Phenobarbital, unlike most other barbiturates (Chapter 13), possesses antiepileptic properties at doses that do not cause excessive drowsiness. Mephobarbital (Mebaral) and primidone (Mysoline) are metabolized to phenobarbital in vivo.

Phenobarbital is the oldest and among the least toxic drugs available for the treatment of *grand mal epilepsy*, focal seizures, and psychomotor epilepsy. This drug is not effective for the control of petit mal and may even worsen this condition.

While phenobarbital is usually well tolerated by patients, common side effects include sedation and dizziness. Chronic administration of this drug is safe and development of a dependent state is rarely a problem. Since abrupt withdrawal may precipitate seizures in epileptic patients, the dosage of this drug should be gradually reduced over a period of many weeks if discon-

Table 18-2   Potential Drug Interactions Involving Antiepileptic Agents

Antiepileptic class/drug	Interacting drug/class	Possible consequences
Barbiturates Phenobarbital	See Table 13-3.	
Hydantoins Phenytoin	Chloramphenicol (Chloromycetin) Dicoumarol anticoagulants Disulfiram (Antabuse) Isoniazid (INH) Oral contraceptives Sulfonamides	Drugs inhibit liver metabolism of phenytoin, causing an increase in plasma levels, potentially increasing its toxicity.
	Salicylates (aspirin) Sulfonamides	High doses of these drugs may displace phenytoin from plasma-binding sites, potentially increasing its toxicity.
	Alcohol (ethanol) Barbiturates (?)	These drugs increase the rate of phenytoin metabolism, which decreases plasma levels and may increase seizure frequency. Barbiturate-induced effects are variable and of questionable clinical significance.
	Folic acid	Phenytoin may induce folic acid deficiency, which may result in megaloblastic anemia. Administration of folic acid may increase rate of metabolism which may increase seizure frequency.
	Tricyclic antidepressants	These drugs may induce seizures, especially in high doses.
	Dexamethasone and corticosteroids Doxycycline (Vibramycin)	Phenytoin increases rate of metabolism of these drugs potentially reducing their clinical effectiveness.

Benzodiazepines
  Clonazepam
  Diazepam
Valproic acid
	Central nervous system depressants
	  Alcohol
	  Antianxiety agents
	  Antidepressants
	    Monoamine oxidase inhibitors
	    Tricyclic antidepressants
	  Antipsychotic agents
	  Barbiturates
	  Narcotics
	  Nonbarbiturate sedative-hypnotics
		Additive CNS depression impairing mental and physical function which may interfere with the safe operation of automobiles or machinery, or engaging in other potentially hazardous activities.

Acetazolamide	Amphetamines Procainamide (Pronestyl) Quinidine	Acetazolamide causes alkalinization of the urine, increasing renal tubular reabsorption of these drugs; this enhances their effects.
	Salicylates	Acetazolamide causes alkalinization of the urine, decreasing renal tubular reabsorption of these drugs; this decreases their effects.
	Phenytoin	Enhanced risk of phenytoin-induced osteomalacia.
	Methenamine	Alkinization of the urine antagonizes the anti-infective activity of methenamine.
Carbamazepine	Monoamine oxidase inhibitor antidepressants	Although interaction remains a theoretical hazard, concurrent administration within 14 days of each other is contraindicated.
	Doxycycline (Vibramycin) Oral anticoagulants	Carbamazepine increases rate of metabolism of these drugs, potentially reducing their clinical effectiveness.

Table 18-2 (Continued)

Antiepileptic class/drug	Interacting drug/class	Possible consequences
	Chloramphenicol (Chloromycetin)	Increased risk of bone marrow depression resulting in potentially fatal blood dyscrasias.
Valproic acid	CNS depressants See Benzodiazepines.	Additive CNS depression.
	Aspirin Warfarin	Valproic acid inhibits the second phase of platelet aggregation. Caution should be exercised when coadministering drugs that modify blood coagulation.

tinuation of treatment is contemplated. In the event that barbiturate allergy or intolerance requires the abrupt termination of phenobarbital, another antiepileptic agent such as phenytoin should be substituted at an equieffective dosage.

Phenytoin

Phenytoin ([*diphenylhydantoin*] Dilantin) is highly effective for the treatment of *grand mal* and psychomotor seizures. Unlike phenobarbital, with which it is often used in combination therapy, phenytoin controls seizures without producing sedation. Phenytoin has been observed to abolish seizures in 60 to 65 percent of grand mal patients and reduce the severity and frequency of seizures in an additional 20 percent.

Recent studies have demonstrated that the antiepileptic effectiveness and toxicity of phenytoin can be correlated with *plasma concentrations* of this drug. Optimal anticonvulsant effects are obtained when drug plasma levels are between 1.0 to 2.0 mg/dl; lower plasma concentrations are generally ineffective, while higher levels are associated with neurotoxicity. Moreover, phenytoin has a long plasma half-life, which, in the absence of gastric distress, permits administration of a single daily dose.

The most common side effects are ataxia, nystagmus, and double vision; excitement and tremors sometimes occur. About 20 percent of all patients experience *gingival hypertrophy*, an overgrowth of the gums. This irreversible problem, most commonly observed in children and young adults, is cosmetically unsightly but does not require termination of drug administration. Regular and vigorous brushing of teeth may be of value in minimizing this condition, with surgical correction sometimes necessary. Other adverse effects that occur less frequently include the appearance of facial hair in females, allergic rashes, and liver disorders. Potential drug interactions involving phenytoin are given in Table 18-2.

Ethosuximide

Ethosuximide (Zarontin) is the drug of choice for the treatment of *petit mal*, completely controlling seizures in 50 percent of the patients and reducing seizure frequency in another 25 percent.

Frequent side effects include gastric upset, loss of appetite, and drowsiness. Blood dyscrasias and liver dysfunction have been reported.

Trimethadione

Formerly the drug of choice for the control of *petit mal* seizures, trimethadione (Tridione) is perhaps less effective and certainly more toxic than ethosuximide. Common side effects include sedation and hemeralopia, a snowy appearance of objects in bright lights, which may be alleviated by the use of sun glasses. Many patients experience a reduction in neutrophils. Less frequent, but potentially life-threatening, are drug-induced allergic reactions and impairments of liver and kidney function. In the opinion of many neurologists, trimethadione should be reserved for the treatment of petit mal seizures only in those patients who cannot tolerate ethosuximide or fail to obtain seizure control with that drug.

Diazepam

Diazepam (Valium), used primarily for the treatment of anxiety (Chapter 16), is employed with great success for the emergency treatment of *status epilepticus*. Effective control of seizures has been observed in 80 to 90 percent of the patients after an intravenous injection. Since the duration of action of this drug is only 30 to 60 minutes, the nurse should exercise extreme vigilance for the reoccurrence of seizures.

GENERAL THERAPEUTIC PRINCIPLES

To date, drugs have proved to be the only effective treatment for the control of seizure disorders. The following general principles are presented to provide the nurse with an understanding of those factors that will permit optimization of the antiepileptic drug therapy.

Prior to the initiation of drug therapy, the EEG recordings or the patient's history (or both) should be used to accurately determine the specific type of epileptic seizure. The use of an inappropriate drug, predicated upon an incorrect diagnosis, will provide the patient with little or no benefit and may increase the frequency and severity of seizures. An attempt should be made to adjust the dosage of these drugs to achieve optimal plasma concentrations, maximizing the control of seizures while minimizing the occurrence of drug-induced toxicity. Many patients benefit from the judicious use of more than one antiepileptic agent.

Among the many possible causes of the unsuccessful treatment of epilepsy include improper diagnosis, inaccurate choice of drugs, or inadequate doses of an appropriate drug; drug-drug interactions (Table 18-2); failure of the patient to take the drug as prescribed; use of alcoholic beverages; lack of rest or the onset of illness.

There appears to be an association between the use of antiepileptic agents (phenobarbital and phenytoin, in particular) and *birth defects*. While over 90 percent of epileptic mothers give birth to normal babies, the incidence of birth defects is two to three times the normal rate. On the other hand, abrupt termination of drug administration may precipitate status epilepticus, jeopardizing the health and well-being of the mother and fetus. Depending upon the frequency and severity of seizures, it may be possible to reduce the drug dosage required to control seizures, especially during the first trimester of pregnancy.

Antiepileptic Drugs:
nursing implications

1. Preparation and education of the family about epilepsy is essential to promote compliance with the treatment regimen. The following directions should be included: carry an identification card or jewelry with pertinent medical information; eat a well-balanced diet; take medication exactly as prescribed; continue close medical supervision while taking antiepileptic drugs; report periods of increased stress and significant drug-induced side effects to physician; take drug(s) with food or liquid to minimize gastro-intestinal distress.

2. Tell a responsible family member how to care for patient during a seizure and what to observe and record.

3. During the initiation of therapy, instruct the patient to avoid operating an automobile or machinery or performing other potentially hazardous tasks requiring mental alertness and physical coordination; these drugs may cause drowsiness and dizziness. These symptoms are dose-related and often disappear with continued drug administration.

4. Advise the patient that alcohol ingestion may interfere with the beneficial effects of the medication or precipitate seizures by decreasing the seizure threshold.

5. Advise the patient to report symptoms that may indicate a hypersensitivity reaction to the drug: rash, fever, severe headache, stomatitis, rhinitis.

6. Have the patient watch for signs that may indicate hematological toxicity: sore throat, easy bruising, petechiae, and nose bleeds.

7. Have the patient watch for signs that may indicate hepatotoxicity: jaundice, dark urine, anorexia, and abdominal pain.

8. Other medication may be prescribed to prevent complications of antiepileptic therapy: folic acid supplement to prevent megaloblastic anemia; vitamin D supplement to prevent hypocalcemia.

9. Instruct the patient to report CNS symptoms that may indicate drug overdosage: nystagmus, diplopia, blurred vision, extrapyramidal disturbances, and increased seizure activity.

10. Caution the patient not to alter prescribed drug regimen. Drug must be gradually withdrawn over a 1- to 3-mo period. Abrupt withdrawal may precipitate seizures.

11. Advise women of childbearing age to discuss potential teratogenic effects of the antiepileptic medication with their physician before becoming pregnant.

12. Observe infants of nursing mothers receiving antiepileptic medication for signs of toxicity.

Phenytoin (Dilantin)

1. Gingival hyperplasia appears most commonly in children and adolescents. This can be minimized by daily brushing with a soft tooth brush, flossing to remove dental plaque, and gum massage.

2. Drug may cause excessive hair on the face and trunk and may cause acne.

Trimethadione (Tridione)

1. Alert the patient or family to recognize and report signs of renal toxicity: edema, urinary frequency, burning on urination, and albuminuria (cloudy urine). Emphasize importance of periodic urine analysis.

2. Hemeralopia (blurred vision in bright light) can be relieved by use of dark glasses.

SUPPLEMENTARY READINGS

Aird, R. B., and D. M. Woodbury, *Management of Epilepsy*. Springfield, Ill.: Charles C Thomas, Publisher, 1974.

Browne, T. R., and J. K. Penry, "Benzodiazepines in the Treatment of Epilepsy," *Epilepsia* **14**: 277–310 (1973).

Conomy, J. P., and J. O. McNamara, "Emergency Management of the Patient with Seizures," *Postgraduate Medicine* **55**: 59–66, 71–74 (1974).

Ferriss, G. S., ed., *Treatment of Epilepsy Today*. Oradell, N. J.: Medical Economics, 1978.

Kutt, H., "Anticonvulsant Blood Levels in the Management of Epileptic Patients," *Clinical Neuropharmacology*, **3**: 1–13 (1978).

Jasper, H. H., A. A. Ward, Jr., and A. Pope, eds., *Basic Mechanism of the Epilepsies*. Boston: Little, Brown & Company, 1969.

Lennox, W. G., and M. A. Lennox, *Epilepsy and Related Disorders*. 2 vols. Boston: Little, Brown & Company, 1960.

Pinder, R. M., R. M. Brogden, T. M. Speight, and G. S. Avery, "Sodium Valproate: A Review of its Pharmacological Properties and Therapeutic Efficacy in Epilepsy," *Drugs* **13**: 81–123 (1977).

Richens, A., *Drug Treatment of Epilepsy*. Chicago: Year Book Medical Publishers, Inc. 1976.

Swift, N., "Helping Patients Live with Seizures," *Nursing '78* **8**(6): 24–31 (1978).

Wiley, L., "Epilepsy Nursing," *Nursing '74* **4**(1): 30–45 (1974).

Woodbury, D. M., J. K. Penry, and R. P. Schmidt, eds., *Antiepileptic Drugs*. New York: Raven Press, 1972.

DRUG TREATMENT OF PARKINSON'S DISEASE

Chapter 19

In recent years dramatic advances have been made in our appreciation of the biochemical and neurophysiological basis for Parkinson's disease. This basic knowledge has led to the introduction and successful use of levodopa for the treatment of this chronic disease of the central nervous system. Prior to considering the drug treatment of parkinsonism, this disease, which afflicts approximately one million Americans, will be briefly examined.

PARKINSON'S DISEASE

Parkinson's disease is readily identified by the appearance of three cardinal symptoms, namely, rigidity, tremor, and bradykinesia. *Rigidity* is the tendency of the body to move as a block, with a loss of spontaneous associated movements in the upper trunk of the body. The parkinsonian *pill rolling tremor* is slow and coarse; it increases when the patient is subjected to stress and diminishes when the individual is engaged in purposeful movements. *Bradykinesia* and *akinesia* are terms that refer to a slowdown or cessation of all voluntary movements, with the result that the patient has great difficulty in initiating such movements. In advanced cases, these represent the most disabling symptoms of the disease and require nursing assistance for the patient.

Other symptoms associated with parkinsonism include mask-like facial expressions ("reptilian stare"), impaired dexterity, disorders of gait (characterized by short, shuffling steps and stooped posture), speech disorders, oculogyric crises (involuntary movements of the eyes), and autonomic dysfunctions, including salivation and excessive sweating.

Etiology of Parkinsonism

While in some cases the cause of this disease is unknown or idiopathic, its etiology has been identified in many patients. Etiological factors include postencephalic parkinsonism, a sequela of the 1917–1925 epidemic of encephalitis lethargica (von Economo's disease); arteriosclerotic parkinsonism; and chemically induced parkinsonism resulting from exposure to high concentrations of carbon monoxide and carbon disulfide (air pollutants) or manganese by mine workers.

With the introduction of potent psychotherapeutic agents for the treatment of mental illnesses in the 1950s, *drug-induced parkinsonism* made its first appearance on a widespread scale. Use of the butyrophenone (haloperidol), thioxanthene (chlorprothixene, thiothixene), and phenothiazine antipsychotic agents (Chapter 15) often produce parkinson-like side effects. The relative incidence of these effects differs among the various phenothiazine drugs; for example, there is a high incidence with fluphenazine,

perphenazine, prochlorperazine, and trifluoperazine, but a relative infrequent incidence with thioridazine. The tricyclic antidepressants and the antihypertensive agent reserpine have also been shown to produce these adverse neurological effects.

Biochemical Basis of Parkinsonism

The *basal ganglia* of the brain control voluntary motor functions and assist in coordination. Normal motor function is modulated by a balance between the excitatory influence of *cholinergic* nerves and the inhibitory influence of *dopaminergic* nerves. Patients with Parkinson's disease have been shown to have a *deficiency of dopamine* in the nigrostriatal neurons serving the striatum. This results in an imbalance of the dopaminergic-cholinergic influences, with the latter predominating.

ANTIPARKINSONISM DRUGS

Pharmacological treatment of parkinsonism restores the normal balance between the opposing cholinergic and dopaminergic influences. The excessive cholinergic influences may be reduced by administration of anticholinergic, muscarinic blocking agents (Chapter 7) or antihistamines that also possess anticholinergic activity (Chapter 53). Conversely, the deficient dopaminergic influences can be increased by administering levodopa, a compound converted to dopamine in the striatum.

Anticholinergic-Antihistaminic Antiparkinsonism Drugs

Prior to the introduction of levodopa in 1970, anticholinergic agents, or drugs with potent central muscarinic blocking properties, were the only compounds available for the treatment of Parkinson's disease.

The belladonna alkaloid scopolamine and newer synthetic anticholinergic agents with fewer peripheral side effects (Table 19-1) produce moderate symptomatic improvement in tremor, rigidity, and akinesia. The number of patients benefited by these drugs and the extent to which these patients improve is significantly less than is observed with levodopa. Unlike levodopa, these drugs are useful for the control of drug-induced parkinsonism.

The clinical benefits conferred by this class of drugs is limited by their atropine-like side effects, including dry mouth, blurred vision, drowsiness, dizziness, constipation, and urinary retention. Antihistamines and ethopropazine (Parsidol, a phenothiazine derivative) are less effective than the synthetic anticholinergic agents; while they produce fewer atropine-like side effects, they cause a higher incidence of sedation. Drug interactions involving these drugs are listed in Table 19-2.

LEVODOPA

Parkinsonism results from a deficiency of the neuronal transmitter, dopamine, in the stri-

Table 19-1   Antiparkinsonism Drugs

Class/generic name	Trade name	Usual oral adult dose (3–4 times daily)	Side effects of drug class	Remarks
Anticholinergics				
Benztropine	Cogentin	0.5–2.5, mg b.i.d., IM, IV: 1–4 mg	Atropine-like: blurred vision, dry mouth, dizziness, drowsiness, constipation, urinary retention. Antihistaminic: dizziness, drowsiness.	Effective drug with anticholinergic, antihistaminic properties for all types of parkinsonism. Long duration of action.
Biperiden	Akineton	1–2 mg	See Benztropine.	Same uses as benztropine.
Cycrimine	Pagitane	1.25–5 mg	See Benztropine.	Ineffective for drug-induced parkinsonism.
Procyclidine	Kemadrin	2–5 mg	See Benztropine.	Same uses as benztropine.
Trihexyphenidyl	Artane, Hexyphen, Pipanol, Tremin	1–5 mg	See Benztropine.	Same uses as benztropine; most widely used anticholinergic antiparkinson drug.
Antihistamines				
Chlorphenoxamine	Phenoxene	50–100 mg	Fewer atropine-like effects, drowsiness, confusion.	Less useful than anticholinergic agents above; effective for all types of parkinsonism.
Diphenhydramine	Benadryl	50 mg	See above; high incidence of drowsiness.	Same as chlorphenoxamine.
Orphenadrine	Disipal	50 mg	No sedation.	Same as chlorphenoxamine.

Table 19-1 (Continued)

Class/generic name	Trade name	Usual oral adult dose (3–4 times daily)	Side effects of drug class	Remarks
Phenothiazine				
Ethopropazine	Parsidol	25–50 mg	Dizziness, drowsiness, rarely agranulocytosis.	Possesses anticholinergic, antihistaminic properties; useful for controlling tremor. Effective for all types of parkinsonism.
Levodopa				
Levodopa [L-Dopa]	Bendopa, Dopar, Larodopa, Levopa, Parda	3–6 gm/o.d.	Nausea, vomiting, abnormal movements of mouth, behavioral changes, hypotension, cardiac arrhythmias, palpitations.	Most effective drug for treatment of parkinsonism, not drug-induced parkinsonism; onset of action several weeks.
Levodopa plus carbidopa	Sinemet	¼ daily dose of levodopa	Lower incidence of nausea, vomiting, and other peripheral effects than levodopa; neurological and behavioral effects may appear earlier and may be more severe.	Terminate levodopa at least 8 h prior to Sinemet; maximum maintenance dose of levodopa achieved more rapidly; can be used with pyridoxine; number of daily doses reduced; more beneficial therapeutic effects.
Miscellaneous				
Amantadine	Symmetrel	100 mg b.i.d.	Hyperexcitability, slurred speech; ataxia, insomnia, hallucinations	Less effective than levodopa, but fewer side effects; more rapid onset of action.
Bromocriptine		25–100 mg o.d.	Similar to levodopa, but less neurological and more behavioral and orthostatic hypotension.	Ergot derivative, dopaminergic stimulant. Somewhat less effective than levodopa; may be used in combination with levodopa. Useful for patients with "on-off" response to levodopa and dyskinesias. Marketed as Parlodel for of amenorrhea-galactorrhea.
Lergotrile			Nausea, vomiting, hypotension, and levodopa-like effects.	Similar to bromocriptine in chemistry, pharmacology, and adverse effects.

Table 19-2   Potential Drug Interactions Involving Antiparkinsonism Drugs

Antiparkinsonism drug/class	Interacting drug/class	Possible consequences
Anticholinergic agents	Amantadine (Symmetrel)	Amantadine potentiates the atropine-like behavioral side effects (confusion, hallucinations) when anticholinergic antiparkinsonism drugs are used in high concentrations.
Anticholinergic agents Antihistamines	Antidepressants Tricyclic Monoamine oxidase inhibitors	Additive anticholinergic side effects; MAOI potentiate side effects of antiparkinsonism drugs with anticholinergic properties.
Anticholinergic agents	Methotrimeprazine (Levoprome)	Possible worsening of parkinsonism symptoms.
Antihistamines	Central nervous system depressants	Additive CNS depression that may interfere with physical or mental performance.
Levodopa	Antidepressants, monoamine oxidase inhibitors	Combination may cause hypertension, flushing, cardiac palpitations.
	Antipsychotic agents Phenothiazines Butyrophenone Reserpine Antidepressants, tricyclics	These drugs block dopamine receptors in the brain producing parkinsonism side effects, thus antagonizing the beneficial effects of levodopa.
	Anticholinergic agents	These drugs decrease gastric emptying time, resulting in increased breakdown of levodopa in the stomach with less available for systemic absorption.
	Diazepam (Valium) Clonidine (Catapres) Methionine Papaverine	These drugs may worsen the parkinsonism syndrome.
	Pyridoxine (Vitamin B_6)	Antagonism of antiparkinsonism effects by increasing the decarboxylation of levodopa to dopamine in the periphery; dopamine cannot enter the brain. Well-established interaction; pyridoxine and vitamin products containing pyridoxine should be avoided by patients taking levodopa. Sinemet can be safely taken with pyridoxine.

atal region of the basal ganglia. Why not replace these deficient stores with dopamine? Unfortunately, oral administration of dopamine fails to cross the blood-brain barrier. By contrast, levodopa, the immediate biochemical precursor of dopamine, does enter the brain and is converted in the nigrostriatal nerve endings by a decarboxylation reaction to dopamine (Figure 19-1).

The beneficial effects of levodopa do not become clearly manifested until this drug is administered on a daily basis for many weeks or months; the patient may require reassurance to continue to take the medication in the absence of rapid and dramatic improvement. Akinesia is the first symptom to show improvement, followed by reductions in rigidity and tremors, as well as other symptoms. Between two-thirds and three-fourths of all parkinsonian patients shown significant improvement, with only 10 percent failing to benefit from this drug. Levodopa does not cure this disease; if drug therapy is terminated, all symptoms return within 2 weeks. Day-to-day variations—and even variations within a day—in the apparent effectiveness of levodopa are observed in a given patient. These variations, sometimes referred to as the *on-off phenomenon*, can be minimized by carefully adjusting the dosage employed to best fit the needs of each patient.

To reduce the high incidence of adverse side effects and obtain maximal therapeutic benefit, it is essential to *gradually* increase the daily dosage and individualize the full dosage administered. The usual initial dose is 0.5 to 1 g daily, divided in two or more doses, given with food. The daily dosage is then gradually increased by increments of not more than 0.75 g every 3 to 7 days as determined by the patient's tolerance to nausea, vomiting, and orthostatic hypotension. With increasing dosage, the patient generally exhibits progressively increasing improvement; for some patients, a significant therapeutic response may require 3 to 6 months. The usual daily maintenance dose ranges from 3 to 6 g taken with food in three or more equally divided and equally spaced doses; total daily dosage should not exceed 8 g. Nursing implications are summarized at the end of this chapter.

Side Effects and Toxicity

Virtually all patients receiving levodopa experience side effects, the intensity of which are dependent on the dose. Some of these adverse effects (nausea, vomiting, orthostatic hypotension) are most evident during the early stages of therapy, while others (abnormal involuntary movements, behavorial disturbances) become evident only after long-term drug administration and often limit the maximum dosage tolerated. The major adverse effects of levodopa are gastrointestinal, cardiovascular, neurological, and behavioral in nature.

Gastrointestinal Almost all patients experience nausea, vomiting, and loss of appetite during the early stages of therapy. These

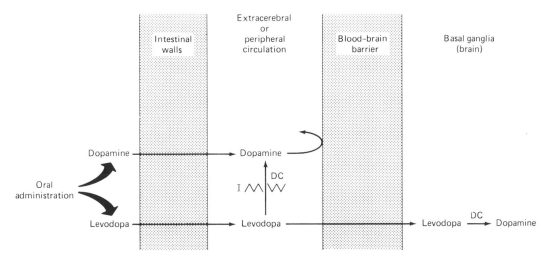

Figure 19-1 Rationale for the Use of Levodopa in the Treatment of Parkinson's Disease. Dopamine when given orally (by mouth) does not cross the blood-brain barrier; levodopa does enter the brain and is converted to dopamine in the basal ganglia by the enzyme dopa decarboxylase (DC). We can prevent the peripheral conversion of levodopa to dopamine with an extracerebral dopa decarboxylase inhibitor (I), which permits more levodopa to enter the brain.

effects may be reduced by increasing the daily dosage more slowly and administering the drug with food. Some patients develop an aversion to coffee, reporting that it has a nauseating aroma and bitter taste.

Cardiovascular   About 30 percent of all patients experience orthostatic hypotension early in treatment, which may cause dizziness or fainting. The nurse should advise the patient to assume a standing position slowly after lying down; tolerance develops to this effect. In a relatively small number of patients, cardiac arrhythmias such as sinus tachycardia and premature ventricular contractions occur. If deemed necessary, propranolol (Inderal) administration may be instituted.

Neurological   The maximum dose tolerated by parkinsonian patients is often limited by the appearance of abnormal involuntary movements of the face (grimacing), mouth (chewing and active tongue movements), neck, and rocking movements of the trunk. These effects are observed in approximately 80 percent of patients receiving the maximal dose for 1 year or more. Tolerance does not develop to these symptoms, and their attenuation can only be accomplished by reducing the daily levodopa dosage. As an inevitable consequence of such a reduction in dosage, the symptoms of Parkinson's disease will increase in severity.

Behavioral   Nervousness, anxiety, agitation, and insomnia are not uncommon during early therapy. Approximately 15 percent of patients experience serious psychiatric disturbances, necessitating a reduction in dosage or drug withdrawal. These effects are variable in nature and include confusion, delirium, depression, psychotic reactions, and hallucinations. The patient's family often requires reassurance that such behavioral changes are associated with drug administra-

tion and do not represent a worsening of the patient's neurological disorder.

Precautions

Levodopa is contraindicated in patients with narrow-angle glaucoma, a history of melanoma, or suspicious undiagnosed skin lesions. It should be used with extreme caution if the patient has severe cardiovascular or pulmonary disease, renal, hepatic or endocrine disease, convulsions, psychoses, neuroses, or wide-angle glaucoma, or has been receiving antihypertensive medication. The safety of levodopa during pregnancy has not been established. Potential drug interactions involving levodopa are presented in Table 19-2.

Carbidopa-levodopa   Levodopa is available in combination with carbidopa, a peripheral (but not central) inhibitor of the decarboxylase enzyme that catalyzes the conversion of levodopa to dopamine. This combination possesses several distinct advantages. Normally, when levodopa is administered alone, more than 99 percent of the total dose is decarboxylated to dopamine in the periphery (and, therefore, cannot reach the brain) and less than 1 percent enters the brain. The peripherally formed dopamine is primarily responsible for the observed gastrointestinal and cardiovascular side effects. Carbidopa plus levodopa (marketed as Sinemet) reduces or eliminates these adverse effects and permits a 75 percent reduction in the dose of levodopa required, since more drug enters the brain (Figure 19-1). Moreover, since these peripheral effects are minimized, the daily dosage of levodopa can be increased more rapidly during the early stages of therapy, and beneficial therapeutic effects may become evident within days. Sinemet appears to increase both the total percentage of patients improved, as well as their degree of improvement; it also reduces the frequency of the on-off phenomenon. When Sinemet is to be given to patients who are being treated with levodopa, levodopa must be discontinued at least 8 hours prior to initiating therapy with the combination.

Amatadine   Amantadine (Symmetrel) is an antiviral drug that has been shown to possess antiparkinsonism activity. While the mechanism of action of amantadine has not been established with certitude, it is thought to act by stimulating the release of dopamine from nigrostriatal neurons. This drug is less effective than levodopa but more effective than the anticholinergic agents. Its beneficial effects are observed within 2 weeks, more rapidly than are those of levodopa, and causes fewer side effects than levodopa or the anticholinergic agents.

Adverse side effects associated with amantadine include hyperexcitability, slurred speech, ataxia, insomnia, and gastrointestinal disorders. The use of amantadine for the prevention of viral disorders will be discussed in Chapter 48.

Antiparkinson Drugs:
nursing implications

Levodopa (Bendopa, Dopar, Larodopa)

1. Significant improvement usually occurs during the second or third week of therapy, but may not occur for 3 or 4 mo in some patients.
2. The rate at which the dosage is increased is determined by the patient's response to the medication and the development of tolerance to its adverse effects. Make accurate observations and report adverse reactions promptly. Total daily dose should not exceed 8 g.
3. Drug should be taken with food to reduce adverse gastrointestinal effects.
4. Caution patients not to take vitamin preparations containing vitamin B_6 (pyridoxine). Vitamin doses greater than 5 mg may reverse the beneficial effects of levodopa.
5. During a period of dosage increase, carefully monitor vital signs. Changes in position should be made slowly to reduce the severity of postural hypotension.
6. Monitor patients for behavioral changes. Depressed patients should be monitored for suicidal tendencies. Elevation of mood may precede objective clinical improvement. Physical activities should be gradually resumed within the limits of other medical problems the patient may have.

Anticholinergic Agents

1. Drug effects are cumulative and therapeutic benefit may not occur for 2 to 3 days.
2. Caution patient about possible drowsiness and blurred vision.
3. Side effects that should be reported by patient are the following: constipation, abdominal pain, and distention, which may indicate paralytic ileus; CNS depression, excitement, or vomiting, which may indicate need for temporary drug withdrawal or reduction in dosage.

SUPPLEMENTARY READINGS

Barbeau, A., and F. H. McDowell (eds.), *L-Dopa and Parkinsonism*. Philadelphia: F. A. Davis Co., 1970.

Bianchine, J. R., "Drugs for Parkinson's Disease; Centrally Acting Muscle Relaxants," in *Goodman and Gilman's The Pharmacological Basis of Therapeutics* (6th ed.), ed. A. G. Gilman, L. S. Goodman, A. Gilman, Chapter 21, pp. 475–495. New York: Macmillan, Inc., 1980.

Bianchine, J. R., and L. Sunyapridakul, "Interactions Between Levodopa and Other Drugs: Significance in the Treatment of Parkinson's Disease," *Drugs* **6**: 364–388 (1973).

Fishbach, F. T., "Easing Adjustments to Parkinson's Disease," *American Journal of Nursing* **78**: 66–69 (1978).

Parkes, D., "Bromocriptine," *Advances in Drug Research* **12**: 247–344 (1977).

Shimomura, S. K., "Parkinsonism," in *Clinical Pharmacy and Therapeutics* (2nd ed.), ed. E. T. Hertindal and J. L. Hirschman. Chapter 39, pp. 581–592. Baltimore: The Williams & Wilkins Company, 1979.

"Symposium on Levodopa in Parkinson's Disease. Clinical and Pharmacological Aspects." *Clinical Pharmacology and Therapeutics* **12**: 317–416 (1971).

NARCOTIC ANALGESICS

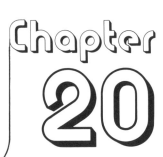

Chapter 20

Opium has held an esteemed place in medicine for thousands of years, and even until the early years of the last century, it was one of the few truly effective and reliable drugs available for the treatment of pain, insomnia, cough, and diarrhea. Today *morphine*, the major active constituent of opium, remains the standard against which all other analgesics are compared for their effectiveness, potency, and safety.

Analgesics—drugs used to relieve pain—are generally categorized as *narcotics* or *nonnarcotics*. The *narcotic agents* are extracted from the opium poppy or are chemical derivatives of morphine; narcotic agents are often referred to as *opiates* or *opioids*. These drugs are effective for the relief of severe pain. Moreover, since the narcotic analgesic agents possess significant abuse potential, they are subject to federal laws controlling their manufacture, distribution, administration, and dispensation. A major challenge facing biomedical scientists is the discovery of analgesic agents that possess the therapeutic effectiveness of morphine but lack its potential for abuse and undesirable side effects.

Aspirin and other *nonnarcotic anal-*

gesics, by contrast, are only effective for the mitigation of mild to moderate pain and are devoid of abuse liability. Apart from their common ability to relieve pain, albeit by a different mechanism of action, the pharmacological properties of narcotics and nonnarcotics bear no other similarities. We shall consider the pharmacology of nonnarcotic agents in Chapter 21.

CLASSIFICATION OF NARCOTIC ANALGESICS

Narcotic agents* may be classified into five categories (Table 20-1): (1) the natural alkaloids of opium, which include morphine and codeine; (2) semisynthetic derivatives of morphine, compounds that are chemical modifications of morphine; (3) synthetic narcotic analgesics, drugs bearing only highly subtle chemical similarities to morphine that are highly potent and possess a high abuse potential; (4) synthetic agents with low potency and a relatively low potential for abuse; (5) narcotic antagonists (Table 20-2), some of which are used as antidotes for the treatment of overdosage by narcotic analgesics and some of which are employed for the treatment of opiate dependence.

 The first four categories of narcotic agents are all employed as analgesic agents for the relief of moderate to severe pain. While differences exist in the potency and duration of action of these drugs (Table 20-1), the general pharmacological properties of these agents are all qualitatively similar to

---

*The term *narcotic* has been loosely used to refer to drugs employed for nonmedical purposes (heroin, cocaine, marijuana); central nervous system depressants; and drugs possessing both sedative and analgesic effects (morphine-like drugs). In this text, the term *narcotic* will be employed only to refer to drugs with morphine-like properties.

morphine. In this chapter, the pharmacology of morphine will be emphasized; the distinguishing characteristics of selected representative narcotic analgesics will then be considered. The narcotic antagonists, the treatment of narcotic dependence, and cough remedies will also be discussed in this chapter.

MORPHINE

Morphine is a naturally occurring alkaloid obtained from the dried juice of the opium poppy plant, *Papaver somniferum;* opium contains 10 percent morphine. The major pharmacological properties of morphine are attributed to its effects on the central nervous system and gastrointestinal tract.

Central Nervous System Effects

This section considers morphine's effects on behavior as well as its analgesic, emetic, and respiratory depressant properties; the effects of this drug and related compounds on cough will be discussed in the last section of this chapter.

Analgesic and behavioral effects
No drug has been developed that is more effective than morphine for the relief of *severe pain*. Morphine rather specifically reduces the patient's awareness of pain and the emotional anguish associated with it without causing the loss of consciousness. Analgesia is accompanied by drowsiness, mental clouding, feelings of tranquility, and euphoria, all of which contribute to the patient's ability to fall asleep readily.

 While the precise mechanism responsible for morphine-induced analgesia has not been determined with certitude, these effects undoubtedly result from an action within the central nervous system, probably in the

Table 20-1 Comparative Properties of Selected Narcotic Analgesics

Generic name (synonym)	Trade name	Usual adult dose, route, and frequency of administration[a]	Distinguishing properties
Natural opium alkaloids			
Paregoric (Camphorated opium tincture)		PO: 5-10 ml 1-4 times daily	Contains opium (equivalent to 0.43 mg morphine/ml), anise oil, benzoic acid, camphor, glycerin, and diluted alcohol (45%). Antidiarrheal agent.
Morphine		SC: 10 mg 4-6 times daily (A) PO: 2-4 mg 3-4 times daily (C)	Undependable absorption orally. Highly effective for relief of severe pain, suppression of cough (antitussive).
Codeine		PO: 30 mg 4-6 times daily (A) PO: 5-10 mg q. 4 h (C)	Useful for relief of mild to moderate pain and as an antitussive. Less sedation and abuse potential than morphine.
Semisynthetic morphine derivatives			
Heroin (diacetylmorphine)			Effective analgesic and antitussive. Very high abuse potential; illegal in United States.
Hydrocodone	Dicodid Hycodan	PO: 5-10 mg 3-4 times daily (C)	Similar to codeine, but more potent and greater abuse liability. Used as antitussive.
Hydromorphone	Dilaudid	PO or SC: 2 mg q. 4 h	Similar to morphine, but more potent, shorter duration of action, less sedation, euphoria, constipation, nausea, and vomiting.
Oxymorphone	Numorphan	SC or IV: 1-1.5 mg. q. 4-6 h	Similar to morphine and hydromorphone.
Synthetic narcotic analgesics			
Meperidine (pethidine, B.P.)	Demerol	PO or IM: 50-100 mg 6-8 times daily	Widely used analgesic, with shorter duration of action than morphine, less sedation, constipation; no antitussive or antidiarrheal activity.

Alphaprodine	Nisentil	SC: 20-40 mg IV: 20 mg	Similar to meperidine; rapid onset and short duration. Used for procedures of short duration, not for chronic pain.
Anileridine	Leritine	SC or IM: 25 mg q. 6 h	Similar to meperidine, about 2 times as potent.
Butorphanol	Stadol	IM: 2 mg q. 3-4 h IV: 1 mg q. 3-4 h	Potent analgesic. Magnitude of respiratory depression not appreciably increased at twice normal analgesic dose; duration of respiratory depression dose-related. Abuse potential relatively low.
Levorphanol	Levo-Dromoran	PO or SC: 2 mg q. 6-8 h	Similar to morphine, but more potent and longer duration of action; less constipation, nausea and vomiting.
Methadone	Dolophine	PO, SC, or IM: 7.5 mg q. 4 h	Analgesic and antitussive, similar to morphine, but longer duration of action and orally active. Used for treatment of narcotic dependence.
Nalbuphine	Nubain	SC, IM, or IV: 10 mg q. 3-4 h	Potent analgesic agent with low abuse potential. Unlike pentazocine and butorphanol, does not increase cardiac work load.
Phenazocine	Prinadol	IM: 2 mg q. 4-6 h	Similar to morphine. Used as preanesthetic, analgesic, in labor and delivery, and relief of severe pain.

Synthetic agents, low potency and relatively low abuse potential

Pentazocine	Talwin	PO: 50 mg q. 3-4 h IM: 30 mg q. 3-4 h	Effective for relief of moderate to severe pain. Abuse potential low, although reported to produce psychological and physical dependence.
Propoxyphene hydrochloride	Darvon		Relief of mild to moderate pain. A 65-mg dose is not more (and probably less) effective than codeine (65 mg) or aspirin (325 mg). Propoxyphene and aspirin (Darvon compound) is an effective analgesic combination. Abuse potential demonstrated.
Propoxyphene napsylate	Darvon-N	PO: 100 mg q. 6 h	

[a]Key to abbreviations: (A) analgesic dose; (C) cough suppressant (antitussive) dose.

Table 20-2 Comparative Properties of Narcotic Antagonists

Generic name	Trade name	Principal therapeutic use(s)	Distinguishing properties
Nalorphine	Nalline	Withdrawn from market in United States.	Possesses narcotic analgesic activity as well as antagonist properties. Unsuitable for use as analgesic because of dysphoric effects. Can produce respiratory depression.
Naloxone	Narcan	Same as nalorphine; narcotic antagonist of choice. Treatment of narcotic-induced respiratory depression; ineffective in reversing respiratory depression induced by nonnarcotic CNS depressants.	Pure narcotic antagonist. Unlike nalorphine, does not produce morphine-like respiratory depression, miosis, analgesia, or sedation.
Naltrexone Cyclazocine		Experimental drugs used for treatment of narcotic dependence.	Orally active and longer duration of action than naloxone.

thalamus and limbic system.* Morphine is useful for the alleviation of almost all types of pain, regardless of its site or origin. It has been clinically observed that narcotic analgesics are more effective in alleviating continuous, dull, aching pain than in relieving pain of a sharp and stabbing nature, such as acute renal or biliary colic.

Respiratory effects Morphine's ability to depress the respiratory centers of the medulla is of considerable toxicological significance. Respiratory failure is the primary cause of death in narcotic overdosage. Large doses of this drug depress the rate of respiration, the minute volume (amount of air passing into and out of the lungs per minute), and the tidal volume (amount of air inspired and expired with each normal breath). Normally, elevated carbon dioxide levels in the blood (pCO_2) serve as a physiological medullary stimulant, causing an increase in the rate of respiration. Morphine depresses the sensitivity of the respiratory centers to this rise in pCO_2.

*Morphine is thought to relieve pain by interacting with opiate receptors, receptors normally activated by endogenous opiates (endorphins). The endorphins are believed to play an important physiological role in pain and other emotional behavior.

Other central effects Narcotics produce constriction of the *pupils*, with some degree of constriction observed in even total darkness. Pinpoint pupils in an individual with respiratory depression is a highly characteristic symptom of morphine poisoning.

Nausea and *vomiting* are common side effects associated with therapeutic doses of narcotic agents. These effects have been attributed to activation of the chemoreceptor trigger zone in the medulla which, in turn, stimulates the vomiting center. Since nausea and vomiting are less frequently observed in bed-ridden patients than ambulatory individuals, a vestibular component may be associated with these effects; tolerance develops with repeated drug administration. *Apomorphine*, a close chemical derivative of morphine, is an extremely potent emetic agent and, as such, is clinically employed for the emergency treatment of poisoning (Chapter 57).

Gastrointestinal Effects

Long before the analgesic effects of opium were recognized, this drug's constipating properties were employed for the treatment of dysentery and diarrhea. The actions of morphine on the smooth muscle of the gastrointestinal tract are highly complex, with *constipation* resulting, in part, from an increase in muscle tone or a reduction in propulsive peristaltic movements, which slow the passage of food and fecal material down the tract. This drug also reduces the patient's responsiveness to normal sensory stimuli associated with the defecation reflex.

Miscellaneous Effects

Therapeutic doses of morphine produce no major alterations in blood pressure, heart rate, or heart rhythms in recumbent patients; hence it is a valuable drug for the relief of pain and anxiety associated with myocardial infarctions. By contrast, orthostatic hypotension and fainting may be observed in ambulatory patients, effects which may be the result of morphine-induced peripheral vasodilation.

Morphine should be used with great caution in patients with asthma because of the ability of this drug to cause contraction of the bronchial smooth muscle (bronchoconstriction).

The tone of the smooth muscle of the urinary tract is altered by morphine. This effect, coupled with a reduction in the perception of the stimuli associated with micturation and stimulation of the release of antidiuretic hormone, all contribute to the urinary retention often observed in patients treated with this drug.

Administration and Therapeutic Uses

Morphine is readily absorbed after intramuscular or subcutaneous injection, with over one-half the injected dose appearing in the bloodstream within 30 minutes. Absorption after oral administration is slow and variable, so this route is rarely employed. By contrast, some narcotic analgesics (codeine, meperidine, methadone) are well absorbed and highly effective when given orally. A summary of the nursing implications associated with the administration of narcotic analgesics appears at the end of this chapter.

Analgesia The most common use of morphine and its derivatives is for the relief of *severe pain*, regardless of cause, which includes acute traumatic injuries, postoperative pain, heart attacks, and terminal cancer. The feelings of tranquility and euphoria, coupled with analgesia, all contribute to providing the patient with relief from suffering. As will be discussed later, chronic use of narcotic analgesics results in tolerance to their analgesic effects, as well as the potential development of a drug-dependent state.

Narcotic analgesics are the mainstay for the relief of chronic pain, for example, terminal cancer. The *Brompton cocktail* has been a very popular orally active analgesic mixture in Great Britain that has been gaining favor in the United States. The specific ingredients and their amounts vary. In Great Britain this mixture contains heroin (diamorphine), a drug that is illegal in the United States. Other mixtures may contain morphine; cocaine (sometimes used to decrease drowsiness and increase alertness); and chlorpromazine (Thorazine) or prochlorperazine (Compazine), included as anti-emetic agents. The bitter taste of morphine is generally masked by using a syrup vehicle containing alcohol and chloroform water.

When a hospitalized patient complains of pain, the nurse must make a careful assessment of its location, quality, intensity, radiation, duration, and timing of onset. Sometimes simply a change in body position, a backrub, or reassurance can relieve the discomfort. When the patient requires medication, it should be administered before the pain becomes severe to provide maximum effectiveness. Some patients do not actively complain of pain but exhibit behaviors manifesting its presence, including distressed facial expressions, vocalization, bodily movements, or more subtle changes in physiological state, such as sweating or increases in pulse, respiratory rate, or blood pressure.

The postoperative analgesic benefits to be derived from morphine therapy must be weighed in terms of its ability to mask the postoperative complications of surgery. The ability of morphine to depress respiration and the cough reflex may predispose the patient to pneumonitis. Moreover, this class of analgesics reduces bowel motility and causes urinary retention, functions often already compromised after abdominal surgery.

The rational use of narcotic analgesics will be discussed in Chapter 24 when the nurse's role in the prevention of drug dependence will be considered.

Diarrhea   One of the frequently encountered side effects associated with the use of all narcotic agents to varying degrees is constipation. This effect serves as the basis for the use of these drugs for the symptomatic treatment of diarrhea. *Paregoric* (camphorated opium tincture) and opium tincture have been used for generations for the treatment of diarrhea in children and adults. The meperidine-related drug *diphenoxylate*, used in combination with atropine (*Lomotil*), is highly effective for the management of acute and chronic diarrhea and is devoid of abuse potential. The management of diarrhea will be discussed in greater detail in Chapter 56.

Dyspnea   Intravenously administered morphine has been found to be highly effective in relieving dyspnea (labored breathing), particularly dyspnea resulting from pulmonary edema and left ventricular failure. Morphine is thought to act by reducing venous return and thereby relieving pul-

monary vascular congestion, which leads to a reduction in pulmonary edema.

Adverse Effects

The most commonly encountered side effects associated with the use of morphine and related narcotic analgesics include nausea and vomiting, orthostatic hypotension, mental clouding, constipation (often necessitating the use of cathartics or enemas), and urinary retention. Depression of both breathing and coughing can predispose the patient to respiratory complications. Allergic reactions to the opiates, resulting from drug-induced release of histamine, may be characterized by urticaria, itching (of the nose in particular), skin rashes, and respiratory distress in asthmatics. If allergic manifestations appear, the opiate should be discontinued and a nonnarcotic analgesic employed. Drug interactions involving the narcotic analgesics are listed in Table 20-3.

Acute Morphine Poisoning

The victim of severe acute opiate poisoning is comatose and cyanotic, has pinpoint pupils, and exhibits a substantial reduction in respiratory rate. Since death most commonly results from respiratory failure, the primary objective of the nurse is to maintain breathing. Specific antagonists have been developed (Table 20-2) which are capable of reversing respiratory depression induced by both natural and synthetic opiates. Intravenous administration of nalorphine (Nalline) or naloxone (Narcan) is capable of restoring respiratory and circulatory function within 1 to 2 minutes. If several doses of these antagonists prove ineffective, the nurse should suspect that the observed respiratory depression has been caused by a central nervous system depressant other than an

Table 20-3   Potential Drug Interactions Involving Narcotic Analgesics

Narcotic agent	Interacting drug/class	Possible consequences
Narcotic agents	Central nervous system depressants Barbiturates Nonbarbiturate sedative-hypnotics Alcohol Antipsychotic (neuroleptic) agents Antihistamines	Sedative effects of narcotic agents may be enhanced when used in combination with central depressant drugs.
	Surgical skeletal muscle relaxants Competitive Depolarizing	Central respiratory depressing effects of narcotics adds to the neuromuscular blockade of muscle relaxants, increasing the risk of respiratory failure.
Meperidine (Demerol)	Antidepressants, monoamine oxidase inhibitors Isocarboxazid (Marplan) Phenelzine (Nardil) Tranylcypromine (Paranate)	Severe and often immediate adverse effects, including excitation, sweating, rigidity, hypertension or hypotension, and coma.
Methadone	Rifampin (Rifadin, Rimactane)	Rifampin appears to stimulate the rate of metabolism of methadone resulting in symptoms of methadone withdrawal.

opiate, such as a barbiturate or nonbarbiturate sedative-hypnotic agent.

OTHER REPRESENTATIVE NARCOTIC ANALGESICS

Codeine

Codeine, the second most important alkaloid naturally derived from the opium poppy, is very widely used as an analgesic and antitussive agent. Its analgesic potency is considerably weaker than morphine: 60 mg of injected codeine produce the same degree of analgesia as 10 mg of morphine. Codeine is frequently administered alone (15 to 60 mg) or in combination with aspirin by oral administration for the relief of moderately severe pain.

The pharmacological effects of codeine closely resemble morphine, but are less intense. Codeine is a less effective analgesic and cough suppressant; it is less constipat-ing and produces less sedation, respiratory depression, nausea, and vomiting. Tolerance to the analgesic effects of codeine develop far less rapidly than morphine, and this drug possesses a lower abuse potential than morphine.

Meperidine

Meperidine (Demerol), a synthetic agent, is among the most extensively employed narcotic analgesics for the relief of severe pain. Meperidine, as morphine, possesses a strong potential for abuse. The pharmacological properties of meperidine differ from those of morphine in several major respects. The analgesic effects of an average subcutaneous dose of morphine (10 mg) persist for 4 to 5 hours. By contrast, meperidine has a shorter duration of action (approximately 2 to 4 hours) and requires ten times the dose (100 mg) to produce equivalent analgesia. This drug lacks the antidiarrheal and antitussive properties of morphine and causes less sedation, nausea, and vomiting. Unlike morphine, meperidine provides effective and reliable analgesia after oral administration. Meperidine is most commonly administered intramuscularly, since subcutaneous injections are irritating to the tissues.

Methadone

Methadone (Dolophine) possesses pharmacological properties similar to morphine, with both drugs equipotent in their abilities to relieve severe pain. While it is also capable of producing respiratory depression, methadone causes less sedation, nausea, and constipation than morphine.

Methadone is an effective analgesic agent that may be administered parenterally or orally; its duration of action is somewhat longer than morphine. Both tolerance and physical dependence develop after chronic use of this drug. The withdrawal syndrome appears more slowly (after 24 to 48 hours) and is of lesser intensity but longer duration than are the symptoms of withdrawal associated with morphine (see page 172). The use of methadone for the treatment of opiate dependence will be considered in a subsequent section of this chapter.

Pentazocine

We have previously noted that a major biomedical research objective is the development of an effective analgesic agent with little or no abuse liability. Pentazocine (Talwin) possesses relatively low potential for abuse when taken orally, and is, therefore, a useful drug for the relief of chronic pain of moderate to severe intensity; tolerance and mild physical dependence have been associated with its habitual use.

Reported adverse effects include nausea, vomiting, diarrhea, dizziness, sedation, and hallucinations. Respiratory depression is rarely encountered with pentazocine and can be counteracted with naloxone, but not nalorphine.

Propoxyphene

Propoxyphene is a synthetic analgesic, given orally exclusively, which has approximately one-half the potency of codeine. Unlike codeine, however, this drug is not an effective cough suppressant.

Among the preparations of this drug that the nurse will commonly encounter are propoxyphene hydrochloride (Darvon), propoxyphene napsylate (Darvon-N), and these propoxyphene salts in combination with aspirin (325 mg) or acetaminophen. The actions and uses of both salts are the same, except that, because of larger molecular weight, a dose of 100 mg of the napsylate is required to produce analgesia equivalent to that produced by 65 mg of the hydrochloride salt.

While therapeutic doses of propoxyphene do not result in drug dependence, the chronic ingestion of 800 mg per day of the hydrochloride may produce mild withdrawal symptoms after abrupt termination of drug administration.

The most common side effects associated with therapeutic doses of propoxyphene include dizziness, sedation, nausea, and vomiting. Acute overdosage is characterized by weakness, confusion, pinpoint pupils, convulsions, respiratory depression, coma, and death; since 20 percent of all fatalities occur within one hour of the overdosage, emergency treatment should be rendered as soon as possible. The narcotic antagonists have been found to be effective for the treatment of respiratory depression induced by propoxyphene. This drug should be employed cautiously, if at all, with alcohol and other central nervous system depressants because of the risk of additive toxicity.

NARCOTIC ANTAGONISTS

By suitable chemical modification of the chemistry of certain narcotic agents, the resulting compounds are capable of antagonizing the effects produced by narcotic analgesics. Nalorphine is an antagonist that retains some morphine-like properties, while naloxone is a pure narcotic antagonist (Table 20-2).

Naloxone

Nalorphine (Nalline), the first clinically developed narcotic antagonist, has many morphine-like properties, including the ability to produce analgesia, respiratory depression, constriction of the pupils, dysphoria, and hallucinations. Naloxone (Narcan), a newer drug, is devoid of morphine-like properties. Unlike nalorphine, it does not cause respiratory depression, sedation, or adverse behavioral aberrations, and is capable of antagonizing poisoning by pentazocine. This narcotic antagonist of choice, when administered intravenously, rapidly and effectively reverses most of the effects of morphine, particularly the coma and respiratory depression observed in acute narcotic poisoning. Naloxone is clinically employed as an antidote for narcotic poisoning, regardless of whether the narcotic is a natural, semisynthetic, or synthetic agent. There is evidence to suggest that a narcotic antagonist acts by displacing the narcotic agonist from opiate receptor sites in the brain. Narcotic antagonists are ineffective in reversing depression induced by alcohol, barbiturate or nonbarbiturate sedative-hypnotics, or other central nervous system depressants.

Administration of narcotic antagonists to narcotic-dependent individuals precipitates an abstinence (withdrawal) syndrome, with symptoms identical to those observed after abrupt cessation of narcotics but that begin within minutes after an injection of the antagonist. Naloxone has been used as a diagnostic agent to ascertain whether an individual is physically dependent upon narcotic agents.

NARCOTIC DEPENDENCE AND ITS TREATMENT

In this section, the pharmacological aspects of narcotic dependence, namely, psychological dependence, tolerance, and physical dependence as well as contemporary treatment approaches to this drug-dependent state, will be considered.

Pharmacological Characteristics of Narcotic Dependence

Psychological dependence Frequent administration of heroin or other narcotics inevitably leads to a compulsive desire on the part of the user to continue to take the drug in order to maintain a state of "well being." The heroin user feels "normal" while under the influence of the drug and "sick" in its absence.

The street user employs narcotic agents to obtain a euphoric high, as well as feelings of tranquility; these latter effects permit the user to temporarily escape from inner anxieties and frustrations. Another compelling factor that perpetuates continued drug usage is the desire to avoid the abstinence syndrome associated with abrupt drug withdrawal.

Despite the fact that tens of thousands of patients are given narcotics each day for therapeutic purposes, documented cases of medically-induced drug dependence are rare.

Nevertheless, these drugs should be judiciously administered, and their use and frequency of administration should be limited to cases that are therapeutically justified.

The street user self-administers narcotic drugs by sniffing or by subcutaneous ("skin popping") or intravenous ("mainlining") injection. Within seconds after an intravenous injection, the pupils are constricted, and a tingling sensation ("rush"), which has been likened to a sexual orgasm, is perceived in the abdomen. The brief euphoric feeling or "high" is followed by a period of tranquility, during which—for a few hours—the user is drowsy and content ("on the nod").

Tolerance After repeated administration of narcotic agents, tolerance rapidly develops to the euphoric, analgesic, and respiratory depressing effects, but not to pupillary constriction or to constipation. The speed with which tolerance is acquired is dependent upon the narcotic agent used, the dosage employed, and the interval between successive doses. Chronic abusers have been reported to be able to survive ten to twenty times the normal lethal dose of morphine (250 mg) during a 24-hour period. Overdosage and death from narcotic poisoning often result from the user inadvertently taking doses in excess of those to which he or she is tolerant. Cross-tolerance develops to all narcotic agents (Table 20-1).

Physical dependence and the abstinence syndrome Chronic administration of narcotics leads to the rapid development of physical dependence. Proof of physical dependence can be demonstrated by the appearance of *abstinence symptoms* observed after abrupt termination of narcotic administration, and the almost immediate suppression of these symptoms when a narcotic agent is readministered. The intensity of the abstinence syndrome is dependent

upon the relative degree of physical dependence. The onset, peak time, and duration of these symptoms varies with the drug used. If we compare meperidine, morphine (or heroin), and methadone, we would observe the following time course for abstinence symptoms, respectively: onset, 3 hours, 8 to 12 hours, and 24 to 48 hours; time of peak symptoms, 8 to 12 hours, 36 to 72 hours, and 3 days; duration of symptoms, 4 to 5 days, 7 to 10 days, and 6 to 7 weeks.

The heroin or morphine abstinence syndrome begins within 8 to 12 hours after the last dose and resembles some of the symptoms commonly associated with influenza, namely, a runny nose, tearing, sweating, yawning, and insomnia. At about 20 hours, gooseflesh (hence the term *cold turkey*), widened pupils, and tremors appear. At the peak of the withdrawal period (48 to 72 hours), the dependent individual suffers from insomnia, weakness, muscle spasms in the legs, chills, intestinal cramps, nausea, vomiting, diarrhea, fever, and elevated blood pressure; in severe cases, delirium and hallucinations may be present. These symptoms abate within 7 to 10 days, even in the absence of treatment. Administration of a narcotic agent at any time during the abstinence syndrome will immediately terminate these symptoms and make the user feel "normal."

Neonatal opiate dependence Heroin and other narcotic agents readily cross the placental barrier and newborn infants of mothers who are chronic users of narcotics have been demonstrated to be physically dependent upon such drugs. The withdrawal syndrome in the infant is characterized by irritability, hyperactivity, tremors, vomiting, a high-pitched cry, sneezing, and respiratory distress. Paregoric, phenobarbital, diazepam (Valium), and chlorpromazine (Thorazine) have been used to treat narcotic withdrawal in neonates.

Treatment of Narcotic Dependence

Successful treatment of narcotic dependence entails far more than achieving a state of drug abstinence for weeks or even months. It has been commonly observed that individuals who have remained drug-free even after extended periods of hospitalization or incarceration return to drug usage in a relatively short period after their return to a familiar neighborhood. Many experts contend that a better understanding of why *relapse* occurs in such individuals holds the key to solving the narcotic dependency problem.

Two basic treatment approaches have been introduced in recent years that have achieved some measure of success; one is psychosocial and the other pharmacological. It is generally accepted that no single approach is best for all individuals; rather an attempt must be made to find the best treatment modality for each person.

Psychosocial approaches Therapeutic treatment communities, such as Synanon, are staffed by health professionals and former addicts. An essential component of these residential programs is the group therapy sessions, in which an attempt is made to rehabilitate the addict to readjust to a drug-free life style. Other programs serve as halfway houses to smooth the otherwise abrupt transition between a prison or hospital and the "real world," which often provides an easy path to readdiction. While many of these programs have been successful in rehabilitating addicts, such structured environments are not suitable for all addicts. Moreover, their facilities are limited and the cost per patient is extremely high.

Pharmacological approaches

Methadone maintenance The most extensively employed treatment approach in the United States is the methadone maintenance program. Ideally used in conjunction with psychotherapy, orally administered methadone is provided to the addict on a daily basis. Methadone prevents the narcotic abstinence syndrome for 24 hours, reduces or eliminates the craving for heroin, and blocks the euphoric effects normally elicited by intravenously administered heroin; it should be noted, however, that if high doses of heroin are injected, methadone blockade of euphoria can be overcome.

While notable successes have been achieved in rehabilitating addicts, enabling them to give up or reduce their illicit use of narcotic agents and permitting them to return to their families or gainful employment, even the staunchest advocates of these programs do not believe methadone to represent the final solution to the narcotic dependence problem. Dependence on methadone develops, and some individuals require the chronic use of this drug for indefinite periods of time.

Methadyl acetate (also referred to as levo-alpha-acetylmethadol (LAAM)), a methadone-like drug, suppresses the narcotic abstinence syndrome for up to 72 hours and is being tested for use in selected patients.

Narcotic antagonists The use of narcotic antagonists represents an alternative pharmacological approach to the treatment of narcotic dependence. Administration of these drugs reduces or prevents the euphoric effects normally elicited by heroin and other narcotics, which should, in theory, result in an extinction of drug-seeking behavior.

Nalorphine and naloxone are effective, but they lack therapeutic utility because of their short durations of action and are not effective orally. Although cyclazocine is capable of antagonizing the euphoric effects of narcotic agents for 24 hours after a single oral dose, this drug causes adverse behavioral side effects. Among the most promising investigational drugs available to date is *naltrexone*, a drug that is active for more than 24 hours after oral administration and lacks significant side effects.

Unlike methadone, the narcotic antagonists have little or no abuse potential. At present, the use of these drugs is under investigation, and their roles in the treatment of narcotic dependence have not been fully assessed.

COUGH REMEDIES

Cough is a protective reflex that serves to clear the respiratory tract of foreign bodies that might otherwise block the airways and obstruct free breathing. The cough reflex may be initiated by mechanical or chemical activation of nerve endings located in the trachea, bronchi, or bronchioles. Such activation triggers an impulse along sensory nerves, which ultimately stimulates the cough center located in the medulla. The cough center activates a sequence of events in the respiratory center and diaphragm that is manifested as a cough.

Depending upon the stimulus initiating it, coughing may be beneficial or harmful and distressing to the patient. A productive cough serves the important function of removing accumulated fluids from the respiratory tract, fluids that may contain entrapped bacteria and dust particles. In general, no attempt is made to suppress a productive cough, and often it is desirable to facilitate such coughing with *expectorants*. A nonproductive cough, by contrast, not only fails to serve the physiological needs of the patient, but may be painful and fatiguing. Such coughs, when not suppressed, often cause irritation of the mucosal linings of the larnyx, pharynx, and trachea and perpetuate the cough reflex cycle. Drugs used to suppress cough are called *antitussives* (Latin *tussis*, "cough"). Cough remedies may contain antitussive or expectorant agents or both (Table 20-4).

Antitussive Agents

Antitussive agents inhibit or suppress the act of coughing by depressing the cough center in the medulla or by blocking the peripheral sensory receptors of the nerves in the bronchial tree responsible for transmitting the tussal impulses to the cough center. Codeine and dextromethorphan act centrally, while benzonatate and other drugs possess both central and peripheral antitussive activity, the latter believed to be of greater importance.

Narcotic agents have long been recognized as the most effective drugs available to suppress cough, but their therapeutic utility is limited by their abuse potential and

Table 20-4   Commonly Employed Antitussives and Expectorants.

Generic name	Trade name	Distinguishing characteristics	Significant adverse effects
Antitussives			
Codeine		Highly effective narcotic agent, with low abuse potential.	Drowsiness, nausea, constipation.
Hydrocodone (dihydrocodeinone)	Dicodid Hycodan	Narcotic antitussive than is more potent than codeine, with greater abuse potential.	Similar to codeine.

Table 20-4   (Continued)

Generic name	Trade name	Distinguishing characteristics	Significant adverse effects
Dextromethorphan	Romilar	Chemically related to levorphanol, but devoid of analgesic and central nervous system depression. Central antitussive properties equal to codeine.	Slight drowsiness and gastrointestinal upset.
Levopropoxyphene napsylate	Novrad	Levo-isomer of propoxyphene (Darvon), devoid of analgesic effects. Effective antitussive, less potent than codeine. No apparent abuse potential.	Nausea and vomiting, lightheadedness, drowsiness, dry mouth.
Noscapine	Nectadon	Natural opium alkaloid, but unlike morphine and codeine, does not produce analgesia, sedation, constipation, and respiratory depression. Devoid of abuse liability.	Minimal drowsiness, headache, nausea.
Benzonatate	Tessalon	Central and peripheral (local anesthetic) antitussive actions.	Minimal; nausea, drowsiness, tightness in the chest, nasal congestion. Temporary local anesthesia of oral mucosa if capsules permitted to dissolve in the mouth.
Expectorants			
Glyceryl guaiacolate (Guaifenesin)		Widely used expectorant, decreases thickness of mucus.	
Terpin hydrate		Employed mainly as a vehicle in elixirs in combination with codeine or dextromethorphan.	
Potassium iodide Sodium iodide		Liquifies thick sputum in chronic bronchitis and bronchial asthma.	Chronic use may result in iodide-induced goiter, hypothyroidism, and other symptoms of iodism (salivation, tearing, running nose, soreness of gums, skin eruptions). Strong salt taste; administer with glassful of water.
Ammonium chloride		Similar to potassium iodide; commonly administered in flavored syrup.	Gastrointestinal upset.
Ipecac syrup		Administered as a syrup to treat bronchitis associated with croup (1-2 ml dose). Effective emetic in children (15 ml) for treatment of poison ingestion (Chapter 57).	

side effects. *Codeine*, the most commonly used narcotic antitussive, is particularly useful for the relief of a painful and nonproductive cough. An effective antitussive dose of codeine is approximately one-quarter to one-half its analgesic dose.

Dextromethorphan (Romilar), the methylated dextro isomer of the narcotic analgesic agent levorphanol (Levo-Dromoran), possesses no analgesic activity, has low potential for abuse, and is not a respiratory depressant. Dextromethorphan is among the most widely used antitussive agents in nonprescription cough remedies. This centrally acting compound approaches codeine in its ability to suppress cough and causes fewer adverse side effects.

Expectorants

Expectorants are drugs that enhance the removal of respiratory tract fluids during the cough reflex. Some compounds stimulate the secretion of these fluids, while others reduce the thickness (viscosity) of mucus, liquifying and facilitating its removal. Commonly employed expectorants include glyceryl guaiacolate, potassium and sodium iodide, ammonium chloride, terpin hydrate, and ipecac.

Narcotic Analgesics:
nursing implications

1. The nurse should account for all narcotics administered or disposed of.
2. The procedure for administering narcotic analgesics should include assessment of the patient's physiological status; evaluation of the patient's emotional reaction to pain; and incorporation of supportive nursing measures including reassurance.
3. Evaluate physiological parameters for signs indicating the patient is experiencing pain: elevated pulse or respiratory rate, restlessness, anorexia, immobility, sweating.
4. Record the time of onset, duration, and quality of pain. Record the relative relief of pain and duration of analgesia after drug administration.
5. Do not withhold medication when it is needed. Maximum analgesic effect is achieved when the drug is administered before the patient experiences maximum pain.
6. Prior to administering narcotic analgesics, note respiratory rate and size of pupils. Respiratory rates of 12 per minute or less and miosis are symptoms of opiate toxicity.
7. Opiates depress cough and sigh reflexes, and thus may cause atelectasis, especially during the postoperative period. Encourage position change, deep breathing, and coughing at regular intervals unless contraindicated.
8. Orthostatic hypotension is most likely to occur in ambulatory patients when moving from the supine to upright position.
9. Monitor fluid intake and output. Urinary retention may result from reduced awareness of bladder stimuli or increased sphincter tone. Offer fluids and encourage the patient to void every 3 to 4 h. Palpate lower abdomen for bladder distention.
10. Check for bowel sounds and abdominal distention during the postoperative period. The constipating effects of opiates can be reduced by increasing the bulk fiber in the diet. Stool softeners may be required.

11. Reassure patient that flushing and increased perspiration are sometimes caused by therapeutic doses. Change linens as needed for patient comfort.

12. These drugs possess high abuse potential. Tolerance, psychological and physical dependence may develop with repeated use. Continually evaluate the patient's need for opiate analgesia and, if indicated, suggest that the physician prescribe a less potent narcotic such as codeine or even a nonnarcotic analgesic.

13. Abrupt withdrawal of drug administration after periods of prolonged administration may result in an abstinence syndrome. The severity of withdrawal symptoms depends upon the duration of drug administration, total daily dose, the specific opiate employed, and the psychological characteristics of the patient.

14. Narcotic antagonists such as naloxone (Narcan) should always be available in case of opiate toxicity. The duration of action of antagonists is generally shorter than the narcotic analgesics. The patient should be carefully monitored for relapse into respiratory depression as the effects of the antagonist dissipate.

SUPPLEMENTARY READINGS

Bickerman, H. A., "Clinical Pharmacology of Antitussive Agents," *Clinical Pharmacology and Therapeutics* **3**: 353–68 (1962).

Braude, M. C., L. S. Harris, E. L. May, J. P. Smith, and J. E. Villarreal, eds., *Narcotic Antagonists*, New York: Raven Press, 1974.

Brogden, R. N., T. M. Speight, and G. S. Avery, "Pentazocine: A Review of its Pharmacological Properties, Therapeutic Efficacy and Dependence Liability," *Drugs* **5**: 6–91 (1973).

Fraser, H. F., and L. S. Harris, "Narcotic and Narcotic Antagonist Analgesics," *Annual Review of Pharmacology* **7**: 277–300 (1967).

Goldstein, A., "Heroin Addiction—Sequential Treatment Employing Pharmacologic Supports," *Archives of General Psychiatry* **33**: 353–358 (1976).

Jaffe, J. H., and W. R. Martin, "Opioid Analgesics and Antagonists," in *Goodman and Gilman's The Pharmacological Basis of Therapeutics* (6th ed.), ed. A. G. Gilman, L. S. Goodman, and A. Gilman, Chapter 22, pp. 494–534. New York: Macmillan, Inc., 1980.

Johnson, J. E., and V. H. Rice, "Sensory and Distress Components of Pain," *Nursing Research* **23**: 203–209 (1974).

Lasagna, L., "The Clinical Effectiveness of Morphine and its Substitutes as Analgesics," *Pharmacological Reviews* **16**: 47–83 (1964).

Maddux, J. F., and C. L. Bowden, "Critique of Success with Methadone Maintenance," *American Journal of Psychiatry* **129**: 100–106 (1973).

Martin, W. R., "Opioid Antagonists," *Pharmacological Reviews* **19**: 463–521 (1967).

McCaffery, M., *Nursing Management of the Patient with Pain*. Philadelphia: J. B. Lippincott Company, 1972.

McCaffery, M., and L. L. Hart, "Undertreatment of Acute Pain with Narcotics," *American Journal of Nursing* **76**: 1586–1591 (1976).

Melzack, R., *The Puzzle of Pain*. New York: Basic Books, Inc., Publishers, 1973.

Miller, R. R., A. Feingold, and J. Paxinos, "Propoxyphene Hydrochloride: A Critical Review," *Journal of the American Medical Association* **213**: 996–1006 (1970).

Murphee, H. B., "Narcotic Analgesics," in *Drill's Pharmacology in Medicine*, ed. J. R. DiPalma, 4th ed., Chapter 18, 19, pp. 324–49, 350–61. New York: McGraw-Hill Book Company, 1971.

Villaverde, M. M., and C. W. Macmillan, *Pain: From Symptom to Treatment*. New York: Van Nostrand-Reinhold Company, 1977.

Wikler, A., ed., "The Addictive States," *Association for Research in Nervous and Mental Disease*, Vol. 46. Baltimore: Wilkins & Wilkins Company, 1968.

NONNARCOTIC ANALGESICS AND ANTI-INFLAMMATORY AGENTS

Chapter 21

This chapter considers drugs that are used extensively to relieve mild to moderate pain, reduce fever, and control inflammatory disorders. Among other drugs included in these discussions will be aspirin, the widely used aspirin substitute acetaminophen, the anti-inflammatory agents phenylbutazone and indomethacin, and drugs used for the treatment of gout.

SALICYLATES

The salicylates are among the oldest classes of drugs that continue to enjoy an unchallenged place in modern therapeutics. Some salicylates, such as salicylic acid and methyl salicylate, are applied externally, while aspirin and sodium salicylate are taken for their systemic effects.

Salicylic Acid and Methyl Salicylate

Salicylic acid, a compound far too irritating to be taken internally, is a common ingredient in nonprescription liquids, ointments, and pads intended for the treatment of corns, calluses, warts, and acne. This drug, called a *keratolytic agent*, softens the epidermal layers of skin, causing them to peel off.

Methyl salicylate or *oil of wintergreen* is a colorless or light yellow liquid with a highly characteristic aroma and the taste of wintergreen. It is the most commonly used external analgesic and counterirritant for the relief of aching pain arising from sore muscles and joints. When rubbed in the skin, it stimulates the flow of blood to the immediate area (*rubefacient effect*), producing a feeling of warmth and the relief of pain. Oil of wintergreen is a potentially dangerous drug that should be kept out of the reach of children. Ingestion of as little as one teaspoonful (5 ml) has been reported to cause fatalities in children.

Aspirin (Acetylsalicylic Acid)

Acetylsalicylic acid was first synthesized in 1899, and since that time it has been among the most widely used therapeutic agents ever developed. Aspirin and sodium salicylate are readily converted to and exist as *salicylate* in the body. Since both drugs have similar analgesic, antipyretic, and anti-inflammatory effects, we shall use the terms *aspirin* and *salicylate* interchangeably. Nursing implications are summarized at the end of this chapter.

Analgesic effects Aspirin is that mysterious "ingredient that doctors recommend most for pain," pain of mild to moderate severity in particular. Clinically, we observe this drug to be more effective for the relief of headache, neuralgia, myalgia, and arthralgia than for acute traumatic injuries or deep-seated visceral pains arising from intestinal cramps or colic. Morphine and related opiates, by contrast, are capable of relieving pain of severe intensity, regardless of its site of origin. Unlike the opiates, tolerance does not develop to the analgesic effects of the salicylates.

The usual effective analgesic dose of aspirin is 650 mg (10 grains or two adult tablets), with maximum relief of pain obtained with three or four tablets.

Normal therapeutic doses of salicylates have no effects on behavior nor do they alter the perception of sensations other than pain. In contrast to the opiates, which relieve pain by an action mediated by central mechanisms, aspirin is generally thought to act peripherally. Bradykinin is thought to be the peripheral chemical mediator of pain and its pain-eliciting effects are enhanced by prostaglandins. The salicylates are believed to relieve pain by inhibiting prostaglandin synthesis.

Antipyretic effects The salicylates effectively reduce fever but do not modify normal body temperature when given in normal therapeutic doses. This antipyretic effect has been attributed to their effects on the thermoregulatory centers in the anterior hypothalamus responsible for loss of body heat. Salicylate-activation of these centers triggers sweating and vasodilation of the cutaneous blood vessels, resulting in heat loss and a reduction in fever. It should be emphasized that these drugs do not remove the cause of fever (that is, the viral or bacterial infection), but provide only symptomatic relief.

While the salicylates are safe and effective antipyretic agents, some authorities argue that antipyretics should not be employed routinely in all cases of low-grade fever. At times the natural rise and fall of fever represents the best diagnostic clue for the physician to follow; fever may also provide an indication of the relative effectiveness of the chemotherapeutic agents prescribed or the appearance of disease complications.

Anti-inflammatory and antirheumatic effects *Inflammation*, a local tissue response to injury, is characterized by redness, heat at the site of inflammation, swelling, pain, and loss of motion. Recent evidence suggests that the naturally occurring *prostaglandins* (long-chain fatty acids widely distributed throughout the body) may be one of the chemical mediators of the inflammatory response.

When administered in high daily doses of 5 to 6 g (15 to 20 tablets), aspirin relieves the pain and reduces the fever, painful swelling, and inflammation associated with such disorders as rheumatoid arthritis and rheumatic fever. Salicylates and other anti-inflammatory agents are thought to produce their beneficial effects, at least in part, by inhibiting the synthesis of prostaglandins. These drugs do not cure chronic inflammatory disorders but provide safe and often highly effective symptomatic relief for the patient.

Miscellaneous effects

Uricosuric effects High daily doses of aspirin (5 g) have uricosuric properties, that is, they increase the urinary excretion of uric acid. Low analgesic doses (1 g daily), by contrast, inhibit uric acid excretion and moreover, interfere with the uricosuric effects of probenecid (Benemid) and sulfinpyrazone (Anturane), drugs used for the treatment of gout.

Blood coagulation   Aspirin, at doses in excess of 3 g daily, has been shown to increase bleeding time. This effect has been attributed to drug-inhibition of prothrombin synthesis, and, more importantly, to a reduction in the ability of platelets to aggregate. In some clinical studies, low doses of aspirin were shown to reduce the incidence of thrombosis (clot formation in blood vessels) postoperatively and decrease the death rate in patients susceptible to or who have previously experienced strokes and heart attacks (Chapter 31).

Patients who are taking coumarin anticoagulants should use aspirin with great caution, if at all. Aspirin can displace these oral anticoagulants from plasma protein binding sites, increasing the levels of pharmacologically active free drug, which may result in potentially dangerous internal bleeding.

Gastrointestinal effects   Notwithstanding the impressions engendered by advertisements, aspirin-induced gastrointestinal upset is not very commonly encountered. The problems of dyspepsia (indigestion), nausea, and vomiting can be reduced by suggesting that the patient take aspirin with food, milk, or a full glass of water.

Approximately 70 percent of all persons taking normal analgesic doses of aspirin suffer a blood loss of 2 to 6 ml, an effect resulting from irritation and ulceration of the gastric mucosa by insoluble salicylate crystals. This painless bleeding, not necessarily associated with gastric upset, may represent a significant problem for patients who are prone to anemia, have a history of peptic ulcers, or who must take high doses of aspirin for extended periods of time.

Metabolic effects   While low doses of salicylates can be safely used by diabetics, high doses (5 to 6 g) have been shown to reduce the blood glucose levels of such patients. Similarly, these doses of salicylates may increase the hypoglycemic effects of sulfonylurea oral hypoglycemic agents.

Side effects and poisoning   While salicylates are relatively nontoxic drugs, each year several hundred individuals die as the result of acute overdosage. This is particularly a problem in children less than 5 years of age who, all too frequently, ingest large numbers of flavored baby aspirins (81 mg or $1\frac{1}{4}$ grains per tablet), mistaking them for candy. The nurse should assume the responsibility to warn parents about the potential hazards associated with leaving medicines within the reach of small children.

Mild cases of chronic aspirin toxicity, called *salicylism*, are characterized by *tinnitus* or ringing in the ears (the most common and reliable symptom of salicylate toxicity), nausea, vomiting, headache, dizziness, and mental confusion. Salicylism may result from the ingestion of large therapeutic doses of these drugs for the treatment of inflammatory disorders.

Symptoms of severe acute salicylate intoxication include rapid and deep breathing, petechial hemorrhages resulting from a depression in prothrombin synthesis, coma, fever, and cardiovascular and respiratory collapse. Complex alterations in the acid-base balance of the body occur, in particular, respiratory alkalosis followed by metabolic acidosis.

Treatment of salicylate poisoning is symptomatic and is predicated upon replacement of lost fluid and electrolytes. The rate of salicylate elimination by the kidney may be increased by alkalinizing the urine with parenteral administration of sodium bicarbonate or lactate. Hemodialysis (the "artificial kidney") has been found to be the most effective method of removing salicylates from the body.

It has been estimated that 0.2 percent of all individuals are *allergic* to aspirin. After taking this drug, such patients may experience skin rashes, swelling of the eyelids, face, and lips, and asthmatic-like symptoms. Individuals with a history of allergic disorders, especially asthma, are more likely to be allergic to aspirin. Potential drug interactions involving salicylates are listed in Table 21-1.

Precautions during pregnancy
Chronic maternal ingestion of aspirin during pregnancy may have adverse effects, including a decreased birth weight, increased stillbirth rate and perinatal mortality, prolonged

duration of pregnancy and parturition, and greater bleeding problems during delivery. For these reasons, nurses should advise their patients not to take aspirin during the last trimester of pregnancy except under the advice and supervision of their physicians.

NONSALICYLATE ANALGESIC-ANTIPYRETIC AGENTS

While the salicylates are very effective and relatively nontoxic analgesic and antipyretic agents, patients suffering form extreme gastrointestinal upset or those who are allergic to these drugs or for whom their use is contraindicated, require alternative agents. A summary of the pharmacological properties of such drugs appears in Table 21-2.

Table 21-1   Potential Drug Interactions Involving Salicylates (Aspirin)

Drug/class	Possible consequences	Mechanism(s) underlying interaction
Coumarin oral anticoagulants 　Dicumarol 　Warfarin (Coumadin, Panwarfin)	Bleeding episodes.	High doses of salicylates (more than 6 g/day) reduce plasma prothrombin levels. Salicylates (more than 2 g/day) interfere with platelet aggregation and clotting. Salicylates may displace coumarin anticoagulants from plasma protein binding sites.
Oral hypoglycemic agents 　Acetohexamide (Dymelor) 　Chlorpropamide (Diabinese) 　Tolazamide (Tolinase) 　Tolbutamide (Orinase)	Enhanced reduction in blood sugar.	Salicylates may displace hypoglycemics from plasma protein binding sites or impair their renal excretion.
Uricosuric agents 　Probenecid (Benemid) 　Sulfinpyrazone (Anturane)	Antagonize antigout effects.	Low doses of salicylates (1–2 g) decrease uric acid excretion.
Ethanol	Increased gastrointestinal bleeding.	Alcohol ingestion produces inflammation of gastric mucosa, while salicylates produce ulceration.
Urinary acidifying agents 　Ammonium chloride 　Ascorbic acid	Increased salicylate toxicity.	Acidification of urine decreases salicylate excretion (Chapter 57).

Table 21-2   Summary of Pharmacological Properties of Analgesic-Antipyretic-Anti-Inflammatory Drugs

Generic name (trade name)	Analgesic-antipyretic	Anti-inflammatory	Uric acid excretion	Therapeutic uses	Usual oral dose	Unique properties
Aspirin Sodium salicylate	Marked.	Marked.	1 g reduced. 5 g increased.	Mild-moderate pain; fever; inflammatory disorders.	325–650 mg q. 4-6 h. Up to 7.8 g daily	Gastrointestinal bleeding and upset; impairment of blood coagulation; allergic disorders.
Salicylamide	Less than aspirin.	Less than aspirin.	No effects.	Used in combination with aspirin or acetaminophen for pain and fever.	650 mg q.i.d.	Ingredient in nonprescription sleep-facilitating products; questionable effectiveness as an analgesic agent.
Acetaminophen (Datril, Tylenol)	Equal to aspirin.	None.	No effects.	Pain and fever.	325–650 mg t.i.d.	Widely used aspirin substitute. Liver damage in high doses.
Phenacetin	Equal to aspirin.	None.	No effects.	Pain and fever.	300 mg q.i.d.	Kidney damage, high doses; methemoglobinemia, hemolytic anemia. Effective but unsafe.
Aminopyrine (Pyramidon)	Equal to aspirin.	Marked.	Slight increase.	Same as aspirin.		Used in Europe. Danger of agranulocytosis limits use.
Mefenamic acid (Ponstel)	Equal to aspirin.	Less than aspirin.	No effects.	Mild to moderate pain; limit use to 7 days; patients over 14 years of age only.	250 mg q. 6 h	Gastrointestinal side effects (diarrhea); headache; blood dyscrasias.
Methotrimeprazine (Levoprome)	Analgesic activity equal to morphine; no antipyretic effects.	None.	None.	Moderate to severe pain. Labor and delivery.	10–20 mg (IM)	Nonaddicting analgesic; intramuscular administration; marked sedation; orthostatic hypotension.

Drug	Analgesic effect	Anti-inflammatory effect	Effect on uricosuric action	Indications	Dosage	Toxicity/Comments
Phenylbutazone (Butazolidin)	Equal to aspirin.	Marked.	Increased.	Rheumatoid arthritis, osteoarthritis, ankylosing spondylitis.	300–600 mg daily	Potentially toxic; gastrointestinal intolerance; edema; blood dyscrasias.
Oxyphenbutazone (Tandearil, Oxalid)	Equal to aspirin.	Marked.	Increased.	Same as phenylbutazone.	300–600 mg daily	Same as phenylbutazone; less gastrointestinal upset.
Indomethacin (Indocin)	Equal to aspirin.	Marked.	Increased.	Same as phenylbutazone.	25 mg t.i.d.	Gastrointestinal, CNS, and visual side effects; headache; blood dyscrasias.
Sulindac (Clinoril)	Equal to aspirin.	Marked.	No effects.	Same as phenylbutazone.	150–200 mg b.i.d. with food.	New drug. Gastrointestinal disorders (pain, upset, nausea, diarrhea), CNS (dizziness, headache), rash. Impairs platelet function.
Ibuprofen (Motrin)	Equal to aspirin.	Less than aspirin.	No effects.	Rheumatoid arthritis, osteoarthritis, mild to moderate pain.	300–400 mg 3–4 times daily	Somewhat less gastrointestinal upset than aspirin. Food delays absorption.
Fenoprofen (Nalfon)	Equal to aspirin.	Less than aspirin.	No effects.	Same as ibuprofen.	300–600 mg q.i.d.	Same as ibuprofen.
Naproxen (Naprosyn)	Equal to aspirin.	Less than aspirin.	No effects.	Same as ibuprofen.	250 mg 2–3 times daily	Same as ibuprofen.
Tolmetin (Tolectin)	Equal to aspirin.	Less than aspirin.	No effects.	Rheumatoid arthritis, osteoarthritis.	600–1,800 mg daily	Same as ibuprofen.
Gold compounds Aurothioglucose (Solganal) Gold Sodium Thiomalate (Myochrysine)	None.	Marked.	No effects.	Rheumatoid arthritis (early active stages).	IM: 10 mg week 1; 25 mg weeks 2 and 3; 50 mg/ week thereafter up to total of 750 mg	Potentially toxic. Treat with BAL (Chapter 57). Variable slow onset and duration; remissions. Skin and blood disorders most common. Contraindicated kidney, liver, blood diseases.

Phenacetin and Acetaminophen

Phenacetin has been used as an analgesic-antipyretic agent for almost 90 years. In the body, phenacetin is biotransformed to acetaminophen, and this metabolite is primarily responsible for the pharmacological effects of phenacetin. Acetaminophen (Datril, Tylenol) is the most widely used analgesic-antipyretic aspirin substitute.

The analgesic and antipyretic activity of acetaminophen and phenacetin are approximately equal to that of aspirin. Unlike aspirin, neither of these drugs possesses anti-inflammatory or antirheumatic properties, nor do they modify the urinary excretion of uric acid or the normal ability of the blood to clot.

Many experts believe that the toxic risks of phenacetin outweigh the beneficial effects of this drug. Among such potential dangers include hemolytic anemia, methemoglobinemia, and, with excessive doses, kidney damage.

Acetaminophen possesses all the beneficial effects of phenacetin but does not cause blood dyscrasias or kidney damage. Moreover, unlike aspirin, it is available in liquid dosage forms (drops, syrup), making it a conveniently administered analgesic-antipyretic for young patients.

Acute acetaminophen overdosage may cause liver damage and failure (*hepatic necrosis*). Symptoms of acute toxicity may occur after the ingestion of about 7 g (approximately twenty-two 325-mg tablets), while 15 to 25 g cause severe liver toxicity and may potentially represent a lethal dose. Symptoms observed during the first few days after drug overdose include loss of appetite, nausea, vomiting, and epigastric distress; later symptoms include encephalopathy, coma, and death, the latter occurring from 2 to 7 days after drug ingestion.

Effective treatment for acetaminophen poisoning is far from satisfactory. Many poison control centers report that oral administration of acetylcysteine (Mucomyst) prevents liver damage. Toxicity can be reduced by promptly emptying the stomach by gastric lavage or with an emetic agent such as syrup of ipecac.

Methotrimeprazine

Methotrimeprazine (Levoprome), a nonaddicting analgesic agent effective for the relief of moderate to severe pain, is chemically related to phenothiazines such as chlorpromazine (Thorazine). The potent analgesic effects of this compound in the absence of respiratory depression, coupled with its ability to relieve anxiety and apprehension, make it a useful drug for obstetrical analgesia, as well as for patients experiencing pulmonary insufficiency.

The major adverse effects, orthostatic hypotension and marked sedation, and the need to administer this drug by intramuscular injection, restrict its use to nonambulatory patients. Its long-term use is not advised because of its potential ability to cause liver dysfunctions and blood dyscrasias.

INFLAMMATORY DISORDERS

Rheumatic disorders affect almost all of us at one time or another during the course of a lifetime. One such disorder, *rheumatoid arthritis*, afflicts 4.5 million Americans, of whom 800,000 are partially disabled and another 200,000 are totally disabled.

Treatment objectives in rheumatic disorders are directed toward the relief of pain, stiffness, joint swelling, and the maintenance of normal joint function. The relatively nontoxic salicylates are often the first choice of physicians for the symptomatic relief of minor rheumatoid disorders and rheumatoid arthritis. Phenylbutazone and indomethacin are widely used drugs for these disorders, but their utility is limited by their potentially severe toxicity. (Nursing implications appear at the end of this chapter.) These drugs should be reserved for patients who fail to adequately respond to the salicylates. Glucocorticoids are also used for the effective treatment of these disorders (Chapter 34).

Phenylbutazone

Phenylbutazone (Butazolidin) is a potent analgesic, antipyretic, and anti-inflammatory agent, but—because of its adverse side effects—its therapeutic applications are limited to inflammatory conditions. This compound also promotes the urinary excretion of uric acid and is employed for the treatment of gout.

This drug has been found to be effective for the treatment of ankylosing spondylitis (inflammation of the vertebratae), rheumatoid arthritis, and acute gouty arthritis attacks. Phenylbutazone reduces the pain, swelling, and inflammation associated with rheumatoid arthritis and increases the patient's ability to move the affected joints. In cases of acute gout (see page 186), this compound usually produces rapid and dramatic relief of pain and inflammation of the joints. Safer drugs are employed chronically to prevent recurring attacks of gout.

Adverse effects and nursing precautions Phenylbutazone is a potentially dangerous drug capable of producing many severe adverse effects in 10 to 45 percent of all patients. Some of these toxic effects include gastrointestinal disorders (nausea, vomiting, activation of peptic ulcers), skin rashes, and disorders of the liver. Edema formation, resulting from salt and water retention, may lead to congestive heart failure and acute pulmonary edema. A variety of serious blood dyscrasias have been caused by this drug, the most dangerous of which are agranulocytosis, aplastic anemia, and leukopenia.

In view of the severe potential dangers associated with the use of phenylbutazone, patients receiving this drug should be under direct medical supervision and should receive periodic blood examinations. Daily dosage of phenylbutazone should not exceed 600 mg. Among the early symptoms of drug-induced toxicity include fever, sore throat or other oral lesions, skin rashes, jaundice, weight gain, and black stools (resulting from gastrointestinal bleeding). Table 21-3 lists some common potential interactions involving phenylbutazone and its active metabolite oxyphenbutazone (Tandearil, Oxalid).

Indomethacin

Indomethacin (Indocin) possesses analgesic, antipyretic, and anti-inflammatory properties. It is effective for the treatment of rheumatoid arthritis, relief of the pain and stiffness associated with osteoarthritis, and for the treatment of acute attacks of gout.

The major adverse effects associated with the use of indomethacin involve the central nervous system and the gastrointestinal tract. Central side effects may include headache, dizziness, visual disturbances, and mental confusion. Gastric irritation and peptic ulcerations are not infrequently observed. This drug is contraindicated in patients with psychiatric disorders, peptic ulcers, gastritis, and ulcerative colitis. Drug interactions involving indomethacin are listed in Table 21-3.

Ibuprofen and Related Drugs

In recent years, ibuprofen (Motrin) and the chemically and pharmacologically related

Table 21-3   Potential Drug Interactions Involving Anti-Inflammatory Agents

Anti-inflammatory agent	Interaction drug/class	Potential consequences
Phenylbutazone (Butazolidin) Oxyphenbutazone (Tandearil)	Oral hypoglycemic agents Acetohexamide (Dymelor) Chlorpropamide (Diabinese) Tolazamide (Tolinase) Tolbutamide (Orinase)	Anti-inflammatory agents interfere with renal excretion of hypoglycemic agents, potentially causing a severe hypoglycemic response in diabetic patients.
Phenylbutazone Oxyphenbutazone Sulfinpyrazone (Anturane) Indomethacin (Indocin)	Oral anticoagulant agents Warfarin Dicumarol Phenprocoumon (Liquamar) Phenindione (Hedulin)	These anti-inflammatory agents may displace the anticoagulants from plasma protein binding sites, thus potentiating the hypoprothrombinemic response and possibly resulting in severe bleeding. This drug combination should be avoided.
Oxyphenbutazone	Methandrostenolone (Dianabol)	This anabolic steroid increases plasma levels of oxyphenbutazone potentially increasing its toxicity.
Indomethacin	Corticosteroids	Increased incidence or severity of gastrointestinal ulceration.

arylalkanoic acid derivatives*, fenoprofen (Nalfon), naproxen (Naprosyn), and tolmetin (Tolectin), have been introduced (Table 21-2). These drugs are effective analgesic, antipyretic, and anti-inflammatory agents. Their major advantage is a lower incidence of gastrointestinal distress than with aspirin.

These drugs are effective for the relief of symptoms associated with rheumatoid arthritis. Ibuprofen and fenoprofen are also useful for the treatment of osteoarthritis. The concurrent use of salicylates and arylalkanoic acid derivatives does not provide therapeutic benefits greater than those observed when aspirin is employed alone and may increase the risk of adverse effects.

The most common adverse effects caused by these drugs include gastrointestinal upset, dizziness, headache, drowsiness, and tinnitus. In most studies, the incidence of gastrointestinal distress has been considerably less than that reported with therapeutically equivalent doses of aspirin or indomethacin. Full assessment of the relative

*Also called propionic acid derivatives.

benefits and risks of these drugs will require additional clinical study.

GOUT

In gout, there is an abnormality of urate metabolism, resulting in an elevation in serum urate levels. In some patients, the observed *hyperuricemia* arises from excessive uric acid production, while in other individuals renal urate excretion is less than normal. The extreme pain associated with gout results from the deposition of urate crystals (tophi) in and around the joints of the large toe, elbow, knee, and ankle, as well as in the renal tubules.

Drugs available for the treatment of gout achieve one of three objectives, namely: terminate an acute attack (colchicine); prevent gouty episodes by increasing the excretion of uric acid with uricosuric agents (probenemid); or prevent attacks by inhibiting the synthesis of uric acid (allopurinol). Nursing implications associated with the administration of these antigout drugs are summarized at the end of this chapter.

An acute attack of gout may be effectively terminated by the administration of colchicine or an anti-inflammatory agent (phenylbutazone, indomethacin) as soon as the symptoms appear.

Colchicine

The use of the meadow saffron, a plant belonging to the lily family, for the treatment of gout dates back to ancient Roman times. Colchicine is an alkaloid obtained from the corm of this plant.

To arrest an acute attack of gout, colchicine (0.5 to 1 mg) is taken every hour until relief of pain occurs (generally 2 to 3 hours) or until the patient experiences nausea, vomiting, or diarrhea. Pain, swelling, and redness generally abate within 12 hours and are absent within 24 to 48 hours. Fewer than 5 percent of all patients with gout fail to obtain benefit from this therapy. Tolerance does not develop to the beneficial effects of colchicine, and this drug is sometimes used prophylactically to minimize the frequency and severity of attacks.

Colchicine is not an analgesic agent nor does it enhance the renal excretion of urates. It is currently believed that colchicine reduces the local production of lactic acid; the presence of this acid is thought to favor the deposition of urate crystals in the joints.

Uricosuric Agents

Probenecid (Benemid) and *sulfinpyrazone* (Anturane) are *uricosuric agents*. Chronic administration of these drugs reduces elevated serum urate levels by promoting uric acid excretion; this effect is accomplished by the ability of these drugs to inhibit the reabsorption of uric acid across the proximal tubules of the nephron. Salicylates interfere with the uricosuric effects of these drugs, and, therefore, aspirin should not be employed concurrently.

While probenecid and sulfinpyrazone are highly effective in preventing acute episodes of gout and gouty arthritis, these drugs lack analgesic and antipyretic properties and are, therefore, ineffective for the relief of pain associated with an acute attack. Daily adult oral doses of probenecid and sulfinpyrazone are 1 to 2 g and 100 to 400 mg, respectively; these doses are given in 2 to 4 divided portions.

Nurses should encourage their patients to maintain a high fluid intake while taking these drugs to reduce the possibility of renal stone formation (urolithiasis) and the occurrence of renal colic.

Allopurinol

Allopurinol (Zyloprim) represents a unique approach to the treatment of gout. This drug, devoid of analgesic, anti-inflammatory, and uricosuric properties, acts by inhibiting the enzyme xanthine oxidase, thus reducing uric acid synthesis. Chronic administration of allopurinol reduces serum urate levels, prevents the formation of new tophi, and mobilizes existing tophi. Since less uric acid is being synthesized when this drug is administered, the potential danger of renal stone formation is reduced. Aspirin, phenylbutazone, indomethacin, or colchicine may be used safely by patients taking allopurinol. The usual daily adult maintenance dose of allopurinol is 300 mg, given once per day.

The principal side effects associated with the use of allopurinol include gastrointestinal upset, skin rashes, fever, leukopenia, and, rarely, reversible liver disorders.

Nonnarcotic Analgesics, Anti-inflammatory, Antigout Agents
nursing implications

Salicylates

1. Ask the patient about history of salicylate hypersensitivity prior to drug administration.
2. Teach the patient and family about nonprescription drugs containing aspirin. Buffered aspirin does not produce more rapid analgesia or less gastrointestinal upset than un-buffered aspirin. Buffered aspirin in effervescent preparations (Alka-Seltzer) is more rapidly absorbed, produces higher plasma salicylate levels, and causes less gastro-intestinal upset than aspirin; the high sodium content of such preparations is contra-indicated for many individuals.
3. Salicylates should be taken at regular specified intervals to obtain maximum anti-inflammatory effects.
4. Teach the patient to recognize that tinnitus is an early sign of toxicity and indicates the need for reduced dosage.
5. Salicylate ingestion is among the most common causes of accidental poisoning in chil-dren less than 5 yr of age. Caution parents to keep all drugs out of the reach of children. Aspirin should not be given routinely to children, nor should it ever be called *candy*. Chil-dren with fever and dehydration are particularly susceptible to toxicity, even from rela-tively small doses.
6. Large doses of aspirin inhibit clotting. Observe patients receiving anticoagulants for bruises or bleeding from the mucous membranes.
7. Observe and teach diabetic patients that salicylates may enhance the hypoglycemic effects of antidiabetic drugs.
8. Because of the potential adverse effects of aspirin on mother and baby, women should be strongly urged not to take aspirin during pregnancy, especially during the last trimester.

Phenylbutazone (Butazolidin)

1. The patient should be advised to discontinue drug and immediately notify the physician upon the appearance of symptoms of potential agranulocytosis (malaise, sore throat, ulcerated mucous membranes) or hypersensitivity reaction (rash, edema, wheezing).
2. A salt-restricted diet may be required because of drug-induced sodium retention.
3. Instruct the patient how to check for edema and to record weight daily.
4. If no improvement is noted within one week, drug should be discontinued. If improve-ment results, dose should be reduced to lowest effective level.
5. Importance of regular and frequent blood tests must be stressed.

Probenecid (Benemid)

1. Advise the patient to continue taking probenecid with colchicine during acute gouty attacks unless directed otherwise by the physician.

2. Aspirin interferes with uricosuric effects of probenecid and should not be used; acetaminophen is an acceptable analgesic.

Allopurinol (Zyloprim)

1. Inform the patient that during initiation of therapy, an increased number of acute gouty attacks may be experienced.

2. A large fluid intake should be maintained to result in urinary excretion of 2 l to reduce risk of kidney damage.

3. Discontinue therapy immediately upon the appearance of a skin rash. Therapy may be reinstituted at a later date, employing a lower dose.

Colchicine

1. Teach the patient to keep drug readily available and the importance of early recognition of prodromal symptoms to reduce severity of attack by early treatment; symptoms include diuresis, mood change, local pruritis, or discomfort in affected joint.

2. Encourage the patient to increase fluid intake during an acute gouty attack to maintain a daily urine output of at least 2 l. This promotes urate excretion and decreases danger of urate crystal deposition in the kidneys and ureters.

3. Explain expected therapeutic response: articular pain and swelling generally decrease within 8-12 h and usually disappear within 24-72 h.

SUPPLEMENTARY READINGS

Atkins, E., and P. Bobel, "Fever," *New England Journal of Medicine* **286**: 27–34 (1972).

Beaver, W. T., "Mild Analgesics: A Review of Their Clinical Pharmacology," *American Journal of the American Medical Sciences* **250**: 576–599 (1965).

Boss, G. R., and J. E. Seegmiller, "Hyperuricemia and Gout," *New England Journal of Medicine* **300**: 1459–68 (1979).

Ferreira, S. H., and J. R. Vane, "New Aspects of the Mode of Action of Nonsteroid Anti-inflammatory Drugs," *Annual Review of Pharmacology* **14**: 57–73 (1974).

Flower, R. J., S. Moncada, and J. R. Vane, "Analgesic-Antipyretics and Anti-Inflammatory Agents; Drugs Employed in the Treatment of Gout," in *Goodman and Gilman's The Pharmacological Basis of Therapeutics* (6th ed.), ed. A. G. Gilman, L. S. Goodman, and A. Gilman, Chapter 29, pp. 682–728. New York: Macmillan, Inc., 1980.

Hudak, C. M., "A Pyramidal Treatment Plan for the Patient With Arthritis," *Nurse Practitioner* **2**(5): 19–23 (1977).

Jozwiak, J. S., "Acetaminophen Overdose," *RN* **41**(12): 56–62 (1978).

Murray, T., and M. Goldberg, "Analgesic Abuse and Renal Disease," *Annual Review of Medicine* **26**: 537–50 (1975).

Roe, R. L., "Drug Therapy in Rheumatic Diseases," *Medical Clinics of North America* **61**(2): 405–418 (1977).

Van Tyle, W. K., "Internal Analgesic Products," in *Handbook of Nonprescription Drugs* (6th ed.), pp. 125–140. Washington, D.C.: American Pharmaceutical Association, 1979.

Villaverde, M. M., and C. W. MacMillan, *Fever: From Symptom to Treatment.* New York: Van Nostrand Reinhold Company, 1978.

CENTRAL NERVOUS SYSTEM STIMULANTS

Central nervous system stimulants or analeptics have been traditionally classified on the basis of their primary site of action, namely, the spinal cord (for example, strychnine), medulla or brain stem (for example, nikethamide), and the cerebral cortex (for example, cocaine, caffeine, amphetamine) (Figure 9-1). The cerebral stimulants are the major drugs of contemporary significance in this class.

SPINAL CORD STIMULANTS

Strychnine, the most important spinal cord stimulant, was extensively employed in the past in low doses as a bitter tonic to stimulate the appetite, as a laxative, as a respiratory and cardiac stimulant for the treatment of overdosage by barbiturates, and as a rat poison. There is a small margin of safety between therapeutic and convulsant doses of this drug. Large doses of this drug produce *convulsions*, arising from the actions of this drug in the spinal cord. Death results from respiratory failure and asphyxia after a series of convulsions. There is no longer a medical justification for the use of this drug.

MEDULLARY (BRAIN STEM) STIMULANTS

These drugs exert direct stimulatory effects on medullary centers, increasing the rate and depth of respiration and minute volume. The medullary stimulants (Table 22-1) have been used for the treatment of respiratory depression induced by barbiturate and nonbarbiturate sedative-hypnotics, alcohol, and narcotic analgesics, and to hasten postoperative recovery periods. In general, doses of these drugs not greatly exceeding those required to stimulate respiration may potentially cause severe convulsions. These analeptic agents have been largely replaced by mechanical respirators, which are equally effective in stimulating respiration and are devoid of convulsive potential.

CEREBRAL STIMULANTS

The most important central nervous system stimulants, when viewed in terms of their contemporary therapeutic and nonmedical uses, are those drugs that stimulate the cerebral cortex. Cerebral stimulants elevate the mood, increase alertness, and suppress

Table 22-1   Representative Medullary and Convulsant Stimulants

Generic name	Trade name	Usual adult dose	Remarks
Pentylenetetrazol	Metrazol	IM: 100–200 mg.	Formerly used as a medullary stimulant and convulsant agent for the treatment of psychiatric disorders; now obsolete.
Picrotoxin			Formerly employed as a respiratory stimulant in barbiturate poisoning; now obsolete.
Nikethamide	Coramine	IV or IM: 2–10 ml of 25% sol.	Respiratory stimulant with weak convulsant properties; rarely used to treat barbiturate overdosage.
Doxapram	Dopram	IV: 2 mg/kg. Repeat in 5 min.	Respiratory stimulant used for treatment of postoperative respiratory depression; increases depth and possibly rate of respiration. Wide margin of safety between respiratory stimulant and convulsant doses. Major adverse effects include hypertension and an increase in heart rate.

Table 22-2   Representative Cerebral Stimulants

Generic name	Trade name	Remarks
Cocaine		After intravenous injection or sniffing, produces rapid but short-lived euphoric excitement, feelings of mental and physical superiority, and often delusions of persecution and hallucinations. Only approved use is as a topically administered local anesthetic agent. Very strong abuse potential.
Caffeine		Pharmacologically active constituent of coffee, tea, cocoa, cola beverages. Mild cerebral stimulant (100–150 mg) and respiratory stimulant (500 mg).
Amphetamine	Benzedrine	Racemic mixture of dextroamphetamine and levoamphetamine, producing central stimulation and more pronounced peripheral effects (hypertension, tachycardia) than dextroamphetamine. Same therapeutic uses as dextroamphetamine.
Dextroamphetamine	Dexedrine	Potent CNS stimulant used for the treatment of hyperkinetic disorders in children, narcolepsy, and short-term management of obesity. Strong abuse potential.
Methylphenidate	Ritalin	Mild CNS stimulant with amphetamine-like effects used for the treatment of hyperkinetic disorders in children and narcolepsy. Nervousness and insomnia are the most common side effects. Abuse potential of this drug has been demonstrated.
Pemoline	Cylert	CNS stimulant but with minimal sympathomimetic effects. Used for treatment of hyperkinetic disorders. Insomnia is the most common side effect. The abuse potential of this recently introduced drug has not been fully assessed.

feelings of fatigue. Cocaine, caffeine, amphetamine, and methylphenidate will be discussed (Table 22-2).

Cocaine

For hundreds of years, the leaves of the coca plant (*Erythroxylon coca*) have been chewed by Peruvian Indians in the Andes Mountains to elevate their spirits, ward off feelings of hunger, and enable them to endure arduous labor for long periods of time. In this chapter, the central stimulating properties of cocaine, the major active constituent of coca, will be considered; the employment of cocaine as a local anesthetic agent, which is the only medically approved use of this drug, is discussed in Chapter 12.

Cocaine is rapidly absorbed after intravenous injection or sniffing ("snorting"). This drug produces intense feelings of euphoric excitement and feelings of mental and physical superiority. These effects, coupled with cocaine-induced paranoid delusions and hallucinations, may result in the performance of antisocial and often violent acts.

Unlike amphetamine, which has a duration of action of several hours after a single injection, cocaine's effects dissipate within 5 to 15 minutes, thus necessitating a subsequent injection to recapture the euphoria. Users often repeat cocaine administration continuously for several days until their drug supply is exhausted. Chronic administration of cocaine does not appear to result in tolerance or physical dependence, but compulsive psychological dependence often develops.

Repeated sniffing of cocaine may cause perforation of the nasal septum resulting from ischemic necrosis, an adverse effect attributed to the vasoconstrictor properties of this drug. In addition to its adverse behavioral changes, high doses may produce tachycardia, palpitations of the heart, fever, abdominal pain, and convulsive seizures. Death is caused by respiratory failure resulting from depression of vital medullary centers.

Caffeine

Caffeine is the most widely used cerebral stimulant. It is a naturally occurring xanthine contained in coffee, tea, cocoa, and the kola nut used to make cola beverages.

Pharmacological effects   With increasing doses, caffeine activates the cerebral cortex, then the medulla, and in toxic doses, the spinal cord. At doses of 50 to 200 mg, the equivalent of one-half to two cups of coffee, caffeine enhances mental alertness and attention span and reduces drowsiness and fatigue. Caffeine is the primary active constituent in nonprescription stimulant products promoted to enhance wakefulness.

Increasing the dosage above 200 mg does not further increase mental and physical performance, but causes nervousness, irritability, tremors, and headache. Larger doses stimulate respiratory centers in the medulla, while toxic doses (larger than 1 g) cause convulsions of the spinal type. Caffeine directly stimulates the myocardium, increasing heart rate and cardiac output, and may also cause arrhythmias. Since caffeine stimulates the flow of pepsin and gastric acid, patients with gastric or duodenal ulcers should avoid or limit their ingestion of coffee.

Chronic administration of large volumes of coffee results in the development of psychological dependence to caffeine, tolerance to its stimulatory properties, and mild physical dependence. The caffeine withdrawal syndrome is characterized by nervousness, irritability, and a pulsating headache.

Therapeutic uses   A caffeine and sodium benzoate injection is sometimes employed as a medullary stimulant in mild cases of respiratory depression. Where severe respiratory depression exists, a mechanical respirator or more potent respiratory stimulatory drugs should be employed. Ergotamine tartrate and caffeine (Cafergot) are used orally (in combination) for the relief of migraine headaches. The beneficial effects of caffeine in this condition have been attributed to its ability to constrict cerebral blood vessels (Chapter 38). Caffeine is the primary active constituent in nonprescription stimulants (NoDoz, Stim 250, Tirend, Vivarin).

Amphetamine

Amphetamine is chemically and pharmacologically similar to ephedrine and other sympathomimetic agents (Chapter 5). While the predominant pharmacological actions of these latter drugs are manifested by peripheral effects, amphetamine acts primarily on the central nervous system. Amphetamine and related drugs (Table 22-2) are among the most potent central stimulants in common medical usage.

Pharmacological effects Therapeutic doses of amphetamine elevate the mood, reduce feelings of fatigue and hunger, increase powers of concentration, bolster self-confidence, and enhance the desire and capacity to carry out work. Performance of simple mental tasks is improved but, while work output is increased, the number of errors associated with the task is not necessarily decreased.

The central stimulatory effects of amphetamine have been attributed to its actions on two brain systems, namely, the ascending reticular activating system (ARAS) and the reward system. Stimulation of the ARAS results in an augmented state of arousal to environmental stimuli, heightening the level of mental and physical activity, and brightening the individual's subjective appraisal of the world. The "flash" or explosive euphoric effect experienced after intravenous amphetamine administration is thought to be the consequence of a profound activation of the reward center.

Amphetamine is an indirect-acting sympathomimetic agent with actions that have been attributed to its ability to stimulate the release of norepinephrine and dopamine from adrenergic nerves, as well as inhibit their reuptake, prolonging their abilities to interact with their respective receptor sites in critical areas of the brain.

Therapeutic uses *Dextroamphetamine* (Dexedrine), the most widely used of the amphetamine-like drugs, has three medically acceptable uses, namely, for the treatment of narcolepsy and hyperkinetic disorders in children and as an appetite suppressant. Nursing implications are summarized at the end of this chapter.

Narcolepsy Narcolepsy is a relatively rare neurological disorder characterized by uncontrollable attacks of sleep, which may occur several times daily; each may be minutes to hours in duration. Dextroamphetamine is highly effective in preventing such attacks of sleep. Tolerance does not appear to develop to this stimulant effect.

Hyperkinetic disorders Hyperkinetic children exhibit such symptoms as intense physical activity and restlessness, aggressiveness and impulsive behavior, a short attention span and easy distraction from the task at hand, and poor school performance, manifested by underachievement and special learning disabilities. It has been estimated that at least 3 percent of American elementary-school children may suffer from hyperkinetic disorders, which many clinicians prefer to designate *minimal brain dysfunction*.

Dextroamphetamine has a paradoxical calming effect in a high proportion of these children, with parents and teachers reporting that drug-treated children present fewer behavioral problems. While tolerance to these beneficial effects does not appear to develop, the benefits obtained after chronic (5-year) drug administration have been recently questioned.

Common side effects observed with the usual therapeutic doses of dextroamphetamine (5 to 10 mg three times daily) are generally minor and include insomnia, loss of appetite, irritability, headache, and gastrointestinal cramps. Chronic use of dextroamphetamine decreases weight gain and growth; these effects can be reduced by using this drug intermittently or discontinuing drug administration during vacation periods. Prior to initiating drug therapy, possible organic causes for the behavioral abnormalities exhibited should be excluded.

Appetite suppression   While obesity has been shown to have social, behavioral, genetic, and physiological determinants, the common factor in virtually all cases is food intake that is in excess of the individual's normal energy requirements. Obesity, in addition to being cosmetically unsightly, is associated with a higher incidence of hypertension, atherosclerosis, coronary artery disease, and diabetes and a reduction in life expectancy.

Dextroamphetamine and pharmacologically related drugs (Table 22-3) are commonly (and, all too often, indiscriminately) employed to suppress appetite, assisting the patient in essential dietary restrictions that are difficult to maintain. Numerous carefully controlled studies have clearly demonstrated that dextroamphetamine is an effective *anorexiant* (appetite suppressant).

Table 22-3   Representative Amphetamine-Like Appetite Suppressants

Generic name	Representative trade name	Usual oral dose	Remarks
Dextroamphetamine	Dexedrine	5 mg t.i.d.	Highly effective appetite suppressant to which tolerance develops within a few weeks. Adverse CNS effects: nervousness, insomnia. Adverse cardiovascular effects low at therapeutic doses: headache, palpitations. High abuse potential.
Methamphetamine (desoxyephedrine)	Desoxyn	2.5–5 mg t.i.d.	Same properties as amphetamine, but greater potency and CNS stimulation, fewer cardiovascular effects.
Benzephetamine	Didrex	25 mg 1–3 times daily	These drugs possess weak amphetamine-like properties and are neither more effective nor cause fewer peripheral side effects. The abuse potential of phenmetrazine and diethylpropion have been documented.
Chlorphentermine	Pre-Sate	65 mg o.d.	
Diethylpropion	Tenuate, Tepanil	25 mg t.i.d.	
Mazindol	Sanorex	1 mg t.i.d.	
Phendimetrazine	Plegine	35–70 mg b.i.d.	
Phenmetrazine	Preludin	25 mg 2–3 times daily	
Phentermine	Wilpo	8 mg t.i.d.	
Fenfluramine	Pondimin	20–40 mg t.i.d.	Although chemically related to amphetamine, this appetite suppressant produces drowsiness and depression rather than stimulation; weak cardiovascular effects. Possible peripheral mechanism of appetite suppression. Gastrointestinal upset common.
Phenylpropanolamine	Diet-Trim Slender-X	25 mg t.i.d.	Most common ingredient in nonprescription appetite suppressants. Pharmacologically similar to amphetamine, but much less potent. Questionable effectiveness at recommended doses. Also used as a nasal decongestant.

The weight loss observed in obese patients taking this drug has been attributed primarily to a reduction in food intake, with an increase in metabolism of fats of minor importance. The appetite suppressing effects of amphetamine are thought to result from a drug-induced inhibition of the feeding center located in the hypothalamus; this drug also depresses the senses of smell and taste, which may contribute to the loss of appetite.

It has been clinically observed that amphetamine produces the greatest weight losses within the first 3 or 4 weeks of continuous therapy. Thereafter, *tolerance* develops, rendering the drug less effective and often resulting in a return to previous undesirable eating habits. To regain the anorexiant effects of amphetamine, as well as its mood elevating properties, some patients increase the dosage taken without consulting their physician, which can lead to the development of state of psychological dependence. Most physicians are aware of these dangers, and, in recent years, have wisely limited the frequency and duration for which they prescribe these drugs. The rapidity with which tolerance develops and the risk of abuse can be substantially reduced by initiating a course of therapy that includes alternating periods of drug use and drug holidays.

No drug developed to date (Table 22-3) is superior to or safer than dextroamphetamine or methamphetamine as an appetite suppressant. With the exception of fenfluramine (Pondimin), all are weak amphetamine-like stimulants, with inherent abuse potential. These drugs are not a cure for obesity but rather serve as a crutch in the initial period during which the patient must adjust to restrictions in caloric intake. Because of the rapid development of tolerance to the appetite suppressing effects of the amphetamines, these drugs should be viewed only as a *short-term aid* in dieting until the patient makes permanent changes in eating patterns.

Side effects, toxicity, and precautions   Side effects observed with the amphetamines include restlessness, anxiety, irritability, insomnia, headache, dryness of the mouth, gastrointestinal disorders, palpitations of the heart, tachycardia, and hypertension.

Acute overdosage of amphetamine produces effects that are an extension of its normal pharmacological effects, including excitement, agitation, hypertension, tachycardia, slurred speech, fever, ataxia, tremors, and a toxic psychosis characterized by hallucinations and delusions of persecution (see below). In cases terminating in death, convulsions and coma occur, with cerebral hemorrhages often noted in postmortem examinations. Treatment of overdosage includes acidification of the urine with ammonium chloride to enhance the rate of urinary elimination and the administration of chlorpromazine (Thorazine) for the management of adverse behavioral effects and the reduction of hypertension.

The amphetamines should not be administered to patients with hypertension, cardiovascular disorders, or hyperthyroidism because their sympathomimetic effects worsen these conditions. Potential drug interactions involving amphetamine and related drugs appear in Table 22-4. These drugs should not be given to individuals with histories of drug abuse.

Misuse and abuse   The amphetamines are widely misused and abused by individuals seeking mood elevation, increased alertness, and reduction in fatigue, and by athletes who become more aggressive when taking these drugs. The nature and extent of the nonmedical use of amphetamine varies widely among individuals, from some regularly taking approximately therapeutic doses by mouth on a daily basis for extended periods of time, to those self-administering massive doses intravenously in sprees.

Table 22-4   Potential Interactions Involving Amphetamine-Like Central Nervous Stimulants

Stimulant	Interacting drug/class	Potential consequences
Dextroamphetamine Methamphetamine	Monamine oxidase inhibitor antidepressants Isocarboxazid (Marplan) Phenelzine (Nardil) Tranylcypromine (Parnate) Furazolidone (Furoxone)	MAO inhibitors block the metabolism of amphetamine, resulting in an increase in blood pressure. Furazolidine also inhibits MAO.
Amphetamines Ephedrine Mephentermine Methylphenidate	Guanethidine (Ismelin)	Amphetamine and related drugs displace guanethidine from binding sites in adrenergic neuron, thus antagonizing its antihypertensive effects.
Amphetamine	Acetazolamide (Diamox) Ammonium chloride Sodium bicarbonate	Urinary acidifying agents such as ammonium chloride and acetazolamide increase the elimination of amphetamine, while sodium bicarbonate, an alkalinizing agent, slows the urinary elimination of amphetamine.

Nursing responsibilities include explanations of the potential physiological and psychological hazards associated with the nonmedical use of amphetamines to such individuals and assist them in identifying alternative means of coping with their problems.

Following an intravenous injection of methamphetamine ("speed" or "meth"), a sudden, overwhelming, pleasurable euphoric feeling ("flash" or "rush") is experienced, during which time the user feels mentally and physically superior. There is an intense fascination with all thoughts and activities, with no interest in food or sleep. Veteran "speed freaks" have been reported to inject 500 mg every 2 to 3 hours continuously for several days without sleep. At the end of a "run," the user falls into a deep sleep for 12 to 18 hours, awakening lethargic and often depressed, with a ravenous appetite.

During the course of a "run," the user often experiences an *amphetamine psychosis*, the clinical symptoms of which are virtually indistinguishable from paranoid schizophrenia that is not drug-induced (delusions of persecution and visual and auditory hallucinations). In addition, the user performs stereotyped, repetitive, purposeless

acts for hours at a time. The amphetamine psychosis generally subsides after the termination of drug administration, although in some instances, the mental aberrations persist for days, weeks, or even months after the last dose. Administration of a phenothiazine (chlorpromazine) or butyrophene (haloperidol) antipsychotic agent effectively controls the amphetamine psychosis.

After chronic administration of amphetamine, *tolerance* is acquired to the peripheral effects of this drug, as well as to the central stimulatory effects that are responsible for excitement and euphoria. By contrast, tolerance does not develop to the amphetamine psychosis. Upon abrupt withdrawal of high doses of amphetamine, the user is greatly fatigued, depressed, and hungry, and exhibits abnormal brain wave recordings associated with rapid-eye movement (REM) sleep suppression. Many investigators have interpreted these symptoms as evidence of an abstinence syndrome associated with the development of physical dependence.

Methylphenidate

Methylphenidate (Ritalin) is chemically and pharmacologically similar to the amphetamines. Therapeutic doses of methylphenidate produce less pronounced effects on the cardiovascular system and less profound central nervous system stimulation, while high doses produce typical amphetamine-like effects and toxic reactions. This drug possesses abuse potential.

This drug has been found to be effective for the treatment of hyperkinetic disorders in children and narcolepsy. Methylphenidate is as effective as amphetamine in the former disorder and may produce less inhibition of growth. Some clinicians prefer using methylphenidate rather than amphetamine for the prevention of daytime sleep attacks of narcolepsy because it has fewer side effects.

Central Nervous System Stimulants: nursing implications

Amphetamines

1. Administer 30-60 min before meals when used for appetite suppression. The last dose should be at least 6 hours prior to the usual time of retiring to prevent insomnia.
2. Instruct the patient on a weight reduction program that drugs are only effective for 4-6 wk when used on daily basis; thereafter, tolerance develops to anorexic effects. The only effective program is one that enables patient to make permanent changes in eating patterns. Assist patient in dietary planning.
3. Amphetamines may mask fatigue that can impair ability to perform potentially hazardous tasks such as driving or operating machinery.
4. Drug should be discontinued if patient exhibits signs of psychological dependence.
5. Instruct the patient about the potential physiological and psychological hazards associated with the nonmedical use of amphetamines.

SUPPLEMENTARY READINGS

Andrews, G., and D. Solomon, eds., *The Coca Leaf and Cocaine Papers.* New York: Harcourt Brace Jovanovich, Inc., 1975.

Appelt, G. D., "Weight Control Products" in *Handbook of Nonprescription Drugs*, APhA Staff Project, 5th ed., pp. 177–183. Washington, D.C.: American Pharmaceutical Association, 1977.

Cantwell, E., ed., *The Hyperkinetic Child: Diagnosis, Management, and Current Research.* New York: John Wiley & Sons, Inc., 1975.

Delacruz, F. F., B. H. Fox, and R. H. Roberts, eds., "Minimal Brain Dysfunction," *Annals of the New York Academy of Sciences* **205**:1–396 (1973).

Hahn, F., "Analeptics," *Pharmacological Reviews* **12**: 447–530 (1960).

Hoebel, R. G., "Pharmacologic Control of Feeding," *Annual Review of Pharmacology and Toxicology* **17**:605–621 (1977).

Kalant, O. J., *The Amphetamines: Toxicity and Addiction*, 2nd ed. Toronto: University of Toronto Press, 1973.

Reichman, F., ed., "Hunger and Satiety in Health and Disease," *Advances in Psychosomatic Medicine* **7**:1–336 (1972).

Saccar, C. L., "Drug Therapy in the Treatment of Minimal Brain Damage," *American Journal of Hospital Pharmacy* **35**:544–552 (1978).

Slater, I. H., "Strychnine, Picrotoxin, Pentylenetetrazol, and Miscellaneous Drugs," in *Drill's Pharmacology in Medicine* (4th ed.), ed. J. R. DiPalma, Chapter 28, pp. 517–532. New York: McGraw-Hill Book Company, 1971.

Smith, D. E., ed., *Amphetamine Use, Misuse, and Abuse*. Boston: G. K. Hall, 1979.

Truitt, E. B., Jr., "The Xanthines," in *Drill's Pharmacology in Medicine* (4th ed.), ed. J. R. DiPalma, Chapter 29, pp. 533–556. New York: McGraw-Hill Book Company, 1971.

Weiss, B., and V. G. Laties, "Enhancement of Human Performance by Caffeine and the Amphetamines," *Pharmacological Reviews* **14**:1–36 (1962).

Whitlock, F. A., et al., *Amphetamines: Medical and Psychological Studies*. New York: MSS Information Corp., 1974.

Zarcone, V., "Narcolepsy," *New England Journal of Medicine* **288**:1156–1166 (1973).

PSYCHOTOMIMETIC AGENTS AND MARIHUANA

Chapter 23

High doses of many pharmacologically diverse compounds are capable of producing hallucinations, sensory illusions, confusion, and bizarre thoughts. Among such drugs are atropine and scopolamine, bromides, lead, cortisone-like steroids, nalorphine, alcohol, and the digitalis glycosides. The disruption of behavior produced by these drugs is, however, generalized and nonspecific and represents only one of many symptoms associated with their toxic effects.

Psychotomimetic agents are compounds that specifically and consistently alter thought and sensory processes as their primary effects in moderate doses in the absence of marked effects on motor or peripheral function. Drugs in this class are sometimes referred to as *hallucinogens*, psychedelics, psychotogens, psychodysleptics, and so forth, where each of these designations has a subtle difference in its meaning from the others.

Interest in these compounds is not restricted to their nonmedical uses and the potential dangers associated with such uses. They are also employed as research tools in an attempt to gain a better understanding of the neurophysiological and neurochemical mechanisms mediating normal behavior, and their behavioral effects may provide insights into the mechanisms underlying the etiology of mental diseases.

This chapter discusses LSD and mescaline, two prototype psychotomimetic agents. Table 23-1 summarizes the properties

Table 23-1   Psychotomimetic Agents

Name	Street name	Source	Route of administration	Pharmacological effects
LSD (Lysergic acid diethylamide)	Acid	Synthetic	Oral	Insight, exhilaration, sensory hallucinations.
Lysergic acid amide	Heavenly blue, Pearly gates	Morning glory seeds	Oral	Drowsiness, perceptual distortions, hallucinations, depersonalization; euphoria may alternate with intense anxiety.
DMT (Dimethyltryptamine)	Businessman's special	Synthetic	Injection	Similar to LSD; shorter duration of action (1–2 h).
Psilocybin; Psilocin		Mexican magic mushroom	Oral	Similar to LSD.
Mescaline	Mesc	Peyote cactus (mescal)	Oral	Similar to LSD; vivid and colorful hallucinations.
DOM (Dimethoxy-methylamphetamine)	STP	Synthetic	Oral	Similar to LSD, effects lasting up to 72 h.
MDA (Methylene-dioxyamphetamine)	Love pill	Synthetic	Oral	Similar to LSD, but milder effects; amphetamine-like euphoria.
Stramonium (Asthmador)		Jimson weed	Inhalation	Disorientation, confusion, hallucinations, atropine-like effects.
Nutmeg (myristicin)		Nutmeg tree	Oral	Euphoria, hallucinations; gastrointestinal distress.
Phencyclidine (Sernyl, Sernylan)	PCP, Hog, Angel dust	Synthetic	Oral, injection	Veterinary anesthetic; euphoric, disorientation, frightening hallucinations; low therapeutic index; often in street drugs.
Marihuana (marijuana)	Grass, weed, pot, dope, hemp	*Cannabis sativa* (hemp plant)	Inhalation, oral	Euphoria, dreamlike state, increased perception.
Tetrahydrocannabinol (THC)		*Cannabis*	Inhalation, oral	Active constituent of marihuana and hashish.

of other compounds in this pharmacologic class. The inclusion of marihuana (also spelled *marijuana*) in this chapter was largely for purposes of convenience. While marihuana does produce hallucinations in high doses, this compound causes euphoria and sedation, as well as other nonbehavioral pharmacological effects, some of which may prove to be of potential therapeutic significance.

LYSERGIC ACID DIETHYLAMIDE (LSD)

The most potent psychotomimetic agent currently available is LSD, with oral doses as low as 0.025 to 0.050 mg (25 to 50 μg) capable of eliciting changes in behavior. This compound is a synthetic agent that is chemically related to the ergot alkaloids (Chapter 38).

Pharmacological Effects

Within 20 to 60 minutes after the ingestion of 100 to 250 μg of LSD, symptoms associated with sympathetic nervous system activation, including pupillary dilation, sweating, tachycardia, and a rise in body temperature, become evident. Fluctuations in mood are common, with feelings of euphoria alternating with dysphoria.

Perceptual sensations are most dramatically altered by LSD, with *synesthesia* (a crossover from one sensory modality to another) frequently reported. Colors become more intense and pulsate and may be "heard." Significant changes in thought processes may occur, with the subject describing participation in a unique experience. Not only does the person now perceive great insight into the world and its problems, but the person can view himself or herself from a distance, a phenomenon called *depersonalization*. The behavioral effects generally persist for 8 to 12 hours, with recovery generally complete by the following day.

While physical dependence apparently does not develop after chronic LSD administration, tolerance to its behavioral effects is observed when 3 or 4 doses are taken at relatively short intervals; after the termination of drug administration, tolerance is rapidly lost. Cross-tolerance has been demonstrated between LSD and mescaline, psilocybin, and psilocin, suggesting that these drugs have a common mechanism of action, but not between LSD and amphetamine or marihuana.

The mechanism underlying the profound effects on behavior of LSD are incompletely understood, but available evidence suggests that this drug may interact with neurons containing serotonin or serotonin receptors in the brain.

Adverse Effects

LSD is a relatively nontoxic compound in humans, and no deaths have been directly attributed to its administration, even in high doses. The adverse behavioral effects produced by this drug, however, are not uncommon. "Bad trips" may be characterized by confusion, extreme anxiety and panic, and marked psychotic states, during which the user may perform acts which jeopardize his or her health and safety.

Flashbacks, a trip in the absence of drug administration, may occur unpredictably weeks or months after the last dose and may be manifested by hallucinations, loss of control, and a panic-stricken feeling.

The most effective treatment of these adverse behavioral effects is to provide the user with friendly and comforting reassurance that the dysphoric feelings will pass. Parenteral administration of short-acting barbiturates or diazepam (Valium) appear to be useful. Many authorities recommend that chlorpromazine (Thorazine) or other antipsychotic agents be avoided, especially when the identity of the psychotomimetic agent has not been clearly established.

Reports have appeared linking the use of LSD to chromosomal breaks in the user and birth defects in the offspring of women using LSD. While the cause and effect relationship of these findings remains controversial, pregnant women should be strongly urged to avoid the use of this drug.

MESCALINE

The peyote cactus (*Lophophora williamsii*) has been used in religious ceremonies by Indians residing in the southwestern United States and northern Mexico. *Mescaline*, an alkaloid extracted from peyote, produces behavioral effects similar to LSD. The most characteristic of these effects are very vivid, colorful, and intense visual hallucinations. A single oral dose produces a hallucinatory state that persists for 5 to 12 hours. Mescaline is the least potent of the commonly employed psychotomimetic agents, approximately 3,000 to 5,000-times less active than LSD. Although mescaline is among the most sought-after street drugs, laboratory analysis of alleged mescaline samples rarely reveals the presence of this compound.

CANNABIS DRUGS (MARIHUANA)

Cannabis sativa, the hemp plant, is a weed that grows freely in many parts of the world, including the entire United States. Several products derived from *Cannabis* are available; they differ in their psychoactive potencies. These differences have been attributed to their concentrations of *delta-9-tetrahydrocannabinol* or *THC*.

Products derived from *Cannabis* are distinguished on the basis of the part of the plant from which they are derived and their method of preparation. *Marihuana* is generally obtained from the leaves and stems of the uncultivated plant, while *hashish* is a resin scraped from the leaves near the flowering tops of the plant. The THC content of hashish is about five times that of the marihuana that is generally available to American users. The average marihuana cigarette ("joint") in the United States contains 2.5 to 5 mg of THC.

Pharmacological Effects

The behavioral effects of *Cannabis* become evident within minutes after inhalation of a cigarette, exert their maximal affects within 10 to 30 minutes, and rarely persist for more than 2 to 3 hours. Low to moderate doses of THC (2.5 to 5 mg) produce minimal physiological changes. The most frequently observed effects include an increase in heart rate and a reddening of the conjunctiva, with these effects temporally coinciding with the onset and duration of the behavioral changes.

The user often experiences a brief stimulatory phase followed by sedation. During the initial phase, subjects may be anxious and restless, experience euphoria, and have a heightened perception of the five senses. Consciousness is altered during the sedative phase, with the subject passing in and out of a dream-like state in which there is a constant and uncontrolled flow of thoughts. Moderate doses of THC may cause rapid fluctuations in mood, more pronounced sensory images, and alterations in normal perceptions of time and distance. At high doses, THC produces a loss of personal identity, fantasies, sensory and mental illusions, disordered thought processes, and hallucinations, which are usually perceived to be pleasant.

Adverse Effects

Cannabis has a very low level of toxicity, and, to date, no documented report has been able to demonstrate lethality directly resulting from an overdose in humans. The major adverse effects are psychological in nature and include the *panic reaction* and an acute psychotic reaction. The former, most frequently encountered by novice *Cannabis* users, is characterized by apprehension, nervousness, and a panic-stricken feeling in which the user feels he or she is losing his or her mind. The panic reaction is short-lived and generally responds favorably to friendly reassurance. The acute psychotic reaction is only occasionally encountered and is manifested by disordered thinking, paranoia, loss of personal identity, and hallucinations.

Chronic, heavy smoking of *Cannabis* may result in impairment of respiratory function, bronchitis, and asthma. Some individuals experience changes in personality and a loss of interest in achievement and the pursuit of long-term goals (amotivational syndrome). Reports suggesting that regular use of *Cannabis* causes teratogenic effects in the developing fetus and impairs male fertility and the immune response (rendering the user more susceptible to infections) remain highly controversial.

Abuse Potential

The magnitude of psychological dependence to marihuana has been shown to be proportional to the frequency of its use. Little or no emotional dependence appears to develop in the occasional user, while such dependency may become quite strong for the "pot head" or very heavy user. Chronic use does not appear to result in the development of marked physical dependence, although, after the abrupt termination of high doses, mild irritability, nervousness, and insomnia have been reported. While experimental evidence suggests that tolerance may be acquired to the effects of *Cannabis*, this issue has not been conclusively resolved to date.

Potential Therapeutic Uses

At present there are no medically approved therapeutic uses of THC. This drug has been reported to reduce intraocular pressure and, therefore, may be of value in the treatment of glaucoma. Other studies suggest that THC may be a useful immunosuppressant, potentially of value for the inhibition of rejection of tissue and organ transplants. In addition, tests are currently being conducted to evaluate the use of this compound or its chemical derivatives for the treatment of hypertension, epilepsy, depression, pain associated with terminal cancer, and anticancer drug-induced nausea and vomiting.

SUPPLEMENTARY READINGS

Braude, M. C., and S. Szara, eds., *Pharmacology of Marihuana*, Volumes 1 and 2. New York: Raven Press, 1976.

Brown, F. C., *The Hallucinogenic Drugs.* Springfield, Ill.: Charles C Thomas, Publisher, 1972.

Cohen, S., and R. C. Stillman, eds., *The Therapeutic Potential of Marijuana.* New York: Plenum Publishing Corporation, 1976.

Dornbush, R. L., A. M. Freedman, and M. Fink, eds., "Chronic Cannabis Use," *Annals of the New York Academy of Sciences* **282**:1–430 (1976).

Efron, D. H., ed., *Ethnopharmacological Search for Psychoactive Drugs.* Washington, D.C.: U.S. Government Printing Office, 1967.

Hoffer, A., "D-Lysergic Acid Diethylamide (LSD): A Review of its Present Status," *Clinical Pharmacology and Therapeutics* **6**:183–235 (1965).

Mechoulam, R., ed., *Marijuana: Chemistry, Pharmacology, Metabolism and Clinical Effects.* New York: Academic Press, Inc., 1973.

Miller, L. L., ed., *Marijuana Effects on Human Behavior.* New York: Academic Press, Inc., 1974.

National Commission on Marihuana and Drug Abuse, First Report, *Marihuana: A Signal of Misunderstanding.* Washington, D.C.: U.S. Government Printing Office, 1972.

Petersen, R. C., ed., *Marijuana Research Findings: 1980.* NIDA Research Monograph 31. Washington, D.C.: U.S. Government Printing Office, 1980.

Silva Sankar, D. V., and 11 other contributors, *LSD—A Total Study.* Westbury, N.Y.: PFD Publications, 1975.

Singer, A. J., ed., "Marijuana: Chemistry, Pharmacology, and Patterns of Social Use," *Annals of the New York Academy of Sciences* **191**:1–269 (1971).

Tinklenberg, J. R., ed., *Marijuana and Health Hazards—Methodological Issues in Current Research.* New York: Academic Press, Inc., 1975.

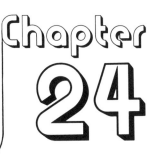

DRUG MISUSE AND ABUSE

Chapter 24

While many share the belief that the non-medical use of drugs is a unique product of the present generation, this practice undoubtedly originated shortly after the discovery of the first drug found to markedly alter mood or behavior. In recent years, we have witnessed a considerable increase in the number of individuals employing drugs for nonmedical purposes. Moreover, while several decades ago such illicit drug usage was predominately limited to the socially and economically disadvantaged, contemporary illicit drug users may be found in all strata of our society.

In the earlier chapters of this third major section of the text, the unique characteristics associated with the use, misuse, and abuse of the central nervous system stimulants, depressants, alcohol, narcotics, and psychotomimetic agents have been considered. The nurse, regardless of practice setting, will encounter individuals who are improperly using these drugs. This chapter is intended to consider some general concepts concerning the nonmedical use of drugs.

SPECTRUM OF DRUG USAGE

Arbitrarily, we might view all drug usage to be placed into one of three categories, namely, drug *use*, drug *misuse*, or drug *abuse*. Attempts to clearly define these terms are obfuscated by the orientation of the author (social, medical, behavioral, legal) as well as by the biases of the author or reader. Moreover, at times it is difficult to draw clear lines of demarcation between these three categories.

Drug use may be considered to be the administration of a drug in conventional therapeutic doses for the treatment of a medical disorder. A simple and generally acceptable definition of *drug abuse* is far more difficult to formulate. One authority defines drug abuse as the "self-administration of any drug in a manner that deviates from the approved medical or social patterns within a given culture." This definition does not take into account dosage or frequency of drug administration or any adverse effects the substance may have on the user. If this definition is adopted, some of the residents of your local community would undoubtedly characterize the use of a single marihuana "joint" to be drug abuse, whereas others would not. Other authors view drug abuse to be the self-administration of any drug to such an extent that it interferes with the health, economic, or social function of the user.

Drug misuse may be considered to be another aspect of the irrational use of drugs; it includes the use or prescribing for use of drugs in the absence of sound medical justification or for the treatment of trivial disorders. The use of a prescribed drug in a manner that deviates from the directions might also be viewed as misuse. In this regard, the prescriber must often share the onus of drug misuse with the patient, with the former possibly more culpable because of a vastly greater appreciation of the inherent risks associated with improper drug usage. The physician who freely prescribes antianxiety agents, hypnotics, stimulants, appetite suppressants, or narcotics in the absence of an adequate examination of the patient is perpetuating the misuse of drugs to the ultimate detriment of the patient in particular and society in general. No less guilty is the physician who prescribes penicillin or other antibiotics for the treatment of a child with a fever of viral origin merely to placate an anxious parent.

The uninformed irrational use of drugs is extremely prevalent and includes the self-administration of a laxative on a daily basis when an individual has failed to have a bowel movement within the past 24 hours; the use of antianxiety agents immediately upon the onset of a mildly stressful situation; and sharing antibiotics remaining from a previous illness with one's family or friends after self-diagnosing the ailment. Depending upon one's perception, smoking and drinking of alcoholic beverages may be categorized as drug use, misuse, or abuse.

CHARACTERISTICS OF DRUG DEPENDENCE

The nurse will commonly encounter the terms *addiction* and *habituation*. To avoid the ambiguities associated with their many definitions, some of which have been contradictory, in 1964 the World Health Organization recommended that these terms be abandoned and that *dependence* be adopted as an all-inclusive designation. Drug dependence is a state of psychic (psychological) dependence or physical dependence or both on a drug, resulting from the use of that drug on a periodic or continuous basis. Furthermore, since the specific characteristics differ for each class of drugs subject to abuse, specific types of drug dependence have been described: for example, dependence of the opiate type, the alcohol-barbiturate type, the amphetamine type, and so forth (Table 24-1).

All types of drug dependence can be differentiated on the basis of three fundamental characteristics: *psychological dependence*, *tolerance*, and *physical dependence* (Table 24-1). While psychological dependence can be modified by subjective factors, tolerance and physical dependence are pharmacological phenomena that are observed in all individuals, regardless of the behavioral state of the user, when certain drugs are chronically administered in sufficiently high doses and at frequent intervals. In an attempt to control illicit drug traffic in 1970, the U.S. Congress enacted the Comprehensive Drug Abuse Prevention and Control Act and established five schedules of controlled substances (Table 24-2).

Table 24-1 Comparative Characteristics of Drugs Subject to Abuse and Misuse

Type of drug dependence	Psychological dependence	Tolerance[a] to		Physical dependence
		Behavioral effects	Normal lethal doses	
Opiate				
Narcotics (Table 20-1)	Strong and rapidly developing.	Marked.	Marked.	Marked; severe, but not life-threatening abstinence syndrome.
Alcohol-Barbiturate				
Ethyl alcohol Barbiturates (Table 13-1) Nonbarbiturates (Table 13-2)	Mild to strong; slowly developing.	Marked.	Little or none.	Intensity dependent upon dosage and duration of drug administration; abstinence syndrome potentially life-threatening.
Cocaine	Strong.	None.	None.	None.
Amphetamine				
Dextroamphetamine Methamphetamine Phenmetrazine Diethylpropion	Moderate to strong.	Marked; not to amphetamine psychosis.	Marked.	Questionable; mild, if at all.
Psychotomimetics				
LSD-like (Table 23-1) Mescaline	Varying degrees.	Marked.	(Low acute toxicity.)	None.
Cannabis				
Marihuana Hashish	Mild to strong.	Mild.	(Low acute toxicity.)	Mild, if at all.
Nicotine				
Tobacco	Varying degrees.	Mild to moderate.	(No acute toxicity as used in tobacco.)	Mild to moderate.
Caffeine				
Coffee Tea	Mild.	Mild to moderate.	(Very low acute toxicity.)	Mild.

[a]Cross-tolerance among members of each drug type, with little or no cross-tolerance between drug types.

Psychological Dependence

Psychological (psychic, emotional) dependence is a state that is said to have developed when an individual feels that drug use must be continued in order to maintain normal well-being. The intensity of psychological dependence may vary from a very mild need to continue to use the drug to an overwhelming and compulsive driving force that takes precedence over all other activities. Factors that are responsible for the initial and continued nonmedical use of drugs will be considered in a later section of this chapter.

The magnitude of psychological dependence is influenced by the specific behavioral

Table 24-2   Summary of Schedule of Controlled Substances
(Comprehensive Drug Abuse Prevention and Control Act of 1970)

Schedule	Accepted medical use in USA	Potential for abuse	Prescription refills	Examples[a]
I (C–I)	None.	High.	℞ illegal.	Heroin, marihuana, LSD.
II (C–II)[b]	Yes.	High.	None.	Morphine, methadone, meperidine, cocaine, amphetamine, amobarbital, pentobarbital, secobarbital, methaqualone.
III (C–III)[b]	Yes.	Some, but less than I and II.	Not more than 5 times and not at all 6 months after ℞ originally written.	Includes nonamphetamine stimulants, depressants, preparations containing only limited quantities of codeine and paregoric.
IV (C–IV)[b]	Yes.	Some, but less than III.	Same as III.	Includes nonamphetamine stimulants, benzodiazepines (diazepam), meprobamate, phenobarbital, chloral hydrate, propoxyphene.
V (C–V)	Yes.	Low and less than IV.	Same as III.	Preparations containing only limited quantities of narcotics; primarily used for treatment of cough and diarrhea.

[a] In accordance with the provisions of the law, substances may be added to or deleted from the schedule or rescheduled.

[b] Prescriptions for drugs in Schedules II, III, and IV must bear the following warning on the container: "Federal Law prohibits the transfer of this drug to any person other than the patient for whom it was prescribed."

effects elicited by the drug, the dose employed, the interval between successive doses, and the duration of repeated drug usage.

Tolerance

Tolerance is said to have developed when, after repeated administration of a given dose, the intensity of the initially experienced effects are diminished. Conversely, when the user must continuously increase the drug dosage in order to maintain the magnitude of the drug's effects when it was first taken, tolerance to the drug exists.

We do not observe tolerance to be an all-or-none phenomenon; that is, it may develop to varying degrees to some drug-induced effects and not at all to others. The nurse will observe that after chronic administration of morphine, a significant degree of tolerance is acquired to its analgesic, sedative, and respiratory depressing effects

(resulting in an increase in the normal lethal dose), but no tolerance is developed to the ability of this drug to produce constipation or constriction of the pupils.

With the development of tolerance to a given drug, *cross-tolerance* may be simultaneously acquired to the drugs in the same pharmacological class and even to other compounds in closely related pharmacological drug classes. For example, with the acquisition of tolerance to morphine, cross-tolerance develops to all other narcotic analgesics, but not to aspirin and other nonnarcotic analgesics. Cross-tolerance is observed to barbiturates, nonbarbiturate sedative-hypnotics, and alcohol.

Physical Dependence

Physical dependence refers to adaptive physiological changes that occur in an individual after repeated drug administration such that "normal" bodily functions are maintained only in the continued presence of the drug. Abrupt drug withdrawal results in adverse changes in physiological function—the *abstinence or withdrawal syndrome*—with specific symptoms that are characteristic for a given pharmacological class of drugs. Administration of that drug or another compound exhibiting *cross-dependence* with the withdrawn drug rapidly terminates the abstinence syndrome.

There are some similarities in the time courses required for the acquisition and loss of tolerance and physical dependence, and theories have been proposed to describe common mechanisms responsible for these phenomena. Nevertheless, tolerance develops to many drugs in the absence of physical dependence.

The development of physical dependence is most commonly associated with psychoactive drugs—to the central nervous system depressants in particular. This phenomenon, however, is not restricted to behaviorally active agents. Chronic administration of laxatives (cathartics) can result in physical dependence, in which case a bowel movement is only achieved when these drugs are taken (Chapter 56).

DRUG-TAKING BEHAVIOR

There are many factors that are responsible for and contribute to an individual's desire to initiate the nonmedical use of drugs and subsequently maintain such behavior on an irregular or continuous compulsive basis. The initial use of an illicit drug may be merely experimental in nature and motivated by curiosity "just to see what it does." For the insecure adolescent, it may represent an act of rebellion against authority, a means of impressing peers, or an attempt to emulate the example set by a local hero or a prominent entertainer or athlete. Some use drugs merely to share a common social experience with friends.

For drug use to continue on a regular basis, it must provide pleasure or reduce the user's actual or imagined mental or physical discomfort. Many members of society use psychoactive drugs to enable them to combat mental or physical fatigue, boredom, depression, insomnia, and anxiety related to satisfying personal needs and aspirations or those imposed by society, their families, or jobs. Drugs are perceived by some of the socially and economically disadvantaged as a vehicle for escape from the misery, pain, frustrations, and injustices confronting them. While some seek drug-induced euphoric excitement, others search for enhanced personal insights to facilitate self-appraisal or to achieve mystical or religious experiences. For those physically dependent upon such drugs as the narcotics, the fear of the extremely unpleasant abstinence syndrome may be sufficiently great to maintain chronic drug usage.

THE NURSE'S ROLE

The nurse can play a critical role in the prevention, treatment, and rehabilitation of individuals who are abusing or misusing drugs. To fully function in this capacity, the nurse must not only maintain an up-to-date understanding of the pharmacology of drugs and their inherent dangers for toxicity and irrational use, but must also be capable of participating in the education and sympathetic treatment of these patients.

The nurse can help reduce the development of drug dependence in hospitalized patients by exercising restraint in the administration of narcotics and hypnotics. If a nonnarcotic agent suffices for the relief of pain, it should be employed in preference to a narcotic. However, for the patient experiencing severe pain that is not responsive to nonnarcotic agents, there is no rational medical justification for withholding narcotics for fear of inducing dependence. As the patient's condition improves and the pain becomes less intense, attempts should be made to gradually reduce the dosage of the opiate and substitute a nonnarcotic agent. In both inpatient and outpatient settings, the nurse should participate in the maintenance of current patient drug records to ensure that patients are not being unnecessarily maintained for protracted periods of time on medications that possess high abuse potential. Open lines of communication should be established with neighborhood pharmacists to preclude the possibility that a given patient is visiting a number of different physicians to obtain multiple prescriptions for the same psychoactive drug.

The nurse should assist the physician and pharmacist in educating patients about the rational use of drugs. While patients may fully understand the benefits to be derived from drug usage, few appreciate the potential dangers that are often associated with their use in the absence of proper medical supervision.

The nurse may be an active participant in the emergency treatment of a patient experiencing acute drug overdosage resulting in life-threatening respiratory depression or cardiovascular collapse. In other situations, the patient may be manifesting drug-induced psychoses or hallucinations. In addition to providing invaluable medical support, the nurse may be called upon to interview the patient or the patient's friends in an attempt to identify the specific drug or drugs taken to initiate the most appropriate therapy.

The nurse may care for a patient who is experiencing an abstinence syndrome after abrupt withdrawal of chronic drug administration. Once again, the nurse may be required to perform a twofold function: to provide immediate medical support and subsequently to facilitate the patient's transition to a drug-free life style. Rehabilitation of the chronic drug user often follows a tortuous path, frequently interrupted by relapses, before recovery is achieved. A sympathetic, reassuring, and supportive nurse can provide the drug user and the user's family with the critical assistance required to enable the patient to continue in the treatment program until full rehabilitation is realized.

SUPPLEMENTARY READINGS

Brecher, E. M., and the Editors of Consumers Reports, *Licit and Illicit Drugs*. Mt. Vernon, N.Y.: Consumers Union, 1972.

Drug Dependence in Pregnancy: Clinical Management of Mother and Child. DHEW Publication No. (ADM) 79–678. Washington, D.C.: U.S. Government Printing Office, 1978.

Dupont, R. I., A. Goldstein, and J. O'Donnell, eds., *Handbook on Drug Abuse*. Washington, D.C.: U.S. Government Printing Office, 1979.

Iverson, L. L., S. D. Iverson, and S. H. Snyder, eds., "Drugs of Abuse," *Handbook of Psychopharmacology* Vol. 12. New York: Plenum Publishing Corporation, 1978.

Kissin, B., J. H. Lowinson, and R. B. Millman, eds., "Recent Advances in the Chemotherapy of Narcotic Addiction," *Annals of the New York Academy of Sciences* **311**: 1–315 (1978).

Lettieri, D. J., M. Sayers, H. W. Pearson, eds., *Theories on Drug Abuse*. NIDA Research Monograph 30. Washington, D.C.: U.S. Government Printing Office, 1980.

Pradhan, S. N., and S. N. Dutta, eds., *Drug Abuse Clinical and Basic Aspects*. St. Louis: The C. V. Mosby Company, 1977.

Richter, R. W., *Medical Aspects of Drug Abuse*. New York: Harper & Row, Publishers, Inc., 1975.

Sapira, J. D., and C. E. Cherubin, *Drug Abuse: A Guide for the Clinician*. New York: American Elsevier, 1976.

Vesell, E. S., and M. C. Braude, eds., "Interactions of Drugs of Abuse," *Annals of the New York Academy of Sciences* **281**: 1–489 (1976).

Section IV

CARDIOVASCULAR DRUGS AND DIURETICS

Chapter 25

INTRODUCTION TO THE CARDIOVASCULAR SYSTEM

Diseases of the cardiovascular system are the most common causes of disability and death in the western world. In Section IV of this textbook, we shall discuss drugs employed for the treatment of cardiovascular disorders.

Included in these discussions will be drugs that favorably alter the rate and force of contractions of the heart (Chapter 26), correct cardiac arrhythmias (Chapter 27), and maintain an adequate blood supply to the heart muscle (Chapter 29). Drugs used to reduce elevated blood pressure and serum lipids are treated in Chapters 28 and 30, respectively. Diuretics, drugs used to enhance the elimination of salt and water, are employed as valuable adjuncts in the treatment of various cardiovascular diseases (Chapter 32). In this section we shall also consider drugs that increase or decrease the rate of blood coagulation (Chapter 31).

To enable the nurse to more fully appreciate these drug-induced effects, it is first necessary to consider the physiology of the cardiovascular system. This chapter is intended to provide a brief overview of the mechanisms by which the heart and blood vessels work together to maintain the normal circulation of blood throughout the body.

OVERVIEW OF THE CARDIOVASCULAR SYSTEM

All living cells require a constant supply of oxygen and nutrients to sustain life. Moreover, these cells require a mechanism that will efficiently remove accumulated waste products. For the unicellular organism this two-way exchange of materials between the environment and the cell is accomplished by the simple process of diffusion. The survival of complex multicellular organisms, however, required the evolution of a more complex transport system that would permit the transfer of materials between individual cells and a far-removed external environment. This transport system is the cardiovascular system.

The *cardiovascular system* consists of a muscular pump, the heart, which propels the blood (containing oxygen, nutrients, and waste materials) around the body through highly specialized blood vessels.

THE HEART

The heart beats continuously at an average rate of 70 times per minute in the adult human, in excess of 2.5 billion times during an average life-span of 70 years. It is essential that the heart continuously function in this manner, because inadequate circulation of only a few minutes duration can result in tissue anoxia, causing irreversible changes that permanently impair the normal function of the brain or other tissues.

The heart consists of four chambers, two above and two below (Figure 25-1). The upper chambers are called the *atria* and the lower ones are called the *ventricles*, with blood flowing from the atria to the ventricles. The right atrium receives blood as it completes its circuit around the body and the right ventricle pumps this blood to the lungs to replenish its supply of oxygen and discharge accumulated carbon dioxide. The freshly oxygenated blood returns from the lungs and enters the left atrium and then the left ventricle. This latter highly muscular chamber ejects the blood into the aorta and on to smaller arteries, which carry the blood to the tissues of the body; the blood is returned to the right atrium by the vena cavae. Capillaries, the smallest blood vessels, connect the arteries and veins, and it is across their single-layer cell membranes that materials are exchanged between the environment and the interior of the individual cells. In summary, it may be said that the right chambers of the heart are concerned with the *pulmonary circulation* and the left chambers with the *systemic circulation* (Figure 25-2). In this section we shall discuss the cardiac cycle and factors that influence heart rate and cardiac output.

Cardiac Cycle

During every minute, the adult heart beats about 70 to 75 times, or once every 0.8 seconds. During this relatively brief period of time, the following mechanical sequence of events, which comprise the *cardiac cycle*, occur: (1) both right and left atria contract simultaneously, forcing the blood into their respective ventricles, which are in a state of relaxation; (2) the blood-filled right and left ventricles contract, expelling the blood into the pulmonary and systemic circulation, respectively; and (3) the atria and ventricles relax. Contraction of the heart is called *systole*, while the period of relaxation is referred to as *diastole*. When the heart rate is increased substantially, the time available for resting and complete refilling is reduced; this results in a decrease in cardiac output, which in time leads to such impairments of cardiac function as those in congestive heart failure.

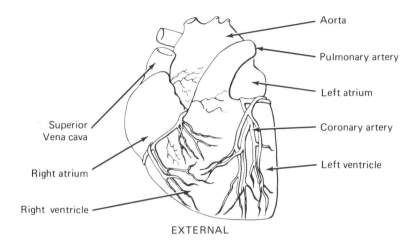

EXTERNAL

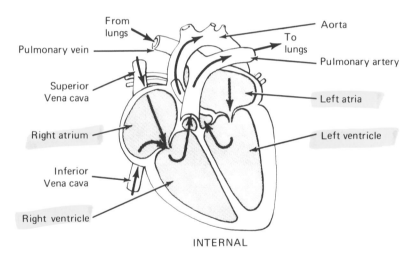

INTERNAL

Figure 25-1   External and Internal Views of the Heart.

Unlike skeletal muscle, cardiac muscle possesses inherent *automaticity*, that is, the initiation of contractions is independent of an external source of stimulation. The *heart beat* originates in a small mass of specialized muscular tissue, the *sinoatrial node* or S-A node (Figure 25-3), which functions as the normal pacemaker of the heart. The S-A node sets the pace for contraction of the heart by initiating electrical impulses that travel through the muscle fibers of the atria and the ventricles. More specifically, this excitatory impulse travels from the S-A node to the atrioventricular node (A-V node) and bundle of His, down the right and left bundle branches, and emerges in the Purkinje fibers, which distribute the impulse to all parts of the ventricles.

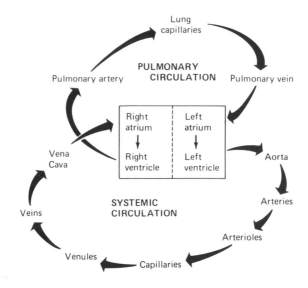

Figure 25-2   Schematic Representation of Pulmonary and Systemic Circulation.

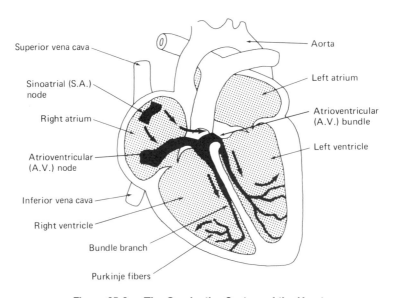

Figure 25-3   The Conductive System of the Heart.

Electrocardiogram An excitatory nerve impulse always precedes the mechanical contraction of the atria and ventricles, and these nerve impulses cause changes in electrical activity that can be detected on the surface of the body with an electrocardiograph. The electrocardiogram (EKG or ECG) serves as a diagnostic record of cardiac function and can be used to assess changes in heart rate or rhythm or in the conduction of electrical activity throughout the cardiac muscle (Figure 25-4). The EKG is frequently employed by nurses and physicians to evaluate the effectiveness of drugs in modifying abnormal cardiac activity, as well as to detect the toxic effects of drugs on the heart.

The normal EKG is composed of a P wave, a QRS complex, and a T wave (Figure 25-4). When the impulse reaches both atria, the latter depolarize electrically, producing a P wave, and contract mechanically, propelling blood into the ventricles. The interval during which the wave of excitation spreads to the A-V node and the ventricles is called the PR interval. When the impulse emerges from the Purkinje fibers, ventricular depolarization occurs, producing a QRS complex; this initiates mechanical contraction of the ventricles and drives blood out of these lower chambers of the heart. Repolarization or recovery of the ventricles is denoted by the T wave. At the end of the T wave, the muscle fibers are ready for the next wave of excitation arising from the S-A node.

Cardiac arrhythmias The normal rhythm of the heart may be altered by disturbances in the pacemaker activity of the

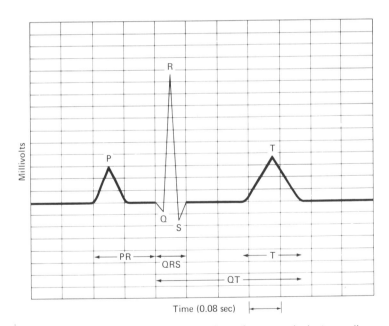

Figure 25-4 Diagrammatic representation of a normal electrocardiogram. Average durations: PR interval, 0.16 seconds; QRS interval, 0.08 seconds; QT interval, 0.36 seconds.

S-A node or by another part of the heart (ectopic focus) usurping the pacemaker function. For example, an irritable focus in the atria, the A-V node, or the Purkinje fibers may begin to generate impulses more rapidly than the S-A node, thus setting a new pace for cardiac contractions. As a result, the atria and ventricles may contract independently and at different rates, interfering with normal cardiac rhythm and causing the heart to become a less efficient or even a totally inefficient pump. The consequences of these arrhythmias vary with their type, some of which may cause death very soon after their initiation.

Heart Rate and Cardiac Output

The resting heart rate and the augmented rate caused by exercise, fever, high ambient temperatures, and emotional stresses are primarily controlled by the *autonomic nervous system.*

The heart is innervated by sympathetic and parasympathetic nerves (Chapter 4) that modify its rate and force of contraction. Parasympathetic nerve fibers supply the S-A and A-V nodes, with some nerve fibers extending to the muscles of the atria. Sympathetic nerves are more extensively distributed throughout the heart muscle, both to the aforementioned areas and to the muscles of the ventricles.

The *vagus* is the only parasympathetic nerve innervating the heart, and its actions are mediated via the release of acetylcholine from its postganglionic (cholinergic) nerve endings. Activation of the vagus nerve causes a slowing of the heart rate (bradycardia) and a reduction in the force of contraction. This parasympathetic cardio-inhibitory effect has been attributed to acetylcholine-induced depression of the S-A and A-V nodes. Activation of the *sympathetic accelerator* nerves results in the opposite effects, namely, an increase in heart rate (tachycardia) and a more powerful force of contraction. These effects are mediated by the release of norepinephrine from sympathetic (adrenergic) nerve endings, a catecholamine that stimulates the S-A node and the heart muscle.

Heart rate is influenced by a finely tuned balance between the inhibitory effects of the parasympathetic (vagus) system and the stimulatory effects of the sympathetic (accelerator) system. Under normal resting conditions, the influence of the vagus predominates. The activity of these autonomic nerves can be modulated by the central nervous system.

Alterations in the normal extracellular concentrations of *potassium*, as the result of disease or drug-induced effects, may result in marked alterations in cardiac function. Excessive potassium levels (hyperkalemia) slows the heart rate, and—in severe cases—can block conduction of the nerve impulse from the atria to the ventricles through the A-V bundle. Hypokalemia greatly increases the risk of fatal cardiac arrhythmias after digitalis administration. Although excessive extracellular concentrations of sodium depress cardiac function, even in severe disease states the alterations in the concentration of this cation are never altered greatly enough to compromise cardiac function. Similarly, while excessive calcium levels cause the heart to enter a state of spastic contraction, such levels are not achieved under physiological conditions. Severe calcium deficiencies cause effects on the heart similar to those observed during hyperkalemia, but the patient succumbs to tetany before effects on the heart are manifested.

Cardiac output, the volume of blood pumped by the heart each minute, is dependent upon the amount of blood expelled by each ventricular contraction (stroke volume) and the heart rate, or

Cardiac output =
(ml/min)

$$\frac{\text{Stroke volume}}{(\text{ml/contraction})} \times \frac{\text{Heart rate}}{(\text{contractions/min})}$$

The normal cardiac output is 5.5 liters per minute, which can be increased up to six times that of resting level by a trained athlete during strenuous exercise. This is accomplished by an increase in heart rate of about three times that of resting rate and a doubling of stroke volume. One physiological mechanism by which stroke volume is enhanced results from increased sympathetic stimulation leading to more forceful ventricular contraction; an increased volume of blood is ejected with each heart beat, enhancing the efficiency of the heart as a pump.

In *congestive heart failure*, the heart beats very rapidly but weakly. This very rapid rate does not permit sufficient time for the ventricles to fill with blood after atrial contraction, and the weak ventricular contraction does not permit the blood to be adequately expelled from this lower chamber.

Blood Supply to the Heart

To maintain normal cardiac function, the heart muscle requires an adequate supply of nutrients and oxygen. The myocardium, unlike most other tissues, does not possess an adequate reserve supply of oxygen. Consequently, at any given moment, the oxygen supply to the myocardium should be at least equal to the amount consumed by the heart muscle during contraction.

The *coronary arteries* (Figure 25-1) normally return 4 to 5 percent of the total cardiac output to the heart. During vigorous physical activity, the coronary blood flow may increase as much as four to six times over resting levels. Decreased oxygen supply to the myocardium results in hypoxia and pain, a disease called *angina pectoris.* Isch-

emia (hypoxia or anoxia) occurs when the oxygen demand exceeds the supply. If the ischemic condition is severe enough to result in tissue anoxia, myocardial infarction (heart attack) results.

CIRCULATION AND REGULATION OF BLOOD PRESSURE

Since the energy requirements of the cells of the body vary greatly during the course of daily activity, adequate circulatory regulation necessitates the transfer of blood flow from relatively inactive cells and tissues to those that are more active. Circulation of blood is accomplished because of gradients or differences in blood pressure among the blood vessels. Blood flows downhill, in effect, from vessels having higher pressure into those vessels with lower pressure. The blood pressure is 100 mm Hg in the aorta, 60 mm Hg in the arterioles, 30 mm Hg in the capillaries, and 10 mm Hg as it enters the veins; upon entering the right atrium, the blood exerts essentially no pressure.

Arterial blood pressure fluctuates with each contraction of the heart. As the blood is ejected from the left ventricle into the aorta, the blood pressure is suddenly increased as the blood enters and swells this elastic artery. The maximum arterial pressure resulting from ventricular contraction, or systole, is called *systolic pressure.* During the relaxation or diastolic phase of the cardiac cycle, blood pressure falls; this is called the *diastolic pressure.* Blood pressure is recorded and expressed as systolic pressure over diastolic pressure; the average normal blood pressure for a college-age student is 120/80. When the arterial blood pressure exceeds 140/90, the patient is said to have *high blood pressure* or *hypertension.* Blood pressure varies with age, sex, and race. The approximate average of the sum of systolic and diastolic pressures represent the *mean blood pressure*, with their difference referred to as *pulse pressure*.

Arterial pressure is directly influenced by the *cardiac output* and the *peripheral resistance* (Figure 25-5). Within certain limits, the faster the heart rate and the greater the force of cardiac contraction, the more elevated will be the arterial pressure. The increase of one or both of these cardiac parameters tends to elevate cardiac output, which increases the volume of blood within the arteries, causing an increase in blood pressure.

Peripheral resistance refers to the opposition or resistance that the walls of the arteries (mainly the arterioles) exert upon the flow of blood. This resistance to flow is inversely related to the diameter of the arterioles; that is, the smaller the diameter, the greater the resistance to blood flow and the higher the blood pressure.

Nerve endings, arising primarily from the *sympathetic* division of the autonomic nervous system, innervate all blood vessels, with the exception of the capillaries. Controlled by the vasomotor center located in the medulla oblongata, these sympathetic nerves are able to modify the activity of the smooth muscle of the arterioles, which control the

degree to which the arterioles are dilated or constricted. Hence the sympathetic nervous system plays a major role in the regulation of blood flow as well as the control of blood pressure. As we shall observe in Chapter 28, many of the antihypertensive agents that the nurse will encounter in practice act by interfering with norepinephrine-induced vasoconstriction. The reduction in arteriolar vasoconstriction resulting from the administration of these drugs reduces peripheral resistance and lowers arterial blood pressure.

SUPPLEMENTARY READINGS

Andreoli, K. G., V. Hunn, D. P. Zipes, and A. G. Wallace, *Comprehensive Cardiac Care: A Text for Nurses and Other Health Professionals* (3rd ed.). St. Louis: The C. V. Mosby Company, 1975.

Antonaccio, M., ed., *Cardiovascular Pharmacology.* New York: Raven Press, 1976.

Bhagat, B. D., *Role of Catecholamines in Cardiovascular Diseases.* Springfield, Ill.: Charles C Thomas, Publisher, 1974.

Brater, D. C., and H. F. Morrelli, "Cardiovascular Drug Interactions," *Annual Review of Pharmacology and Toxicology* 17: 293–309 (1977).

Burch, G. E., and T. Winsor, *A Primer of Electrocardiography* (6th ed.). Philadelphia: Lea & Febiger, 1972.

Cranefield, P. F., *The Conduction of the Cardiac Impulse.* New York: Futura Publishing Co., 1975.

Debarry, P., L. P. Jefferies, and M. R. Light, "Teaching Cardiac Patients to Manage Medications," *American Journal of Nursing* 75: 2,191–93 (1975).

Gordon, F. S., "Geriatric Medications: Tailoring Cardiovascular Therapy to the Patient," *RN* **41**(3): 56–61 (1978).

Guyton, A. C., C. E. Jones, and T. G. Coleman, *Circulatory Physiology: Cardiac Output and its Regulation* (2nd ed.). Philadelphia: W. B. Saunders Company, 1973.

Langer, G. A., and A. J. Brady, *The Mammalian Myocardium.* New York: John Wiley & Sons, Inc., 1974.

Montcastle, V. B., ed., Part VII, "The Circulation," *Medical Physiology* (13th ed.). Vol. 1. St. Louis: The C. V. Mosby Company, 1974.

Scheinman, M. M., ed., "Symposium on Cardiac Emergencies," *Medical Clinics of North America,* **63**(1): 1–299 (1979).

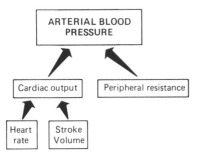

Figure 25-5 Major Factors Modifying Arterial Blood Pressure.

DIGITALIS AND RELATED CARDIAC GLYCOSIDES

Chapter 26

The medical properties of digitalis were first reported by the English physician-botanist William Withering in 1785. Almost 200 years later, it remains the drug of choice for the treatment of congestive heart failure and is among the most frequently prescribed drugs in the United States. In our discussions in this chapter, the term *digitalis* will be used to refer to the leaf or to selected cardioactive chemicals derived from the leaves of the purple foxglove, *Digitalis purpurea*, as well as to other naturally occurring compounds with similar pharmacological properties.

These digitalis-like compounds are chemically classified as *glycosides*. A glycoside is a chemical which, when hydrolyzed, breaks down into a sugar and a nonsugar (aglycone). The aglycone fraction of the digitalis glycosides contains a steroid nucleus; it is this latter fraction of the glycoside that is responsible for the effects of digitalis on the heart. The sugar portion of the molecule is not required for the cardioactive properties of the drug but increases its ability to cross cell membranes.

Although all digitalis-like drugs are generally thought to have an identical mechanism of action on the heart, major differences exist among these compounds with respect to their relative absorption into the blood stream after oral administration, as well as in their onsets and durations of action (Table 26-1, page 218). Because of the low margin of safety associated with the therapeutic use of this class of drugs, it is essential that the nurse appreciate these differences. The general pharmacological properties of the digitalis glycosides will now be discussed.

The last section of this chapter discusses the pharmacology of dobutamine, a sympathomimetic amine used for the short-term treatment of congestive heart failure.

PHARMACOLOGICAL ACTIONS ON THE HEART

The primary effects of digitalis on the heart are two-fold. First, this drug has a *positive inotropic effect*, that is, it stimulates the force of contraction of the heart muscle; the therapeutic utility of digitalis in the treatment of congestive heart failure is predicated upon this effect. Second, this agent both directly and indirectly *modifies the formation and*

Table 26-1 Comparative Properties of Representative Digitalis Preparations

Generic name (Selected trade name)	Absorption from gastrointestinal tract	Onset of action (IV)	Peak effect	Half-life in normal patients	Usual digitalizing dose/24 h	Usual daily oral maintenance dose	Principal route of elimination	Distinguishing characteristics
Digitalis leaf (Digifortis)	20–40%	2–6 h (oral)	12–24 h	4–6 days	1 g, P.O.	0.1 g	Renal.	Powdered leaf available for oral administration as capsule, tablet, and tincture. Contains mixture of cardiac glycosides, with digitoxin the most important. Use largely replaced by purified glycosides digoxin, digitoxin.
Digitoxin (Crystodigin, Purodigin)	90–100%	0.5–2 h	4–12 h	4–6 days	1.2–1.6 mg, P.O. 1 mg, IV	0.1–0.2 mg	Liver; renal elimination of metabolites.	Slow onset, long duration of action. Advisable to avoid in patients with liver disease. Available as tablet, pediatric elixir, and solution for injection.
Digoxin (Lanoxin)	50–75%	15–30 min	1–5 h	36 h	1.25–1.5 mg, P.O. 0.75–1.5 mg, IV	0.25–0.50 mg	Renal.	Most widely used cardiac glycoside; available as tablet, pediatric elixir, and solution for injection.
Deslanoside (Cedilanid-D)	Unreliable.	10–30 min	1–2 h	33 h	0.8 mg, IV		Renal.	Used for rapid digitalization only.
Ouabain [G-Strophanthin]	Unreliable.	5–10 min	0.5–2 h	21 h	0.3–0.5 mg, IV		Renal.	Employed only intravenously. Most rapid onset and shortest duration of action. Use limited to unusual situations when immediate digitalization is essential.

conduction of electrical impulses in the myocardium, generally resulting in a reduction in heart rate; these latter effects make digitalis useful for the treatment of cardiac supraventricular arrhythmias.

Inotropic Effects

By virtue of a direct effect on the myocardium, digitalis causes the heart to beat more forcefully, more completely, and with more efficient utilization of available nutrients.* Digitalis administration increases the cardiac output of patients with congestive heart failure to levels that approach normal. This positive inotropic effect is also observed in patients with normal cardiac function, but cardiac output is rarely increased.

The precise mechanism responsible for these positive inotropic effects has not been established with certainty. One widely accepted theory suggests that digitalis interferes with the movement of sodium and potassium across the cell membrane of the heart muscle and increases the concentration of intracellular calcium.

Effects on Heart Rate and Electrophysiological Parameters

The ability of digitalis to modify heart rate and conduction are important both therapeutically as well as toxicologically.

At therapeutic doses, digitalis has modest effects on the heart rate of normal individuals, yet is capable of producing a significant reduction in cardiac rate in patients with congestive heart failure. This effect is secondary to, and associated with, the ability of this drug to enhance cardiac output.

*Epinephrine enhances the force of myocardial contraction, but because it also augments heart rate and the expenditure of energy resources, it is not useful for the treatment of congestive heart failure.

The *electrophysiological* effects of digitalis underlie its ability to modify the conduction velocity of impulses, the refractory period, and the automaticity of cardiac cells.

The *conduction velocity* of nerve impulses is slowed by all doses of digitalis, in particular, atrioventricular conduction at the A-V node and bundle of His; these effects are manifested on the EKG by a prolongation of the PR interval. At low doses this response has been attributed to a drug-induced increase in *vagal* activity and can be blocked by atropine; at higher doses this depression of A-V conduction appears to result from the direct effects of this drug on the heart.

The influence of digitalis on the *refractory periods* of various parts of the heart are markedly different. The A-V refractory period is prolonged, an effect that is responsible for the beneficial effects of this drug in the management of atrial fibrillation. Toxic doses increase the refractory period and depress A-V conduction to such an extent that complete heart block may occur.

Excessive levels of digitalis increase the *automaticity* of all cardiac tissues capable of self-excitation, and this effect may result in the appearance of ectopic arrhythmias. The Purkinje fibers of the ventricles are particularly sensitive to these effects of digitalis.

THERAPEUTIC USES

The primary therapeutic uses of the digitalis glycosides are for the management of congestive heart failure and for cardiac supraventricular arrhythmias.

Congestive Heart Failure

The patient with congestive heart failure (a disorder also referred to as *cardiac decompensation*) exhibits a weak but rapid heart beat, cardiac output that is less than normal, and impaired systemic circulation. Impaired blood flow to the kidney contributes to the reduction in urine output and the resulting edema. Incomplete emptying of the heart during ventricular systole in time leads to enlargement of the heart and an increase in venous pressure. Pulmonary edema and shortness of breath (dyspnea) are commonly observed.

Digitalis taken alone or in combination with diuretics is the treatment of choice for the management of congestive heart failure. The beneficial effects have been attributed primarily to its positive inotropic effects in the absence of increased energy expenditures by the myocardium. The drug-induced enhanced force of ventricular contraction increases the expulsion of blood from the heart, thereby augmenting cardiac output and improving systemic circulation and renal plasma flow. Urinary output is enhanced, edema dissipates, and breathing improves; diuretics are commonly employed to facilitate the removal of excessive body fluids. With the reduction in heart rate that results indirectly from an increase in cardiac output, the ventricles fill more completely during diastole; the size of the enlarged heart decreases and begins to return to normal and venous pressure falls.

Cardiac Arrhythmias

Digitalis has been found to be effective for the management of a variety of supraventricular arrhythmias, in particular, atrial fibrillation, atrial flutter, and paroxysmal atrial tachycardia.

In cases of *atrial tachycardia*, the atria beat 150 to 250 times per minute with normal A-V conduction. The ventricles, bombarded by impulses, respond by weakly and inefficiently contracting, with the pumping effectiveness of the heart often reduced by 25 percent. This condition causes palpitations, patient discomfort, and may, in time, result in cardiac failure. Digitalis slows the rate of ventricular contractions by depressing conduction and prolonging the refractory period of the A-V node. This drug does not alter fibrillation of the atria.

In *atrial flutter*, ectopic atrial pacemakers discharge at a rate of 250 to 350 times per minute; some degree of A-V block is usually present, varying from 2:1 to 4:1. Digitalis slows the rate of ventricular contractions by increasing the degree of A-V block and converts the flutter to fibrillation. Withdrawal of digitalis after fibrillation has developed often results in the return of a normal sinus rhythm. Some authorities consider synchronous D.C. (direct current) cardioversion to be the initial treatment of choice for atrial flutter.

Paroxysmal atrial tachycardia is associated with sudden increases in the heart rate from 95 to 150 beats per minute; the origin of this disorder is in the atrium, but not the S-A node. These attacks are often disabling and may be hazardous if prolonged in duration. Digitalis proves useful in this disorder and may act by increasing vagal activity. Caution should be exercised prior to administering digitalis because paroxysmal atrial tachycardia may be the consequence of severe digitalis poisoning.

DIGITALIS PREPARATIONS AND THEIR ADMINISTRATION

While all digitalis glycosides exert qualitatively similar effects on the heart, the available products markedly differ with respect to the degree to which they are absorbed from the gastrointestinal tract after oral administration. The onset of action, time to peak effect, and duration of action also differ among these drugs (Table 26-1).

If possible, the oral route of administration should be employed. Intravenous administration should be reserved for emergencies or when the patient cannot tolerate this drug by mouth. Nursing implications associated with digitalis administration are summarized at the end of this chapter.

Digitalization

The therapeutic objective in the treatment of congestive heart failure is to administer a sufficient amount of digitalis until the signs and symptoms of this disorder have disappeared; this is called *digitalization*. After the total loading dose has been administered, maintenance doses are given to replace drug losses from the body resulting from renal elimination or liver metabolism and inactivation. Rapid or slow digitalization may be employed.

Rapid digitalization, a procedure commonly employed in acutely ill hospitalized patients, involves administration of the total loading dose of a digitalis glycoside (usually digoxin) within a 24-hour period. In this method the maximum therapeutic effect is rapidly achieved and the symptoms of toxicity are more readily observed and can be correlated with the body concentrations of drug; this permits the determination of a safe and optimal total body store of drug to fit the unique requirements of the patient. Once digitalization has been accomplished, maintenance doses are administered. The specific dose given is dependent upon the digitalis glycoside to be employed, the total body dose that can be safely administered, and the rate of drug elimination from the body; this last factor is influenced by *renal function*. While diminished renal function does not require adjustments in the digitalizing dose, appropriate reductions must be made in the maintenance doses employed to prevent drug cumulation and poisoning.

In *slow digitalization* the patient is placed on a maintenance dose, rather than a large loading dose, from the outset. Primarily employed for the nonacute patient with normal kidney function, this procedure does not require continuous patient monitoring and is, therefore, suitable for use in an ambulatory individual. The major disadvantage associated with slow digitalization is the protracted period of time required to attain the maximum body stores of drug necessary to produce the desired therapeutic effect.

DIGITALIS TOXICITY

Of all the drugs in common medical usage, the therapeutic index of the digitalis glycosides is among the lowest. Studies conducted in animals reveal that therapeutic doses are equivalent to 60 percent of the toxic dose, and this toxic dose is approximately 40 percent of the lethal dose. Approximately one out of every five patients taking digitalis exhibit signs and symptoms associated with drug-induced toxicity. From these facts the nurse may validly conclude that extreme caution must be exercised when administering these highly potent and potentially dangerous drugs. Noncardiac and cardiac symptoms are associated with digitalis overdosage and poisoning.

Gastrointestinal symptoms, including loss of appetite, nausea, vomiting, painful abdominal cramps, and diarrhea, are among the earliest signs of digitalis toxicity. Other noncardiac symptoms of toxicity are extreme fatigue, weakness in the extremities, visual disturbances (abnormal colors, blurred vision), and behavioral aberrations such as nightmares, agitation, and hallucinations. In about one-half of all cases, these noncardiac symptoms precede the adverse effects on the heart.

Cardiac symptoms, the most serious adverse effects associated with overdosage, are arrhythmias or increasing heart failure. *Arrhythmias* may be of virtually any type, with the most commonly encountered including ventricular premature beats, atrial and ventricular tachycardia, and sinoatrial and atrioventricular block. Ventricular tachycardia represents a particularly ominous sign because it may be followed by ventricular fibrillation, the most frequent cause of death resulting from digitalis overdosage.

The nurse should be cognizant of the *factors that predispose patients to digitalis toxicity*, the most common of which is *hypokalemia*; excessive potassium losses are often caused by diuretics, frequently administered with digitalis. These factors and potentially adverse digitalis-drug interactions are summarized in Tables 26-2 and 26-3, respectively.

Treatment of Digitalis Toxicity

If the digitalis-induced arrhythmia does not threaten the patient's life, digitalis withdrawal may be the only treatment necessary. Ventricular arrhythmias may be effectively

Table 26-2   Factors Predisposing Patients to Digitalis Toxicity

Factor	Mechanism underlying enhanced toxicity
Electrolyte imbalances	
Hypokalemia.	This is the most common cause of digitalis toxicity in previously well-managed patients. Since potassium inhibits the excitability of the heart, subnormal serum or myocardial levels increase the risk of digitalis-induced enhanced ectopic pacemaker activity, potentially resulting in arrhythmias. Common causes of excessive potassium loss include: drugs, diuretics in particular (Table 26-3); loss of large volumes of body fluids resulting from diarrhea or vomiting; and inadequate electrolyte intake.
Hypomagnesemia.	Deficiencies of serum magnesium have been associated with increased digitalis toxicity. Hypomagnesemia may result from long-term administration of magnesium-free fluids (hyperalimentation); amphotericin B and diuretics (Table 26-3); chronic alcoholism; and fluid loss associated with vomiting.
Age	Premature infants and neonates (less than one month of age) and elderly individuals may be more susceptible to the effects of digitalis (digitoxin) because of undeveloped or impaired renal function, respectively, and, therefore, do not excrete this drug or its metabolites at normal rates, resulting in cumulative toxicity.
Disease	
Impaired renal function.	Reduced ability to excrete digitalis glycosides or their metabolites.
Impaired liver function.	Digitoxin is metabolized extensively by the liver to biologically active and inactive metabolites. Although not demonstrated clinically to date, impaired hepatic function might increase serum levels of digitoxin. Digoxin is almost completely excreted, virtually unchanged, by the kidney.
Hypothyroid function.	Hypothyroid patients require lower than normal doses of digitalis glycosides because their ability to metabolize and excrete these drugs is reduced.
Other diseases.	An increased incidence of digitalis toxicity has been observed in patients with advanced cardiac disease (cardiomyopathies, hypertrophic subaortic stenosis), cor pulmonale and chronic pulmonary diseases.

Table 26-3 Potential Drug Interactions Involving Digitalis Glycosides

Interacting drug/class	Potential consequences

Amphotericin B (Fungizone)
Diuretics, potassium-wasting
   Acetazolamide (Diamox)
   Furosemide (Lasix)
   Ethacrynic acid (Edecrin)
   Chlorthalidone (Hygroton)
   Thiazide diuretics
      Chlorothiazide (Diuril)
	By increasing the loss of potassium (inducing hypokalemia), these drugs increase the risk of digitalis toxicity.

Quinidine	Administration of quinidine can cause an increase in serum digoxin levels in stabilized patients.
Succinylcholine (Anectine, Quelicin)	Potentiates the cardiac effects of digitalis, increasing risk of ventricular irritability, potentially resulting in arrhythmias.

Sympathomimetic agents
   Epinephrine (Adrenalin)
   Isoproterenol (Isuprel)
   Ephedrine
	Employed alone, these drugs may cause ectopic pacemaker activity—additive risk when employed with digitalis.

Cholestyramine (Questran) Colestipol (Colestid) Neomycin Metoclopramide (Reglan) Propantheline (Pro-Banthine)	Inhibit the gastrointestinal absorption of digitoxin or digoxin, thereby reducing plasma levels and potentially reducing therapeutically beneficial effects.

managed by the oral administration of *potassium chloride*, a drug that tends to reduce myocardial excitability. In severe cases, or when the patient is unable to take drugs by mouth, potassium may be administered by slow intravenous infusion. Potassium should be withheld in patients exhibiting hyperkalemia, complete heart block, or impaired renal function.

Almost all antiarrhythmic agents have been employed for the management of these arrhythmias, and these drugs are indicated in life-threatening cases. Intravenous lidocaine (Xylocaine) or phenytoin (Dilantin) are considered preferable to quinidine, propranolol (Inderal), or procainamide (Pronestyl) because the latter drugs may precipitate complete heart block in patients with A-V block. The pharmacology of these antiarrhythmic agents will be discussed in Chapter 27.

NURSING RESPONSIBILITIES ASSOCIATED WITH DIGITALIS ADMINISTRATION

The nurse should regularly assess the patient's general appearance and color, the presence of edema and tachypnea, and—when possible—pulmonary rales and ventricular gallop sound. Accurate records of body weight and fluid intake and output should also be maintained to evaluate the effectiveness of the prescribed medication.

Prior to administering *each* dose of digitalis, the nurse should carefully examine the patient for signs and symptoms associated with digitalis toxicity. These symptoms include loss of appetite in a patient with a normally good appetite, fatigue, lassitude, nausea, or visual disturbances. The EKG and pulse should be monitored to ascertain whether any alterations in heart rate or rhythm are present. If the apical pulse rate falls below 60 beats per minute for an adult patient or less than 90 to 110 per minute for a child, the next dose of digitalis is generally withheld until the physician has been consulted.

Extreme care must be exercised in checking the labels of bottles containing digitalis preparations to ensure that the proper drug and strength are being administered. Because some of these drugs have similar names (digoxin, digitoxin), errors can readily occur. The digitalis glycosides are extremely potent drugs possessing a dangerously low margin of safety. Serious adverse effects may occur if 0.2 mg tablets are administered instead of the prescribed 0.1 mg tablets. Calculation of doses should be meticulously checked and rechecked to preclude errors arising from misplaced decimals such as 1.0 mg instead of 0.1 mg.

The nurse should participate in the education of the patient about the nature of congestive heart disease. The patient must be instructed to restrict salt intake to prevent problems with edema. It should be clearly understood that the ultimate treatment objective is to abolish the disabling symptoms and improve the quality of the patient's life. Digitalis does not cure this disease, and the patient must continue to take the prescribed medication, as directed, for a lifetime and remain under regular medical supervision. Symptoms associated with digitalis toxicity should be described to the patient and a responsible family member. Upon the appearance of these signs, the patient should immediately consult the physician prior to taking the next scheduled dose. Other nursing implications appear at the end of this chapter.

DOBUTAMINE

It will be recalled from Chapter 5 that the sympathomimetic amine isoproterenol (Isuprel) increases both the force and rate of cardiac contractions, causes general vasodilation, and causes a reduction in mean blood pressure. These effects result from β-adrenergic activation. Dobutamine (Dobutrex), an isoproterenol-like drug, is a direct-acting positive inotropic agent with relatively mild chronotropic, hypertensive, arrhythmogenic, and vasodilatory effects.

Dobutamine is used for inotropic support in the short-term management of patients with congestive heart failure due to depressed contractility resulting from either organic heart disease or cardiac surgical procedures. The usual rate of intravenous infusion is 2.5 to 10 μg/kg/min as required to increase cardiac output; on occasion up to 40 μg/kg/min may be employed. Patients with atrial fibrillation having a rapid ventricular response should be administered a digitalis preparation prior to dobutamine.

The most common adverse effects associated with dobutamine administration are increased heart rate, blood pressure, and ventricular ectopic activity. Less frequent side effects are nausea, headache, anginal pain, nonspecific chest pain, palpitations, and dyspnea. This drug is contraindicated in idiopathic hypertropic subaortic stenosis. Dobutamine is unstable in alkaline solutions.

Digitalis Glycosides:
nursing implications

1. Check and recheck dosage calculations; even small errors may be of critical importance.
2. Take the apical pulse of the adult for 1 full minute prior to drug administration, noting the rate, rhythm, and quality. If rate is 60 or below or a change in rhythm is noted, withhold the drug and report to the physician. If a cardiac monitor is being used, observe for arrhythmias.
3. Observe for early signs of digitalis intoxication: fatigue, weakness, anorexia, salivation, nausea, vomiting, diarrhea, irritability, apathy, headache, visual disturbances, and facial pain.
4. Observe for CNS effects, especially in elderly individuals: confusion, anxiety, and hallucinations.
5. During digitalization, it is essential to check laboratory reports and know normal serum values of digitalis, potassium, magnesium, and calcium.
6. Hypokalemia increases risk of digitalis toxicity. Symptoms include anorexia, paresthesia, drowsiness, mental depression, polyuria, cardiac irritability, muscle weakness, hypoactive reflexes, postural hypotension, and dyspnea.
7. Monitor fluid balance carefully: ascertain intake and output ratio; weigh patient daily under standard conditions; assess extremities for edema; and auscultate lungs for rales.
8. Infants and elderly patients are more sensitive to actions of digitalis and more susceptible to toxicity. In children cardiac arrhythmias are more reliable signs of early toxicity than vomiting, diarrhea, or neurological signs.
9. Arrange for public health agency referral if adequate home supervision is not available.
10. Teach the patient or a responsible family member how to monitor drug effects and provide written instructions including how and when to check pulse; daily weight; diet and fluid restrictions, if required; toxic symptoms which must be reported; and graduated physical activity program.
11. Emphasize to the patient that regular medical supervision is essential, and that other medications should not be taken without consulting the physician.
12. Dietary planning must be individualized and include specific sodium restriction; reduced caloric intake if weight reduction is recommended; foods rich in potassium to be eaten; instructions as to whether a salt substitute would be appropriate or harmful; foods and nonprescription drugs with a high sodium content that should be avoided.

SUPPLEMENTARY READINGS

Albeit, S., J. Fiedler, T. Landau, and I. Rubin, "Recognizing Digitalis Toxicity," *American Journal of Nursing* 77: 1935–45 (1977).

Binnion, P. F., "Drug Interactions with Digitalis Glycosides," *Drugs* 15: 369–80 (1978).

Doherty, J. E., and J. J. Kane, "Clinical Pharmacology of Digitalis Glycosides," *Annual Review of Medicine* 26: 159–71 (1975).

Elenbaas, R. M., "Congestive Heart Failure," in *Clinical Pharmacy and Therapeutics* (2nd ed.), ed. E. T. Herfindal and J. L. Hirschman. Chapter 18, pp. 272–89. Baltimore: The Williams & Wilkins Company, 1979.

Fisch, C., and B. Surawicz, ed., *Digitalis.* New York: Grune & Stratton, Inc., 1969.

Hoffman, B. F., and J. T. Bigger, Jr., "Digitalis and Allied Cardiac Glycosides," in *Goodman and Gilman's The Pharmacological Basis of Therapeutics* (6th ed.), ed. A. G. Gilman, L. S. Goodman, and A.Gilman. Chapter 30, pp. 729–60. New York: Macmillan, Inc., 1980.

Lee, K. S., and W. Klaus, "The Subcellular Basis for the Mechanism of Inotropic Action of Cardiac Glycosides," *Pharmacological Reviews* **23**: 193–261 (1971).

Lindenbaum, J., "Bioavailability of Digoxin Tablets," *Pharmacological Reviews* **25**: 229–38 (1973).

Marks, B. H., and A. M. Weissler, ed., *Basic and Clinical Pharmacology of Digitalis.* Springfield, Ill.: Charles C Thomas, Publisher, 1972.

Mason, D. T., "Digitalis Pharmacology and Therapeutics: Recent Advances," *Annals of Internal Medicine* **80**: 520–30 (1974).

Rasmussen, S., R. J. Noble, and C. Fisch, "The Pharmacology and Clinical Use of Digitalis," *Cardiovascular Nursing* **11**(1): 23–28 (1975).

Smith, T. W., and E. Haber, "Digitalis," *New England Journal of Medicine* **289**: 945–52, 1010–15, 1063–72, 1125–29 (1973).

ANTIARRHYTHMIC DRUGS

Chapter 27

Antiarrhythmic drugs are clinically employed to prevent or control disturbances of normal cardiac rhythm. Since these arrhythmias arise from aberrations in the electrophysiological events that are responsible for normal mechanical contraction of heart muscle, we shall first examine the basis for these disturbances in rhythm and then consider the general mechanisms by which drugs in this therapeutic class correct these abnormalities.

ELECTROPHYSIOLOGICAL BASIS FOR ARRHYTHMIAS AND DRUG EFFECTS

As you will recall from Chapter 25, electrical impulses normally arise in the sinoatrial node, spread rapidly through the atria along specialized conducting tissues to the atrioventricular node, and culminate in contraction of the ventricles. Most of the commonly observed arrhythmias (Table 27-1) are thought to result from disorders in the automaticity of cardiac muscle or as a consequence of abnormalities in the normal conduction of nerve impulses.

Under certain circumstances, sites in the myocardium exhibit greater than normal *automaticity*, generating impulses at a higher frequency than the S-A node, and assume the pacemaker function; such sites, referred to as abnormal or *ectopic pacemakers*, cause an abnormal sequence of contractions in different parts of the heart. Arrhythmias that result from disorders in impulse formation can be managed by drugs that are capable of depressing the automaticity of cardiac muscle; this property is possessed by all commonly employed antiarrhythmic drugs (Table 27-2). The antiarrhythmic actions of digitalis were discussed in the last chapter.

Certain cardiac arrhythmias, such as atrial flutter and atrial fibrillation, are thought to result from disturbances in the normal *conduction of nerve impulses*. A *circus movement* is said to occur when an impulse originates in one part of the heart muscle, spreads in a circular (circus) pathway through the heart and returns to restimulate the originally excited muscle in a continuous manner. Disorders of this type appear to be associated with a reduction in the conduction velocity of the nerve impulse and a greatly shortened refractory period (that time during which the heart muscle is nonresponsive to restimulation by an impulse). Drugs capable of modifying the conduction velocity and the refractory period are useful in abolishing such circus movements. Table 27-2 summarizes the comparative properties of commonly employed antiarrhythmic drugs on the electrophysiological properties of the heart and their therapeutic applications.

While arrhythmias may be intermittent (paroxysmal) or sustained, all adversely affect the ability of the heart to function as an effective pump. The clinical selection of drugs in this class continues to be empirical, with no single drug always effective in the management of a given arrhythmia (Table 27-1). In some cases, the lack of severity of the cardiac disturbance do not justify the potential dan-

Table 27-1   Common Cardiac Arrhythmias and Favored Treatments

Arrhythmia	Characteristics	Treatment
Paroxysmal atrial tachycardia.	Episodic increase in atrial rate to 150-250 beats/min.	Digitalis, quinidine, procainamide
Atrial flutter.	Ectopic pacemaker discharging at rate of 250-350 times/min; A-V block usually present.	Digitalis, D.C. cardioversion, propranolol
Atrial fibrillation.	Irregular atrial activity at rates of 350-600 times/min, with ventricular rates of 130-170 times/min.	Digitalis, D.C. cardioversion, quinidine, procainamide
Ventricular tachycardia.	Life-threatening emergency with ventricular rate of 150-250 beats/min.	Lidocaine Phenytoin[a]
Ventricular fibrillation.	Life-threatening major cause of death after myocardial infarction.	Lidocaine Potassium chloride[a]

[a] Treatment of digitalis-induced ventricular arrhythmias.

Table 27-2   Comparative Effects of Commonly Employed Antiarrhythmic Drugs

Drug (Selected trade names)	Auto-maticity	Conduction velocity	Refractory period	Inotropic effects	Therapeutic uses[a]	Remarks
Quinidine salts (Cardioquin, Cin-Quin, Quinaglute)	↓	↓	↑	↓	AF, AFT, PST, PS, VT	Contraindicated: complete A-V block, thrombocytopenic purpura. Caution: incomplete A-V block. Not used to treat digitalis toxicity.
Procainamide (Pronestyl)	↓	↓	↑	↓	Same as quinidine	Pharmacological effects similar to quinidine; Less effective than quinidine for AF, AFT.
Disopyramide (Norpace)	↓	↓	↑	↓	VA, VT	Pharmacological effects similar to quinidine. Anticholinergic side effects.
Lidocaine; lignocaine (Xylocaine for Cardiac Arrhythmias)	↓	0	↓	0	VA	Local anesthetic used as intravenous antiarrhythmic agent for emergency treatment of ventricular arrhythmias in cardiac surgery or myocardial infarctions; CNS depression.
Phenytoin (Dilantin)	↓	↑	↓	0	PAT	Antiepileptic agent used for treatment of PAT associated with digitalis toxicity.
Propranolol (Inderal)	↓	↓	↓	↓↓	AF, AFT, PAT	β-adrenergic blocking agent, with use restricted to cases where adrenergic mechanisms responsible for arrhythmias. Produces marked cardiac depression. May cause bronchospasms in asthmatic patients.
Bretylium tosylate (Bretylol)	↑	0-↑	↑	0	VA, VT	Used for life-threatening disorders that fail to respond to other drugs. Tendency to decrease blood pressure.

[a] Key to abbreviations: AF = atrial fibrillations; AFT = atrial flutter; PAT = paroxysmal atrial tachycardia; PS = premature systoles; PST = paroxysmal supraventricular tachycardia; VA = ventricular arrhythmias; VT = ventricular tachycardia.

gers of the drug, and medication may be withheld.

We shall now discuss the properties of commonly used antiarrhythmic agents, emphasizing quinidine, the prototype agent in this therapeutic class. Nursing implications associated with the use of commonly employed antiarrhythmic agents appear at the end of this chapter.

QUINIDINE

Quinidine, an isomer of the antimalarial drug quinine, was the first compound found to possess therapeutically useful antiarrhythmic properties. This drug continues to enjoy widespread usage, but must be employed with caution because of its potential toxicity.

Antiarrhythmic Actions

Quinidine *depresses the heart*, an effect attributed to its ability to decrease myocardial excitability, reduce the conduction velocity of impulses, and prolong the refractory period of the heart (Table 27-2).

This drug depresses the *automaticity* of the S-A node, as well as of ectopic pacemakers. The latter are more sensitive to the depressing effects of quinidine, thus permitting the normal pacemaker to regain control over impulse formation. By direct effects on the atria, A-V node, and ventricles, quinidine slows the *conduction velocity* at which impulses spread throughout the myocardium. Varying degress of heart block may occur if this drug is not used cautiously in patients with conduction defects. Quinidine also prolongs the *refractory period*, rendering the myocardium nonresponsive to impulses generated at excessive frequencies.

Therapeutic Uses

The primary therapeutic uses of quinidine are for the prevention or control of such cardiac arrhythmias as atrial fibrillation and flutter, paroxysmal supraventricular tachycardia, ventricular tachycardia, and premature systoles. The usual starting dose of quinidine hydrochloride is 200 to 400 mg at 5- to 8-hour intervals spaced evenly for several days; maintenance doses range from 100 to 400 mg every 4 to 6 hours.

Adverse Effects and Precautions

Quinidine is a potentially dangerous drug with sudden fatalities associated with its use. Adverse effects may be sufficiently severe that up to 30 percent of patients taking this drug on a maintenance basis may have to discontinue its use.

Like quinine and the salicylates (aspirin), high doses of quinidine cause *cinchonism*, a toxic syndrome characterized by ringing of the ears (tinnitus), nausea, vomiting, diarrhea, and dizziness. *Thrombocytopenic purpurea* is a rare but serious allergic disorder resulting from quinidine administration. Typically, petechial hemorrhages appear in the buccal mucous membranes several weeks after the initiation of drug administration. The nurse should frequently inspect the oral cavity for early signs of this adverse reaction. A history of this disorder represents a contraindication to the use of this drug.

Quinidine may cause potentially severe and often life-threatening *cardiotoxic* effects, including ventricular tachycardia and arrhythmias and heart block. The ventricular tachycardia results from the atropine-like effects of quinidine on the vagus nerve. Prior administration of digitalis glycosides, or drugs that increase vagal activity, prevent this problem. The risk of ventricular fibrillation increases with the size of the dose of quinidine administered.

Quinidine is contraindicated in patients with complete heart block and should be used with extreme caution in patients exhibiting incomplete heart block. This drug depresses atrioventricular and intraventricular impulse conduction, actions which may result in cardiac arrest in patients with pre-existing conduction defects. The dose of quinidine should be reduced in patients with renal disease.

The nurse should frequently monitor the blood pressure of patients taking this drug. Large doses of quinidine may cause a reduction in blood pressure, an effect resulting from peripheral vasodilation.

Potential quinidine-drug interactions are summarized in Table 27-3 at the end of this chapter.

Preparations and Their Administration

Quinidine may be administered orally and by intramuscular and intravenous injection; the oral route is safer and should be employed, if possible. The nurse should caution patients taking tablets or capsules not to chew these preparations because this drug has a very *bitter taste.* After oral administration, peak effects may be observed within 1 to 3 hours and persist for 6 to 8 hours. Among the salts of quinidine available for oral administration are the sulfate, the gluconate (Quinaglute), and the polygalacturonate (Cardioquin). Quinidine gluconate is the salt most commonly employed for intravenous injection and should be infused at a very slow rate, highly diluted in isotonic dextrose solution. The EKG and blood pressure should be frequently monitored for evidence of drug-induced arrhythmias or marked hypotension.

PROCAINAMIDE

Procainamide (Pronestyl), a drug chemically related to the local anesthetic procaine (Chapter 12), has pharmacological actions and therapeutic uses that are very similar to those of quinidine (Table 27-2). The most favorable results with this drug have been obtained in the treatment of ventricular arrhythmias, except those resulting from digitalis toxicity; in these latter cases, procainamide has proved to be unreliable. Since procainamide depresses conduction, it should not be given to patients with conduction defects; reduction of the QRS interval by more than 30 percent should alert the nurse to drug-induced toxicity.

Like quinidine, procainamide is capable of causing ventricular tachycardia and a marked reduction in blood pressure after large intravenous doses. Extracardiac side effects include nausea, loss of appetite, vomiting, diarrhea, flushing, and hallucinations. Hypersensitivity reactions are often characterized by chills, fever, joint pain, and skin rashes.

For the treatment of ventricular arrhythmias, the usual initial oral dose is 500 mg to 1 g every 2 hours; maintenance doses are given every 4 to 6 hours.

LIDOCAINE

Lidocaine (Xylocaine), among the most extensively employed local anesthetic agents* (Chapter 12), is now commonly used in coronary care units for the *emergency treatment*

*Lidocaine hydrochloride solutions containing epinephrine or preservatives are intended for use as local anesthetics and should not be administered intravenously for the treatment of arrhythmias.

of ventricular arrhythmias associated with cardiac surgery or resulting from myocardial infarction. Lidocaine, only effective when administered parenterally, has a very rapid onset of antiarrhythmic action after intravenous injection and a short duration of action after the termination of drug administration; these time-response parameters make lidocaine an extremely useful drug in an intensive care unit when minute-by-minute control of ventricular arrhythmias is deemed essential. Intravenous doses of 0.5 to 1.5 mg/kg are often given at 3- to 5-minute intervals to a total of 200 to 300 mg. The actions of this drug on the electrophysiological events in the heart as well as its therapeutic uses differ somewhat from quinidine and procainamide (Table 27-2); lidocaine is not useful for the management of atrial flutter or fibrillation or supraventricular arrhythmias.

Drowsiness is a very commonly encountered side effect associated with lidocaine administration; this effect may prove beneficial in the management of patients with acute myocardial infarctions. Other early signs of lidocaine toxicity include dizziness, numbness of the lips and tongue, and speech disturbances. Since reports of lidocaine-induced *convulsions* are common, the nurse should ensure that diazepam (Valium) or an ultrashort-acting barbiturate is available for immediate intravenous administration.

PHENYTOIN

Phenytoin (Dilantin), long employed for the treatment of epilepsy (Chapter 18), is employed as an antiarrhythmic agent exclusively for the control of paroxysmal atrial tachycardia caused by digitalis toxicity. Intravenous doses of 50 to 100 mg may be given at 10-minute intervals until the desired response is achieved or toxic effects appear. Initial oral doses are 1 g on the first day, reduced to 400 to 500 mg by the fourth day. It is currently undergoing clinical investigation for potential use for the management of other cardiac arrhythmias. This drug should be used with extreme caution in patients exhibiting heart block. Rapid intravenous infusion can result in hypotension and complete heart block.

PROPRANOLOL

Propranolol (Inderal) is a β-blocking agent (Chapter 6) with marked effects on the heart. This drug competitively antagonizes the effects of catecholamines released from sympathetic nerves. In addition, propranolol has direct effects on the heart, decreasing both the conduction velocity and the refractory period; this drug causes a pronounced *reduction in cardiac rate* (Table 27-2). Its ability to reduce ischemic injury may prevent arrhythmias associated with myocardial infarction.

Propranolol is employed clinically to control supraventricular tachycardias and ventricular arrhythmias. The usual oral dose is 10 to 30 mg three to four times daily. It is capable of antagonizing the ability of endogenous catecholamines to increase myocardial contractility, and, therefore, should be used with great caution in patients with heart failure. The nurse should administer propranolol with care in asthmatic patients because of the risk of causing bronchospasms. Potential drug interactions involving propranolol are summarized in Table 27-3.

Table 27-3   Potential Adverse Drug Interactions Involving Antiarrhythmic Drugs

Antiarrhythmic agent	Interacting drug/class	Possible consequences
Quinidine	Digitalis glycosides	Quinidine may increase the serum levels of digoxin.
	Tubocurarine (Tubarine)	Quinidine use in immediate postoperative period in patients receiving tubocurarine during surgery may result in recurarization and respiratory paralysis.
	Warfarin (Coumadin, Panwarfin)	Quinidine causes mild hypoprothrombinemia, which can be additive with warfarin's anticoagulant effects—potentially resulting in serious bleeding.
	Barbiturates Phenytoin (Dilantin)	Drugs stimulate rate of metabolism of quinidine.
	Acetazolamide (Diamox) Antacids Sodium bicarbonate	These drugs alkalinize the urine, which reduces secretion of quinidine, increasing serum levels and potential risk of toxicity.
Lidocaine	Phenytoin (Dilantin)	Epileptics receiving phenytoin and lidocaine may experience severe cardiac depression.
Lidocaine Procainamide Propranolol	Tubocurarine Succinylcholine	These drugs may enhance the the neuromuscular blockade produced by these skeletal muscle relaxants.
Propranolol	Insulin Oral hypoglycemic agents	There is increased risk of hypoglycemia in diabetic patients receiving these drugs in combination.
	Digitalis glycosides	Digitalis-induced bradycardia may be enhanced by propranolol.
	Isoproterenol (Isuprel) Epinephrine (Adrenalin)	The β-adrenergic blocking actions of propranolol may antagonize the antiasthmatic effects.
	Methyldopa (Aldomet) Antidepressants, monoamine oxidase inhibitors	Combination can result in marked hypertensive response.

DISOPYRAMIDE

Disopyramide (Norpace), a newly approved antiarrhythmic drug, has pharmacological properties similar to quinidine and procainamide. After oral administration, this drug is rapidly and completely absorbed. This drug is effective in the treatment of ventricular arrhythmias, suppressing premature beats and tachycardia. In some studies, disopyramide has proved useful in conditions refractory to conventional therapy.

The usual adult dosage is 400 to 800 mg daily, given orally in four divided doses, following an initial loading dose of 300 mg. This dose should be reduced in patients with renal insufficiency. Therapeutic effects are generally observed within 30 minutes to 3 hours after the initial dose.

The most common adverse effects associated with administration of this drug result from its *anticholinergic properties* and include dry mouth and urinary hesitancy; urinary retention, although relatively uncommon, is the most serious potential danger caused by this drug.

Antiarrhythmic Drugs: nursing implications

1. Patients getting IV antiarrhythmic drugs should receive continuous EKG monitoring and frequent checks of blood pressure (B.P.) and heart and respiratory rates.
2. Observe cardiac monitor for depression of cardiac activity such as prolongation of the PR interval, widening of the QRS complex, or an increase in arrhythmia.
3. If a potentially lethal arrhythmia develops or an adverse reaction to the drug occurs, be prepared to discontinue the drug, administer emergency drugs, and use emergency resuscitative techniques, including defibrillation.
4. Advise the patient of need for regular follow-up appointments to assess cardiac status and laboratory tests for drug-induced changes.
5. Teach the patient or a responsible family member the purpose of the drug and how to monitor the drug effect including specific dosage schedule, symptoms to report, recommended physical activity, and diet and weight control. The patient should be advised to avoid excessive caffeine, alcohol, smoking, heavy meals, and nonprescription drugs unless first approved by the physician.

Procainamide (Pronestyl)

1. Treatment of atrial arrhythmias with procainamide is usually preceded by digitalization. The increased atrial contraction may be sufficient to dislodge atrial mural thrombi with subsequent pulmonary embolism. Be alert for symptoms of pleuritic chest pain, tachypnea, tachycardia, hypotension, and cough.
2. Monitor IV infusion to be certain that dose does not exceed 25-50 mg/min. Keep patient supine and check B.P. very frequently. If diastolic pressure falls 15 mm Hg or more, drug should be discontinued.

3. Have levarterenol (Levophed) or dopamine (Intropin) available to manage excessive hypotensive response.

4. Instruct patient on oral therapy to report symptoms of renal dysfunction such as dysuria, hematuria, oliguria; agranulocytosis such as sore mouth, throat, or gums, fever, respiratory infection, unexplained bleeding or bruising; and lupus erythematosus such as polyarthralgia, fever, myalgia, skin lesions.

Quinidine

1. A test dose should be administered prior to initiating therapy to determine whether patient exhibits drug idiosyncrasy.

2. Observe cardiac monitor for absence of P waves or a pulse rate over 120, both indications for discontinuing drug.

3. Monitor vital signs every 1-2 h during acute treatment and daily for hospitalized patients receiving oral therapy.

4. Observe the patient for hypersensitivity reaction manifested by respiratory difficulty or skin eruptions.

5. Have drugs available for emergency treatment of adverse reactions: sodium lactate for cardiotoxicity; vasoconstrictors for hypotension.

6. Advise the patient to immediately notify physician of disturbance in vision, tinnitus, palpitations, shortness of breath, or feelings of faintness.

Lidocaine (Xylocaine)

1. Observe for adverse CNS effects: drowsiness, confusion, paresthesia, visual disturbances, excitement, or behavioral changes.

2. Observe for twitching or tremors, which may precede convulsions. Resuscitation equipment and emergency drugs should be immediately available for management of convulsions or respiratory depression.

3. Lidocaine hydrochloride solutions containing epinephrine or preservatives should not be used to treat arrhythmias. Vial should be labeled "For Cardiac Arrhythmias."

Propranolol (Inderal)

See the nursing implications for adrenergic blocking agents in Chapter 6.

SUPPLEMENTARY READINGS

Anderson, J. L., D. C. Harrison, P. J. Moffin, and R. A. Winkle, "Antiarrhythmic Drugs: Clinical Pharmacology and Therapeutic Uses," *Drugs* **15**: 271–309 (1978).

Bigger, J. T., Jr., "Arrhythmias and Antiarrhythmic Drugs," *Advances in Internal Medicine* **18**: 251–81 (1972).

Krone, R. J., and R. E. Kleiger, "Prevention and Treatment of Supraventricular Arrhythmias," *Heart and Lung* **6**: 79–88 (1977).

Krone, R. J., R. E. Kleiger, and G. O. Oliver, "Treatment of Chronic Ventricular Arrhythmias," *Heart and Lung* **6**: 68–78 (1977).

Levitt, B., J. S. Borer, and A. Sarapa, "The Clinical Pharmacology of Antiarrhythmic Drugs, Part I: Lidocaine and Procainamide; Part II: Quinidine,

Propranolol, Diphenylhydantoin, and Bretylium," Cardiovascular *Nursing* **10**, 5, 6: 23–26, 27–31 (1974).

Manzi, C. C., "Cardiac Emergency—How to Use Drugs and CPR and Save Lives," *Nursing '78* **8**, 3: 30–39 (1978).

Mason, D. T., and others, "Antiarrhythmic Agents, I. Mechanisms of Action and Clinical Pharmacology; II. Therapeutic Considerations," *Drugs* **5**: 261–91, 292–317 (1973).

Resnekov, L., ed., "Symposium on Cardiac Rhythm Disturbances I & II," *Medical Clinics of North America* **60**, 1, 2: 1–386 (1976).

ANTIHYPERTENSIVE DRUGS

Chapter 28

The antihypertensive drugs that are currently available do not correct the underlying pathophysiological factors responsible for hypertension, but rather relieve the symptoms by several different mechanisms, prevent complications, and prolong the lives of the patients. While agreement is lacking among clinicians about the relative merits of initiating therapy in mildly hypertensive patients with a favorable prognosis, the therapeutic benefits derived from the treatment of moderate to severe hypertensives is unquestioned. This chapter begins with an overview of hypertension.

HYPERTENSION

Hypertension is the most common disorder of the cardiovascular system, with recent estimates suggesting that at least 25 million Americans have elevated blood pressure. Severe and persistent hypertension causes extensive adverse effects on the tissues of the body, particularly on the heart, arteries, kidneys, and brain. Hypertension places greater demands on the heart, eventually resulting in hypertrophy of this organ. The coronary blood flow fails to keep pace with the increased demands for oxygen, and angina pectoris or myocardial infarction may result. Atherosclerosis progresses more rapidly in hypertensive people, increasing the risk of coronary artery disease. The blood vessels in the kidneys and brain are weakened by chronic hypertension; this weakness, in time, may lead to rupture of these vessels. Damage to the kidneys and impairment of renal function is a common complication of untreated hypertension. A *cere-*

brovascular accident (stroke, apoplexy) is a rupture of blood vessels within the cranial cavity that causes damage to the brain.

Classification and Etiology of Hypertension

Hypertension is generally classified as primary (essential) or secondary hypertension. *Secondary hypertension* is said to be present when the cause of the elevation in blood pressure can be identified and is secondary to or the result of an underlying disorder such as kidney disease, hyperthyroidism, pheochromocytoma, or drugs (for example, oral contraceptives). Correction of the underlying cause very often results in the *cure* of the hypertensive state.

About 85 to 90 percent of all cases of high blood pressure are of unknown etiology and are called *primary* or *essential hypertension*. While essential hypertension can be controlled with the available drugs, it cannot be cured. The nurse should educate the patient about this very fundamental fact. Drugs must be taken for a lifetime even when the patient is asymptomatic.

Patients with essential hypertension often manifest extensive *constriction of the arterioles*, resulting in an increase in peripheral vascular resistance. Although arteriolar vasoconstriction has not been directly demonstrated to result from aberrations in *vasoconstrictor catecholamines*, many of the effective antihypertensive agents currently employed in the management of this disorder have been demonstrated to inhibit central sympathetic function, prevent the release of catecholamines, or deplete their stores in peripheral adrenergic nerve endings. It has also been suggested that essential hypertension may be caused by an increase of *sodium* and calcium in the smooth muscle of blood vessels or a decrease in smooth muscle content of cyclic AMP (an endogenous vasodilator substance). A sodium-restricted diet and the use of diuretic agents that promote the excretion of sodium both reduce elevated blood pressure.

Studies conducted in recent years point to the possible involvement of the *renin-angiotensin system* in some hypertensive disorders. Reductions in arterial blood pressure or low levels of plasma sodium stimulate the secretion of the enzyme *renin* from the kidneys. This enzyme is involved in the formation of the hormone *angiotensin II*, the most potent vasoconstrictor and pressor substance known. In addition to increasing arterial blood pressure, by virtue of its ability to cause arteriolar vasoconstriction, angiotensin II causes the release of aldosterone. This adrenocortical hormone causes a reduction in the excretion of salt and water, resulting in an increase in blood volume and blood pressure (Chapter 34). Catecholamines have been shown to stimulate renin secretion by an interaction with β-adrenergic receptors. While the available evidence suggests that the renin-angiotensin system contributes to some hypertensive states, it remains to be determined how extensive and to what magnitude this system is involved in essential hypertension.

DRUG TREATMENT OF ESSENTIAL HYPERTENSION

The ideal antihypertensive agent should be capable of maintaining blood pressure within normal limits in both supine and erect body positions without reducing cardiac output or interfering with circulation of blood to such vital organs as the brain, heart, and kidneys.

The primary sites of action of antihypertensive agents are depicted in Figure 28-1. While subsequent discussions of these drugs

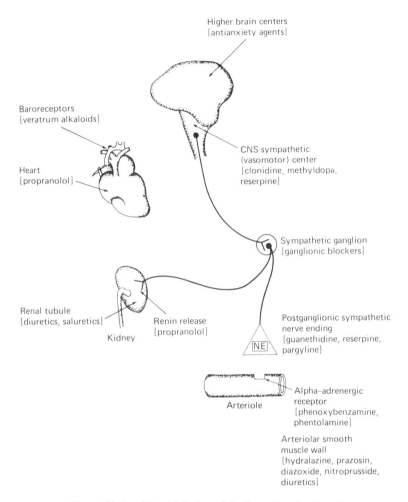

Higher brain centers
[antianxiety agents]

Baroreceptors
[veratrum alkaloids]

CNS sympathetic
(vasomotor) center
[clonidine, methyldopa,
reserpine]

Heart
[propranolol]

Sympathetic ganglion
[ganglionic blockers]

Renal tubule
[diuretics, saluretics]

Renin release
[propranolol]

Kidney

Postganglionic sympathetic
nerve ending
[guanethidine, reserpine,
pargyline]

NE

Arteriole

Alpha-adrenergic
receptor
[phenoxybenzamine,
phentolamine]

Arteriolar smooth
muscle wall
[hydralazine, prazosin,
diazoxide, nitroprusside,
diuretics]

Figure 28-1   Sites of Action of Antihypertensive Agents.

emphasize the major mechanisms responsible for their antihypertensive effects, in many instances secondary actions contribute to the observed beneficial effects.

We shall now discuss centrally acting drugs, ganglionic blocking agents, drugs acting at sympathetic nerve endings, direct vasodilators, and diuretics used for the treat-ment of hypertension. Therapeutic consid-erations associated with the use of these drugs for the management of hypertension will be outlined in the last section of this chapter. A summary of nursing implications associated with the use of commonly em-ployed antihypertensive agents appears at the end of this chapter.

Centrally Acting Drugs

The *vasomotor center*, located in the pons and medulla oblongata of the brain stem, transmits impulses through the spinal cord to sympathetic vasoconstrictor fibers, which innervate all the blood vessels of the body. This center is normally active and its impulses maintain a partial state of contraction in the blood vessels, a state called *vasomotor tone*. The level of activity of this system is controlled by central and peripheral influences.

Higher centers of the brain, including the hypothalamus and cerebral cortex, control the activity of the vasomotor center and influence the degree of arteriolar vasoconstriction and blood pressure. In the periphery, blood flow and arterial blood pressure are controlled by circulatory reflexes, the most important of which is the *baroreceptor reflex*. An increase in arterial blood pressure stretches the walls of the major arteries in the chest and neck which, in turn, excites the stretch receptors located in the carotid sinus and aortic arch. Signals are transmitted from these receptors to the vasomotor center and reflex signals are sent back to the heart and blood vessels, causing a slowing of the heart rate, dilation of the blood vessels, and a reduction in blood pressure to normal. A decrease in blood pressure causes the opposite effects.

Centrally acting drugs employed for the treatment of hypertension include the sedatives and agents that reduce sympathetic function by their direct or indirect effects on the vasomotor center.

Sedative and antianxiety agents such as the barbiturates (phenobarbital and butabarbital) and the benzodiazepines (chlordiazepoxide, diazepam) do not possess specific antihypertensive properties. Their depressant actions on the higher brain centers produce calming effects that serve to reduce anxiety, which may be responsible for mild hypertension in some patients.

Methyldopa and clonidine are thought to lower blood pressure by mechanisms that result in a depression of sympathetic function in the central nervous system. Available evidence does not permit us to exclude the possibility that the peripheral actions of these drugs may contribute to these hypertensive effects. The veratrum alkaloids reflexly inhibit central sympathetic function by sensitizing baroreceptors.

Methyldopa   It was formerly believed that the antihypertensive effects of methyldopa (Aldomet) resulted from its ability to inhibit the biosynthesis of norepinephrine in peripheral sympathetic (adrenergic) nerves. While such a peripheral action may contribute to the observed reduction in elevated blood pressure, recent studies suggest that the primary site of action of methyldopa is in the central nervous system. The actions of this drug are thought to be mediated via its metabolite *α-methylnorepinephrine*.

Methyldopa is a useful drug for the chronic management of essential hypertension and may also be administered intravenously for the management of hypertensive emergencies. Renal blood flow and glomerular filtration is maintained in patients with *impaired renal function;* thus this drug is useful for the control of hypertensive disorders in individuals with chronic kidney disease. The average daily oral dose is 1 g.

Drowsiness, sedation, and weakness are common side effects associated with the early use of methyldopa. Other adverse effects include depression, dry mouth, nasal stuffiness, gastrointestinal upset, sexual impotence, fever, and liver function abnormalities. The incidence and severity of postural hypotension is less than that observed with guanethidine (see page 241). Retention of salt and water, leading to edema and weight gain, is common if a diuretic is not co-administered with methyldopa. Rare allergic reactions include hemolytic anemia, hepatitis, and drug fever. Potential drug interactions involving methyldopa are summarized in Table 28-5, page 246.

Clonidine Clonidine (Catapres), a newly introduced drug, is thought to produce hypotension and bradycardia primarily by a central mechanism that may result from activation of central α-adrenergic receptors that cause inhibition of sympathetic nerve activity in the vasomotor center. This drug has also been shown to act peripherally by inhibiting the release of norepinephrine from sympathetic nerves and renin from the kidneys. Following intravenous administration of clonidine, a short-lived pressor response is noted, followed by a prolonged reduction in blood pressure accompanied by a reduction in heart rate.

Very common side effects caused by clonidine include sedation, dry mouth, orthostatic hypotension, impotence, and constipation; salt and water retention occur during the first few days of treatment, but generally do not persist. Abrupt discontinuation of clonidine administration often results in restlessness, irritability, an increase in heart rate, and a rebound elevation in blood pressure. If the drug is to be withdrawn, the dose should be gradually reduced. Since clonidine is a relatively new drug, a complete assessment of its potential benefits and adverse effects has not been accomplished to date. Daily oral doses range from 0.4 to 2 mg.

Veratrum alkaloids The veratrum alkaloids (obtained from the green and white hellebore plants, *Veratrum viride* and *Veratrum album*) reduce heart rate and arterial blood pressure by reflexly inhibiting central sympathetic function. These drugs, including alkavervir (Veriloid) and cryptenamine (Unitensen), sensitize baroreceptors in the carotid sinus and aortic arch, resulting in reflex inhibition of the vasomotor center in the brain stem.

Although effective in their abilities to reduce elevated blood pressure, use of these drugs is associated with a high incidence of nausea and other adverse effects. The low margin of safety of the veratrum alkaloids has caused them to fall into disfavor, and they are rarely employed.

Ganglionic Blocking Agents

Drugs capable of interrupting transmission of nerve impulses at the autonomic ganglia were among the earliest compounds found to be effective antihypertensive agents. *Ganglionic blocking agents* compete with acetylcholine for cholinergic nicotinic receptor sites at the autonomic ganglia (Chapter 4), thereby inhibiting transmission of nerve impulses from preganglionic neurons to both sympathetic and parasympathetic postganglionic neurons.

Blockade of postganglionic *sympathetic* nerve transmission prevents arteriolar vasoconstriction, producing a profound reduction in blood pressure. This is the desired therapeutic effect, and the ganglionic blockers are among the most potent antihypertensive agents available. Normally, when the patient assumes a standing position after lying down, a sympathetically mediated vasoconstrictor reflex is activated, permitting the maintenance of adequate blood flow to the brain. Ganglionic blockers prevent this compensatory vasoconstriction, resulting in orthostatic hypotension and sometimes fainting. This *orthostatic hypotension* is one of the adverse side effects caused by many antihypertensive drugs and is particularly pronounced with the ganglionic blocking agents.

Precautions and side effects The nurse should advise the patient to rise slowly from a lying position to a sitting position and to a standing position to reduce the incidence of fainting associated with *orthostatic hypotension.* Patients should also be cautioned against standing without movement for prolonged periods of time to prevent pooling of blood in the legs. Hot baths should be avoided by a patient taking these drugs because such heat promotes peripheral vasodilation and hypotension.

Reduction in nerve transmission to postganglionic *parasympathetic* nerves also results in many adverse side effects, including dry mouth, constipation, urinary retention, blurred vision, and the inability to accommodate the muscles of the eye for close vision.

Because of the high incidence of distressing side effects and the discovery of equally effective and more specific antihypertensive agents, the ganglionic blocking agents are now rarely used for the chronic management of essential hypertension. Their contemporary use is primarily restricted to the treatment of hypertensive emergencies when it is imperative to reduce blood pressure rapidly (Table 28-1). They are also employed for the treatment of patients who fail to respond to other classes of antihypertensive medications.

Ganglionic blockers are contraindicated in pyloric stenosis, cerebral arteriosclerosis, coronary insufficiency, recent myocardial infarction, or glaucoma. These drugs should be employed cautiously in elderly patients and those with renal impairment.

Drugs Acting at Sympathetic Nerve Endings

Antihypertensive agents with their primary site of action at sympathetic (adrenergic) nerve endings may act via several separate and distinct mechanisms, including depletion of norepinephrine and blockade of the release of this neurotransmitter substance. In these cases, one observes a reduction in effective norepinephrine concentrations released by sympathetic nerve endings in response to nerve impulses and, as a consequence, a decrease in sympathetically mediated vasoconstriction. In marked distinction to the ganglionic blocking agents, these drugs do not interfere with the transmission of nerve impulses in postganglionic parasympathetic neurons and, therefore, do not adversely modify the normal function of cells

Table 28-1 Comparative Properties of Ganglionic Blocking Agents

Generic name	Trade name	Distinguishing properties
Mecamylamine hydrochloride	Inversine	Unlike other drugs in this class, well absorbed after oral administration. Adverse central effects include tremors, delusions, hallucinations; same peripheral adverse effects. Administered orally only as antihypertensive agent at a maintenance dose of 7.5 mg t.i.d.
Trimethaphan camsylate	Arfonad	Rapid onset and short duration of action (5 min) after intravenous infusion. Used only to induce hypotension of brief duration for surgical procedures to prevent excessive bleeding and during diagnostic procedures to improve visualization. Respiratory depression and tachycardia are potential adverse effects. Doses by intravenous infusion range from 0.2 to 5 mg/min.

innervated by acetylcholine. Hence these drugs are more specific in their abilities to reduce elevated blood pressure.

Reserpine   Reserpine is the major alkaloid derived from the Indian snakeroot *Rauwolfia serpentina.* Originally introduced as an antipsychotic agent, at present it is principally employed for the treatment of hypertension. This drug and related *rauwolfia* alkaloids (Table 28-2) are commonly employed for the management of mild essential hypertension, very often used in combination with a thiazide diuretic.

Actions   The hypotensive effects of reserpine have been attributed to its ability to deplete norepinephrine from peripheral sympathetic nerve endings. This drug alters the ability of nerve-ending storage granules to retain norepinephrine. As a consequence, the concentration of this neurotransmitter in nerve endings is reduced; less is then available for release to produce constriction of the arterioles.

Reserpine also produces marked effects on the central nervous system. The ability of this drug to cause depletion of norepinephrine and serotonin from certain areas of the brain is generally thought to be responsible for the *tranquilizing* or calming properties associated with this drug. The central actions of reserpine may contribute to its hypotensive effects.

Adverse effects   With reserpine-induced reduction in sympathetic activity, there is a disruption of the normal physiological balance between opposing sympathetic and parasympathetic effects, resulting in a predominance of the latter. This imbalance is manifested by a variety of adverse side effects including nasal congestion and stuffiness, visual disturbances, bradycardia, diarrhea, and an increase in gastric acid secretion leading to the possible formation of new or aggravation of preexisting peptic ulcer. The nurse may also observe that previously alert and cheerful patients become lethargic, apathetic, and depressed after taking this drug. Other side effects include fluid retention, weight gain, and a reserpine-induced parkinsonism state. Drug interactions

Table 28-2   Comparative Properties of Reserpine and Related Drugs

Generic name	Selected trade names	Source	Distinguishing properties (usual oral daily maintenance dose)
Rauwolfia serpentina	Raudixin	Powdered whole root containing all alkaloids.	Antihypertensive-calming properties attributed to reserpine, which accounts for approximately 50% of total activity of product. Only used orally (50–300 mg).
Reserpine	Serpasil, Sandril, Rau-Sed, Reserpoid	Natural alkaloid obtained from *Rauwolfia.*	Used orally, alone or in combination with thiazide diuretics, for treatment of mild hypertension and with potent antihypertensive agents for severe hypertension. Intravenous reserpine employed for hypertensive emergencies (0.1–0.25 mg).
Deserpidine	Harmonyl	Natural alkaloid.	Similar to reserpine, used orally only (0.25–0.50 mg).
Rescinnamine	Moderil Cinnasil	Natural alkaloid.	Similar to reserpine, used orally only. Sedation and bradycardia less pronounced than reserpine (0.25 mg).

involving reserpine are summarized in Table 28-5.

Guanethidine Guanethidine (Ismelin) is a potent drug useful for the management of severe hypertension. This drug is believed to lower blood pressure by two different mechanisms. Guanethidine depletes peripheral stores of norepinephrine presumably by preventing its reuptake and causing its slow release; this reserpine-like action is less rapid than is the one observed after reserpine administration. A second and far more important action is the ability of guanethidine to effectively prevent the release of norepinephrine in response to a nerve impulse. Drugs acting by this latter mechanism are referred to as *adrenergic neuron blocking agents*.

The onset of the antihypertensive effects of guanethidine is *slow*, with maximum reductions in blood pressure not observed until 2 or 3 days after the initiation of oral drug administration at a dose of 10 mg. Doses are usually increased at weekly intervals until optimal therapeutic benefit is obtained; the average maintenance dose is 25 to 50 mg, given once daily. This drug has a long duration of action, with its antihypertensive effects persisting for at least 1 week after the discontinuation of drug administration.

The most frequently encountered side effect is *postural hypotension*, which is generally manifested by dizziness when the patient arises from bed in the morning. Other common side effects include diarrhea, bradycardia, fatigue, nasal stuffiness, failure to ejaculate (without altering erection), and weight gain caused by salt and water retention; this latter adverse effect can be minimized by co-administration of a thiazide diuretic. Unlike reserpine, methyldopa, and clonidine, guanethidine does not cross the blood-brain barrier and, therefore, does not cause sedation or depression. Potential drug interactions involving guanethidine are summarized in Table 28-5.

Pargyline We have previously discussed the use of *monoamine oxidase inhibitors* as antidepressant agents in Chapter 17. Pargyline (Eutonyl) is another member of this pharmacological class that possesses antihypertensive effects. The mechanism of action of the antihypertensive effects for pargyline is not clear, but does not appear to be the direct result of its ability to inhibit the enzyme monoamine oxidase.

While pargyline is an effective drug for the treatment of moderate and severe hypotension, its severe side effects and potential drug interactions severely limit its therapeutic usefulness. Among the common side effects observed after pargyline administration are weight gain (which may or may not be associated with fluid retention), dry mouth, gastrointestinal disturbances, drowsiness, and nervousness. Adverse drug interactions may occur after the concurrent use of pargyline with sympathomimetic amines, sedatives, antihistamines, antidepressants, narcotics, and hypoglycemic agents. These drug interactions and food interactions (wine, beer, cheese) were summarized in Table 17-2 (page 141).

The initial oral dose of pargyline is 25 mg which may be increased at weekly intervals.

Adrenergic Receptor Blocking Agents

In Chapter 6 we discussed the pharmacology of antagonists of norepinephrine at its α- and β-adrenergic receptor sites. Since norepinephrine-induced activation of α-receptors produces arteriolar vasoconstriction, it might be assumed that α-*adrenergic blocking agents* such as phenoxybenzamine (Dibenzyline) or phentolamine (Regitine) might be useful for the treatment of essential hypertension. Results with these drugs have been generally disappointing because of the high incidence of reflex tachycardia, palpitations, and orthostatic hypotension.

β-adrenergic blocking agents The β-adrenergic blockers propranolol (Inderal), metoprolol (Lopressor), and nadolol (Corgard) have recently been approved for use as antihypertensive agents in the United States. It has been suggested that β-blockers exert their antihypertensive effects by one or more of the following mechanisms: (1) by competitively antagonizing catecholamines at peripheral sites (the heart) resulting in a reduction in cardiac output; (2) by a central action reducing the sympathetic outflow to the periphery; and (3) by blocking renin release, which inhibits angiotensin II synthesis.

Propranolol is primarily employed in combination with other drugs (thiazide diuretics, hydralazine) for the management of essential hypertension. It inhibits the reflex cardiac stimulation caused by hydralazine. It will be recalled from Chapter 6 that propranolol nonselectively blocks both β_1- and β_2-adrenergic receptors, the latter action resulting in pronounced bronchoconstriction in patients with bronchial asthma and other obstructive respiratory disorders. The blocking actions of metoprolol are relatively selective for the β_1-receptors in the heart.

Potential drug interactions involving propranolol and nadolol (Table 6-2, page 61) and adverse effects were given in Chapter 6. The initial oral antihypertensive dose of 20 mg four times daily may be increased by 20 mg increments to 80 mg four times daily.

Adverse side effects associated with metoprolol administration are generally mild and transitory and include fatigue, drowsiness, depression, diarrhea, shortness of breath, and bradycardia. The usual maintenance dose of metoprolol is 100 mg twice daily. Nadolol has a long duration of action which permits once a day administration. The usual dosage range in hypertension is 80 to 320 mg given a single daily dose.

Direct Arteriolar Vasodilators

Drugs in this class act directly on the smooth muscle of the arteriolar wall, causing vasodilation; this reduces peripheral vascular resistance.

Hydralazine Hydralazine (Apresoline), in addition to its ability to reduce elevated blood pressure by its direct vasodilatory effects, also causes reflex stimulation of heart rate and cardiac output. These latter effects, if not antagonized, could offset the beneficial reduction in peripheral vascular resistance and negate the antihypertensive effects of this drug. Hence, propranolol is frequently co-administered with hydralazine to counteract hydralazine-induced increases in the rate and force of myocardial contraction.

A high incidence of adverse side effects is associated with the use of hydralazine; some of the most common include headache, cardiac palpitations, dizziness, loss of appetite, nausea, and sweating. The first three of these effects are less pronounced when propranolol is co-administered.

Administration of hydralazine must be discontinued upon the appearance of drug fever, urticaria, skin rash, polyneuritis, gastrointestinal bleeding, or symptoms of coronary insufficiency. Chronic administration of this drug at daily doses of 200 mg or more can result in an acute rheumatoid state or a syndrome closely resembling disseminated lupus erythematosus. The latter syndrome may persist for many years and may require treatment with glucocorticoids, which, in turn, can further complicate hypertension. The potential usefulness of hydralazine for the management of moderate to severe hypertension is greatly limited by its side effects. The concurrent use of other antihypertensive drugs permits the use of hydralazine at lower doses, resulting in a reduction in these adverse effects. Initial daily doses begin at 20 to 80 mg, with the usual maintenance dose of 100 to 200 mg employed.

Minoxidil (Loniten) has pharmacological properties similar to those of hydralazine but appears to be more potent and effective. This drug also causes salt retention and tachycardia, effects that can be controlled by concurrent administration of a thiazide diuretic and propranolol, respectively. At present, minoxidil is being tested in combination with propranolol for the management of severe hypertension that is not responsive to other antihypertensive medications.

Common adverse effects include salt and water retention, an increase in heart rate (worsening or precipitating anginal attacks), pericardial effusion, and hypertrichosis (excessive hairiness), which is reversible. The usual daily maintenance dose is 10 to 40 mg administered as a single dose or in divided doses.

Prazosin Prazosin (Minipress) reduces elevated blood pressure primarily by producing direct relaxation of peripheral arterioles and thereby decreasing total peripheral resistance. Unlike hydralazine, the antihypertensive effects of prazosin are unaccompanied by clinically significant changes in cardiac output, heart rate, renal blood flow, or glomerular filtration rate.

This new drug, indicated for the management of mild to moderate hypertension, may be employed alone as the initial drug or may be used with diuretics or other anti-

hypertensive agents. The usual adult oral dose is 1 mg three times daily; dosage may be increased gradually to a daily total of 20 mg which is generally administered in two divided doses.

The most common adverse effects—in order of frequency—are dizziness, headache, drowsiness, lack of energy, weakness, cardiac palpitations, and nausea. In most instances these side effects disappear with continued drug administration. Nurses should advise their patients to rise slowly since prazosin may cause orthostatic hypotension with resulting syncope; more common than loss of consciousness are dizziness and lightheadedness.

Diazoxide Diazoxide (Hyperstat I.V.) is chemically related to the thiazides but is devoid of diuretic activity. After intravenous injection of 300 mg, this drug produces a dramatic reduction in blood pressure within 5 minutes, making it among the most valuable drugs currently available for the emergency treatment of *hypertensive crisis.*

Once the antihypertensive effect has been manifested, it generally persists for from 2 to 12 hours. After each intravenous injection, nurses should carefully monitor blood pressure until it has stabilized. Repeated drug administration at 2- to 12-hour intervals will generally maintain reductions in the hypertensive condition until the oral medication becomes effective. The use of diazoxide is not usually required for more than 4 or 5 days.

This drug commonly causes salt and water retention, effects that can be controlled by administration of the thiazide diuretics. The most unusual side effect produced by diazoxide is hyperglycemia. When diazoxide is to be used in diabetics or patients with a family history of diabetes, or when repeated injections are required, the nurse should carefully monitor the blood sugar levels.

While this hyperglycemic response is generally mild and blood sugar levels return to normal in the absence of treatment, susceptible patients may require the administration of insulin or other hypoglycemic agents.

Sodium nitroprusside Sodium nitroprusside (Nipride) is another direct-acting arteriolar vasodilator that is useful for the short-term management of hypertensive crisis.

Adverse effects include nausea, agitation, and muscle twitching. It is essential that the nurse continuously monitor the blood pressure and drug flow rates of patients receiving intravenous infusions of nitroprusside; the maximum dose should not exceed 800 μg/minute. Dyspnea, cyanosis, and cardiovascular collapse have been reported to result when blood pressure is permitted to fall too markedly. Patients with renal impairment are more susceptible to the toxic effects of this drug.

Nitroprusside is extremely sensitive to *decomposition in light;* this decomposition may be recognized by a change in the color of drug solution from reddish-brown to blue. To reduce the rate of drug breakdown, the nurse should wrap the infusion bottle with an opaque material such as aluminum foil. The nurse should only administer *freshly prepared* solutions, discarding any that are more than 4 hours old.

Antihypertensive Diuretics (Saluretics)

Diuretics are drugs that promote the excretion of water in the urine, whereas *saluretics* enhance the excretion of both sodium and water. Orally active saluretics, the *thiazide* derivatives in particular, are among the most frequently employed drugs for the treatment of hypertension.

When used alone, the thiazides possess only weak antihypertensive effects and are useful only for the treatment of mild hypertension. More important, however, is the use of these drugs in combination with more potent antihypertensive agents for the treatment of moderate to severe hypertension in patients with normal renal function. By augmenting the hypotensive effects of other drugs, these latter drugs may be employed in lower doses, thereby reducing the incidence and severity of their adverse side effects. In addition, saluretics antagonize sodium and water retention caused by many antihypertensive agents (reserpine, hydralazine, methyldopa, guanethidine). Excessive salt and fluid retention significantly contribute to refractoriness (tolerance) to nondiuretic antihypertensive drugs.

Arterial blood pressure is strongly influenced by the *plasma volume*. During the early phases of thiazide administration, one observes a reduction in plasma volume and a decrease in cardiac output. After several weeks of continuous diuretic administration, plasma volume and cardiac output return to predrug levels but the beneficial hypotensive effects are sustained. Thus, it would appear that the antihypertensive effects of these drugs cannot be explained simply on the basis of a reduction in extracellular fluid volume. It has been suggested that saluretics may cause alterations in the concentrations of salts in the smooth muscle walls of the arterioles, which results in increased vasodilation.

Common thiazide saluretics used for the treatment of hypertension include chlorothiazide (Diuril) and hydrochlorothiazide (Esidrix, HydroDiuril, Oretic); representative nonthiazides include chlorthalidone (Hygroton), quinethazone (Hydromox), furosemide (Lasix), and spironolactone (Aldactone). The pharmacology, adverse effects, and drug interactions involving the diuretics and saluretics will be discussed in detail in Chapter 32.

THERAPEUTIC CONSIDERATIONS

The choice of the most appropriate antihypertensive medication(s) for a given patient depends upon a variety of factors, two of which include the severity of the hypertensive state and the co-existence of other medical problems. Since it is far beyond the scope of this text to discuss these factors in detail, we shall only briefly examine each.

The *severity of hypertension* is gener-

Table 28-3   Classification and Treatment of Hypertension of Varying Severity

Hypertensive classification	Diastolic blood pressure (mm Hg)	Clinical symptoms	Possible drug treatments (Maintenance doses)
Mild	90–105	Asymptomatic, with no tissue or organ damage.	(1) No medication with minimal adverse prognostic factors. (2) Hydrochlorothiazide (50 mg b.i.d.) and/or reserpine (0.25 mg daily).
Moderate	105–130	Asymptomatic or symptomatic with some evidence of tissue or organ damage.	Hydrochlorothiazide and one of the following: (1) Methyldopa (0.5–1 g daily) (2) Hydralazine (100–200 mg daily) (3) Propranolol (variable doses)
Severe	130–140	Symptomatic with damage to heart, kidneys, optic fundi.	Hydrochlorothiazide and one of the drugs listed for moderate hypertension and/or: (1) Guanethidine (25–50 mg daily) (2) Clonidine (0.15–0.90 mg daily)
Hypertensive crisis	over 140	Medical emergency with moderate to severe tissue damage.	Parenteral administration of one of the following when immediate reduction in blood pressure is essential. (1) Diazoxide (300 mg) (2) Nitroprusside (0.03–0.09 mg/min)

Table 28-4   Associated Medical Problems Influencing the Choice of Antihypertensive Disorders

Medical disorder	Drug	Rationale for caution or contraindication
Cerebrovascular diseases Depression	Reserpine Methyldopa	The central effects of these drugs may cause adverse behavioral effects, confusion, and enhanced depression.
Coronary artery disease	Hydralazine	Myocardial stimulation increases work load placed on the heart; may produce angina attack.
Congestive heart failure	Propranolol	Blockade of sympathetic influences on the heart increasing the force of contraction.
Atrioventricular conduction defects	Propranolol	Drug-induced depression of A-V conduction resulting in heart block.
Diabetes mellitus	Thiazine diuretics Furosemide	In prediabetics, thiazides may cause hyperglycemia and glycosuria. In diabetics, these diuretics may antagonize the hypoglycemic effects of antidiabetic agents.
Hyperuricemia (gout)	Thiazide diuretics Chlorthalidone	Diuretics increase serum urate levels, which may result in acute gouty arthritis.
Renal insufficiency	Guanethidine Thiazide diuretics	Decrease in renal blood flow. Aggravation of renal impairment.
Asthma	Propranolol	Increased risk of bronchoconstriction.

ally assessed by evaluating the patient for the presence of tissue damage and monitoring diastolic blood pressure (Table 28-3). As you will note from this table, successful therapy often requires the utilization of more than one drug. Multiple drugs are employed to maximize the potential benefits and to minimize the incidence and severity of side effects. If the patient is asymptomatic or experiencing only minor discomfort from the hypertensive state, the patient may perceive that the drug-induced side effects are more distressful than the potential benefits to be derived from drug treatment; this may result in the patient failing to take the prescribed medication. *Patient noncompliance* is a major problem in the management of hypertension. The nurse should assume an important role in educating the patient about the nature of hypertension, its potential consequences if improperly treated, and the importance of taking medication according to the prescribed dosage schedule.

Prior to prescribing drugs for the hypertensive patient, the physician must ascer-

Table 28-5   Potential Drug Interactions Involving Antihypertensive Agents

Antihypertensive agent	Interacting drug/class	Potential consequences
Methyldopa Reserpine	Pargyline Monamine oxidase inhibitor inhibitor antidepressants	Possible headache, severe hypertension, hallucinations.
Methyldopa Guanethidine	Levarterenol (norepinephrine)	Marked enhancement of pressor response to levarterenol.
Methyldopa Reserpine Guanethidine	Methotrimeprazine (Levoprome)	Orthostatic hypotension and decrease in blood pressure.
Clonidine	Tricyclic antidepressants	Antihypertensive effects of clonidine may be antagonized by tricyclics.
Reserpine Clonidine	Levodopa	Possible antagonism of antiparkinsonism effects of levodopa.
Guanethidine	Amphetamines Ephedrine Methylphenidate (Ritalin) Phenylephrine Tricyclic antidepressants Monoamine oxidase inhibitor antidepressants Phenothiazines	Antihypertensive effects of guanethidine may be antagonized, with loss of control of blood pressure.
Pargyline	Other antihypertensive agents except thiazides See Table 17-2 (page 141) for monoamine oxidate inhibitor antidepressants.	Possible headache, severe hypertension. See Table 17-2 (page 141).
Propranolol	See Table 6-2 (page 61).	See Table 6-2 (page 61).
Diazoxide	Hydralazine (Apresoline)	Severe hypotensive reaction.
Diazoxide	Thiazide diuretics	Enhanced hyperglycemic response to diazoxide.
	Coumarin anticoagulants	Possible increased anticoagulation.
Diuretics Saluretics	See Table 32-3 (page 273).	See Table 32-3 (page 273).

tain whether the patient has other *health problems* that may be worsened by the administration of certain antihypertensive drugs. Table 28-4 summarizes the potential adverse effects that antihypertensive drugs may have on selected common associated medical disorders.

Since certain drugs may elevate blood pressure, it is essential that a careful drug history be determined. If oral contraceptives are responsible for the observed hypertension, this medication should be discontinued, and an alternative form of contraception be employed. Since obesity or a high salt intake contributes to hypertension in many patients, blood pressure may return to normal levels by instituting a weight reduction program and a low salt diet.

Antihypertensives: nursing implications

1. Orthostatic hypotension develops most often when therapy is initiated or dosage is increased. Caution the patient to change position slowly, dangle legs for several minutes before standing, avoid hot baths or showers, and avoid prolonged standing.
2. The patient should be cautioned to lie down or sit down with head low if feeling faint or dizzy.
3. Take the patient's blood pressure (B.P.) in lying, sitting, and standing positions during periods of dosage adjustment.
4. Monitor fluid intake and output and check for reduction in urine volume. Weigh the patient under standardized conditions and check for edema.
5. Watch for signs of tolerance which may occur during the second or third month of therapy with some antihypertensive drugs.
6. Teach the patient or a responsible family member the purpose of the drug and how to monitor drug effects. Include specific dosage schedule; symptoms to report; recommended physical activity, diet, and weight control; things to avoid, including excess caffeine, alcohol, smoking, and nonprescription drugs without consulting the physician. Urge patient to keep return appointments and take medication as directed.

Methyldopa (Aldomet)

1. Reversible hepatotoxicity may develop in 8–10 wk and is an indication to discontinue medication. Symptoms include chills, fever, headache, pruritis, anorexia, rash, enlarged liver, and positive Coombs test.
2. Sedation and drowsiness occur during first few days of therapy but disappear with continued use or dosage reduction.

Guanethidine (Ismelin)

1. Observe for diarrhea, bradycardia, or edema; all are indications that medication should be discontinued.

2. Caution the patient to avoid stress, which can precipitate acute cardiovascular collapse.

3. Drug may sensitize the patient to some sympathomimetic agents found in nonprescription cold remedies, potentially resulting in hypertensive crisis. Caution the patient to consult with the physician or pharmacist prior to taking nonprescription medications.

Reserpine

1. Mental depression is a serious adverse effect that may lead to attempted suicide. Instruct patient and a responsible family member to report early signs of depression: altered sleep patterns, anorexia, personality changes, sexual impotence, and self-deprecation.

2. Have a sympathomimetic agent (ephedrine) available in case of overdose.

Hydralazine (Apresoline)

1. Complete blood counts, lupus erythematosus (LE) cell preparation and antinuclear antibody tests are advised before and periodically during therapy.

2. If the patient develops arthralgia, fever, chest pain, or malaise, the LE prep test is indicated.

3. Vitamin B_6 (pyridoxine) may be prescribed for peripheral neuritis.

Diuretics

See nursing implications for the diuretics in Chapter 32.

SUPPLEMENTARY READINGS

Capell, P. T., and D. B. Case, *Ambulatory Care Manual for Nurse Practitioners*, pp. 34–48. Philadelphia: J. B. Lippincott Company, 1976.

Giblin, E., "Controlling High Blood Pressure," *American Journal of Nursing* **78**: 824–32 (1978).

Kaplan, N. M., *Clinical Hypertension*, 2nd ed. Baltimore: Williams & Wilkins Company, 1978.

Kelly, K. L., "Beta Blockers in Hypertension: A Review," *American Journal of Hospital Pharmacy* **33**: 1284–90 (1976).

Koch-Weser, J., "Diazoxide," *New England Journal of Medicine* **294**: 1271–74 (1976).

Long, M. L., and others, "Hypertension—What Patients Need to Know," *American Journal of Nursing* **76**: 765–80 (1976).

McMahon, F. G., *Management of Essential Hypertension*. Mount Kisco, N.Y.: Futura Publishing Company, 1978.

Oparil, S., and E. Haber, "The Renin-Angiotensin System," *New England Journal of Medicine* **291**: 389–401, 446–57 (1974).

Page, L. B., and J. J. Sidd, "Medical Management of Primary Hypertension," *New England Journal of Medicine* **287**: 960–66, 1018–23, 1074–81 (1972).

Palmer, R. F., and K. C. Lesseter, "Sodium Nitroprusside," *New England Journal of Medicine* **292**: 294–97 (1975).

Perloff, D. ed., "Syndrome on Hypertension," *Medical Clinics of North America* **61**(3): 463–700 (1977).

Ram, C. V., "Newer Antihypertensive Drugs—Pharmacology and Therapeutics in Critical Care," *Heart and Lung* **6**: 679–84 (1977).

Scriabine, A., and C. S. Sweet, eds., *New Antihypertensive Drugs*. New York: Spectrum Publications, 1976.

Veterans Administration Cooperative Study Group on Antihypertensive Agents, "Effects of Treatment on Morbidity in Hypertension: Results in Patients with Diastolic Blood Pressures Averaging 115 through 129 mm Hg," *Journal of the American Medical Association* **202**: 1,028–34 (1967).

Veterans Administration Cooperative Study Group on Antihypertensive Agents, "Effects of Treatment on Morbidity in Hypertension: II. Results in Patients with Diastolic Blood Pressures Averaging 90 through 114 mm Hg," *Journal of the American Medical Association* **213:** 1143–52 (1970).

Wollam, G. L., R. W. Gifford, Jr., and R. C. Tarazi,

"Antihypertensive Drugs: Clinical Pharmacology and Therapeutic Use," *Drugs* **14:** 420–60 (1977).

Woosley, R. L., and A. S. Nies, "Guanethidine," *New England Journal of Medicine* **295:** 1053–57 (1976).

Chapter 29

ANTIANGINAL DRUGS

Coronary artery disease, the major cause of death in western nations, results from an inadequate blood supply to the heart muscle. Atherosclerosis of the coronary arteries reduces coronary blood flow and decreases oxygen delivery to the myocardium.

Angina pectoris, one common type of coronary artery disease, is clinically characterized by extreme substernal pain, which may remain localized or may radiate to the shoulders or arms. This pain occurs when the oxygen requirements of the myocardium temporarily exceed the available supply. Anginal attacks are usually precipitated by exercise or activities that increase the work of the heart muscle and its demands for oxygen. Anxiety-provoking events, cold environments, or eating heavy meals are other common causes. Such events cause a release of epinephrine and

norepinephrine, which stimulate the heart, and result in a greater consumption of oxygen by the myocardium. Pain generally persists for 3 to 5 minutes; it dissipates when the patient rests.

The major aim in the management of angina is reduction of the attack frequency and severity to permit the patient to live a normal life. While the prophylactic use of drugs may assist in the achievement of this objective, the patient must be instructed to avoid or minimize those activities that precipitate anginal attacks.

Drugs used for the treatment of angina act by dilating the coronary arteries or by reducing cardiac work. Nitroglycerin and related nitrites have been the mainstay of drug treatment, with propranolol also of value in the management of this disorder.

NITROGLYCERIN
AND THE NITRITES

Many nitrites and nitrates are capable of re-laxing smooth muscle; the muscles in the walls of the coronary arteries are particularly sensitive to the dilating effects of these drugs. Upon evaluation of the comparative properties of these antianginal drugs, collectively referred to as *nitrites*, we observe that they differ primarily with respect to their route of administration, rate of onset, and duration of action (Table 29-1). Apart from their longer duration of action, there is no clinical evidence that any of these drugs are superior to nitroglycerin for the treatment or prevention of anginal attacks.

Nitroglycerin (Glyceryl Trinitrate)

Nitroglycerin was found to be an effective antianginal agent approximately 100 years ago and continues to remain the drug of choice for the management of this cardio-vascular disorder. This drug and related nitrites can produce relaxation of many smooth muscles (biliary tract, bronchi, uterus), but in therapeutic doses their predominant effects are on the smooth muscle of the coronary arteries.

Effects on the heart Within minutes after placing a 0.3- to 0.6-mg tablet of nitroglycerin under the tongue (*sublingual* administration), the patient begins to experience relief from the pain associated with an acute anginal attack. Moreover, when taken prior to exercise or stress, this drug reduces the susceptibility of the patient to an attack.

In the past, nitroglycerin's antianginal effects were attributed to its ability to produce *coronary vasodilation.* By virtue of its ability to relax arterial smooth muscle and reduce the resistance exerted by the walls of the coronary arteries, it was thought to increase blood flow

and the supply of oxygen to the myocardium. It is now generally believed that the beneficial effects of nitroglycerin result from a drug-induced reduction in cardiac work that *decreases the oxygen requirements* of the heart. This reduction in cardiac work involves peripheral vasodilation, decreased venous return to the heart, and a reduction in the peripheral resistance against which the heart must work.

Adverse effects and tolerance The major adverse effects observed after administration of the nitrites represent extensions of their cardiovascular effects, in particular, vasodilation. *Headache*, often severe in intensity, is the most common side effect encountered during the early days of drug therapy. Other frequently reported side effects include dizziness, weakness, flushing of the face and skin, and postural hypotension, which is worsened by ingestion of alcoholic beverages.

Within several days after the initiation of nitrite administration, *tolerance* develops to drug-induced headache as well as to the beneficial antianginal effects; hence it is usually necessary to increase the dosage requirements of patients receiving these drugs on a continuous basis.

A number of sustained release nitrite preparations are available; it is reported that they have durations of action of 12 hours. Clinical studies have failed to demonstrate the effectiveness of such preparations, which may be the consequence of the rapid development of tolerance. Within several days after the discontinuation of nitrite administration, both the beneficial effects and their abilities to produce headaches are restored.

Administration and drug stability Nitroglycerin is absorbed from the mucous membranes of the mouth and from the skin and can, therefore, be effectively administered sublingually and topically, respectively. Nurses should inform patients that sublingual

Table 29-1   Comparative Properties of Antianginal Drugs

Generic name	Selected trade names	Route of administration	Onset	Duration	Use[a]	Remarks (usual adult dose)
Amyl nitrite	———	Inhalation.	30 sec	3-5 min	A	Inhalation of liquid contents of crushed ampule (pearl) 2-3 times; flushing and headache common. Infrequently used.
Nitroglycerin (glyceryl trinitrate)	Nitrostat	Sublingual.	3 min	15-30 min	A, P	Terminate or prevent attack. Readily deteriorates in light, heat, or moisture. Store in dark glass container (0.3-0.6 mg PRN).
	Nitro-Bid Nitrol	Topical.	30-60 min	3 h	P	Application of 1-2 inches of ointment to skin (commonly chest, abdomen) to prevent attacks, particularly at night.
Isosorbide dinitrate	Isordil Laserdil	Sublingual. Chewable.	2-5 min	2-4 h	A, P	Terminate or prevent attacks (2.5-10 mg PRN). Long duration of action.
	Sorbitrate	Oral.	15-30 min	4-6 h	P	Prevent attacks (10 mg q.i.d.)
Erythrityl tetranitrate	Cardilate	Sublingual. Chewable.	5 min	2-4 h	A, P	Terminate or prevent attacks (5-10 mg PRN or t.i.d.).
		Oral.	15-30 min	4 h	P	Prevent attacks. Tolerance develops with repeated use.
Pentaerythritol tetrantirate	Peritrate P.E.T.N.	Oral.	15-30 min	4-5 h	P	Similar to erythrityl tetranitrate. Sustained release preparations available, but not recommended (10-40 mg q.i.d.).
Propranolol	Inderal	Oral.	30 min	6 h	P	Effective drug for prevention of attacks. Acts by reducing oxygen requirements of heart. Often used in combination with nitrites. (40 mg q.i.d.)

[a] Abbreviations: A = arrest acute anginal attack; P = prevent or reduce severity of attacks.

tablets taken orally (swallowed) are relatively ineffective because of rapid breakdown and inactivation by the liver. Should a single sublingual tablet prove to be ineffective in terminating an acute anginal attack within 5 minutes, one or two additional doses may be taken at 5-minute intervals. Moreover, this drug may be taken prophylactically prior to activities known to precipitate attacks in the patient; when so employed, it exerts its protective effects for approximately 30 minutes.

The nurse should educate the patient about the importance of properly storing nitroglycerin tablets. This drug readily breaks down when exposed to light, heat, or moisture and is volatile, causing tablets to lose their potency. Tablets should be stored in dark, airtight, *glass* containers; plastic containers should not be utilized. If a tablet fails to produce a burning sensation when placed under the tongue, it is very likely to be of substandard potency and a fresh supply of tablets should be obtained.

PROPRANOLOL

Exercise enhances sympathetic nerve activity causing an increase in the force and rate of cardiac contractions; this leads to greater oxygen consumption by the heart muscle and precipitation of an anginal attack in susceptible individuals. The β-adrenergic blocking agents propranolol (Inderal) and nadolol (Corgard) antagonize these sympathetically mediated responses. While coronary blood flow is usually decreased after their administration, this is offset by a marked reduction in the oxygen requirements of the myocardium.

Chronic administration of propranolol decreases the frequency of anginal attacks. Therapy is generally initiated with daily doses of 40 mg, with maintenance doses ranging from 160 to 400 mg per day. The usual maintenance dose of nadolol is 80 to 240 mg daily. Sublingual nitroglycerin is frequently provided for the management of acute attacks. Abrupt withdrawal of propranolol may cause a worsening of angina, especially in patients with severe coronary artery disease. Hence it is deemed wise to gradually reduce the dose of this drug over a 1- to 2-week period when contemplating discontinuation of therapy.

The adverse effects and precautions associated with the use of this drug were discussed in Chapter 6, with potential drug interactions summarized in Table 6-2 (page 61).

ETHANOL

For many years, some physicians have recommended that their patients consume *moderate* amounts of alcoholic beverages for the treatment of coronary artery disease and to relieve anginal pains. Moreover, recent clinical studies suggest that individuals who consume moderate volumes of alcohol have a lower incidence of myocardial infarction and angina than nondrinkers. Available evidence reveals that ethanol's ability to relieve anginal pains is probably not the result of coronary vasodilation, but more likely a consequence of its central sedative effects.

Antianginal Drugs:
nursing implications

Nitroglycerin (sublingual tablets)

1. Instruct the patient to sit down upon the first signs of anginal pain, place tablet under the tongue, and allow it to dissolve.

2. If pain is not relieved within 5 min, repeat dose up to a maximum of 3 tablets. If pain is not relieved within 15 min, advise patient to call physician or obtain assistance in being taken to the emergency room.

3. Instruct patient on care of sublingual tablets. They should be stored in a cold place in a dark, airtight, glass bottle. Carry a small supply at all times. Tablets lose potency in containers made of metal, plastic, or cardboard. Tablets that fail to produce a burning or stinging sensation when placed under the tongue have lost their potency and should be replaced by fresh tablets.

4. Teach patient expected effect and side effects of drug. Transient headache is common. Postural hypotension may be reduced by changing position slowly and avoiding prolonged standing. Acute hypotension may occur if alcohol is ingested too soon after drug. Advise the patient to report blurred vision or dry mouth which are indications for drug withdrawal.

5. Patients must learn to identify factors which precipitate anginal pain and avoid them: emotional distress, heavy meals, smoking, extreme temperatures, excessive caffeine, and excessive or increased exercise.

Propranolol (Inderal)

See the nursing implications for adrenergic blocking agents in Chapter 6.

SUPPLEMENTARY READINGS

Allendorf, E. E., and others, "Teaching Patients About Nitroglycerin," *American Journal of Nursing* **75:** 1168–70 (1975).

Angelakos, E. T., "Coronary Vasodilators," in *Drill's Pharmacology in Medicine* (4th ed.), ed. J. P. DiPalma, Chapter 39, pp. 809–23. New York: McGraw-Hill Book Company, 1971.

Charlier, R., *Antianginal Drugs.* New York: Springer-Verlag, 1971.

Epstein, S. E., and others, "Angina Pectoris: Patho-physiology, Evaluation, and Treatment," *Annals of Internal Medicine* **75:** 263–96 (1971).

Gensini, G. G., ed., *The Study of the Systemic Coronary and Myocardial Effects of Nitrates.* Springfield, Illinois: Charles C Thomas, Publisher, 1972.

McGregor, M., "Drugs for the Treatment of Angina Pectoris," in *Clinical Pharmacology*, Vol. 2. *International Encyclopedia of Pharmacology and Therapeutics*, Section 6, ed. L. Lasagna, pp. 377–403. Oxford: Pergamon Press, Inc., 1966.

Parratt, J. R., "Recent Advances in the Pathophysiology and Pharmacology of Angina," *General Pharmacology* **6:** 247–51 (1975).

ANTILIPEMIC DRUGS

Atherosclerosis is principally a disease of large- and medium-sized arteries in which deposits of *lipids* line the walls of these vessels, causing degenerative changes and impairment of blood flow. Major complications of atherosclerosis include myocardial infarction, coronary arterial disease (angina), cerebral arterial diseases (leading to stroke and senility), peripheral arterial diseases (resulting in poor circulation to the extremities, with the potential development of gangrene), hypertension, and kidney disease.

HYPERLIPIDEMIA AND CHOLESTEROL

While the exact cause or causes of atherosclerosis remain an enigma, it would appear that certain *risk factors* contribute to its etiology. Some of these factors include diet, particularly one that results in high serum cholesterol levels, obesity, cigarette smoking, lack of physical exercise, hypertension, emotional stress, and hereditary influences.

Cholesterol is contained in the diet and is also biosynthesized by many tissues of the body. It is a key intermediate compound for the biosynthesis of the male and female sex hormones, the adrenocorticosteroid hormones (aldosterone and cortisol), and for the manufacture of bile acids and salts required for the digestion and absorption of fats. Approximately 80 to 90 percent of the body's cholesterol is ultimately converted to bile salts.

To date, considerable research effort has been devoted to evaluating the role of lipids (triglycerides, free fatty acids, and cholesterol) in the etiology of atherosclerosis. No direct cause and effect relationship has as yet been clinically established between *hyperlipidemia* (elevated serum lipid levels) and atherosclerosis, nor has it been demonstrated that a reduction in elevated lipid levels significantly retards the progression of the atherosclerotic state or other cardiovascular disorders.

ANTILIPEMIC DRUGS

The antilipemic drugs now used to reduce the serum levels of cholesterol inhibit the absorption or biosynthesis of this lipid or increase the rate of its metabolism and elimination.

Sitosterols

Sitosterols, plant sterols obtained from wheat, corn, rye, rice, and soy, act by reducing the intestinal absorption of dietary cholesterol. The ability of sitosterols (Cytellin) to reduce serum cholesterol has not been clearly established in a clinical setting.

Clofibrate

Clofibrate (Atromid-S) is among the most effective drugs currently available for the reduction of total serum lipids, triglycerides in particular, and to a lesser extent, cholesterol. While the exact mechanism of action of clofibrate is not known, it is generally believed to inhibit the biosynthesis of cholesterol and may also speed the rate of the removal of lipids from the circulation. Several weeks of continuous drug administration are required before demonstrable reductions in serum lipids are observed. The usual daily dose is 2 g.

This drug should be used as adjunctive therapy to diet and other measures intended for the reduction of elevated serum cholesterol levels. Obese patients should be advised to reduce weight and increase physical activity within their capabilities. Serum lipid levels should be determined during the first few months of clofibrate administration, and the drug should be withdrawn after 3 months if the therapeutic response is not adequate.

Apart from nausea and abdominal upset, clofibrate is generally well tolerated. This drug is contraindicated in patients with impaired liver or kidney function. Clofibrate should be used cautiously in patients receiving oral coumarin anticoagulants. This drug is capable of increasing the anticoagulant effects of the coumarins by a mechanism that may involve their displacement from plasma protein binding sites. To prevent the risk of bleeding, prothrombin times should be monitored and the dose of the anticoagulant reduced if necessary.

Nicotinic Acid (Niacin)

High doses of nicotinic acid (1.5 to 6 g daily) reduce serum levels of cholesterol by a mechanism thought to involve inhibition of its synthesis. The clinical utility of this compound is severely limited by a high incidence of such unpleasant side effects as flushing, pruritis (itching), and gastrointestinal upset; impairment of liver function has been reported.

Thyroid Hormones

It has been recognized for many years that *thyroid function* influences serum lipid levels. Hyperthyroid patients have low serum lipid levels, whereas patients with depressed thyroid function have elevated levels. While the natural thyroid hormones (for example, levothyroxin) increase the rate at which cholesterol is broken down into bile acids, these compounds cause palpitations of the heart, may precipitate angina, and cause nervousness, insomnia, and weight loss.

Dextrothyroxine (Choloxin), a synthetic thyroxine analog, appears to be an effective drug, yet it may increase the risk of coronary disease. This drug should not be employed in patients with a history of heart disease and hypertension. Dextrothyroxine increases blood sugar levels in diabetic patients. The initial daily oral dose is 1 mg, which may be increased by 1-mg increments until a maximum daily dose of 8 mg is reached.

Probucol

Probucol (Lorelco) is a new drug capable of lowering serum cholesterol levels by mechanisms that have not been clearly established. Among the postulated mechanisms are inhibition of cholesterol transport from the intestines, inhibition of cholesterol biosynthesis at an early stage, or enhancement of the elimination of bile salts and cholesterol in the feces.

Reductions in serum cholesterol levels are generally observed within 2 to 4 weeks after the initiation of therapy, with maximal effects requiring up to 7 weeks.

The usual dose of probucol is 500 mg given twice daily with the morning and evening meals. The adverse effects are generally mild to moderate, of short duration, and seldom require that the drug be discontinued. The most frequently encountered side effects involve the gastrointestinal tract and include diarrhea, flatulence, abdominal pain, nausea, and vomiting.

Ion-Exchange Resins

Cholestyramine (Questran) is a nonabsorbable ion-exchange resin that binds bile acids in the intestinal tract and increases their elimination in the feces. The continuous elimination of bile acids results in the increased conversion of cholesterol to bile acids, causing a reduction in the serum levels of cholesterol. While little change is generally observed in serum triglycerides, cholesterol levels fall markedly during the early weeks of cholestyramine administration but rise rapidly after discontinuation of drug therapy.

The resin has an unpleasant sandy or gritty quality and should not be taken dry. Nurses should advise patients to mix this drug with liquids. Common side effects include nausea and constipation; the latter is minimized when the patient is encourage to maintain a high fluid intake. The usual dose of this resin is 4 g three to four times daily before meals and at bedtime.

Colestipol (Colestid) is an ion-exchange resin that has pharmacological properties, adverse side effects, and drug-interactions similar to those of cholestyramine. The usual daily dose of this compound is 15 to 30 g in two to four divided doses. It is recommended that colestipol be administered in beverages, soups, cereals, or crushed fruits.

Drug interactions These ion-exchange resins have been reported to bind to many drugs in the intestine, preventing their absorption. Such drugs include penicillin and tetracycline antibiotics, coumarin derivative anticoagulants, digitalis glycosides, thyroid hormones, and fat-soluble vitamins, especially vitamin K. Nurses should recommend that patients take their orally administered drugs 1 hour before or 4 hours after these medications.

Antilipemic Drugs:
nursing implications

1. These drugs should only be employed after dietary and weight-control methods to reduce cholesterol and triglyceride levels have been attempted without success.
2. Serum cholesterol and lipid levels should be determined frequently during the first few months of therapy. If the response is inadequate within 3 mo, the drug should be discontinued.

Clofibrate (Atromid-S)

1. This drug increases the effects of oral anticoagulants. Observe such patients for bleeding or bruising.

2. Instruct the patient to report flu-like symptoms: malaise, muscle soreness, aching, weakness.

3. Discontinue the drug if serum transaminase or other liver function tests are abnormal.

4. Monitor diabetics closely; the drug may cause hyperglycemia and glycosuria.

Cholestyramine (Questran)

1. The drug must be dissolved before administration. Mix in vehicle to mask unpleasant taste and texture.

2. Supplemental water-miscible forms of vitamins A and D should be taken during long-term therapy. Chronic drug use may increase bleeding tendency. Advise patient to report bleeding, bruising, or tarry stools. Treat with parenteral vitamin K.

3. Constipation can be a serious problem that can be managed with a high bulk diet, increased fluids, and stool softeners.

4. Other drugs should be taken at least 1 h before or 4 h after cholestyramine to avoid interference with the absorption of these drugs.

SUPPLEMENTARY READINGS

Civin, H., and others, "Diet vs. Drugs in Hyperlipidemia," *Patient Care* **10**: 20-59 (1976).

Coronary Drug Project, "Clofibrate and Niacin in Coronary Heart Disease," *Journal of the American Medical Association* **231**: 360–81 (1975).

Fredrickson, D. S., J. R. Goldstein, and M. S. Brown, "Familial Hyperlipoproteinemias," in *The Metabolic Basis of Inherited Disease* (4th ed.), eds. J. B. Stanbury, J. B. Wyngaarden, and D. S. Fredrickson, pp. 604-55. New York: McGraw-Hill Book Company, 1978.

Havel, R. J., and J. P. Kane, "Drugs and Lipid Metabolism," *Annual Review of Pharmacology* **13**: 287–308 (1973).

Holmes, W. L., R. Paoletti, and D. Kritchevsky, eds., "Pharmacological Control of Lipid Metabolism," *Advances in Experimental Medicine and Biology* **26**: 1–359 (1972).

Lees, R. S., and D. E. Wilson, "The Treatment of Hyperlipidemia," *New England Journal of Medicine* **284**: 186–95 (1971).

Levy, R. I., "The Effect of Hypolipidemic Drugs on Plasma Lipoproteins," *Annual Review of Pharmacology and Toxicology* **17**: 499–510 (1977).

Ross, R., and J. A. Glomset, "The Pathogenesis of Atherosclerosis," *New England Journal of Medicine* **295**: 369–77, 420–25 (1976).

ANTICOAGULANT AND COAGULANT DRUGS

Chapter 31

Blood clotting represents an important defense mechanism of the body to prevent excessive internal or external hemorrhage. *Thrombus* (clot) development within a blood vessel, however, may lead to an obstruction of blood flow to tissues. In the absence of clot breakdown or the availability of collateral circulation, the thrombus may cause infarction and necrosis of such tissues. *Emboli* that break off from the original clot may lodge in vital areas of the body, such as the lungs, with potentially lethal consequences.

In other situations, we observe a failure in normal blood clotting. Minor injuries in such individuals may result in excessive and even life-threatening hemorrhaging.

Prior to our discussion of anticoagulant and coagulant drugs, we shall first consider the basic mechanisms underlying the formation and resolution (breakdown) of blood clots.

BLOOD CLOT FORMATION AND RESOLUTION

Clotting Mechanisms

When a small blood vessel is cut or damaged, the injury initiates a series of events

leading to the formation of a clot which, by sealing off the vessel, prevents further blood loss; this is called *hemostasis*. The clot consists of blood platelets and fibrin.

The sequence of events culminating in fibrin formation are presented in Figure 31-1, with the names of the blood clotting factors given in Table 31-1. The formation of a blood clot occurs in three stages: (1) the formation of activated factor X; (2) the conversion of prothrombin to thrombin by the action of activated factor X; and (3) the conversion of fibrinogen to fibrin by thrombin.

Factor X, a prothrombin-converting substance, can be activated by an intrinsic or extrinsic pathway (Figure 31-1). The *intrinsic pathway* is initiated with the activation of factor XII by contact with an appropriate surface (glass or, within the body, the collagen fibers underlying the endothelium in blood vessels). Via a series of interrelated reaction steps, activated factor X is formed. In the presence of lipids from blood platelets, calcium, and factor V, activated factor X catalyzes the conversion of prothrombin to thrombin. The *external pathway* involves the direct activation of factor X by tissue thromboplastin, a substance released from the walls of damaged

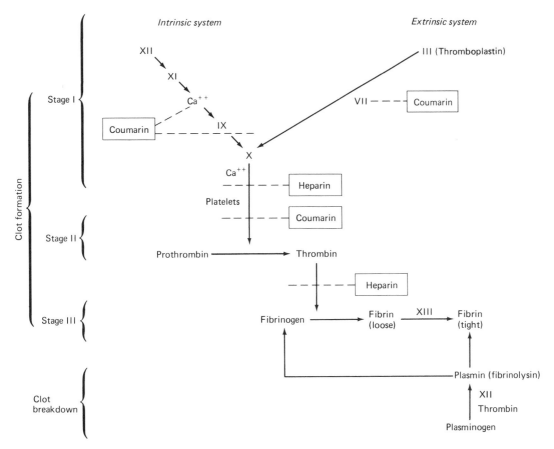

Figure 31-1   Summary of Mechanisms Involved in Clot Formation and Breakdown and the Sites of Anticoagulant Action.

Table 31-1   Blood Clotting Factors

Factor I	Fibrinogen.
Factor II	Prothrombin.
Factor III	Tissue thromboplastin.
Factor IV	Calcium.
Factor V	Proaccelerin; labile factor; accelerator globulin.
Factor VI	No longer recognized as a clotting factor.
Factor VII	Proconvertin; stable factor: serum prothrombin conversion accelerator (SPCA).
Factor VIII	Antihemophilic factor (AHF): antihemophilic globulin (AHG).
Factor IX	Plasma thromboplastin component (PTC): Christmas factor.
Factor X	Stuart-Prower factor.
Factor XI	Plasma thromboplastin antecedent (PTA).
Factor XII	Hageman factor.
Factor XIII	Fibrin-stabilizing factor.

blood vessels; this reaction involves factor VII.

Anticlotting Mechanisms

The tendency of blood to clot within the living organism is normally counterbalanced by reactions that prevent clot formation within blood vessels and that promote the breakdown of clots once they are formed. These *fibrinolytic systems* cause the breakdown of fibrin, fibrinogen, and factors V and VIII by the enzyme *plasmin* or *fibrinolysin* (Figure 31-1). Plasmin is formed from its biologically inactive precursor plasminogen by activators including factor XII and thrombin.

ANTICOAGULANTS

Anticoagulant compounds are available that prevent blood from coagulating both *in vitro* and *in vivo*. As can be noted from Figure 31-1, free *calcium* ions are required for clotting. In the test tube, clotting can be prevented in freshly drawn blood by the addition of sodium oxalate, which forms an insoluble salt with calcium, or by the chelating agent ethylenediaminetetraacetic acid (EDTA) or sodium citrate, compounds which bind calcium ions. *Sodium citrate* is used as an anticoagulant for the storage of blood. Heparin prevents clotting both in vivo and in vitro, while the coumarin and indandione derivatives are only active in vivo.

Heparin

Heparin is chemically characterized as a mucopolysaccharide that possesses highly acidic properties. It is a naturally occurring substance that is stored primarily in tissue mast cells. Commercial heparin, obtained from the lungs of domestic animals used for human food consumption, is sold under many trade names including Heprinar, Liquaemin Sodium, and Panheprin.

Actions Heparin prevents blood clotting by (1) inhibiting the conversion of prothrombin to thrombin by thromboplastin (*antithromboplastin action*); (2) antagonizing the ability of thrombin to catalyze the conversion of fibrinogen to fibrin (*antithrombin action*); and (3) decreasing the agglutination or clumping of platelets by reducing their adhesiveness.

In addition to its anticoagulant actions, heparin also has interesting effects on plasma lipids. After the ingestion of a meal rich in fats, the plasma becomes cloudy with fat particles. Within minutes after the injection of very small doses of heparin, the cloudiness of the hyperlipemic plasma disappears. This effect appears to result from a breakdown of triglycerides (fats) into smaller particles. The physiological significance of these observations has yet to be determined.

Administration and therapeutic uses
Heparin is not therapeutically effective after oral administration. Aqueous solutions of sodium heparin are generally administered intravenously or subcutaneously, with the dosage calculated as units of heparin. After a single intravenous dose of 5,000 units (approximately equivalent to 50 mg), the onset of anticoagulation is virtually immediate, with maximum effects observed within 5 to 10 minutes. In the absence of a second dose, clotting time will return to normal within 3 to 4 hours. Since the response of patients may be variable, the nurse should check clotting times two to three times daily to preclude overdosage. Clotting time should be maintained at 25 to 30 seconds or two to three times the normal duration of clot formation.

When immediate anticoagulation is required, such as in cases of arterial occlusion, heparin is the drug of choice. This drug is employed clinically to prevent clotting during transfusions, to prevent the development of postoperative clots or the extension of existing clots, and for the treatment of phlebitis, thrombophlebitis, and pulmonary embolism. It is also used as an anticoagulant for blood samples submitted for laboratory analysis. Heparin does not dissolve clots.

Toxicity Toxicity of heparin results from *overdosage* and is manifested by bleeding from open wounds and mucous membranes. Because of the short duration of action of this drug, treatment generally requires only a reduction in dosage or the frequency of subsequent injections. If the hemorrhaging must be arrested, the specific antagonist *protamine sulfate* may be administered intravenously. Protamine has an immediate onset of action and a duration of action of 2 hours; it is capable of neutralizing the anticoagulant effects of heparin on a milligram for milligram basis.

Adverse effects other than bleeding are rarely encountered with the use of heparin. Administration of large doses for periods of 6 months have been reported to cause osteoporosis in humans. The nurse should exercise caution when administering heparin subcutaneously to prevent superficial bleeding and hepatoma formation. Other nursing implications are summarized at the end of this chapter.

Coumarin Derivatives

In 1941, a coumarin compound was found to be responsible for a hemorrhagic disorder in cattle after their ingestion of improperly cured sweet clover. This compound, *bishydroxycoumarin*, and chemically related agents have subsequently been employed as clinically useful anticoagulants. The properties of the coumarin derivatives and heparin are quite dissimilar and are compared in Table 31-2.

Actions While heparin exerts its maximal anticoagulant effects within minutes after its administration, the coumarin derivatives require 1 or more days to manifest their peak therapeutic effects (Table 31-3). The coumarins *prolong prothrombin time* by inhibiting the synthesis of prothrombin and factors VII, IX, and X by the liver. The synthesis of these compounds requires

Table 31-2   Comparison of Heparin and Coumarin-Indandione Anticoagulants

Characteristics	Heparin	Coumarins-Indandiones
Anticoagulant activity	In vivo, in vitro.	In vivo.
Mechanisms of anticoagulant action	Antithromboplastin. Antithrombin. Decrease platelet aggregation.	Inhibition of formation of prothrombin and factors VII, IX, X.
Route of administration	Parenteral.	All oral. Sodium warfarin: oral and parenteral.
Peak effects	Immediate.	12–18 h
Duration of action	3-4 h	1–14 days
Laboratory tests to control dose	Lee-White clotting time.	Prothrombin time.
Treatment of overdose	Protamine.	Vitamin K. Fresh whole blood.
Therapeutic use	Immediate anticoagulation.	Long-term anticoagulation.
Cost daily treatment	High.	Low.

Table 31-3 Comparative Properties of Coumarin and Indandione Derivatives

Generic name	Selected trade names	Onset of action	Peak effects	Duration of action	Daily oral doses (mg)		
					Day 1	Day 2	Maintenance
Coumarin Derivatives							
Dicumarol (Bishydroxycoumarin)		24–48 h	3–5 days	4–14 days	200–400	100–200	25–150
Warfarin sodium[a]	Coumadin Sodium Panwarfin	2–12 h	1.5–3 days	4–5 days	25–50	10–15	2.5–10
Warfarin potassium	Athrombin-K	2–12	1–1.5 days	4–5 days	25–50	10–15	2.5–10
Phenprocoumon	Liquamar	24–36 h	2–3 days	7–14 days	18–30	10	0.75–6
Indandione Derivatives							
Phenindione	Hedulin	2–8 h	1.5–3 days	4–5 days	300	200	100
Anisindione	Miradone	2–8 h	1–2 days	1–3 days	300	200	25–250

[a]Can be administered orally or by intramuscular or intravenous injection.

vitamin K, and it is generally believed that the coumarin derivatives act by blocking the utilization of vitamin K in the formation of these blood clotting factors by the liver. Conversely, vitamin K antagonizes the anticoagulant effects of the coumarins and is used as an antidote for the treatment of overdosage by these drugs.

Administration and therapeutic uses

The coumarin derivatives are well absorbed after oral administration and, therefore, are usually administered orally. Sodium warfarin is the only member of this class that can be given by injection. The primary differences among the coumarin drugs are their time courses of actions (Table 31-3). To hasten the onset of anticoagulation, a higher loading dose is administered for the first 48 hours, followed by smaller maintenance doses.

These drugs are clinically employed for the prevention and treatment of venous thrombosis and pulmonary embolism, the treatment of atrial fibrillation with embolization, and as an adjunct in the treatment of coronary occlusion.

Considerable variation is observed among patients in their response to the coumarins, and it is necessary to determine an optimal dose for each patient. Dosage is generally adjusted to prolong the *one-stage prothrombin time test* from 12 seconds to 20 to 25 seconds. Prolongation of prothrombin times greater than these markedly increase the risk of internal hemorrhaging.

Toxicity

Overdosage of the coumarins results in marked *hypoprothrominemia*, which can cause the death of the patient as the result of massive bleeding. To preclude this possibility, the nurse should carefully monitor laboratory reports of prothrombin times. Nurses should regularly check patients for signs of hemorrhaging, including bleeding from the gums and nose, petechiae, and the presence of blood in the urine and stools.

Treatment of overdosage may be counteracted by *fresh whole-blood transfusions*, which provide deficient coagulation factors dependent on vitamin K. Intravenous administration of *phytonadione* (vitamin K_1; Mephyton) is a highly effective antidote of coumarin-induced hypoprothrombinemia and is capable of returning prothrombin times to safe levels within 6 hours. Vitamin K is ineffective in reversing the anticoagulant effects of heparin.

Precautions and drug interactions

Coumarin derivatives are contraindicated in patients with bleeding disorders, blood dyscrasias, ulcerative lesions of the gastrointestinal tract, severe liver disease, and recent operations on the brain or spinal cord. Other nursing implications are summarized at the end of this chapter.

Drug interactions involving the coumarin oral anticoagulants are potentially life threatening and have been well documented in the clinical literature (Table 31-4). Interactions involving these drugs result primarily from alterations in their rates of metabolism and their displacements from plasma protein binding sites.

Alterations in metabolism Coumarin anticoagulants are metabolized and inactivated by microsomal enzymes located in the liver. *Enzyme inducers*, drugs capable of enhancing the activity of these microsomal enzymes, can profoundly alter the magnitude of the normal anticoagulant effects.

Barbiturates, in particular *phenobarbital*, are among the most potent enzyme inducers in common therapeutic use. Three potential therapeutic problems can result from the interaction of phenobarbital with a coumarin derivative such as warfarin.

Table 31-4   Potential Drug Interactions Involving Oral Anticoagulants

Mechanism underlying interaction	Interacting drug/class	Potential consequences
Inhibition of coumarin absorption	Cholestyramine (Questran)	Binds to coumarins, decreased intestinal absorption, decreased plasma levels, increased prothrombin times.
Enzyme induction	Barbiturates Carbamazepine (Tegretol) Cimetidine (Tagamet) Ethchlorvynol (Placidyl) Glutethimide (Doriden) Griseofulvin (Fulvicin, Grifulvin, Grisactin) Phenytoin (Dilantin) Rifampin (Rifadin, Rimactane)	Stimulated metabolism of coumarins, decreased plasma levels.
Mechanisms not established	Adrenocorticosteroids Oral contraceptives.	Reduced anticoagulant response.
Displacement of plasma-protein binding	Antidiabetic agents tolbutamide (Orinase) Chloral hydrate (Noctec) Diazoxide (Hyperstat I.V.) Ethacrynic acid (Edecrin) Mefenamic acid (Ponstel) Phenytoin (Dilantin) Phenylbutazone (Butazolidin) Oxyphenbutazone (Tandearil)	Displacement of coumarins from albumin binding sites, increased free coumarin plasma levels, increased risk of bleeding.
Enzyme inhibition	Allopurinol (Zyloprim) Chloromycetin (Chloramphenicol) Disulfiram (Antabuse)	Inhibition of coumarin metabolism by liver, increased plasma levels, decreased prothrombin times, increased risk of bleeding.
Inhibition of vitamin K synthesis or absorption	Chloramphenicol (Chloromycetin) Cholestyramine (Questran)	Reduction in synthesis of blood clotting factors, increased risk of bleeding.
Inhibition of synthesis or increased breakdown of clotting factors	Anabolic steroids Clofibrate (Atromid-S) Dextrothyroxin (Choloxin) Salicylates (aspirin) Quinidine Thyroid hormones	Decreased levels of endogenous clotting factors, increased risk of bleeding.
Ulcerogenic agents	Indomethacin (Indocin) Phenylbutazone (Butazolidin) Salicylates (aspirin)	Increased risk of gastrointestinal bleeding.
Mechanisms not established	Ethanol Glucagon Antithyroid agents propylthiouracil	Increased sensitivity to anticoagulant effects of coumarins.
Potentiation of antidiabetic agents	Tolbutamide (Orinase) Chlorpropamide (Diabinese)	Coumarins appear to inhibit metabolism of these antidiabetic agents, increasing their abilities to reduce blood sugar levels.

If the administration of both drugs is initiated at the same time, phenobarbital will enhance the rate of warfarin metabolism and inactivation, thus reducing the anticoagulant effects normally produced by that dose of warfarin. This problem can be readily overcome by increasing the dose of warfarin. A second problem may be observed in the patient receiving maintenance doses of warfarin who is subsequently given phenobarbital. Within 2 to 5 days after the initiation of the barbiturate, as a consequence of enzyme induction the effective plasma levels of warfarin will be reduced, prothrombin times will be shortened, and the risk of clot formation will be increased. The last problem, which may result in severe hemorrhaging, may occur when a chronically administered barbiturate is discontinued and the maintenance dose of warfarin not reduced. The enzyme-inducing effects of phenobarbital dissipate within 2 to 3 weeks after the last dose. In the absence of its inductive effects, plasma levels of warfarin increase, thereby increasing the hypoprothrombinemic effect and enhancing the risk of bleeding. This last situation is most commonly observed in the patient who has received a barbiturate for sedation during a period of hospitalization. Upon discharge from the hospital, the barbiturate is discontinued without a reduction in the dose of warfarin. To preclude the occurrence of these three problems, nonbarbiturate sedative-hypnotics might be preferred, such as diazepam (Valium) or flurazepam (Dalmane). Table 32-4 lists other enzyme inducers.

Plasma-protein binding displacement Oral anticoagulants are highly bound to the plasma-protein albumin. Warfarin is plasma-protein bound to the extent of 97 percent, with only 3 percent unbound and available to prevent coagulation. Drugs such as phenyl-butazone (Butazolidin) possess greater affinity for albumin binding sites than warfarin and displaces warfarin when the two drugs are administered concurrently. If phenylbutazone were to displace only 3 percent of the bound warfarin, the plasma levels of free warfarin would double, potentially resulting in fatal bleeding.

The oral anticoagulants are potentially dangerous drugs. The nurse should very carefully monitor the patient's drug records prior to the initiation of anticoagulant drug administration to prevent adverse drug interactions. Similarly, caution must be exercised before the addition or deletion of medications to patients receiving maintenance doses of anticoagulants. The nurse should advise ambulatory patients to consult with their physicians or pharmacists prior to taking any new drugs. Table 31-4 summarizes potential interactions involving anticoagulants.

Indandione Derivatives

The indandione derivatives (Table 31-3, page 262) have pharmacological properties similar to those of the coumarins (Table 31-2, page 261). In addition to the potential danger of bleeding caused by overdosage of these drugs, hypersensitivity reactions including blood disorders (agranulocytosis) and liver and kidney damage have been reported. Many clinicians believe that this class of oral anticoagulants should be reserved for patients who cannot tolerate the coumarin derivatives.

FIBRINOLYTIC (THROMBOLYTIC) AGENTS

Whereas the anticoagulants prevent clot formation, *fibrinolytic agents* are employed to *hasten* the dissolution of blood clots, thus reopening blood vessels after their occlusion to prevent tissue necrosis from occurring.

Fibrinolysin (Thrombolysin), administered by intravenous drip, is recommended for the treatment of phlebothrombosis, thrombophlebitis, pulmonary embolism, and thrombosis of arteries. Repeated administration of this drug may result in severe allergic reactions. Streptokinase (Streptase) and urokinase (Abbokinase) are also used to promote dissolution of clots in deep veins of patients with acute thrombophlebitis. The potential clinical benefits of these drugs must be carefully weighed against the risk of inducing spontaneous bleeding.

Inhibitors of thrombus formation

Excessive aggregation of blood platelets, with subsequent thrombus formation (a clot in a blood vessel), may be of great significance in the etiology of cerebrovascular accidents (stroke), myocardial infarction (heart attack), and postoperative complications after cardiovascular surgery. The controversial results of early clinical trials suggest that aspirin and sulfinpyrazone, when taken on a daily, long-term basis, may inhibit thrombus formation. Low doses of aspirin have been shown to reduce the incidence of thrombosis postoperatively and decrease the death rate in patients susceptible to or who have previously experienced strokes and heart attacks. The antigout drug sulfinpyrazone (Anturane) has been suggested to possibly reduce the incidence of heart attacks in patients who had previously experienced one such episode. The future role of aspirin and other inhibitors of thrombosis in the management of cardiovascular disorders remains to be determined.

COAGULANTS (HEMOSTATICS)

It is often necessary to hasten coagulation to limit blood loss during operations or from wounds. Hemorrhage may be controlled at the site of bleeding by such physical measures as the application of pressure or cold. Placing a large surface area of gauze or cotton at the bleeding site stimulates clot formation and solidifies the clot. Removal of these materials, however, may result in new tissue damage and renewed bleeding.

Gelatin sponge (Gelfoam) or oxidized cellulose (Oxycel, Surgicel) can be employed as dressings and are absorbed from their site of administration within several days. Fibrin foam is used as a mechanical barrier to facilitate the clotting process.

Aminocaproic acid (Amicar), administered orally or by slow intravenous drip, is used to control serious bleeding associated with certain surgical procedures. This drug inhibits activation of plasminogen and blocks the action of plasmin (Figure 31-1). Rapid intravenous injection may cause hypotension, bradycardia, and cardioarrhythmias.

Localized oozing of blood from capillaries can often be arrested by the local application of *vasoconstrictors* (epinephrine, norepinephrine) or *astringent agents* that precipitate blood proteins. The latter drugs, including ferric chloride, alum, and tannic acid, are less effective than the vasoconstrictor drugs.

Anticoagulants:
nursing implications

Heparin

1. Anticipate that each dose of heparin will be ordered individually after the prothrombin time has been evaluated by the physician.

2. Observe the patient for signs of bruising or bleeding in urine, stools, and gums. Instruct patient to report active bleeding or prolonged menstrual periods in females.

3. Heparin may have a diuretic effect beginning 36–48 h after initial dose. Encourage the patient to eat potassium-rich foods.

4. Administration of oral anticoagulant usually overlaps heparin for 3–5 days while heparin dosage is being reduced.

5. Reassure patients with alopecia that it is only temporary and reversible.

Coumarin-type

1. Prior to initiating therapy, reliability of the patient should be established. Periodic blood tests and strict adherence to the treatment schedule is essential.

2. Vitamin K should be available to reverse excess bleeding. Patient may be advised to carry vitamin K at all times to be used for treatment of spontaneous hemorrhage. Parenteral vitamin K and whole blood transfusion may be necessary for severe bleeding.

3. Instruct the patient and a responsible family member to discontinue the drug and report the following symptoms of agranulocytosis: fatigue, sore throat, and fever; of hepatitis: dark urine, jaundice, and pruritis.

4. Warn the patient to avoid use of prescription or nonprescription drugs without consulting the physician.

SUPPLEMENTARY READINGS

Biggs, R., ed., *Human Blood Coagulation, Haemostatis, and Thrombosis*. Oxford: Blackwell Scientific Publications, 1972.

Ehrlich, J., and S. S. Stivala, "Chemistry and Pharmacology of Heparin," *Journal of Pharmaceutical Sciences* 62: 517–44 (1973).

Genton, E., M. Gent, J. Hirsh, and L. A. Harker, "Platelet-Inhibiting Drugs in the Prevention of Clinical Thrombotic Disease," *New England Journal of Medicine* 294: 1174–78, 1236–40, 1296–300 (1975).

Jaques, L. B., *Anticoagulant Therapy: Pharmacological Principles*. Springfield, Illinois: Charles C Thomas, Publisher, 1965.

Koch-Weser, J., and E. M. Sellers, "Drug Interactions With Coumarin Anticoagulants," *New England Journal of Medicine* 285: 487–98, 547–58 (1971).

Lowe, G. D. O., and D. H. Lawson, "Clinical Use of Hemostatic Agents," *American Journal of Hospital Pharmacy* 35: 414–22 (1978).

Moore, K., "How Patient Education Can Reduce the Risk of Anticoagulation," *Nursing '77* 7(9): 24–29 (1977).

O'Reilly, R. A., and P. M. Aggeler, "Determinants of the Response to Oral Anticoagulant Drugs in Man," *Pharmacological Reviews* 22: 35–96 (1970).

Sherry, S., and A. Scriabine, ed., *Platelets and Thrombosis*. Baltimore: University Park Press, 1974.

Weiss, H. J., "Platelet Physiology and Abnormalities of Platelet Function," *New England Journal of Medicine* 293: 531–41, 580–88 (1975).

Zbinden, G., "Evaluation of the Thrombogenic Effects of Drugs," *Annual Review of Pharmacology and Toxicology* 16: 177–88 (1976).

DIURETICS AND SALURETICS

Saluretics are drugs that enhance urine output by increasing the loss of sodium, chloride, and water from the body. Such drugs have widespread clinical applications for the management of edema associated with premenstrual tension, congestive heart failure, nephrosis and other kidney diseases, cirrhosis of the liver, and as a valuable adjunct in the treatment of hypertension. *Diuretics*, on the other hand, are drugs that predominantly promote the loss of water from the body. Drugs in this class (diuretics and saluretics) augment diuresis by different mechanisms. Prior to considering the pharmacology of these drugs, we shall first examine the basic elements of renal physiology.

RENAL PHYSIOLOGY

The kidneys serve two major physiological functions. They are primarily responsible for the elimination of most of the end products of bodily metabolism and they control the volume and composition of the body fluids. Each kidney contains over one million *nephrons*, each of which is capable of forming urine. The nephron (Figure 32-1) consists basically of a *glomerulus*, from which fluid is filtered, and a long *tubule*, in which the filtered fluid is converted to urine and eventually eliminated from the body. Let us now consider the component parts and function of the nephron in somewhat greater detail.

The Nephron

Blood enters the glomerulus through the afferent arteriole and exits via the efferent arteriole. The glomerulus consists of a network of capillaries. Pressure of the blood in the glomerulus results in the *filtration* of water, most of the essential constitutents of the extracellular fluid, and waste products. Proteins, protein-bound drugs, and other substances are not filtered. The filtrate flows first into the *proximal* tubule, located in the cortex of the kidney, and then into the *loop of Henle*, which extends into the kidney medulla. Ascending from the loop of Henle, the fluid passes into the *distal tubule*, which is in the kidney cortex, to the *collecting duct* and then empties into the *renal pelvis* for ultimate removal from the body (Fig. 32-1). The nephron normally reabsorbs, and thus returns to the blood, 99 percent of the glomerular filtrate, with only 1 percent excreted as urine.

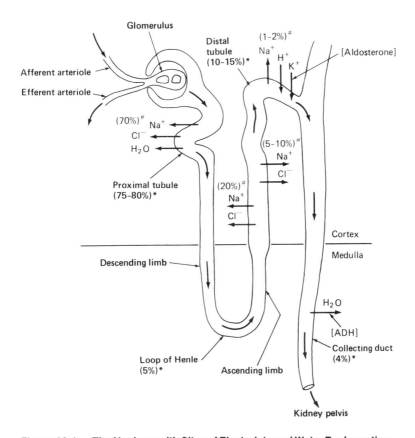

Figure 32-1   The Nephron with Sites of Electrolyte and Water Reabsorption.

Water and Electrolyte Reabsorption

Approximately 75 to 80 percent of the electrolytes and water filtered by the glomerulus are reabsorbed in the *proximal tubule* and returned to the blood stream. Sodium is actively transported across the walls of the proximal tubules, with chloride and water following by a passive process. While it would appear that inhibition of salt and water reabsorption in the proximal tubules should represent a major site of action of diuretic and saluretic drugs, this is not the case; inhibition of distal tubular transport mechanisms results in a far greater urine output.

As the filtrate enters the *descending limb of the loop of Henle*, water is reabsorbed and the remaining fluid becomes more concentrated (hypertonic). Sodium and chloride are reabsorbed to the extent of 20 to 30 percent as the fluid passes up the *ascending limb of the loop of Henle*. Since this segment of the tubule does not permit the reabsorption of water, the fluid becomes more dilute (hypotonic).

In the *distal tubule*, and under the influence of the mineralocorticoid hormone *aldosterone*, sodium and chloride are reabsorbed and potassium or hydrogen ions added to the fluid. The exchange of sodium and hydrogen ions represents an important mechanism by which the kidneys help maintain the acid-base balance of the body. Water reabsorption occurs primarily in the *collecting duct*, a transport process mediated by the *antidiuretic hormone* (ADH), a hormone released from the posterior pituitary gland (neurohypophysis).

DIURETICS AND SALURETICS

Diuretic and saluretic drugs may act by one or more of the following mechanisms: (1) increase the rate of glomerular filtration (xanthines); (2) inhibit the reabsorption of sodium by a direct action on the kidney tubules (mercurials, thiazides, furosemide, ethacrynic acid); (3) inhibit sodium reabsorption by an osmotic action (mannitol); (4) inhibit the exchange of sodium ions for hydrogen ions (carbonic anhydrase inhibitors); (5) inhibit the action of aldosterone (spironolactone); and (6) inhibit the release of antidiuretic hormone (ethyl alcohol). For the purpose of the ensuing discussion, the term *diuretic* will be used to include the saluretics. Nursing implications associated with the administration of diuretics are summarized at the end of this chapter.

Organomercurial Diuretics

With the introduction of orally active, highly potent, and less toxic drugs, the once popular organomercurial diuretics find limited clinical applications in modern therapeutics.

Effects and therapeutic uses Organomercurials act by inhibiting the reabsorption of sodium, chloride, and water in the ascending limb of the loop of Henle and in the proximal tubule. The loss of potassium is less than that observed with other classes of diuretics. These drugs cause far greater diuresis when the pH of the urine is acidic. The acid-forming salt *ammonium chloride*, a compound itself possessing modest diuretic properties, is often employed with the organomercurials, potentiating their diuretics effectiveness by virtue of its ability to acidify the urine.

The organomercurials are employed for the treatment of edema associated with the nephrotic syndrome, cirrhosis of the liver, and portal obstruction. They are less effective than ethacrynic acid or furosemide (see page 274) in relieving edema secondary to congestive heart failure.

Administration Organomercurials (Table 32-1) must be parenterally administered, usually by the intramuscular route. The intravenous route should be avoided because of the potential danger of cardiac toxicity.

Within 1 to 2 hours after an intramuscular injection of an organomercurial agent, an increase in urine flow becomes evident, an effect that may persist for 12 to 24 hours. Fluid losses equivalent to 2.5 percent of the total body weight are average responses.

Table 32-1   Organomercurial Diuretics

Generic name	Trade name	Usual dose	Remarks
Mercaptomerin sodium	Thiomerin	IM or SC: 125 mg daily	Solutions, once prepared, are unstable and must be refrigerated.
Mersalyl with theophylline	Salyrgan-Theophylline	IM: 1 ml once or twice weekly	Solution contains theophylline to enhance absorption.
Merethoxylline procaine	Dicurin	IM or SC: 0.5-2 ml daily	Procaine added to reduce discomfort when mercurial is injected into tissues; also contains theophylline.

Toxicity and precautions   The incidence of adverse side effects associated with the organomercurials is relatively low. Cardiac toxicity is only observed after intravenous injection. Manifestations of allergic reactions to this drug class include flushing of the face, gastrointestinal disorders, itching, urticaria, fever, and chills. Organomercurials are contraindicated in patients with renal insufficiency, acute nephritis, or a history of hypersensitivity to the mercurial ion.

Carbonic Anhydrase Inhibitors

Inhibition of the enzyme carbonic anhydrase in the renal tubule decreases the amount of hydrogen ions available for exchange with sodium. These excess sodium ions, as well as potassium, bicarbonate, and water, are consequently retained in the tubule and excreted in an alkaline urine.

Acetazolamide (Diamox), the most commonly used carbonic anhydrase inhibitor, is a relatively nontoxic drug. The therapeutic utility of this and related drugs is limited by low potency and the rapid development of tolerance to their diuretic effects within 48 hours after initiation of therapy. The usual oral dose of acetazolamide is 250 to 375 mg administered once daily.

In addition to acetazolamide, other members of this class include dichlorphenamide (Daranide, Oratrol), ethoxzolamide (Cardrase, Ethamide), and methazolamide (Neptazane). These drugs are primarily employed for the treatment of *glaucoma* (Chapter 7); they decrease intraocular pressure by reducing the rate of production of aqueous humor.

Thiazide Diuretics

The *thiazide* or *benzothiadiazide diuretics*, discovered two decades ago in search of more potent carbonic anhydrase inhibitors, are the most widely used class of diuretic agents. These drugs are employed for the treatment of a wide variety of edematous conditions, as well as for the management of hypertension. While differences exist among the thiazides with respect to their time courses of action and potencies (Table 32-2), none of these drugs is safer nor produces significantly greater diuresis at equivalent therapeutic doses than chlorothiazide (Diuril), the first drug developed in this class.

Effects   The thiazides enhance the elimination of sodium, chloride, potassium, and water by inhibiting the active reabsorption of sodium and chloride ions at the distal tubule. Their abilities to inhibit carbonic anhydrase appear to be of limited therapeutic significance. Thiazides do not alter the acid-base balance and, unlike the organomercurials and carbonic anhydrase inhibitors, their diuretic effectiveness is not modified by changes in the pH of the urine. While the mechanism underlying their antihypertensive effects is not well understood, it may involve alterations in the ionic balance in the smooth muscle walls of the arterioles.

Therapeutic uses   The clinical popularity of the thiazides may be attributed to their high degree of diuretic effectiveness after oral administration, their relatively short onset of action (2 hours), their continued diuretic effectiveness even after extended periods of drug administration, and a relatively low order of toxicity. Although the thiazides are capable of producing electrolyte imbalances, the detrimental consequences of such imbalances can be minimized if the nurse judiciously maintains proper precautions.

The thiazides are most often the first class of drugs employed in the management of *hypertension*, used either alone or in combination with other antihypertensive medications (Chapter 28).

They are generally highly effective drugs for the treatment of edema associated

Table 32-2 Comparative Properties of the Thiazide Diuretics

Generic name	Selected trade names	Peak effect (h)	Duration of action (h)	Usual daily oral dose (mg)
Chlorothiazide	Diuril	4	6-12	500-1,000
Hydrochlorothiazide	Esidrix HydroDiuril Oretic	4	6-12	50-100
Bendroflumethiazide	Naturetin	6-12	18-24	2.5-5
Benzthiazide	Aquatag Exna	4-6	12-18	50-100
Cyclothiazide	Anhydron	7-12	18-24	1-2 (every other day)
Hydroflumethiazide	Diucardin Saluron	3-4	24	50-100
Methyclothiazide	Enduron Aquatensen	6	24	2.5-10
Polythiazide	Renese	6	36	1-4
Trichlormethiazide	Metahydrin Naqua	6	24	2-4
Metolazone[a]	Zaroxolyn	2	12-24	5-10
Quinethazone[a]	Hydromox	6	18-24	50-100
Chlorthalidone[a]	Hygroton	2	48-72	100 (daily or every other day)

[a] These drugs are chemically not thiazides, but they have diuretic properties resembling thiazides.

with congestive heart failure, cirrhosis of the liver, premenstrual tension, pregnancy, various types of renal abnormalities (nephrotic syndrome, glomerulonephritis, and chronic kidney failure), and drug-induced edema (estrogens, glucocorticoids, and antihypertensive agents).

Chlorothiazide and related drugs produce a paradoxical *reduction* in urinary output (by as much as 50 percent) in patients with *diabetes insipidus*; this hormonal disease, resulting from a deficiency of ADH, is characterized by extreme diuresis. It has been suggested that these drugs act by decreasing the glomerular filtration rate and causing the increased reabsorption of the filtrate by the proximal tubules; less filtrate is available for reabsorption at distal reabsorption sites and, therefore, less water is available for excretion.

Adverse effects and precautions

Many of the adverse effects associated with thiazide administration result from electro-lyte imbalances (hypokalemia and hyponatremia) or a fall in blood pressure. Early signs of electrolyte abnormalities include dryness of the mouth; thirst; weakness; lethargy; muscle cramps, pains, or fatigue of muscles; and oliguria and gastrointestinal disturbances. The nurse should know and watch for these signs of electrolyte imbalance.

Plasma potassium levels should be regularly monitored in patients receiving thiazides for prolonged periods of time. Reduction in plasma potassium markedly increases the susceptibility of patients to digitalis toxicity (Chapter 26). To compensate for excessive diuretic-induced loss of potassium, potassium chloride is often co-administered with these drugs. Enteric-coated tablets of this salt should be avoided because of the danger of gastrointestinal ulceration; solutions of potassium chloride (Kaochlor, Kay Ciel) are preferred when replacement is required. Potassium-rich foods are listed in the last section of this chapter.

Uric acid levels in the plasma are

Table 32-3 Potential Drug Interactions Involving Diuretics

Diuretic	Interacting drug/class	Potential consequences
Thiazides Chlorthalidone Ethacrynic acid Furosemide	Digitalis glycosides	Diuretic-induced reductions in plasma potassium increase the risk of digitalis toxicity.
Thiazides Ethacrynic acid Furosemide	Corticosteroids	Corticosteroids cause loss of plasma potassium, an effect that may be enhanced when these drugs are coadministered with diuretics.
Thiazides Ethacrynic acid Furosemide	Lithium carbonate (Eskalith, Lithane, Lithonate)	These diuretics increase lithium reabsorption by kidney tubules, increasing plasma levels, which may increase risk of lithium toxicity.
Thiazides	Uricosurics Probenecid (Benemid) Sulfinpyrazone (Anturane)	These diuretics increase plasma levels of uric acid, which may precipitate acute attacks of gout in susceptible patients, thus potentially reducing effects of uricosurics.
Thiazides Ethacrynic acid Furosemide	Sulfonylurea oral antidiabetic drugs Insulin	Thiazides, and to a lesser extent ethacrynic acid and furosemide, increase blood glucose levels in diabetics, thereby antagonizing the hypoglycemic effects of these drugs with potential loss of diabetic control.
Thiazides Furosemide	Muscle relaxants, surgical	Potentiated neuromuscular blockade.
Thiazides	Chlorpropamide (Diabinese)	Chlorpropamide may potentiate the ability of the thiazides to reduce plasma sodium levels.
Ethacrynic acid Furosemide	Aminoglycoside antibiotics Neomycin Streptomycin Gentamicin (Garamycin) Kanamycin (Kantrex)	These diuretics and the aminoglycoside antibiotics, when administered individually, are potentially ototoxic. Since this risk may be increased when these drugs are used in combination, alternative diuretics (thiazides) should probably be employed.
Furosemide	Cephalosporin antibiotics Cephaloridine (Loridine) Cephalothin (Keflin)	Furosemide, and perhaps ethacrynic acid, may increase the potential for cephalosporin-induced kidney toxicity.
Ethacrynic acid	Warfarin	Ethacrynic acid can potentially displace warfarin from plasma protein binding sites, increasing the risk of bleeding.
Spironolactone Triamterene	Potassium chloride Ammonium chloride	These diuretics cause potassium retention; hyperkalemia may result if potassium supplements are administered.

frequently increased, and, in susceptible individuals, acute attacks of gout may be precipitated. Uricosuric drugs (Chapter 21) counteract this thiazide-induced effect without reducing their diuretic effectiveness.

These diuretics may increase blood glucose levels in prediabetics and worsen preexisting *diabetes mellitus*. This may necessitate an increase in the dose of insulin or other antidiabetic agent to maintain optimal control of blood sugar levels.

Thiazides should be employed with great caution in patients with severe liver or renal dysfunction, as these drugs may cause an unpredictable worsening of such disorders. Potential adverse drug interactions involving the thiazides are summarized in Table 32-3.

Ethacrynic Acid and Furosemide

Ethacrynic acid (Edecrin) and furosemide (Lasix), the most powerful diuretics in common therapeutic use, have a common spectrum of pharmacological effects. Both drugs have a rapid onset of diuretic action after oral administration and both inhibit sodium and chloride reabsorption in the ascending loop of Henle ("loop diuretics"). Their effects are independent of changes in the acid-base balance of the urine.

Therapeutic uses These drugs cause marked diuresis even in patients who have responded maximally to other diuretics including the thiazides. They are useful for the treatment of edema of cardiac, liver, or renal origin. Therapeutic indications include edema associated with congestive heart failure, cirrhosis of the liver, and nephrotic syndrome. Their use should generally be reserved for patients who fail to respond to thiazides. In addition, these drugs are useful as adjuncts for the management of hypertensive crises, particularly when acute pulmonary edema or renal failure is present, and a rapid and massive reduction in extracellular fluid volume is deemed essential.

Both drugs may be administered orally or intravenously. After oral administration, diuresis begins within one hour, reaching peak effects within 2 hours; ethacrynic acid has a longer duration of action (6 to 8 hours) than furosemide (4 to 6 hours). Diuresis occurs within minutes after intravenous administration and exhibits peak effects within 30 minutes. Usual daily doses of these drugs is from 40 to 50 up to 200 mg.

Adverse effects and precautions The primary adverse effects associated with the administration of ethacrynic acid and furosemide arise from the excessive and rapid loss of fluid and electrolytes, potassium in particular. Symptoms associated with such losses include weakness, dizziness, hypotension, and circulatory collapse. These drugs are highly potent diuretics and should only be employed under close supervision. These drugs are capable of increasing urate and glucose levels in susceptible patients.

Ototoxicity, resulting in temporary hearing losses, has been reported after the use of ethacrynic acid and, to a lesser degree, with furosemide. This relatively rare adverse effect appears to be associated with only these two diuretics. Other side effects include gastrointestinal disturbances, blood disorders, and skin rashes. Potential adverse drug interactions associated with these diuretics appear in Table 32-3.

Spironolactone and Triamterene

Spironolactone (Aldactone) and triamterene (Dyrenium) are often called *potassium-sparing diuretics*. Rarely employed alone, these compounds are most frequently used with other diuretics to prevent excessive potassium depletion.

Effects Spironolactone is an *aldosterone antagonist* at the distal tubule; it antagonizes the aldosterone-mediated sodium-potassium exchange, resulting in a reduction in sodium reabsorption and retention of potassium. Triamterene is not a true aldosterone antagonist, but promotes sodium loss while conserving potassium.

Therapeutic uses and adverse effects When employed alone, spironolactone and triamterene are relatively weak oral diuretic agents. They are employed with other diuretics to enhance sodium loss while preventing excessive plasma potassium depletion. These drugs should not be employed in patients with hyperkalemia.

Adverse effects associated with spironolactone administration include lethargy, drowsiness, headache, mental confusion, gastrointestinal disturbances, and skin rashes. Similar effects are observed with triamterene but are generally less severe. High doses of spironolactone have been shown to cause benign tumors in rats; it is not clear what relationship these findings have to humans.

Osmotic Diuretics

Osmotic diuretics are drugs that are readily filtered by the glomerulus but are reabsorbed by the kidney tubules to only a very limited extent. When administered in large doses, these drugs are retained in the tubules, promoting excretion of water.

Mannitol, a sugar alcohol, is the most widely used osmotic diuretic. Intravenous administration of hypertonic solutions (5 to 20 percent) of mannitol (Osmitrol) is used to promote diuresis in acute renal failure before irreversible renal failure has been established. It is also employed to reduce intraocular pressure and cerebrospinal fluid pressure before, during, and after surgery. This drug should not be administered to patients with advanced renal failure or congestive heart disease.

Urea may be administered intravenously to reduce elevated intracranial pressure resulting from brain tumors or head injuries.

Xanthine Diuretics

The naturally occurring xanthines, namely caffeine, theobromine, and theophylline, all possess modest diuretic activity, with theophylline the most potent member of this class.

Theophylline and *aminophylline* (theophylline ethylenediamine) increase cardiac output and renal plasma flow, enhancing the rate of glomerular filtration. In addition, these drugs may also have a direct effect on the kidney tubules that results in a reduction in the reabsorption of sodium and chloride.

Intravenous administration of aminophylline enhances the diuretic effect of the organomercurials. The xanthines are not very effective diuretics and have limited clinical applications in modern therapeutics.

NURSING PRECAUTIONS ASSOCIATED WITH DIURETIC ADMINISTRATION

With the clinical availability of new and highly potent diuretic agents, the nurse must exercise great care to avoid complications arising from drug-induced extreme losses in fluids and electrolyte imbalances. Electrolyte disturbances may readily occur when fluid losses are excessive or occur too rapidly, or when the diuretic promotes excessive excretion of essential electrolytes, such as potassium and sodium.

To prevent these potential dangers, the nurse should maintain records of fluid intake and urine output in hospitalized patients. The nurse should instruct ambulatory patients to maintain weight records determined at a fixed time during the day (for example, prior to breakfast). Increased body weight or leg pitting upon the application of pressure potentially suggest the development of tolerance to the diuretic medication.

With the exception of spironolactone and triamterene, all other commonly employed diuretics cause potassium loss. To counteract potential depletion of this essential electrolyte, patients should be advised to increase their intake of such potassium-rich products as oranges, bananas, apricots, dates, and grapefruit juice.

Nurses should recommend that ambulatory patients take diuretics in the morning rather than the evening, thus precluding the possibility of nighttime diuresis and inter-ference with sleep. Other nursing implications are summarized below.

Diuretics:
nursing implications

1. Administer drug early in the day to avoid sleep disturbance due to nighttime diuresis.
2. Monitor fluid balance: weigh the patient daily under standard conditions; measure abdominal girth in patients with ascites.
3. Assess the patient for fluid retention: check for dependent edema; auscultate lungs for rales.
4. Monitor serum electrolytes, urine, and blood urea nitrogen (BUN) in patients receiving large doses or therapy over long periods of time.
5. Observe the patient for signs of electrolyte imbalance: anorexia, nausea, vomiting, thirst, dizziness, headache, paresthesia, drowsiness, and mental confusion.
6. Observe the patient for signs of hypersensitivity reaction: sore throat, rash, and jaundice.
7. Instruct the patient how to minimize postural hypotension: move slowly from lying to sitting position; sit down or lie down if feeling weak.
8. Observe the patient for diuretic-induced potentiation of other drugs: antihypertensives may excessively reduce blood pressure (B.P.); electrolyte loss may enhance risk of digitalis cardiotoxicity.
9. Monitor B.P. and pulse in patients with impaired cardiac function. Cardiac output may be reduced from diuretic-induced hypovolemia. Changes in serum potassium may potentiate digitalis toxicity and precipitate cardiac arrhythmias.
10. Monitor diabetics for hyperglycemia. Diuretics may precipitate symptoms in mild or latent diabetics.
11. Instruct the patient to report joint pain. Diuretics may precipitate acute gouty attacks in susceptible patients.
12. Teach the patient or a responsible family member the purpose of the drug and how to monitor drug effects including the amount of fluid loss and weight loss anticipated; diet, with specific information on amount of sodium and potassium to be included; specific directions for use of potassium supplement, if ordered; and signs and symptoms to be reported to the physician.

Thiazides

1. Observe the patient for signs and symptoms of hypokalemia: anorexia, nausea, vomiting, paresthesia, mental confusion, muscle weakness, paralytic ileus, hypoactive reflexes, and cardiac arrhythmias.

2. Caution patient against alcohol ingestion because of risk of severe hypotension when taken with thiazides.

3. Caution patients not to eat licorice, because it can cause severe hypokalemia.

Ethacrynic Acid (Edecrin) *and Furosemide* (Lasix)

1. These drugs cause rapid diuresis, which may result in electrolyte imbalance. Excessive diuresis, loss of more than 2 lb (1 Kg) daily, hematuria, oliguria, or sudden diarrhea are indications for drug discontinuation.

2. Observe the patient closely during IV administration. Excessive diuresis can produce dehydration, hypotension, peripheral vascular collapse, and thromboembolic complications due to hemoconcentration.

3. Instruct the patient to report early signs of ototoxicity: vertigo, tinnitus, or fullness in the ears. Hearing loss may be temporary or permanent. Hearing impairment is usually associated with renal insufficiency, uremia, rapid IV injection of high doses, or concurrent administration of other ototoxic drugs such as the aminoglycoside antibiotics.

4. Consult the physician regarding allowable salt intake, which is usually liberalized to prevent hyponatremia and hypochloremia.

Spironolactone (Aldactone) *and Triamterene* (Dyrenium)

1. In general, avoid potassium supplements with these potassium-sparing diuretics.

2. Observe the patient for symptoms of hyperkalemia: irritability, nausea, intestinal colic and diarrhea, weakness, dyspnea, difficulty speaking, and cardiac arrhythmias.

3. Gynecomastia may occur with spironolactone and may persist after drug withdrawal.

SUPPLEMENTARY READINGS

Goldberg, M., "The Renal Physiology of Diuretics," in *Renal Physiology. Handbook of Physiology*, eds., J. Orloff and R. W. Berliner, Sect. 8, p. 1003–31. Washington, D.C.: American Physiological Society, 1973.

Jacobson, H. R., and J. P. Kokko, "Diuretics: Sites and Mechanisms of Actions," *Annual Review of Pharmacology and Toxicology* **16:** 201–14 (1976).

Kemp, G., and D. Kemp, "Diuretics," *American Journal of Nursing* **78:** 1006–10 (1978).

MacLeod, S. M., "The Rational Use of Potassium Supplements," *Postgraduate Medicine* **57:** 123–28 (1975).

Manzi, C., "Edema—How to Tell if it's a Danger Signal," *Nursing '77* **7**(4): 66–70 (1977).

Mudge, G. H., "Diuretics and Other Agents Employed in the Mobilization of Edema Fluid," in *Goodman and Gilman's The Pharmacological Basis of Therapeutics* (6th ed.), eds., A. G. Gilman, L. S. Goodman, and A. Gilman, Chapter 36, pp. 892–915. New York: Macmillan, Inc., 1980.

Papper, S., "Renal Failure," *Medical Clinics of North America* **55:** 335–57 (1971).

Reidenberg, M. M., *Renal Function and Drug Action.* Philadelphia: W. B. Saunders Company, 1971.

Renkin, E. M., and R. R. Robinson, "Glomerular Filtration," *New England Journal of Medicine* **290:** 785–92 (1974).

Section V

THE HORMONES AND VITAMINS

Chapter 33

INTRODUCTION TO THE ENDOCRINE SYSTEM

Control and maintenance of a constant internal environment, *homeostasis*, in the face of often marked changes occurring in the external environment and within the organism is accomplished by the cooperative activities of the nervous system and the endocrine system. The endocrine system acts via chemical messengers called *hormones*.

Normal health requires that optimal amounts of these hormones be released. Excessive or inadequate amounts of hormones can often severely disrupt the homeostatic balance, causing extensive adverse effects to the individual. Naturally occurring hormones or their synthetic derivatives are clinically employed for the management of endocrine disorders resulting from a hor-

monal deficiency; this is a classical example of *replacement therapy*. Conversely, other drugs may be used to reduce the synthesis or antagonize the actions of hormones when the endocrine disease results from an excessive secretion of these chemicals. Some hormones, most notably the glucocorticoids, are employed for the treatment of a broad spectrum of disorders lacking an endocrinological etiology; several hormones find extensive use as diagnostic agents.

This chapter is intended to provide an overview of the endocrine system and the hormones. In particular, we shall examine the general physiological functions of hormones and the mechanisms responsible for control of their release. In the subsequent chapters in this section, we shall consider the physiology and pharmacology of specific endocrine glands and their hormones.

HORMONES

The *endocrine glands* release hormones directly into the blood for transport to their target cells or organs, where they exert their actions. Although some of these chemical messengers, such as growth hormone and thyroid hormone, influence the functional activity of cells throughout the body, most hormones act selectively on specific tissues.

Physiological Functions and Mechanisms of Hormonal Action

Hormones control the functional activity of their target tissues. Many hormones provide this control by regulating the rate of chemical reactions within the cell or by selectively modifying the permeability of cell membranes to essential nutrient substances, electrolytes, and water. Growth, maturation, and reproduction of the organism are also under hormonal control. In addition, some of the activities of the autonomic and central nervous systems and certain behavioral patterns are subject to hormonal influences. While many of these activities can be carried out in the absence of the endocrine system, under such conditions the rates at which these functions are carried out are far too slow (or, in rare instances, too rapid) to efficiently serve the needs of the organism and thereby maintain homeostasis.

Hormones accomplish many of their effects by two general mechanisms, namely, via activation of cyclic AMP or by increasing protein synthesis; these two mechanisms are often interdependent.

Cyclic AMP-mediated effects   In recent years it has been recognized that many hormones act indirectly on their target cells via the intracellular mediator substance cyclic adenosine-3′,5′-monophosphate, or *cyclic AMP*. The following sequence of events is believed to occur. The hormone, or "first messenger," interacts at the membrane of the target cell with a receptor that is specific for each individual hormone. The hormone-receptor interaction activates *adenylate cyclase*, an enzyme present in the cell membrane. Adenylate cyclase immediately thereafter catalyzes the conversion of intracellular adenosine triphosphate (ATP) to cyclic AMP. Depending upon the specific target cell, the "second messenger," cyclic AMP, initiates physiological functions normally associated with that hormone. Such effects include enzyme activation, vitalization of protein synthesis, alterations in the permeability of the cell membrane, changes in muscle tone, or initiation of glandular secretions.

Protein synthesis induced by steroid hormones   Steroid hormones released by the adrenal gland, ovaries, or testes are capable of increasing intracellular protein synthesis. The steroid hormone enters the cell and binds to a specific cytoplasmic receptor protein; both enter the nucleus of the cell, where they activate specific chromosomal genes to form messenger RNA. The newly formed messenger RNA enters the cytoplasm and promotes the formation of new protein molecules. These proteins are probably enzymes that catalyze specific functions of the cell.

Regulation of Hormone Release

The rate of release of many hormones from endocrine glands is carefully regulated by influences arising from within the central

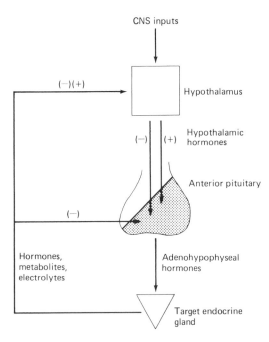

CNS inputs

(−)(+)

Hypothalamus

(−)   (+)   Hypothalamic hormones

Anterior pituitary

(−)

Hormones, metabolites, electrolytes

Adenohypophyseal hormones

Target endocrine gland

Figure 33-1   Hypothalamic-Pituitary-Endocrine Gland Interrelationships.   Hypothalamic releasing (+) or inhibitory (−) factors control release of adenohypophyseal hormones which influence secretion of hormones by endocrine glands. Excessive circulating levels of hormones, metabolites, or electrolytes inhibit additional release of hypothalamic or adenohypophyseal hormones by a negative feedback system.

nervous system, as well as by the levels of that hormone or other endogenous substances within the blood (Figure 33-1).

Classically, the *anterior pituitary gland* or *adenohypophysis* has been viewed as the master gland responsible for controlling the functional activity of many of the individual endocrine glands. It is now known that the anterior pituitary gland is the target of controlling excitatory and inhibitory hormones released from the *hypothalamus* (Figure 33-2).

The hypothalamus receives stimuli from the external environment, from other parts of the central nervous system, and from the internal body environment. Changes in

levels of hormones, biochemicals, electrolytes, and water in the body are carried by the blood to the hypothalamus (Figure 33-1). In response to these stimuli, specific hypothalamic hormones or trigger substances are released in order to maintain homeostasis. These hypothalamic hormones increase or inhibit the secretion of hormones from the anterior pituitary gland, which, in turn, directly influence the release of hormones from many endocrine glands (Figure 33-2).

THE PITUITARY GLAND

The pituitary gland, or *hypophysis*, is located at the base of the brain and is connected to the hypothalamus by the hypophyseal stalk. Anatomically and functionally, the hypophysis consists of three lobes: the anterior pituitary (adenohypophysis), the posterior pituitary (neurohypophysis), and the intermediate lobe (Figure 33-2).

Anterior Pituitary Gland

The anterior pituitary gland releases at least six hormones that serve to regulate the growth and metabolism of target tissues; some of these *tropic hormones* influence the release of hormones from target endocrine glands (Table 33-1).

As you might anticipate, alterations in the functional activity of the adenohypophysis cause profound changes in the homeostatic balance of the body. To illustrate this point, let us outline some of the many consequences of pituitary insufficiency (panhypopituitarism), a condition resulting from disease or surgical removal of the pituitary gland. The adrenal cortex atrophies, reducing the release of corticosteroids, decreasing the resistance of the patient to stress, and causing disruptions in the fluid, electrolyte, carbohydrate, and fat balance in the

Table 33-1 The Adenohypophyseal Hormones

Hormone	Physiological functions	Disorders from adenohypophyseal abnormalities[a]	Clinical uses
Somatotropin (STH) or growth hormone (GH) [Asellacrin]	Promotes growth of all body tissues; influences carbohydrate, protein, and fat metabolism.	Giantism ($\uparrow$) Acromegaly ($\uparrow$) Dwarfism ($\downarrow$) Diabetogenic ($\uparrow$)	Hypopituitary dwarfism [IM: 1 ml (2 I.U.) three times weekly for 6-month periods].
Corticotropin or adrenocorticotropic hormone (ACTH)	Stimulates growth of adrenal gland and production and release of hormones from the adrenal cortex; hormones affect metabolism of carbohydrates, proteins, fats and mineral balance (Chapter 34).	Cushing's disease ($\uparrow$) Addison's disease ($\downarrow$)	Adrenal insufficiency (diagnosis); therapeutic uses have been largely replaced by glucocorticoids (Chapter 34).
Thyrotropin or thyroid-stimulating hormone (TSH)	Controls synthesis and release of thyroid hormones (Chapter 35).	Secondary hypothyroidism ($\downarrow$)	Differentiation of primary (thyroid) and secondary (pituitary) hypothyroidism (diagnosis).
Prolactin	With other hormones, initiates and maintains lactation after childbirth; also causes sodium and water retention.	Forbes-Albright syndrome-tumor ($\uparrow$) (hyperprolactenemia-galactorrhea-amenorrhea syndrome)	————
Gonadotropins 1. Follicle-stimulating hormone (FSH)	Females: Stimulates growth of and estrogen secretion by ovarian follicles. Males: Stimulates sperm formation (Chapter 37).	Infertility ($\downarrow$) Reproductive disorders ($\downarrow$)	Crude gonadotropin preparations available containing FSH and LH; used to induce ovulation in infertile females.
2. Luteinizing hormone (LH)	Females: Stimulates ovarian follicles, ovulation, and production of estrogen and progesterone (sex hormones) by corpus luteum. Males: Stimulates testes to produce testosterone (sex hormone) (Chapter 37).		Human chorionic gonadotropin (HCG) secreted by placenta; used to treat cryptorchidism and in pregnancy tests.

[a]($\uparrow$) Increase and ($\downarrow$) decrease in secretion of adenohypophyseal hormones.

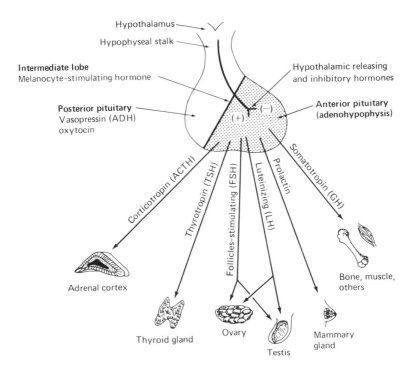

Figure 33-2   The Hypothalamus, Hypophyseal Hormones, and the Target Endocrine Glands and Tissues of the Adenohypophyseal Hormones.

body. Atrophy of the gonads of the female prevents ovulation, causes cessation of the menstrual cycle, and adversely affects the female secondary sex characteristics. Reductions in thyroid function render the patient mentally and physically sluggish. We shall examine the physiological functions of these and other endocrine glands in the subsequent chapters in this section.

Posterior Pituitary Gland

The posterior pituitary gland secretes two hormones, vasopressin and oxytocin. After the synthesis of these small protein molecules by cells in the hypothalamus, they travel down nerve fibers, terminating in the neurohypophysis, and are released in response to appropriate stimuli.

Vasopressin (antidiuretic hormone)

Vasopressin, or antidiuretic hormone (ADH), increases the permeability of the kidney tubules (the collecting ducts in particular) to water, thereby increasing the reabsorption of water and preventing its excessive loss in the urine (Chapter 32).

This hormone is employed clinically for the symptomatic treatment of pituitary diabetes insipidus, a disorder caused by an ADH deficiency and characterized by extreme urinary excretion (polyuria).

Unsuitable for oral administration, vasopressin is given by intramuscular or

Table 33-2   Comparative Properties of Vasopressin Preparations

Generic name	Trade name	Usual adult dose	Distinguishing characteristics
Vasopressin injection	Pitressin	IM or SC: 5-10 U.S.P. units (0.25–0.5 ml) 3-4 times daily	Sterile solution in water containing synthetic vasopressin or from posterior pituitary glands from which oxytocin has been removed.
Vasopressin tannate	Pitressin tannate	IM: 2.5-5 U.S.P. units (0.5-1 ml) q. 1–3 days	Long-acting vasopressin preparation suspended in peanut oil; may cause pain and sterile abscesses at injection site. Should never be given intravenously.
Posterior pituitary		Insufflation of 5–20 U.S.P. units t.i.d.	Powder containing dried posterior pituitary gland (vasopressin and oxytocin). Intranasal irritation, respiratory distress, allergic reactions may occur.
Lypressin (lysine-8-vasopressin)	Diapid	1–2 sprays in one or both nostrils q. 6 h	Effective synthetic product with no marked undesirable systemic effects; no allergic reactions reported.
Desmopressin	DDAVP	1 spray (0.1 ml) b.i.d.	Effective synthetic product with longer duration of action and lower incidence of adverse effects than other products. Headache most common side effect. Drug of choice for pituitary diabetes insipidus.

subcutaneous injection or by nasal insufflation of a powder or spray. A comparison of the available vasopressin preparations is given in Table 33-2.

Injection of large doses of vasopressin causes *vasoconstriction*, manifested by facial pallor. More serious, however, is constriction of the coronary arteries, which may precipitate acute attacks of angina pectoris in susceptible individuals; this compound is contraindicated in such patients. Women may experience uterine menstrual-like cramps after vasopressin administration.

Oxytocin   Oxytocin is clinically employed to induce labor in pregnant females and to decrease hemorrhage after delivery of the placenta; it plays a physiological role in milk letdown. The properties of oxytocin will be discussed in greater detail in Chapter 38.

Intermediate Lobe

Melanocyte-stimulating hormone (MSH) is the major hormone secreted by the intermediate lobe of the pituitary gland. In fish, amphibia, and reptiles, MSH participates in the control of skin coloration, causing a darkening of the skin. The precise functional role of this hormone in humans has not been established.

SUPPLEMENTARY READINGS

Berson, S. A., and R. S. Yalow, *Peptide Hormones.* New York: American Elsevier Publishing Co., 1973.

Fisher, L., ed., *Neuroendocrine Integration: Basic and Applied Aspects.* New York: Raven Press, 1975.

Krueger, J. A., and J. C. Ray, *Endocrine Problems in Nursing. A Physiological Approach.* St. Louis: The C. V. Mosby Company, 1976.

Lock, W., and A. V. Shally, ed., *The Hypothalamus and Pituitary in Health and Disease.* Springfield, Ill.: Charles C Thomas, Publisher, 1972.

Pastan, I., "Cyclic AMP," *Scientific American* **227**(2): 97–105 (1972).

Sachs, B. A., ed., "The Brain and the Endocrine System," *Medical Clinics of North America* **62**(2): 227–426 (1978).

Spencer, R. T., *Patient Care in Endocrine Problems.* Philadelphia: W. B. Saunders Company, 1973.

Tepperman, J., *Metabolic and Endocrine Physiology*

(3rd ed.). Chicago: Year Book Medical Publishers, Inc., 1973.

Thomas, J. A., and M. G. Mawhinney, *Synopsis of Endocrine Pharmacology.* Baltimore: University Park Press, 1973.

Tixier-Vidal, A., and M. G. Farquhar, *The Anterior Pituitary.* New York: Academic Press, Inc., 1975.

Ville, D. B., *Human Endocrinology: A Developmental Approach.* Philadelphia: W. B. Saunders Company, 1975.

Williams, R. H., ed., *Textbook of Endocrinology* (5th ed.). Philadelphia: W. B. Saunders Company, 1974.

ADRENOCORTICAL STEROIDS

Chapter 34

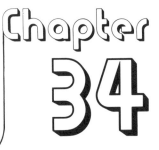

The mammalian *adrenal glands*, perched as small caps on top of each kidney, consist of two functionally distinct parts: the *adrenal cortex*, the outer and larger portion of the gland, surrounding the *adrenal medulla*. The latter, inner portion of the gland is part of the sympathetic nervous system and releases catecholamines, which enable the organism to successfully cope with a "fight or flight" situation (Chapter 5). While a functional adrenal medulla is not absolutely essential for the maintenance of life, destruction of the adrenal cortex results in death within 2 weeks in the absence of treatment.

The glucocorticoid hormones of the

adrenal cortex are widely employed for the treatment of hormonal deficiencies, as well as for the management of a variety of non-endocrine disorders—including those with an inflammatory and allergic etiology.

CLASSIFICATION OF ADRENOCORTICAL STEROIDS

Steroid hormones naturally secreted by the adrenal cortex and synthetic derivatives of such hormones are collectively referred to as *adrenocortical steroids* or *corticosteroids*.

Table 34-1   Relative Activity of Adrenocortical Steroids

Natural adrenocortical steroids	Relative activity	
	Mineralocorticoid	Glucocorticoid
Aldosterone	10,000	50
Desoxycorticosterone	100	1
Corticosterone	15	50
Cortisol	10	150

Cholesterol is the common precursor of these natural compounds.

The adrenocortical steroids are of three major types. (1) *Adrenal androgens* are normally of limited physiological importance; however, certain tumors of the adrenal gland can evoke marked secretion of these sex hormones, resulting in masculinization of female patients. These disorders are collectively called the *adrenogenital syndrome*. (2) The *mineralocorticoid aldosterone* has profound effects on the electrolyte and water balances of the body and is essential for life. (3) *Glucocorticoids* such as *cortisol*, or hydrocortisone, exert their major effects on carbohydrate, protein, and fat metabolism and also have anti-inflammatory and antiallergic actions.

The biological properties of the glucocorticoids and mineralocorticoids are not mutually exclusive for a given compound; that is, naturally occurring glucocorticoids possess mineralocorticoid activity and vice versa. Table 34-1 compares these overlapping activities. Synthetic derivatives of the endogenous glucocorticoids possess extremely potent anti-inflammatory properties, with minimal secondary effects on electrolyte and water balances.

CORTICOTROPIN

Corticotropin—or adrenocorticotropic hormone, abbreviated ACTH—secreted by the anterior pituitary gland, is essential for the synthesis of the adrenocortical steroids and is required for the maintenance of the structure and function of the adrenal cortex. This pituitary hormone also controls cortisol release.

Secretion of corticotropin is regulated by the *corticotropin-releasing factor* (CRF), a hypothalamic hormone. Emotional or physical stress activates CRF, as do low blood levels of cortisol. Conversely, elevated levels of cortisol transmit messages to the anterior pituitary or hypothalamus, which supress additional release of corticotropin and CRF, respectively. This negative feedback system regulates the circulating levels of cortisol.

In addition to modulating the release of cortisol from the adrenal cortex, corticotropin also stimulates the growth and development of this endocrine gland and enhances the rate at which glucocorticoids and, to a lesser extent, mineralocorticoids are biosynthesized. Prolonged suppression of corticotropin release results in adrenal cortical atrophy. We shall return to the clinical significance of this point when we discuss the adverse effects associated with the chronic therapeutic use of glucocorticoids.

Therapeutic Uses

The biological effects of corticotropin administration are mediated by cortisol and will be discussed in a later section of this chapter.

Corticotropin is rapidly inactivated after oral administration and is generally given by intramuscular or intravenous injection. Slow intravenous injection of corticotropin is *diagnostically* employed for differentiating whether adrenal insufficiency is primary (that is, failure of the adrenal cortex) or secondary (consequence of anterior pituitary dysfunction). Significant elevations (twofold or threefold) in plasma cortisol or 24-hour urinary 17-hydroxycorticosterone levels over a 2- to 3-day period during corticotropin administration is indicative of a functionally active adrenal gland.

Cosyntropin (Cortrosyn), a synthetic subunit of corticotropin, is currently being employed for this diagnostic purpose because it is less allergenic than the natural hormone. Plasma levels of cortisol are assessed 30 to 60 minutes after intramuscular or intravenous injection of cosyntropin. This drug cannot be employed to replace the therapeutic uses of corticotropin discussed later.

Corticotropin has been found to be clinically superior to the glucocorticoids for the treatment of severe myasthenia gravis (Chapter 7). The repository gel preparation of this hormone (Acthar Gel) is generally administered intramuscularly once daily for 10 to 20 days. During the course of corticotropin administration, muscle strength actually decreases to such an extent that mechanical support of respiration is often required. Within days after the termination of drug administration, muscle strength returns to normal. Remissions of the myasthenic state persisting for several months in duration have been obtained.

Abrupt cessation of corticotropin injections result in adverse reactions that are attributed to adrenal insufficiency (see page 294). Allergic reactions may occur with repeated administration of this hormone; these allergic reactions are not associated with glucocorticoid administration.

MINERALOCORTICOIDS

While the glucocorticoids permit us to better withstand stress, their continued secretion is not essential; mineralocorticoids, by contrast, are required for the survival of the individual. Aldosterone is the most important mineralocorticoid secreted by the adrenal cortex, with corticosterone and desoxycorticosterone assuming far less physiological importance. Desoxycorticosterone is the only endogenous mineralocorticoid available for clinical use.

Aldosterone

The primary physiological function of aldosterone is to conserve the sodium stores of the body. This hormone enhances the reabsorption of sodium in the kidney tubules, preventing the excessive loss of this electrolyte in the urine. Secondary effects associated with sodium reabsorption include the retention of chloride and water and the loss of potassium (Chapter 32).

While corticotropin plays a critical role in regulating the secretion of cortisol, this pituitary hormone has only a modest influence on the release of aldosterone. Factors promoting the release of aldosterone include low plasma sodium levels, resulting from a sodium-restricted diet or the use of diuretic agents, as well as a reduction in blood volume and blood pressure that might result from excessive bleeding. You will recall from Chapter 25 that a reduction in blood pressure activates the release of the enzyme renin from the kidneys, and this enzyme catalyzes the formation of angiotensin II. The latter compound stimulates the release of aldosterone from the adrenal cortex, promoting the conservation of sodium, chloride, and water and elevating the blood pressure.

Aldosterone-associated disorders

Primary aldosteronism   Excessive secretion of aldosterone causes edema, a condition associated with congestive heart failure, certain kidney diseases, cirrhosis of the liver, and toxemia of pregnancy. In *primary aldosteronism*, a tumor of the adrenal cortex secretes excessive aldosterone. Although edema is not marked, there are slight elevations in plasma sodium and pronounced reductions in plasma potassium. This condition is clinically characterized by muscle weakness, tetany or muscle spasms, and some degree of hypertension. The aldosterone antagonist *spironolactone* (Aldactone) is used to treat this disorder; it prevents aldosterone-induced retention of sodium and promotes the conservation of potassium (Chapter 32).

Addison's disease   This disorder results from the inability of the adrenal cortex to produce sufficient quantities of mineralocorticoids and glucocorticoids. An aldosterone deficiency causes marked fluid and electrolyte losses, resulting in a marked reduction in the volume of extracellular fluid. Cardiac output is reduced, with shock and death ensuing within 4 days to 2 weeks after the complete cessation of aldosterone secretion.* Desoxycorticosterone (Percorten) and fludrocortisone (Florinef), the latter a potent synthetic mineralocorticoid, are used to treat Addison's disease, as we shall discuss shortly.

The consequences of glucocorticoid deficiency are also witnessed in Addison's disease. The absence of cortisol prevents the patient from maintaining adequate blood glucose levels between meals, and proteins and fats are not mobilized from tissue storage sites to provide energy. These biochemical defects cause the patient to experience extreme weakness and fatigue. Resistance to stress is also diminished, with cardiovascular collapse and death sometimes resulting from normally minor traumatic or infectious conditions. For these reasons, glucocorticoids are generally administered to such patients. Patients with this disease must understand the nature of their condition and how to avoid complications, in particular the necessity of avoiding or minimizing stress.

---

*President John F. Kennedy was among the most notable patients with Addison's disease.

Desoxycorticosterone

Desoxycorticosterone is a naturally occurring mineralocorticoid possessing very little glucocorticoidal activity (Table 34-1, page 285). Preparations of this hormone are clinically available for intramuscular injection (as a solution in oil), as pellets for subcutaneous implantation, and as tablets for buccal administration. The usual daily maintenance dose of this drug for the treatment of Addison's disease is 1 to 5 mg.

Large doses of desoxycorticosterone may cause edema, resulting in congestive heart failure or pulmonary congestion. Excessive losses of potassium may cause muscle weakness and cardiac abnormalities. Since chronic administration of this hormone has been observed to cause hypertension in many patients, nurses should periodically monitor the patient's blood pressure.

In recent years, fludrocortisone (Florinef) has become the mineralocorticoid of choice for the treatment of Addison's disease. This synthetic drug is highly potent and can be taken orally. The usual daily dose of this drug is 0.05 to 0.1 mg.

GLUCOCORTICOIDS

The glucocorticoids are very widely used therapeutic agents; they are most commonly employed for the treatment of topical and systemic inflammatory and allergic disorders. At the time of their clinical introduction three decades ago, limitless therapeutic potential was ascribed to this drug class. With the realization that the chronic use of these drugs is associated with a high incidence of often serious side effects, the glucocorticoids are no longer the recipients of unrestrained praise; nevertheless, they still occupy a significant place in modern therapeutics.

The most important natural glucocorticoid is *cortisol*, a hormone commonly referred to as *hydrocortisone*.

Physiological Effects

The glucocorticoids exert diverse biological effects, many of which influence the functional activity of tissues throughout the body. Cortisol secretion is enhanced by *stresses* arising from widely differing causes. By mechanisms that have not been clearly established to date, cortisol permits us to resist the adverse influence of stress, undoubtedly by its general effects on cellular processes rather than by any highly specific effect.

Metabolic effects   Cortisol may produce two different types of effects on metabolic reactions, effects that are dose-related. In the absence of cortisol release, some biochemical reactions proceed at rates that are not optimal to serve the needs of the organism. Administration of small physiological doses of cortisol (20 mg daily) enables such reactions to occur at rates that preserve the homeostatic balance of the body; this has been called a *permissive action*. Large pharmacological doses of cortisol, far in excess of those quantities normally secreted by the adrenal cortex, produce exaggerated effects similar to those observed in Cushing's disease, a disorder resulting from excessive release of glucocorticoids.

One of the primary effects of glucocorticoids is the stimulation of gluconeogenesis, the biosynthesis of glucose from amino acid precursors. While blood glucose levels rise, cortisol prevents the tissue uptake and utilization of this sugar to supply energy requirements. Elevations in blood glucose activate a compensatory release of insulin from the pancreas. In patients with Cushing's disease, diabetes-like symptoms often develop as a consequence of glucocorticoid-induced inhibition of glucose uptake by tissues. For these reasons, cortisol is said to have an *anti-insulin effect*.

Cortisol increases the catabolism (breakdown) of proteins, reduces the rate of protein synthesis, an *anti-anabolic effect*, and enhances the excretion of amino acids. Large doses of cortisol inhibit the growth of children. In both children and adults, muscle weakness, osteoporosis (thinning of the bones) with an increased tendency for fracturing, and an impairment of wound healing are also observed; all of these adverse effects are caused by protein catabolism. High doses of glucocorticoids also increase the disposition of fats in the face ("moon face") and upper back ("buffalo hump"), symptoms characteristically observed in Cushing's disease.

Cortisol possesses some mineralocorticoid activity, but less than aldosterone (Table 34-1, page 285). Thus, it should not be surprising that administration of this hormone causes retention of sodium and edema formation and hypertension. These salt-retaining effects are markedly reduced with the newer synthetic glucocorticoids (Table 34-2).

Anti-inflammatory, antiallergic, and Immunosuppressant effects   Glucocorticoids are very extensively used for the clinical management of *inflammatory disorders*, both within the body and on its exterior surfaces. *Inflammation* is characterized by pain, swelling, heat, redness, and loss of function. Cortisol and related drugs are highly effective in supressing these symptoms of inflammation but do not correct its underlying cause. The precise mechanism of this anti-inflammatory effect is highly complex. Among the actions suggested to be involved include stabilization of lysosomes, inhibition of the migration of polymorphonuclear leukocytes and the functions of fibroblasts, and antagonism of the increased capillary permeability associated with inflammatory processes.

These hormones are valuable drugs for the management of disorders associated with *hypersensitivity* (allergic) reactions and the

Table 34-2   Comparison of Selected Systemic Adrenocorticosteroids

Generic name	Selected trade names	Anti-inflammatory		Salt-retaining activity (hydro-cortisone = 1)	Routes of adminis-tration[a]
		Relative potency (hydro-cortisone = 1)	Equiv-alent doses mg (oral)		
Mineralocorticoids					
Desoxycorticosterone	DOCA, Percorten	0	———	100	I, P
Fludrocortisone	Florinef	10		125	O
Glucocorticoids					
Cortisone	Cortone	0.8	25	0.8	O, I
Hydrocortisone (cortisol)	Cortef, Hydrocortone, Solu-Cortef	1	20	1	O, I
Prednisone	Meticorten, Deltasone, Paracort, Delta-Dome	4	5	0.8	O
Prednisolone	Delta-Cortef, Hydeltrasol, Meticortelone, Sterane	4	5	0.8	O, I
Methylprednisolone	Medrol, Depo-Medrol, Solu-Medrol	5	4	0.5	O, I
Triamcinolone	Aristocort, Kenacort	5	4	0	O, I
Paramethasone	Haldrone	10	2	0	O
Dexamethasone	Decadron, Hexadrol	25–30	0.75	0	O, I
Betamethasone	Celestone	30	0.6	0	O, I

[a] Abbreviations: I = injection; O = oral; P = pellets for implantation.

immunological responses of the body, such as the rejection of tissue grafts. Cortisol does not appear to modify the titer of circulating antibodies (IgG or IgE), nor does it alter antigen-antibody interactions, the release of chemical mediators of hypersensitivity reactions, or interfere with the normal processes associated with the development of cell-mediated immunity. It would appear that these compounds prevent or suppress the inflammatory responses resulting from hypersensitivity reactions.

Reduction in the numbers of circulating eosinophils and lymphocytes and a decrease in the size of lympoid tissue are observed after glucocorticoid administration.

Healing of wounds may be delayed because corticosteroids suppress immune responses and retard granulation tissue.

Synthetic Glucocorticoids

The natural hormone *cortisone* was the first corticosteroid employed for the management of rheumatoid arthritis because of its anti-inflammatory effect. While this drug proved to be clinically effective, sodium retention—leading to edema formation—hyperglycemia, osteoporosis, and other adverse effects were associated with its usage. Alterations in the chemical structure of cortisone have lead to the clinical introduction of many glucocorticoids possessing highly potent anti-inflammatory effects with little or virtually no sodium-retaining properties (Table 34-2); to date, it has not been possible to dissociate the desired anti-inflammatory effects from adverse effects on carbohydrate and protein metabolism. Apart from potency differences, all the synthetic glucocorticoids have the same spectrum of pharmacological properties and many similar undesirable effects, and they can often be used interchangeably at equivalent doses.

Administration and Therapeutic Uses

Glucocorticoids are rapidly and completely absorbed from the gastrointestinal tract after oral administration and are, therefore, commonly given by mouth. Some members of this class are injected intramuscularly, intravenously, intradermally, or into joints, while others are applied locally to the conjunctival sac of the eye or on the skin (Tables 34-2 and 34-3).

General therapeutic considerations
These drugs have extremely broad clinical applications and are currently employed for the diagnosis and management of scores of medical disorders (Table 34-4). With the ex-

ception of several relatively unusual disorders resulting from an inadequate secretion of adrenocortical steroids, such as Addison's disease, the vast majority of the clinical applications of these drugs are not predicated upon replacement of a hormonal deficiency. Furthermore, these drugs have not been demonstrated to cure any disease, but rather provide only symptomatic relief to the patient.

The following critical factors must be taken into consideration prior to the initiation of glucorticoid therapy. In the absence of specific contraindications prohibiting their use, large doses may be safely administered for several days. The incidence and severity of adverse effects and the magnitude of pituitary and adrenocortical suppression increase when therapy is continued for prolonged periods of time (months) and the dose exceeds the equivalent of the daily cortisol secretion (20 mg); the equivalent doses of synthetic glucocorticoids are given in Table 34-2.

Whenever possible, an attempt should

Table 34-3   Selected Topical and Ophthalmic Anti-Inflammatory Adrenocorticoids

Generic name	Selected trade names	Routes of administration[a]
Cortisone	———	Op
Hydrocortisone	Cortef, Cortril, Cort-Dome, Hytone	Op, T
Prednisolone	Econopred, Hydeltrasol, Meti-Derm, Metreton	Op, T
Methylprednisolone	Medrol	T
Triamcinolone	Aristoderm, Kenacort,	T
Dexamethasone	Decadron, Decaderm, Maxidex, Hexadrol	Op, T
Betamethasone	Celestone, Diprosone, Valisone	T
Amcinonide	Cyclocort	T
Desonide	Tridesilon	T
Diflorasone	Florone	T
Flumethasone	Locorten	T
Fluocinolone	Synalar, Fluonid	T
Fluocinonide	Lidex, Topsyn	T
Flurandrenolide	Cordran	T
Fluorometholone	Oxylone	T
Halcinonide	Halog	T

[a] Key to abbreviations: Op = ophthalmic solutions, suspensions, or ointments; T = topical creams, ointments, or sprays.

Table 34-4 Selected Therapeutic Uses of Glucocorticoids

Endocrine Disorders	Status asthmaticus
Primary or secondary adrenocortical insufficiency	Contact dermatitis
Congenital adrenal hyperplasia	Atopic dermatitis
	Serum sickness
Rheumatic Disorders	Drug hypersensitivity reactions
Rheumatoid arthritis	
Osteoarthritis	*Respiratory Diseases*
Acute gouty arthritis	Sarcoidosis
	Fulminating or disseminated pulmonary tuberculosis
Collagen Diseases	Aspiration pneumonitis
Systemic lupus erythematosus	Hyaline membrane disease
Acute rheumatic carditis	
Polymyositis	*Gastrointestinal Diseases*
Polyarteritis nodosa	Ulcerative colitis
	Celiac sprue
Skin Diseases	Enteritis
Pemphigus	
Erythema multiforme (Stevens-Johnson syndrome)	*Hematologic Diseases*
Exfoliative dermatitis	Thrombocytopenia
Severe psoriasis	Acquired (autoimmune) hemolytic anemia
Severe seborrheic dermatitis	Erythroblastopenia (RBC anemia)
Eye Diseases	*Neoplastic Diseases*
Allergic conjunctivitis	Leukemias and lymphomas (adults)
Iritis and iridocyclitis	Acute leukemia (children)
Posterior uveitis	Breast cancer
Choroiditis	
Sympathetic ophthalmia	*Miscellaneous Uses*
Allergic blepharitis	Nephrotic syndrome
Keratitis	Cerebral edema
	Organ transplantation
Allergic Diseases	Differential diagnosis of hypercorticism and
Allergic rhinitis	Cushing's disease
Bronchial asthma	

be made to employ alternate-day therapy for patients requiring high doses and prolonged treatment. This dosing schedule appears to cause considerably less suppression of adrenal function than consecutive-day therapy. After administering the glucocorticoid in divided daily doses to control the symptoms during the early phase of therapy, the total daily dose is given in the morning for about 1 week. Thereafter, the patient takes twice the daily dose on alternate mornings. Patients should be warned that the severity of their symptoms may worsen on drug-free days and

be advised that this dosing schedule reduces the long-term adverse effects associated with glucocorticoid administration and subsequent withdrawal.

Therapeutic Indications Three general medical problems are responsive to glucocorticoid administration, namely, chronic nonfatal conditions, acute exacerbations, and acute self-limiting disorders.

Chronic nonfatal conditions Disorders of this type, such as rheumatoid arthritis and bronchial asthma, do not present a direct threat to the patient's life. In general, glucocorticoid therapy is initiated when the patient fails to respond to safer, more conservative treatment measures. Steroids are often given at the smallest effective doses, in combination with conventional nonsteroidal medications. In many instances the dose of glucocorticoid employed will provide only partial symptomatic relief. At frequent intervals, the daily dose of steroid should be gradually reduced until the lowest effective dose is employed.

Acute exacerbations These conditions are characterized by acute episodes of chronic nonfatal diseases (rheumatoid arthritis) or fatal diseases (pemphigus, disseminated lupus erythematosus). Large doses of glucocorticoids are given at the outset and are gradually reduced when the acute exacerbation of the nonfatal disease is brought under control. In lethal diseases, these large doses are maintained for long periods of time or for the remainder of the patient's life. In these latter conditions, the dangers of adrenal insufficiency and the adverse effects induced by steroid administration are considered to be less critical than permitting the disease to continue uncontrolled.

Acute self-limiting disorders The most impressive clinical benefits of glucocorticoid administration are observed in patients who require a short-term course of therapy for the management of acute inflammatory disorders of the skin and eye. When administered properly, the dangers associated with the systemic effects of these drugs are minimal.

In the subsequent paragraphs of this section, we shall briefly consider selected aspects of some of the general clinical uses of glucocorticoids.

Replacement therapy Intravenous infusion of hydrocortisone succinate in a saline-glucose solution may prove life-saving in the emergency treatment of *acute adrenal insufficiency*. After the patient has stabilized, this drug is given intramuscularly. *Chronic adrenal insufficiency* (Addison's disease) is commonly managed by the oral administration of fludrocortisone and cortisone.

Rheumatoid disorders Glucocorticoids are capable of producing dramatic symptomatic relief of the signs of inflammation observed in *rheumatoid arthritis*. Stiffness and tenderness of the joints and muscles dissipate, with improved joint mobility observed within days after the initiation of therapy; steroid-induced elevations in mood are noted and appetite increases. In view of the chronic nature of this and related rheumatoid disorders and the need to continue steroid administration for long periods of time or even a lifetime, the benefits versus the risks associated with these drugs may be carefully evaluated prior to using them. It is generally accepted that other modes of therapy should be first tried, including rest, physical therapy, salicylates, indomethacin, and gold salts (Chapter 21). The maintenance doses of steroids are intended to control—but usually not to eradicate—the symptoms of rheumatoid arthritis. Intra-articular (within the joints) injections of these hormones are often used to arrest acute attacks of gouty arthritis and osteoarthritis.

Collagen diseases The *connective tissue* or *collagen diseases* are a group of disorders with common or overlapping clinical or histological features. These common histological characteristics include widespread inflammatory changes to connective tissues and blood vessels. Among these collagen diseases and their sites of inflammation are rheumatoid arthritis (joints), rheumatic fever (heart), polyarteritis nodosa (small and medium-sized arteries), disseminated lupus erythematosus (connective tissue in many parts of the body), and polymyositis (muscle). All of these diseases are serious and disabling, and some are lethal. Glucocorticoids are able to provide symptomatic relief in these disorders, reduce disability, and, in some instances, prolong survival time.

Skin diseases A wide variety of skin disorders often show dramatic improvement after systemic, intralesional, or topical steroid administration. Topical preparations are available as creams, ointments, lotions, and aerosol sprays (Table 34-3, page 290). *Percutaneous penetration* of steroids may be increased by as much as ten times by *occlusion* of the topically administered drug with an impermeable film such as plastic wrap. While occlusion markedly enhances clinical effectiveness, it also increases the risk of systemic drug absorption, potentially resulting in adrenal atrophy (suppression) and other adverse effects. This risk is increased when these drugs are applied in large quantities, or to extensive skin surfaces, or over prolonged periods of time. Nurses should advise patients not to wear plastic occlusions for longer than 12 hours each day. If extensive lesions are to be treated, a sequential approach might be employed, treating one area of the body at a time. Patients should be instructed to apply only a thin film of these topical preparations on the effected area; the use of excessive amounts increases the dangers of systemic toxicity and is uneconomical.

The nurse should inspect lesions between dressings for the development of infection. If detected, suitable antifungal or antibacterial drugs should be administered; in the absence of a prompt response to these drugs, steroid administration should be terminated until the infection is controlled.

Systemically administered glucocorticoids are very useful for the control of *pemphigus*, a relatively uncommon disorder characterized by blisters of the skin and mucous membranes. In the absence of treatment, the mortality rate is greater than 90 percent. Steroid therapy has reduced the mortality rate by one-half and has enabled patients to live a more comfortable life.

Eye diseases Glucocorticoids are commonly used to treat inflammatory diseases of the eye and to prevent corneal scarring, which, in many instances, can preserve the vision of the patient. Therapeutically effective concentrations are achieved in the aqueous humor after conjunctival instillation. Chronic administration of these drugs increases intraocular pressure in normal patients and those with glaucoma. Intraocular pressure should be regularly monitored in patients applying these drugs to the eye for periods exceeding 2 weeks.

Allergic diseases The symptoms associated with such allergic disorders as hay fever, serum sickness, drug hypersensitivity reactions, angioneurotic edema, and anaphylaxis are effectively controlled by systemic glucocorticoid administration. Antihistamines (Chapter 53) should be tried initially in less severe allergic disorders, while in life-threatening conditions (anaphylaxis, angioneurotic edema), therapy should initiated with subcutaneous administration of epinephrine (Chapter 5).

Use of glucocorticoids should be reserved for those cases of bronchial asthma that fail to respond to bronchodilator sympathomimetics (Chapter 5) or other conventional types of antiasthmatic therapy (Chapter 54). In some instances, low doses of steroids are used in combination with these standard drugs. *Beclomethasone* (Vanceril), self-administered by inhalation, causes minimal systemic effects normally associated with other drugs in this class and little adrenocortical suppression (Chapter 54).

Neoplastic disorders   Prednisone, a glucocorticoid, is employed in combination with other anticancer drugs for the treatment of *acute lymphocytic leukemia* and *lymphomas*. The beneficial effects of the steroids have been attributed to their ability to cause atrophy of lymphoid tissues. Glucocorticoids are also used in the treatment of *breast cancer*. The use of glucocorticoids as anticancer drugs is discussed in Chapter 51.

Adverse Effects

The administration of small doses of the glucocorticoids, equivalent to the amounts normally secreted by the adrenal cortex, rarely causes adverse effects. By contrast, the chronic use of these drugs at doses only slightly in excess of these physiological levels will eventually lead to adverse effects that compromise the health of the patient. These adverse effects may be the consequence of abrupt drug withdrawal or the chronic use of high doses.

Acute adrenal insufficiency   Rapid reduction or abrupt discontinuance of the dosage of glucocorticoids often causes a *corticosteroid withdrawal syndrome* characterized by fever, muscle and joint pain, and feelings of fatigue. Such symptoms may be erroneously interpreted as an exacerbation of the rheumatoid condition.

It will be recalled from our earlier discussion of the mechanisms that control cortisol release that when optimal circulating plasma levels of cortisol are present, a negative feedback message is transmitted to the hypothalamus or anterior pituitary gland, which results in a termination of corticotropin secretion. Chronic administration of cortisol or synthetic glucocorticoids has a similar inhibitory effect on corticotropin release, resulting in a temporary atrophy of the adrenal cortex. If, after abrupt discontinuation of glucocorticoid administration, the patient is subjected to a severe stress such as an operation, the temporarily nonfunctional adrenals are incapable of secreting additional cortisol to maintain the homeostatic balance. Unable to successfully respond to the stress, the patient may die as the result of acute adrenal insufficiency and cardiovascular collapse.

Patients should be advised to be alert for the early symptoms of acute adrenal insufficiency, including fatigue, muscle weakness, joint pain, fever, anorexia, nausea, and signs of orthostatic hypotension (dizziness, fainting, or dyspnea).

When patients no longer require chronic corticosteroid administration, drug withdrawal should be accomplished slowly. As a general rule, the daily dose of prednisone (or an equivalent glucocorticoid) may be reduced by 10 percent every 2 weeks until the symptoms can be controlled with a single 20-mg dose taken each morning. At weekly intervals, the daily dose is then reduced by 2.5 mg increments until a dose of 10 mg is reached; this dose can be discontinued within 1 or more months.

Withdrawal from oral maintenance corticosteroids, with the corresponding return of the patient's own basal adrenocortical secretion of cortisol, may not be complete for as long as 1 year. During this time, the patient should be strongly urged to carry an identification card or wear a bracelet or tag indicating possible adrenal insufficiency and need for corticosteroids during periods of acute stress, trauma, infection, or prior to and after operations.

Chronic glucocorticoid administration   Cushing's disease results from the excessive secretion of corticosteroids. Chronic administration of glucocorticoids at doses in excess of their normal levels produces a condition called *iatrogenic Cushing's syndrome*. This condition is characterized by a round and puffy face (moon face), edema, fat deposition on the back (buffalo hump), acne, easy bruisability, thinning of the skin, purplish thread-like marks on the face, hypertension, muscle weakness, and masculinization of female patients. Other undesirable effects of long-term, high-dose glucocorticoid administration include hyperglycemia, increased susceptibility and decreased resistance to infections, activation of peptic ulcers, osteoporosis, and adverse behavioral changes.

Precautions and Contraindications

Diabetes mellitus may develop in susceptible individuals during the course of steroid therapy, and, therefore, periodic tests should be given to detect elevated blood glucose levels (hyperglycemia). This condition can generally be controlled by diet or insulin administration and does not necessitate discontinuation of steroid therapy. Similarly, these drugs are not contraindicated in diabetic patients.

Susceptibility to infections is increased by these drugs; moreover, the symptoms of an infectious disorder such as fever may be masked by glucocorticoid administration. Once the infection is diagnosed, vigorous treatment with antibiotics or other antimicrobial agents should be initiated without discontinuing steroid therapy. Glucocorticoids are contraindicated in the presence of viral and fungal infections that are resistant to available chemotherapeutic agents.

Notwithstanding the life-saving effects of steroids in the treatment of fulminating pulmonary tuberculosis, these drugs are generally contraindicated in patients with a history of tuberculosis because of their potential ability to reactivate healed lesions. Should steroid therapy be essential in such patients, physicians commonly prescribe antitubercular drugs prophylactically; periodic chest x-rays and sputum studies should be ordered to determine whether the tubercular disorder has been reactivated.

Peptic ulceration, with hemorrhage and perforation, is sometimes observed in patients chronically receiving glucocorticoids for the management of rheumatoid arthritis and other disorders. To minimize the possibility of this potentially dangerous condition, nurses should advise patients to take their medication with meals or milk; antacids are often co-administered with the steroids.

Diets rich in protein and potassium should be recommended to prevent drug-induced muscle weakness and wasting (*myopathy*); the highest incidence of myopathy is observed with triamcinolone and dexamethasone. Wound healing is often delayed in patients receiving these drugs. *Osteoporosis*, with potential fractures of the vertebrae, is a frequent complication of systemic glucocorticoid therapy, with particular risk for postmenopausal women. Periodic spinal x-rays should be taken; evidence of this adverse effect is justification for discontinuance of therapy. Upon early signs of mineral depletion, physicians may recommend protein-rich diets (100 g or more daily) and calcium and vitamin D supplements.

While patients with a history of psychiatric disorders are most likely to experience behavioral disorders with steroids, such problems also have been observed in emotionally stable individuals. Euphoria and mania are most commonly observed, with mood swings to a depressive phase and suicidal tendencies not uncommon. The nurse should look for changes in mood or for evidence of psychotic reactions in patients taking these drugs and report such changes to the physician. Triamcinolone produces sedation and depression rather than euphoria. These behavioral aberrations are reversible and usually dissipate upon reduction of steroid dosage or drug withdrawal.

Potential drug interactions involving

Table 34-5   Potential Drug Interactions Involving Corticosteroids

Interacting drug/class	Potential consequences
Barbiturates (phenobarbital) Phenytoin (Dilantin)	These drugs appear to enhance the metabolism of corticosteroids, probably as the result of induction of liver drug metabolizing enzymes. This may produce a reduction in steroid effect resulting in a worsening of asthmatic or Addisonian symptoms.
Indomethacin (Indocin) Salicylates (aspirin)	Both drugs may increase the incidence and severity of gastrointestinal ulceration caused by each.
Salicylates (aspirin)	Corticosteroids may increase the risk of salicylate toxicity (salicylism) by displacing aspirin from plasma protein binding sites.
Antidiabetic Agents Insulin Oral hypoglycemic agents	The ability of glucocorticoids to increase blood glucose levels may antagonize the beneficial effects of these drugs in the management of diabetes. An increase in the dosage of these antidiabetic agents may be required.
Amphotericin B (Fungizone) Ethacrynic acid (Edecrin) Furosemide (Lasix) Thiazide diuretics	Additive enhancement of potassium depletion resulting in hypokalemia.
Anticoagulants, oral Coumarin	Antagonism of anticoagulation in some studies while enhancement of anticoagulation and gastrointestinal ulceration in other studies.

the corticosteroids are summarized in Table 34-5. Nursing implications are summarized at the end of this chapter.

INHIBITORS OF ADRENOCORTICAL STEROID BIOSYNTHESIS

Attempts have been made to find drugs that inhibit the biosynthesis of adrenocortical steroids for the nonsurgical management of adrenal tumors. *Mitotane* (Lysodren), a compound chemically similar to the insecticide DDT, has been found to provide symptomatic relief in the treatment of inoperable cancer of the adrenals (Chapter 51). Aminoglutethimide, an investigational drug, has been shown to decrease the excessive secretion of cortisol in adrenal tumors. It is not useful for the treatment of Cushing's disease, which

results from excessive release of corticotropin from the pituitary gland.

Metyrapone (Metopirone) is the most widely used inhibitor of corticosteroid biosynthesis. While it has not proved to be useful for the management of excessive steroid release from adrenal tumors, it is clinically employed as a *diagnostic agent* to evaluate the ability of the anterior pituitary to release corticotropin. Administration of metyrapone inhibits cortisol biosynthesis, normally leading to a compensatory increase in corticotropin synthesis and release, which in turn augments the secretion of steroids by the adrenal cortex; this rise in steroids can be readily determined by measuring 17-hydroxycorticosteroids in the urine before and after drug administration. This rise is not observed in patients with hypothalamic or pituitary lesions that impair the synthesis or release of corticotropin.

Adrenocorticosteroids:
nursing implications

1. Emphasize the need for regular medical supervision when taking these drugs.

2. Advise the patient to carry a card identifying the drug being taken, the exact dose, and the physician to be contacted in the event of emergency.

3. The patient should be alert for early symptoms of acute adrenal insufficiency: fatigue, muscle weakness, joint pain, fever, anorexia, nausea, or signs of othostatic hypotension including dizziness, fainting, or dyspnea.

4. Alternate-day therapy may be instituted for patients requiring long-term therapy to prevent suppression of the adrenal cortex and deficiency symptoms when the drug is withdrawn. Patient should understand the reason for slow drug withdrawal. Provide support and reassurance if the symptoms increase during period of drug dosage reduction.

5. Instruct the patient to report signs and symptoms of diseases that could be masked by adrenocorticosteroids (infections and inflammatory conditions).

6. Wound healing will be slow because the drug retards granulation tissue.

7. Instruct the patient to take drug with meal and report signs of gastric distress. Be alert for tarry stools (melena) or anemia, which are early signs of otherwise undetectable gastric bleeding.

8. Monitor fluid balance and daily weights. Increase in B.P. and fluid retention may occur within 2 wk of initiation of drug. Dietary sodium restriction and potassium supplements may be necessary.

9. Check the patient for muscle weakness and wasting, signs of negative nitrogen balance.

10. The patient should be protected against and warned to avoid falls because drugs may cause osteoporosis and increased susceptibility to fractures.

11. Patients receiving long-term therapy should be evaluated for hyperglycemia and glycosuria because of diabetogenic potential of drugs.

12. Observe the patient for and report signs of Cushing's syndrome resulting from excessive endogenous or exogenous adrenocorticosteroids: rounding of face, acne, muscle weakness, hirsutism, hypertension, osteoporosis, edema, amenorrhea, striae and thinning of skin, ecchymosis, impaired glucose tolerance, negative nitrogen balance, alkalosis, and behavioral disturbances.

14. Observe the patient for signs of muscle rigidity or convulsions in children since drugs may lower seizure threshold. An increase in steroid dose may be required in epileptic patients receiving phenobarbital or phenytoin (Dilantin) since these drugs stimulate metabolism of steroids.

SUPPLEMENTARY READINGS

Azarnoff, D. L., ed., *Steroid Therapy*. Philadelphia: W. B. Saunders Company, 1975.

Baxter, J. D., "Glucocorticoid Hormone Action," *Pharmacology and Toxicology B* **2**: 605–59 (1976).

Blount, M. and A. B. Kinney, "Chronic Steroid Therapy," *American Journal of Nursing* **74**: 1626–31 (1974).

Bond, W. S., "Toxic Reactions and Side Effects of Glucocorticoids in Man," *American Journal of Hospital Pharmacy* **34**: 479–85 (1977).

Byyny, R. L., "Withdrawal from Glucocorticoid Therapy," *New England Journal of Medicine* **295**: 30–32 (1976).

Cope, C. L., *Adrenal Steroids and Disease* (2nd ed.). Philadelphia: J. B. Lippincott Company, 1972.

Glaz, E., and P. Vecsei, *Aldosterone*. Oxford: Pergamon Press, Inc., 1971.

Grant, I. W. B., D. M. Harris, and P. Turner, eds., "Proceedings of a Symposium on Beclomethasone Dipropionate Aerosols—April 1977," *British Journal of Clinical Pharmacology* **4** (Suppl. 3): 251S–302S (1977).

Grieco, M. H., and P. Cushman, Jr., "Adrenal Glucocorticoids After Twenty Years. A Review of their Clinically Relevant Consequences," *Journal of Chronic Diseases* **22**: 637–711 (1970).

Melby, J. C., "Clinical Pharmacology of Systemic Corticosteroids," *Annual Review of Pharmacology and Toxicology* **17**: 511–27 (1977).

Rheumatism Review Committee, "Rheumatism and Arthritis," *Annals of Internal Medicine* **59**: 1–125 (1963).

Ross, E. J. "Aldosterone and its Antagonists," *Clinical Pharmacology and Therapeutics* **6**: 65–106 (1964).

Temple, T. E., and G. W. Liddle, "Inhibitors of Adrenal Steroids Biosynthesis," *Annual Review of Pharmacology* **10**: 199–218 (1970).

Thompson, E. B., and M. E. Lippman, "Mechanism of Action of Glucorticoids," *Metabolism* **23**: 159–202 (1974).

Thorn, G. W., ed., "Symposium on the Adrenal Cortex," *American Journal of Medicine* **53**: 529–700 (1972).

THYROID HORMONE AND ANTITHYROID DRUGS

The *thyroid hormone* manufactures and secretes *thyroxine* and *triiodothyronine*, hormones that have a profound influence on the rate of cellular metabolism and also play an important role in normal growth and development. The critical importance of the thyroid gland in maintaining the homeostatic balance of the body can be readily appreciated when we examine disorders associated with inadequate and excessive hormonal secretions. These disorders, *hypothyroidism* and *hyperthyroidism*, can be effectively managed by replacement with thyroid hormones or administration of antithyroid drugs, respectively.

PHYSIOLOGY OF THE THYROID GLAND

In this section, we shall discuss the biosynthesis of the thyroid hormones, factors that control their release, and their normal physiological functions.

Biosynthesis of Thyroid Hormones

Biosynthesis of the thyroid hormones occurs in four steps: (1) iodide trapping; (2) oxidation of iodide to free iodine; (3) attachment of iodine to the amino acid tyrosine to form iodinated tyrosine derivatives; and (4) coupling of two iodotyrosine molecules to form thyroxine and triiodothyronine (Figure 35-1).

Small, but adequate, supplies of *iodide* are generally provided by the diet and are contained in drinking water, seafood, and soil in coastal regions in which leafy vegetables are grown. Such dietary sources of iodide are inadequate in certain geographic regions, such as the midwestern United States; in the past, thyroid deficiencies were endemic in these areas. Inadequate natural sources of iodide can be readily supplemented by use of *iodized table salt;* in the United States, 0.1 g of iodide is contained in each gram of salt.

By an extremely efficient active transport process, the thyroid gland is capable of concentrating the body's iodide. This *iodide trapping* accounts for the ability of the normally functioning thyroid gland to concentrate iodide to levels 20 to 50 times those present in the plasma.

After having gained access to the thyroid follicular cells, iodide is *oxidized to iodine*, which is then attached to the amino acid tyrosine to form monoiodotyrosine and

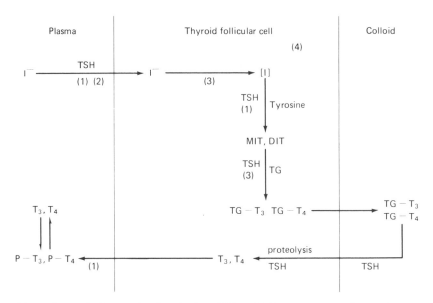

Figure 35-1. Pathways for Synthesis of Thyroid Hormones and Sites of Drug Action. Abbreviations: I^- = dietary iodide; [I] = iodine; MTI = monoiodotyrosine; DIT = diiodotyrosine; T_3 = triiodothyronine; T_4 = thyroxine; TSH = thyrotropin (thyroid-stimulating hormone); TG = thyroglobulin; P = plasma proteins. **Sites of inhibition by drugs:** (1) excess iodide (potassium iodide); (2) perchlorate; (3) thioamides; (4) radioactive iodine (^{131}I).

diiodotyrosine. The final step in the biosynthesis of thyroid hormones involves the coupling of two diiodotyrosine molecules to form tetraiodothyronine or *thyroxine* (T_4) or the coupling of one molecule of monoiodotyrosine and diiodotyrosine to form *triiodothyronine* (T_3). Normally, the ratio of thyroxine to triiodothyronine is about 3:1. These hormones are stored in the colloid of the glandular follicles as part of a large glycoprotein *thyroglobulin*.

Control of Release

Thyroglobulin is too large to pass across the cell membranes of the follicles and enter the bloodstream. By the action of proteolytic enzymes, thyroglobulin is broken down, freeing the thyroid hormones and permitting them to enter the circulation. In euthyroid individuals, the daily secretion rates of thyroxine and triiodothyronine are 70 μg and 25 μg, respectively; T_3 is three to four times more potent than T_4.

Less than 0.1 percent of the total thyroxine found in the plasma is free and available to exert its biological effects. Approximately 85 percent is bound to *thyroxine-binding globulin*, with the remainder bound to thyroxine-binding prealbumin. Less than 0.5 percent of the total plasma triiodothyronine is free, with the remainder plasma-protein bound, although less strongly than thyroxine.

The functional activity of the thyroid gland is controlled by the anterior pituitary hormone *thyrotropin* (thyroid-stimulating hormone, TSH), which in turn is controlled by hypothalamic TSH-releasing hormone. In the absence of either hormone, the thyroid gland atrophies. Normal thyrotropin secretion increases the mass of the cells of the thyroid gland (hypertrophy), augments iodide trapping, and stimulates thyroid hormone synthesis and the rate of stored hormone release into the circulation. The rate of thyrotropin secretion is controlled by the levels of circulating hormones, with even slightly elevated levels reducing the release of this pituitary hormone by a negative feedback mechanism.

Physiological Effects

Thyroid hormones increase the *metabolic rate* of most of the cells of the body, augmenting the rate at which foods are utilized to provide the energy needs of the body. Carbohydrate and fat metabolism are increased, as in oxygen consumption (basal metabolic rate). Normal body growth and development of the central nervous system require a normally functioning thyroid gland.

THYROID DISORDERS

The most commonly encountered disorders associated with thyroid function are goiter, hypothyroidism, and hyperthyroidism.

Goiter

In some thyroid disorders, the gland becomes enlarged, producing an obvious swelling in the neck. This endocrine gland enlargement, called *goiter*, may occur in patients with excessive, deficient, or normal secretion of thyroid hormones.

Simple goiter refers to a condition in which a normal thyroid gland fails to produce an adequate quantity of hormones to meet the body's needs, such as during puberty or pregnancy. In an attempt to satisfy these increased hormonal demands, the pitu-

itary gland secretes additional thyrotropin, which leads to glandular hypertrophy. Goiter is endemic in those geographic regions where dietary iodide intake is inadequate or when substances are ingested that interfere with the utilization of iodide to synthesize thyroid hormones; such *goitrogenic* substances have been found in turnips, cabbages, and kales.

Adult patients with simple goiter are usually euthyroid, but they may exhibit a reduction in urinary iodide excretion and elevated radioactive iodide uptake.

Hypothyroidism

Thyroid deficiencies may be manifested at birth or during infancy (*cretinism*) or in the adult (*myxedema*). Cretinism is caused primarily by a failure of the thyroid gland to develop; myxedema may result from a hypothalamic or pituitary gland disorder, surgical removal of the thyroid gland or inhibition of its normal function by chemicals or irradiation, or from an inadequate dietary intake of iodide.

Cretinism The cretin usually remains undiagnosed for the first 3 to 6 months after birth. Characteristic symptoms include puffy features with a swollen tongue, lack of facial expression, yellow, cold, and dry skin, poor appetite, sluggishness, a distended abdomen and umbilical hernia, and a reduced body temperature and pulse rate. In the absence of thyroid hormone replacement therapy, irreversible mental retardation may result, as well as a marked reduction in the rate of body growth and development.

Myxedema During the early phases of adult hypothyroidism, called *myxedema* or *Gull's disease*, symptoms may be few or absent. Early patient complaints include lethargy, sleepiness, constipation, or weight gain, which is often associated with menstrual disorders. In more advanced cases, the patient's problems include fatigue, intolerance to cold, coarse and sparse hair, brittle nails, and thick, dry skin with the absence of sweating; the face is often puffy and speech is slow.

Hypothyroid patients metabolize drugs more slowly than normal and are, therefore, more sensitive to drug overdosage. Since the usual doses of barbiturates and narcotics may cause severe respiratory depression in these patients, they are usually administered at one-half their normal doses.

Hyperthyroidism

Hyperthyroidism or *thyrotoxicosis*, caused by excessive hormone secretion, is primarily manifested by an increased rate of metabolism, with cardiovascular and neuromuscular abnormalities. The most common type of hyperthyroidism is *Graves' disease*, an autoimmune disorder characterized by toxic (hyperthyroid) diffuse goiter and the presence of the serum gamma globulin long-acting thyroid stimulator (LATS).

The most prominent symptom seen in Graves' disease is *exophthalmos* (protrusion of the eyeballs) with retraction of the upper lids; hence, this disease is sometimes referred to as *exophthalmic goiter.* Other symptoms include warm and moist skin, sweating, weight loss, increased sensitivity to heat and intolerance to cold, fine tremors, menstrual disorders, diarrhea, extreme nervousness, and emotional instability. Alterations in *cardiac function* are the most dangerous consequences of untreated hyperthyroidism and include tachycardia and cardiac arrhythmias, which may lead to cardiac failure. These cardiovascular effects have been attributed to the ability of the thyroid hormones to sensitize the cardiac β-receptors to the actions of the endogenously released catecholamines.

TREATMENT OF HYPOTHYROIDISM AND GOITER

Natural or synthetic preparations of thyroxine or triiodothyronine (Table 35-1) are used to treat hypothyroidism and for conditions in which it is desirable to suppress the secretion of thyrotropin (for example, goiter). Most physicians prefer using thyroid tablets because they are highly effective and the least expensive form of therapy; the latter is of importance since patients generally employ these drugs for a lifetime.

In the management of myxedema, dosage is gradually increased at 2-week intervals until an optimal dose is found or until adverse effects appear. The only potentially hazardous effects are those involving the cardiovascular system and include anginal pain and cardiac palpitations; a rise in pulse rate is among the earliest symptoms of thyroid overdosage. Other, less severe, side effects include nervousness, insomnia, sweating, and weight loss. Potential drug interactions involving the thyroid hormones are given in Table 35-3 (page 306); nursing implications are summarized at the end of this chapter.

It is essential that therapy be instituted immediately after cretinism has been diagnosed in an infant to prevent irreversible mental retardation. With prompt therapy soon after birth, it may be possible for the patient to achieve normal physical and mental development. Adult doses of thyroid hormone are given to children by 5 years of age with no major adverse effects resulting.

The treatment objective in *simple goiter* (thyroid enlargement in the absence of hyperthyroidism) is the effective suppression of thyrotropin secretion. In many cases, a substantial or even total regression in the size of the thyroid gland has been observed. Favorable responses are noted within weeks

Table 35-1 Thyroid Preparations[a]

Generic name	Selected trade names	Composition	Usual daily oral adult dose	Peak effects	Duration of action	Distinguishing characteristics
Thyroid tablets	Thyrar	Powdered gland of cow or pig; T$_4$ and T$_3$.	60–180 mg	1–3 wk	3 wk	Most widely used thyroid preparation; least expensive. Precise T$_4$ and T$_3$ content not known, but generally uniform potency. Deterioration under poor storage conditions.
Thyroglobulin	Proloid	Purified extract of pig gland; T$_4$ and T$_3$.	60–180 mg	1–3 wk	3 wk	Similar to thyroid, but more expensive.
Levothyroxine Sodium (T$_4$)	Synthroid Levoid	Synthetic T$_4$.	0.1–0.2 mg, PO or IV	1–3 wk (oral)	3 wk	Widely used drug of known potency. Highly variable absorption after oral administration; 0.1 mg levothyroxine equal 65 mg thyroid.
Liothyronine Sodium (T$_3$)	Cytomel	Synthetic T$_3$.	50–100 μg (0.050–0.10 mg)	1–3 days	5–6 days	Drug of choice when rapid onset required. Short duration necessitates administration several times daily. Expensive; 25 μg liothyronine equal 65 mg thyroid.
Liotrix (T$_4$ and T$_3$)	Euthyroid Thyrolar	Synthetic T$_4$ and T$_3$ in ratio of 4:1.	Liotrix-"2"	1–3 wk	3 wk	Known ratio of T$_4$ to T$_3$. Expensive, with no proven advantages.

[a]T$_4$ = thyroxine (tetraiodothyronine); T$_3$ = triiodothyronine.

after thyroid hormone therapy is initiated, with maximum benefit requiring many months of continuous therapy. While *endemic goiter*—resulting from a deficiency of dietary iodide—responds favorably to thyroid hormones, most clinicians prefer to treat this condition by supplementing iodide intake.

MANAGEMENT OF HYPERTHYROIDISM

Three modes of therapy are currently employed for the treatment of hyperthyroidism: (1) the use of antithyroid drugs, which inhibit the synthesis of thyroid agents, and adjuncts to therapy that are used to manage some of the symptoms of this disorder; (2) radioactive iodine, which damages the thyroid gland; and (3) surgical removal of all or part of the thyroid gland. *Surgery (thyroidectomy)* is preferred in children and pregnant females, but not in elderly patients or those with cardiovascular diseases that render such individuals poor surgical risks.

Antithyroid Drugs

In our discussion of antithyroid drugs, we shall consider the thioamides that inhibit thyroid hormone synthesis and the iodides.

Table 35-2   Antithyroid Drugs

Generic name	Trade name	Usual adult oral dose	Distinguishing characteristics
Propylthiouracil		300–600 mg daily in divided doses.	Skin rash, agranulocytosis. See nursing implications at the end of this chapter.
Methylthiouracil	Methiocil	200 mg daily in divided doses.	Higher incidence of side effects than propylthiouracil. No longer used in the United States.
Methimazole	Tapazole	15–30 mg daily in divided doses.	Widely used antithyroid drug; incidence of agranulocytosis less than propylthiouracil.
Carbimazole	Neo-mercazole		Very widely used in Great Britain, but not available in the United States.
Strong Iodine Sol. (Lugol's solution)		2–5 gtts (0.1–0.3 ml) t.i.d. 10–14 days preoperatively.	Aqueous solution containing 5% iodine and 10% potassium iodide.
Potassium Iodide Sol. (Saturated solution potassium iodide; SSKI)		Same dose as Lugol's solution.	Aqueous solution containing 1 g of potassium iodide per ml. May be used as a substitute for Lugol's sol.
Propranolol	Inderal	10–40 mg q.i.d.	Not really an antithyroid agent; provides symptomatic relief. Manages tachycardia and arrhythmias in hyperthyroidism. Short-term use preoperatively and prior to and after radioactive iodine.
Sodium Iodide I 131	Iodotope I-131 Oriodide-131 Theriodide-131	4–5 mCi orally.	Used for patients over 30 yr; contraindicated during pregnancy. Safe and highly effective in Graves' disease. Disadvantages: high incidence of hypothyroidism.
Potassium perchlorate			Effective antithyroid drug that acts by interfering with iodide trapping. Rarely used because of risk of aplastic anemia.

Propranolol has been recently approved for use as an adjunctive drug in the management of hyperthyroidism (Table 35-2).

Thioamides Propylthiouracil, methimazole, and other members of a class of antithyroid drugs chemically classified as *thioamides* (Table 35-2), act by interfering with the oxidation of iodide to iodine, the attachment of iodine to tyrosine, and the coupling of iodinated tyrosine molecules, thus preventing the synthesis of thyroxine and triiodothyronine (Figure 35-1). In the absence of the negative feedback inhibitory influence of circulating thyroid hormones, thyrotropin secretion increases, leading to an enlargement of the thyroid (goiter).

After the initiation of therapy, improvement is not clearly manifested for several days to 2 or more weeks until the thyroxine stores in the thyroid gland are depleted. Clinical improvement is exhibited by a reduction in sweating, tremors, basal metabolic rate, and pulse rate. Approximately one-half the patients receiving these drugs on a continuous basis for one year will experience a remission of symptoms that may persist for several years; the remaining patients require additional courses of therapy to remain free of symptoms.

In addition to the use of thioamides for the treatment of Graves' disease, these drugs are employed to prepare hyperthyroid patients for subtotal thyroidectomy. Drug therapy is continued until a euthyroid state is achieved; thereafter, iodide is given 7 to 10 days preoperatively. Pretreatment with these drugs reduces the hazards associated with this surgical procedure.

The most severe adverse effect caused by propylthiouracil and methimazole administration is *agranulocytosis*. This potentially fatal blood dyscrasia occurs in one of 500 to 1,000 patients receiving these drugs. Patients should be advised to stop drug therapy on the appearance of sore throat and fever and immediately contact their physicians. Skin rash is the most frequently encountered side effect; joint pain and stiffness, nausea, and headache may occur occasionally.

Iodide The class containing iodides is the oldest class of drugs employed for the management of thyroid disorders; these drugs are capable of producing the most rapid reduction in elevated thyroid activity and hormone blood levels. Symptoms of hyperthyroidism improve within 24 hours, with maximum beneficial effects observed after 10 to 15 days of drug therapy. Several weeks thereafter, the symptoms of hyperthyroidism return to their initial intensity, despite continuation of drug therapy; therefore, the iodides are not suitable for long-term management of thyrotoxicosis.

The high therapeutic doses of iodide are believed to control disease symptoms by inhibiting the synthesis of thyroid hormones and by suppressing their release from the thyroid gland.

Iodide preparations (Table 35-2), the most important of which is *Lugol's solution* (Strong Iodine Solution), is employed preoperatively mainly to prepare patients for thyroidectomy. Minor adverse effects caused by iodide administration include inflammation of the salivary gland, rhinitis, headache, conjunctivitis, and gastritis.

Propranolol With the realization that the thyroid hormones enhance the effects of endogenously released catecholamines, adrenergic blocking agents have been used to control the cardiovascular and neuromuscular symptoms associated with hyperthyroidism. Propranolol has been found to control tachycardia, arrhythmias, and tremors. This drug is generally employed on a short-term basis in combination with conventional antithyroid drugs prior to thyroidectomy and to provide symptomatic control of hyperthyroidism until the beneficial effects of radioactive iodine treatment occur. The adverse effects and potential drug interactions associated with propranolol are discussed in Chapter 6.

Radioactive Iodine

The radioactive isotope of iodine, I-131, like stable (nonradioactive) iodine, is taken up from the blood stream by the thyroid gland, attaches to tyrosine to form the thyroid hormones, and is stored in the colloid of the follicles. This isotope emits beta rays, which damage and even completely destroy, the thyroid gland while causing virtually no injury to surrounding tissues. The gamma rays emitted by radioactive iodine can be quantified by external detectors to assess the functional state of the thyroid gland.

Therapeutic uses   Radioactive iodine (radioiodine) is employed for the treatment of hyperthyroidism in adults and, in lower (tracer) doses, is used as a diagnostic agent for assessment of thyroid disorders.

Hyperthyroidism   Radioiodine is most useful for the treatment of Graves' disease in patients over 30 years of age, those not contemplating reproduction, individuals with heart disease, or those who have not satisfactorily responded to antithyroid drugs or who have relapsed after total thyroidectomy.

The symptoms of hyperthyroidism are gradually reduced over a 2- to 3-month period after a single oral or intravenous dose of I-131 (4 to 5 mCi). Over one-half of the patients are cured, with most of the remainder favorably responding to a second dose administered three months after the first. To hasten the control of this disorder, antithyroid drugs or propranolol may be administered.

The major disadvantage attendant with the use of this isotope is the development of _hypothyroidism;_ this has been estimated to occur in 70 percent of patients so treated after 10 years. Some clinicians recommend that replacement therapy with thyroid hormone be initiated shortly after radioiodine administration. Because of the high probability of hypothyroidism and carcinogenic potential, this treatment approach is not advised for use in children or adults under 30 years of age; it is also contraindicated during pregnancy.

Diagnostic uses   The ability of the thyroid gland to take up tracer doses of radioiodine (5 to 10 μCi) serves as the basis

Table 35-3   Potential Drug Interactions Involving Thyroid Hormones

Interacting drug/class	Potential consequences

Oral anticoagulants
    Coumarins
    Indandiones
	Thyroid hormones enhance ability of oral anticoagulants to depress activity of vitamin K dependent clotting factor. Increased risk of bleeding has been clinically demonstrated. Reduction in dose of anticoagulant may be required.

Cholestyramine resin (Questran) Colestipol (Colestid)	These resins bind thyroid in the intestines, impairing its absorption. At least a 4-h interval should elapse between administration of these drugs.

Antidiabetic agents
    Insulin
    Oral hypoglycemic drugs
	Thyroid hormone therapy may increase the dosage requirements of antidiabetic agents.

Phenytoin (Dilantin)	Phenytoin is capable of displacing thyroid hormones (thyroxine) from plasma protein binding. Potential risk of thyroid-induced adverse cardiovascular effects after intravenous phenytoin.

for its use in the diagnosis of thyroid disorders. In myxedema, only a small fraction of the isotope is taken up by the thyroid, while most of the administered drug is excreted in the urine. The glands of hyperthyroid patients, by contrast, retain a much larger proportion of radioiodine, with only small amounts excreted.

Thyroid Hormones and Antithyroid Drugs: **nursing implications**

Thyroid hormones

1. Teach the patient the expected therapeutic response and the importance of taking the drug regularly as prescribed. Initial doses are generally small and gradually increased.
2. Observe the patient for therapeutic effects: weight loss, improved appearance of skin and hair, and increased mental alertness.
3. Instruct the patient to report symptoms of thyroid excess: excessive weight loss, palpitations, leg cramps, nervousness, diarrhea, abdominal cramps, headache, insomnia, and intolerance to heat.
4. Hypothyroid patients exhibit increased sensitivity to barbiturates and narcotics and require lower doses.
5. Observe the diabetic patient for hyperglycemia. Increased dosage of antidiabetic drugs may be required.
6. The effects of oral anticoagulants may be potentiated by thyroid. Instruct such patients to report bruising or bleeding.

Propylthiouracil

1. Teach the patient the expected therapeutic response, explaining the nature of the slow improvement anticipated over 2-3 wk.
2. Observe the patient for therapeutic effects: weight gain and reduced pulse rate. Return to euthyroid state may require several months.
3. Instruct the patient to monitor clinical response by recording pulse daily and weight 2-3 times weekly. Sudden weight gain or tachycardia indicate inadequate clinical response.
4. Patients in remission should continue to regularly monitor their pulses and weights and report signs of recurrent hyperthyroidism: tremor, anxiety, increased pulse rate, or weight loss.
5. Instruct the patient to report symptoms of drug overdosage which develop insidiously: contraction of muscle bundles when pricked, mental depression, nonpitting edema, or intolerance to cold.
6. Instruct the patient to discontinue medication and report symptoms of agranulocytosis to the physician: sore throat, fever, rash.

SUPPLEMENTARY READINGS

Burrows, G. N., ed., "Symposium on Current Concepts of Thyroid Disease," *Medical Clinics of North America* **59**(5): 1043–1277 (1975).

DeGroot, L. J., and J. B. Stanbury, *The Thyroid and its Diseases* (4th ed.). New York: John Wiley & Sons, Inc., 1975.

Greep, R. R., and E. B. Astwood, ed., *Thyroid, Handbook of Physiology*, Sec. 7, Vol. 3. Baltimore: The Williams & Wilkins Company, 1974.

Hallal, J., "Thyroid Disorders," *American Journal of Nursing* **77**: 417–32 (1977).

Liberti, P., and J. B. Stanbury, "The Pharmacology of Substances Affecting the Thyroid Gland," *Annual Review of Pharmacology* **11**: 113–42 (1971).

Mills, L. C., "Drug Treatment in Thyroid Disease," *Seminars in Drug Treatment* **3**:377–402 (1974).

Selenkow, H. A., and F. Hoffman, ed., *Diagnosis and Treatment of Common Thyroid Diseases*. Amsterdam: Excerpta Medica, 1971.

Spaulding, S. W., "Hypothyroidism: Early Diagnosis and Treatment," *Primary Care* **4**: 79–88 (1977).

Stanbury, J. B., and P. L. Kroc, ed., *Human Development and the Thyroid Gland*. New York: Plenum Publishing Corporation, 1973.

Werner, S. C., and S. H. Ingbar, ed., *The Thyroid* (3rd ed.). New York: Harper & Row, Publishers, Inc., 1971.

INSULIN, ORAL HYPOGLYCEMIC DRUGS, AND GLUCAGON

Chapter 36

Diabetes mellitus is a very common disease. Approximately 2 percent of all Americans have diabetes, with its prevalence as high as 10 percent among individuals over 60 years of age. Six decades ago, the prognosis for a diabetic child was almost certain death prior to maturity. Although not capable of producing a cure, insulin administration has enabled the diabetic to live a long life enjoying, for the most part, reasonable health.

In this chapter, we shall discuss insulin and its role in the etiology of diabetes; gluca-gon, an insulin antagonist, will also be considered. Oral hypoglycemic agents, widely employed by many diabetic patients, will be examined as well.

PHYSIOLOGY OF INSULIN

In 1921–1922 the Canadians F. G. Banting and C. H. Best demonstrated that an extract obtained from the pancreas had beneficial therapeutic effects in diabetic dogs and humans. *Insulin* was extracted from the pancreas in pure form in 1926, and its precise chemical structure was established in 1954. This hormone is a *protein* consisting of two linked chains, with a total of 51 amino acids. Insulin must be administered by injection; if taken orally, this protein is broken down and inactivated in the gastrointestinal tract.

In addition to serving as an exocrine gland, secreting pancreatic juice containing enzymes for the digestion of foods, the *pancreas* also secretes two hormones. The endocrine activities of the pancreas are carried out by the *islets of Langerhans*, a small group of cells representing only 1.5 percent of the total weight of this organ. The alpha cells secrete *glucagon*, while the beta cells manufacture, store, and secrete *insulin;* these mutually antagonistic hormones participate in fuel utilization and fuel storage, respectively.

Metabolic Effects of Insulin

Insulin's primary physiological function is the *conservation* of all the metabolic fuels that supply the energy needs of the body. To accomplish this objective, we shall observe that this hormone exerts profound effects on the metabolism of carbohydrates, fats, and proteins. Conversely, in the absence of adequate insulin secretion (such as in the diabetic patient), marked disturbances occur in the storage and metabolism of these endogenous compounds.

Carbohydrates Insulin is the principal hormone controlling carbohydrate metabolism. The most prominent effect observed after insulin injection is a rapid reduction in blood glucose levels. This *hypoglycemic effect* results from insulin enhancement of glucose transport across cell membranes, thus permitting this sugar to enter the cell. The most important sites of this action are

skeletal muscle and adipose (fat) tissue; by contrast, glucose can enter the brain, kidney, and red blood cells even in the absence of insulin.

Once glucose enters the cell, insulin is required for its biochemical conversion to glycogen, the normal storage form of this sugar. Large amounts of glycogen are stored in the liver and muscle, and when the energy requirements of the body are increased (such as during exercise), glycogen is broken down and glucose becomes available.

Fats and proteins In addition to being immediately utilized as a source of energy or being stored as glycogen, glucose can be converted to *triglycerides* (esters of glycerol and fatty acids) which are stored in adipose tissues. Insulin is not only required for triglyceride synthesis, but it also inhibits lipase, an enzyme which catalyzes the breakdown of triglycerides to free fatty acids. The major cause of death in uncontrolled diabetes, ketosis, results from aberrations in fat metabolism causing acidosis.

Lack of insulin decreases the rate of protein synthesis and augments the breakdown of proteins to amino acids. Insulin increases the transport of amino acids into cells and promotes the incorporation of amino acids into proteins. Abnormalities in protein metabolism in the diabetic result in delayed wound healing and failure of children to grow at a normal rate.

Control of Insulin Secretion

The rate of insulin release is primarily dependent upon the concentration of *blood glucose*. A rise in blood glucose, as might be observed after food ingestion, activates the rate of insulin secretion, while below normal glucose levels, as between meals, inhibit the rate of insulin release. Subnormal blood sugar levels stimulate the secretion of *epi-*

nephrine from the adrenal medulla and *glucagon* from the pancreas. These hormones, acting via the second messenger cyclic AMP (Chapter 33), promote the breakdown of glycogen to glucose (glycogenolysis).

DIABETES MELLITUS

Two major types of diabetes mellitus are recognized: juvenile-onset (ketosis-prone) and maturity-onset (nonketogenic). *Juvenile-onset diabetes* may occur at any age, but usually makes its appearance—often abruptly—during childhood or adolescence. Insulin synthesis and secretion are virtually absent; when this disease is fully established, beta-cell function is totally lost. This type of diabetes is severe in intensity, difficult to control, and commonly complicated by ketosis.

Maturity-onset (adult-onset) diabetes, the type observed in about 85 percent of all diabetics, is a gradually developing disorder, usually occurring after 35 years of age; the incidence is higher in women. While these patients have functionally active beta cells containing insulin, there appears to be an impairment in its secretion, manifested by a delay in hormone release when blood glucose levels are elevated. Maturity-onset diabetes is generally mild and stable, very rarely associated with ketosis, and, in many patients, can be managed by diet and control of obesity with or without the use of hypoglycemic agents; however, approximately 20 to 30 percent of maturity-onset diabetics are unstable (brittle) and require insulin administration.

Clinical Manifestations of Diabetes

Untreated diabetes mellitus is clinically manifested by hyperglycemia, glycosuria, polyuria, and polyphagia, as well as by feelings of fatigue and loss of weight. Ketosis and acidosis may occur in poorly controlled patients, particularly in the juvenile and unstable adult types. We shall now consider the underlying basis for these symptoms, which result from a decrease in glucose metabolism and an increase in fat and protein metabolism.

Normally, the body manages its glucose frugally. Some is immediately expended to provide energy, while the remainder is stored as glycogen or triglycerides for subsequent utilization; very little glucose is excreted in the urine. The diabetic is incapable of adequately utilizing or conserving glucose. In the absence of insulin, glucose is not transported across cell membranes but remains in the blood, resulting in *hyperglycemia*. When blood sugar levels exceed 180 mg/dl, the excess is excreted in the urine (*glycosuria*). Sugar acts as a diuretic agent, and accompanying its excretion is the loss of large volumes of water (*polyuria*); this excessive water loss causes cellular dehydration and creates extreme feelings of thirst, resulting in the consumption of large volumes of liquids (*polydipsia*). Notwithstanding high blood glucose levels, the diabetic is unable to utilize this sugar intracellularly as a source of energy; hunger (*polyphagia*), weakness, and loss of weight result. Moreover, lack of insulin increases protein breakdown and impairs the rate of protein synthesis from amino acids, thus further contributing to weight loss.

The initial problems confronting the diabetic result from aberrations in carbohydrate metabolism, but disturbances in *fat metabolism* are often ultimately responsible for the morbidity and mortality in the uncontrolled patient. Approximately 30 to 40 percent of dietary glucose is normally stored as fats in the form of triglycerides. Less than 5 percent of this sugar is so stored by the diabetic, resulting in very high levels of free fatty acids. These free fatty acids are metabolized to ketone bodies (*ketosis*), which alters the acid-base balance of the body and causes *acidosis*. In the absence of prompt treatment, *ketoacidosis* may result in unconsciousness (*diabetic coma*) and death. Diabetic coma is sometimes mistaken for severe alcohol intoxication; however, rather than having the smell of alcohol on the breath, the diabetic often—but not always—has the odor of the ketone, acetone.

Nursing Responsibilities

One of the major nursing responsibilities for the care of the diabetic involves educating the patient about the general nature of this disorder and the need for chronic treatment. In addition, the nurse should instruct the patient in self-care including: recognition of the early symptoms of hyperglycemia and hypoglycemia and how to manage them; urine testing for the presence of glucose; proper administration of insulin or oral hypoglycemic agents or both; dietary instructions; and personal hygiene, including care of the feet and skin. Nursing implications associated with diabetes and insulin administration are summarized at the end of this chapter.

INSULIN TREATMENT OF DIABETES

In this section, we shall consider the therapeutic uses of insulin, differences among the available insulin preparations, and potential adverse effects associated with its administration.

Therapeutic Uses of Insulin

Insulin is clinically employed for the chronic management of diabetes mellitus and for the emergency treatment of diabetic ketoacidosis and coma.

Chronic management of diabetes mellitus   The most common therapeutic use of insulin is for the symptomatic management of diabetes, when this disorder cannot be controlled by modifications in diet only. While insulin may be employed effectively in all types of diabetes, it is required in juvenile-onset and in unstable maturity-onset types. The objective in therapy is to maintain fasting blood glucose levels (60 to 100 mg/dl) or plasma/serum levels (70 to 115 mg/dl) within normal limits, which is associated with minimal physiological and degenerative changes, and maintains a sense of well-being in the patient.

Although the average daily dose of insulin is 40 to 60 units, each diabetic patient must employ that dose which best fulfills his or her unique requirements. This dose is determined by many factors that are subject to daily variations, including the level of endogenously secreted insulin, diet, level of exercise, and other concurrently existing illnesses or stresses. The patient must understand that determination of daily insulin requirements is essential for the maintenance of good health and well-being. Inadequate insulin doses will not completely control the disease symptoms, while excessive amounts will produce an exaggerated reduction in blood sugar (hypoglycemic reaction) with potentially fatal consequences. The patient should understand completely that insulin does not cure diabetes but must be employed for a lifetime to replace the insufficient amounts of insulin secreted by the pancreas.

While insulin provides symptomatic relief and reduces the acute risks associated with this hormonal disorder, the *chronic complications* of diabetes continue. These chronic problems include degenerative changes to the blood vessels, kidneys (diabetic nephropathy), eyes (diabetic retinopathy, the third most common cause of blindness in the United States), and nervous system (neuropathy). Reduced blood flow to the extremities causes slow wound healing, infections, ulceration, and, in advances cases, gangrene. The diabetic has a higher than normal risk of atherosclerosis and coronary artery disease. At this time, it has not been clearly established whether insulin's control of blood sugar within normal limits protects the patient against the development of these chronic complications.

Diabetic ketoacidosis and coma

Failure to satisfactorily control diabetes or the development of refractoriness to insulin may result in severe dehydration and ketoacidosis, which is clinically manifested by coma, circulatory failure and, in the absence of emergency treatment, death. Successful management involves intravenous and subcutaneous insulin administration and replacement of fluid and electrolyte losses with isotonic sodium chloride and potassium supplementation. Patients may require 1000 units of insulin or more during the first 24 hours of treatment to reduce the extreme hyperglycemia. Clinical responses are evaluated by monitoring the decline in plasma glucose and ketone levels.

Insulin Preparations and their Administration

Commercial insulin preparations, obtained from the pancreas of beef and pigs, are supplied in 10 ml vials containing 40, 80, and 100 units/ml; these preparations are referred to as U-40, U-80, and U-100, respectively. In the coming years, only U-100 insulin will be available in an attempt to (1) reduce the risk of patient error associated with the availability of preparations having different concentrations and syringes having dual calibrations; (2) reduce the injection volume required; and (3) make the dosage and dilutions metric for ease in calculations. Concentrated

solutions of insulin injection (regular insulin) are available (containing 500 units/ml) for emergency use in the treatment of ketoacidosis and for patients requiring very large doses of this hormone because of the development of resistance.

Available preparations

Preparations of insulin are classified as fast-, intermediate-, or long-acting according to their onset, time of peak activity, and duration of their effects on blood sugar after subcutaneous injection (Table 36-1).

Regular insulin has a rapid onset and short duration of action. This preparation, administered 20 to 30 minutes prior to meals, must be given 2 or 3 times daily and produces large fluctuations in blood glucose levels between doses. The main uses of this preparation are restricted to the emergency treatment of ketoacidosis and in patients whose insulin requirements change rapidly, such as during acute infections or during a postoperative recovery period. This is the only insulin preparation that may be safely given by intravenous administration.

With the addition of zinc and the protein protamine to insulin (*protamine zinc insulin suspension*), insulin is slowly released from the site of injection into the blood. This preparation is slow in onset (4 to 6 hours) but maintains its hypoglycemic effects for over 24 hours after a single injection. The primary disadvantage of this preparation is the danger of hypoglycemia during the night. For the severely diabetic patient, the onset of this product may be too slow. To overcome this difficulty, 2 to 3 units of regular insulin may be mixed and co-administered with one unit of protamine zinc insulin suspension. *Isophane insulin suspension* (*NPH insulin*) has time-response effects on blood glucose similar to this mixture, namely, a relatively rapid onset of action (1 to 2 hours) and a moderately long duration of action (18 to 28 hours).

Table 36-1   Comparative Properties of Insulin Prepartions

Official (U.S.P.) name (common name)	Trade name	Onset of action (h)	Time of peak effect (h)	Duration of action (h)	Remarks
Fast-Acting Insulin Types					
Insulin Injection (Regular Insulin)	Iletin	0.5–1	2–4	4–8	Only type safe intravenously; no protein modifier.
Prompt Insulin Zinc Suspension	Semilente	0.5–1	4–6	10–14	No protein modifier; deep subcutaneous injection.
Intermediate-Acting Insulin Types					
Globin Zinc Insulin Injection	Globin Zinc Insulin	1–2	6–10	18–24	Contains protein globin; deep subcutaneous injection.
Isophane Insulin Suspension (Isophane Insulin; Isophane Insulin Injection)	NPH Insulin NPH Iletin	1–2	6–10	18–28	Contains protein protamine; mix carefully before using.
Insulin Zinc Suspension (Lente Insulin)	Lente Iletin	2–4	10–12	18–28	No protein modifier; deep subcutaneous injection.
Long-Acting Insulin Types					
Protamine Zinc Insulin Suspension (Protamine Zinc Insulin)	Protamine Zinc and Iletin	4–6	10–14	over 36	Contains protein protamine; mix carefully before using.
Extended Insulin Zinc Suspension	Ultralente Iletin	6–8	10–14	over 36	No protein modifier; deep subcutaneous injection.

Administration   All insulin preparations should be *refrigerated* but not frozen. Insulin suspensions should be carefully mixed, but not shaken, immediately prior to withdrawal of the required dose.

The nurse should instruct the patient or a member of the family on the proper technique associated with *subcutaneous* drug administration. Loose connective tissues, generally in the arms, thighs, buttocks, or abdomen are the preferred sites of injection. Since insulin may be irritating and the diabetic is more susceptible than the normal individual to infection, sites of injection must be rotated and ideally should not be used more frequently than once a month.

Overdosage and Adverse Effects

The nurse should participate in the instruction of the diabetic to prevent the occurrence of *hypoglycemic reactions.* The importance of not missing meals and the avoidance of wide fluctuations in diet must be emphasized, and the patient must be aware of the symptoms of hypoglycemia.

Early signs of hypoglycemia include feelings of hunger and weakness, sweating, nausea, and nervousness. In more advanced stages, the patient will experience mental confusion, incoherent speech, double vision, loss of consciousness (insulin coma), and convulsions. A severe and prolonged hypoglycemic reaction, if untreated, can result in permanent brain damage or death. Patients should be advised to carry lump sugar or hard candy or to take a liquid containing carbohydrates at the first signs of hypoglycemia. Moreover, such individuals should be urged to carry cards that identify them as diabetics. Unconscious patients may be treated with intravenous injections of glucose (dextrose) solutions or with glucagon (see page 317).

Local allergic reactions to insulin, including itching, redness, and swelling at the site of injection, are often observed during the early days of treatment. These responses generally subside spontaneously, although in some cases it may be necessary to select a different brand of insulin.

Potential drug interactions involving insulin are given in Tables 36-3 and 36-4 (page 316) and nursing implications are summarized at the end of this chapter.

ORAL HYPOGLYCEMIC DRUGS

While insulin has dramatically altered the prognosis for diabetic patients, this hormone must be injected one or more times daily to control blood sugar levels. The *oral hypoglycemic agents* were developed as a simple and more acceptable alternative to insulin. Nevertheless, since very basic differences exist between these drugs and insulin, the nurse should never consider these drugs to be "oral insulin substitutes" that can be employed interchangeably with insulin.

There are two major classes of oral hypoglycemic agents, namely, the biguanides and the sulfonylureas; the latter is the only class now available for general use in the United States (Table 36-2).

Biguanides

Phenformin (DBI, Meltrol) is the only biguanide that has been approved for the treat-

Table 36-2   Comparative Properties of Oral Hypoglycemic Agents

Generic name	Trade name	Peak effect (h)	Duration of action (h)	Adult usual oral daily dose (maximum safe dose)	Distinguishing characteristics
Sulfonylureas					
Tolbutamide	Orinase	4–6	6–12	1500 mg (3 g)	Generally drug of first choice; lowest incidence of side effects. Useful in renal impairment. Short duration of action.
Acetohexamide	Dymelor	3	12–24	750 mg (1.5 g)	Highest incidence of gastrointestinal side effects. Apart from longer duration of action, no advantages over tolbutamide.
Tolazamide	Tolinase	4–6	10–14	250 mg (1 g)	Similar to tolbutamide.
Chlorpropamide	Diabinese	10	up to 60	250 mg (750 mg)	Among the most effective sulfonylureas with the longest duration of action and highest incidence of adverse effects.
Biguanide					
Phenformin	DBI Meltrol	4	12, for extended release capsule.	100 mg (200 mg)	Effective hypoglycemic agent but withdrawn from general usage in the United States because of risk of fatal lactic acidosis.

ment of diabetes in the United States. The hypoglycemic effects of this drug have been attributed to an extrapancreatic effect, namely, to its ability to promote the uptake of glucose by skeletal muscle. This drug does not lower blood sugar levels in nondiabetic patients.

While clinically effective, phenformin was withdrawn from the general American market in 1977 because of the high risk of the potentially fatal *lactic acidosis.* This drug may be obtained from the manufacturer for use in selected patients. Phenformin has been used for the treatment of stable maturity-onset diabetes and, when used in combination with insulin, may also be effective in managing juvenile and brittle maturity-onset types. The usual dose of phenformin (when employed alone) is 50 to 100 mg in two divided doses.

The most common side effects involve the gastrointestinal tract and include a metallic taste, anorexia, nausea, and vomiting. These effects may be reduced by advising the patient to take this drug with meals.

Sulfonylureas

The sulfonylurea oral hypoglycemic agents are chemically related to the antibacterial sulfonamides (Chapter 42). The members of this class have similar actions and therapeutic indications, and differ primarily with respect to their potency, onset, and duration of action (Table 36-2).

The hypoglycemic effects of the sulfonylureas have been attributed to their abilities to stimulate the release of insulin from the beta cells of the pancreas. In the absence of a pancreas, or in diabetics where there is a total absence or gross deficiency of insulin secretion (juvenile-onset), these drugs are ineffective and should not be employed. These drugs are therapeutically indicated for the management of stable maturity-onset diabetes.

Toxicity The overall incidence of adverse effects to the sulfonylureas is less than 10 percent, with chlorpropamide (Diabinese) having the highest incidence and tolbutamide (Orinase) the lowest. Side effects that are common to all members of this class include gastrointestinal disturbances (loss of appetite, nausea, abdominal cramps, and diarrhea), weakness, headache, tinnitus, allergic skin reactions, and blood disorders. A disulfiram-type reaction (Chapter 14) has been observed when alcoholic beverages are used by patients taking sulfonylureas.

The risk of prolonged hypoglycemia, which may occur nocturnally, is generally less with oral drugs than with insulin. This effect, most frequently seen after chlorpropamide, is rarely caused by such short-acting drugs as tolbutamide.

The sulfonylureas are contraindicated during pregnancy because of their potential adverse effects on the fetus and in the presence of renal glycosuria because of the danger of fatal hypoglycemia. Potential drug interactions that may result in an antagonism of the antidiabetic effects of tolbutamide and related drugs are given in Table 36-3 (page 316); drug interactions that may potentiate their hypoglycemic response are summarized in Table 36-4 (page 316). Nursing implications are summarized at the end of this chapter.

UGDP controversy In 1970 a report appeared that was initially intended to evaluate the effectiveness of antidiabetic therapy in preventing or reducing the incidence of vascular disease in diabetic patients. Eight hundred noninsulin-requiring patients at twelve different university-based diabetic clinics (University-Group Diabetes Program or UGDP) were compared for up to an eight-year period; patients received one

Table 36-3   Potential Interactions of Antidiabetic Agents with Drugs that Produce Hyperglycemia[a]

Interacting drug/class	Mechanism underlying antagonism of antidiabetic effect
Corticosteroids	Intrinsic hyperglycemic effect of corticosteroids.
Dextrothyroxine (Choloxin)	Possible intrinsic hyperglycemic effect of thyroid hormone analog.
Diazoxide (Hyperstat I.V.)	Produces clinically significant hyperglycemia.
Epinephrine (Adrenalin)	Decreases glucose uptake by tissues and increases glycogen breakdown to glucose.
Guanethidine (Ismelin)	Mechanism unknown.
Oral contraceptives	May impair glucose tolerance.
Rifampin (Rifadin, Rimactane)	Stimulates tolbutamide metabolism.
Thiazide diuretics	Increases blood glucose in diabetics and prediabetics. Easily reversible; increased dose of antidiabetic agents rarely required.
Thyroid hormone	See dextrothyroxine.

[a]Interaction may result in a loss of antidiabetic control, which might require increased dosage requirements of antidiabetic agents. Unless otherwise stated, interaction potentially involves insulin and sulfonylurea oral hypoglycemic agents.

Table 36-4   Potential Interactions of Antidiabetic Agents with Drugs that Produce or Increase Risk of Hypoglycemia[a]

Interacting drug/class	Mechanism underlying enhanced hypoglycemia
Alcohol (Ethanol)	1. Acute alcohol ingestion, especially by alcoholics, may modify carbohydrate metabolism of diabetics, resulting in hypoglycemia (hyperglycemia has been reported in a few studies). 2. Chronic alcohol ingestion may increase the rate of tolbutamide metabolism. 3. Chlorpropamide and others may provoke a disulfiram-type reaction when taken with alcohol (flushing, headache, and so on).

Anabolic steroids
    Methandrostenolone (Dianabol)
    Testosterone
	Hypoglycemic effects in diabetics, not normal patients. May also inhibit metabolism of oral hypoglycemic agents.

β-Adrenergic blockers Propranolol (Inderal)	Blocks homeostatic response to hypoglycemia.
Chloramphenicol (Chloromycetin)	Inhibition of tolbutamide metabolism.
Coumarin oral anticoagulants	Inhibition of metabolism of sulfonylurea agents. Clinically significant.
Monoamine oxidase inhibitor antidepressants	May cause significant drop in blood glucose at therapeutic doses, possibly blocking homeostatic response to hypoglycemia. Clinically significant.
Phenylbutazone (Butazolidin)	Inhibits tolbutamide metabolism and displacement from plasma-protein binding. Interferes with urinary excretion of active metabolite of acetohexamide. Clinically significant.
Salicylates (aspirin)	Moderate to large doses (5-6 g) have intrinsic effect on carbohydrate metabolism resulting in hypoglycemic response in diabetics.
Sulfonamides	Inhibits sulfonylurea metabolism or displacement from plasma-protein binding. Established for sulfaphenazole (Sulfabid—no longer available in United States). Possible interaction with sulfamethazine, sulfisoxazole (Gantrisin), and sulfamethizole (Thiosulfil).

[a]Interaction may result in pronounced hypoglycemic reaction and diabetic coma. A reduction in the dosage of antidiabetic agents may be required.

of the following treatments: diet and placebo, insulin, tolbutamide, or phenformin. It was unexpectedly observed that the incidence of cardiovascular mortality was highest in those patients receiving tolbutamide and phenformin.

The results of this study have been interpreted by many investigators to indicate that: (1) the combination of diet and tolbutamide is no more effective than diet alone in prolonging life or preventing nonfatal complications; and (2) tolbutamide and diet may be less effective than diet alone or than diet and insulin in reducing cardiovascular mortality. On the basis of this study, the American Diabetes Association has advised that attempts be made to use diet to manage maturity-onset diabetes in the absence of ketosis. If control is not achieved with diet, they suggest that insulin be used rather than oral hypoglycemic agents because insulin is more effective and probably is safer.

The appearance of the UGDP report has generated considerable—and often heated—comment both supporting and refuting these conclusions. More recent studies suggest that users of the oral hypoglycemic agents have a higher incidence of cardiac arrhythmias and myocardial infarction than diabetics who are being managed with diet alone. Whether or not the conclusions of the UGDP report are valid, it is generally accepted that *proper diet* and *weight reduction* are of critical importance in the successful management of maturity-onset diabetes.

GLUCAGON

The protein hormone *glucagon* physiologically acts to increase blood sugar levels between meals and during periods of hypoglycemia thus making available a source of energy. This *hyperglycemic effect* is accomplished by activating liver glycogen breakdown and stimulating glucose synthesis from amino acid starting materials. Thus, while insulin serves to store fuels, glucagon activates fuel mobilization.

The primary therapeutic use of glucagon is for the treatment of *insulin-induced hypoglycemia* when a solution of glucose (dextrose) is not available. A return to consciousness should be observed within 20 minutes after subcutaneous administration of glucagon hydrochloride (1 mg). In the absence of a favorable response, glucose should be intravenously administered without delay. Glucagon is ineffective in raising blood sugar levels once liver glycogen has been depleted, such as after a hypoglycemic reaction of long duration. Patients receiving glucagon should remain under very close medical supervision; within 1.5 hours after a single injection, blood sugar will fall to normal or even hypoglycemic levels. To preclude the risk of the patient returning to a diabetic coma, glucose should be given orally or by injection.

Diazoxide

Diazoxide is employed intravenously for the treatment of hypertensive crisis (Chapter 28). *Orally* administered diazoxide (Proglycem) is therapeutically used to increase blood glucose levels in hypoglycemic conditions. The hyperglycemic effects of this drug have been attributed to its ability to inhibit insulin release from the pancreas, as well as to decrease the utilization of glucose by peripheral tissues.

Diazoxide is clinically indicated for the management of hypoglycemia resulting from excessive insulin secretion from islet-cell tumors or extrapancreatic malignancies in adults and children. The hyperglycemic effect begins within 1 hour after drug administration and, in patients with normal kidney function, generally persists no longer than 8 hours. The usual daily dose is 3 to 8 mg/kg in 2 or 3 equal, divided doses every 8 to 12 hours. Dosage must be individualized, based upon the severity of the hypoglycemic condition, blood glucose level, impairment of renal function, and the clinical response of the patient.

The most prominent side effect is *fluid retention* resulting from a reduction in sodium and water excretion. This drug should be used cautiously in patients with compromised cardiac reserve because it may precipitate congestive heart failure; fluid retention usually responds favorably to diuretic administration. Unlike intravenously administered diazoxide (Hyperstat I.V.), changes in blood pressure are not marked with the oral preparation. The latter product may increase pulse rate and serum uric acid levels. Thiazide diuretics (Chapter 32) may intensify the hyperglycemic and hyperuricemic effects of diazoxide.

Overdosage of diazoxide causes marked hyperglycemia, which may be associated with ketoacidosis. These effects respond to insulin administration and restoration of the fluid and electrolyte balance.

Insulin and Oral Hypoglycemic Drugs:
nursing implications

1. Teach the patient and a responsible family member the nature of diabetes mellitus; the cause, symptoms, prevention, and treatment of hypoglycemia and ketoacidosis; the importance of following the diet and maintaining optimal body weight; the exercise program; and personal hygiene to prevent infections and peripheral vascular complications.

2. Emphasize importance of regular followup visits for blood sugar evaluation and adjustment of medication, if necessary.

3. Instruct the patient to carry a card identifying the individual as a diabetic, the name of the physician to be contacted in case of emergency, and the dose and identity of the antidiabetic medications used.

4. Teach dietary management including weight control; use of diabetic exchange lists; and time for ingestion of food relative to time of peak drug action.

5. Observe the patient for symptoms of hypoglycemia: headache, fatigue, drowsiness, lassitude, tremors, nausea, sweating, and nervousness. Promptly administer rapidly absorbed carbohydrate and notify the physician.

6. Treat patients with severe hypoglycemia with IV glucose (10–50%) or glucagon. As soon as patient is fully conscious, oral carbohydrate should be given.

7. Advise the patient to carry candy or lumps of sugar at all times for management of hypoglycemic reactions.

8. Teach patient to watch for signs of hyperglycemia: thirst, polyuria, drowsiness, flushed dry skin, decreased blood pressure, and fruity odor to breath.

9. Diabetic ketoacidosis is a medical emergency treated with IV insulin. It is precipitated

by infection, illness, emotional stress, surgery, or pregnancy. During treatment, monitor fluid intake and output, blood pressure, urinary sugar, and acetone.

Insulin

1. Teach the patient and a responsible family member the action of insulin, its administration and storage, and adjustment of dosage, if necessary, in relation to sugar urine tests, illness, change in activity, diet, travel, or pregnancy.

2. If insulin is temporarily unavailable, instruct the patient to decrease food intake by one-third and drink large amounts of noncaloric fluids. Insulin should be used as soon as possible to return to the normal dosing schedule and diet.

3. In event of illness, advise the patient to continue insulin use and drink noncaloric fluids liberally. If unable to eat the prescribed diet, replace it with liquid carbohydrate. Test urine for sugar and acetone four times daily and consult the physician for adjustments in insulin dosage.

4. Juvenile diabetics are more susceptible to insulin shock and diabetic coma than adult-onset diabetics. Observe the patient closely for infection or emotional disturbances which may increase insulin requirements.

5. Activity and insulin requirements vary inversely, that is, insulin requirements decrease when the patient is physically active.

Oral Hypoglycemic Agents

1. Observe the patient carefully during first week to evaluate therapeutic response.

2. Instruct the patient to report side effects: pruritis, jaundice, skin rash, dark urine, fever, sore throat, or diarrhea.

3. Patients who become hypoglycemic after use of long-acting drugs should be closely monitored for 3-5 da.

4. With long-acting hypoglycemic agents, observe the patient for mild CNS symptoms and report changes in sleep patterns, frequent nightmares, night sweats, or morning headaches to the physician.

5. Patients receiving oral agents should be taught how to administer insulin because it may be required during periods of extreme stress or illness.

6. Instruct the patient to monitor weight and note ratio of fluid intake to output. Weight gain should be reported.

7. Caution patient that alcohol intolerance (flushing, pounding headache, or tachycardia) may occur and last 1-4 h.

SUPPLEMENTARY READINGS

Ehrlich, R. M. "Diabetes Mellitus in Childhood." *Primary Care* **1**: 613-24 (1974).

Elenbaas, R. M., and P. J. Forni, "Management of Insulin Allergy and Resistance," *American Journal of Hospital Pharmacy* **33**: 491-97 (1976).

Guthrie, D. W., *Nursing Management of Diabetes Mellitus.* St. Louis: C. V. Mosby Company, 1977.

Hussar, D. A., "The Hypoglycemic Agents—Their Interactions," *Journal of the American Pharmaceutical Association* NS **10**: 619–24 (1970).

Karam, J. H., S. B. Matin, and P. H. Forsham, "Antidiabetic Drugs after the University Group Diabetes Program (UGDP)," *Annual Review of Pharmacology* **15**: 351–66 (1975).

Larner, J., "Insulin and Oral Hypoglycemic Drugs; Glucagon," in *Goodman and Gilman's The Pharmacological Basis of Therapeutics* (6th ed.), ed. A. G. Gilman, L. S. Goodman, and A. Gilman, Chapter 64, pp. 1497–1523. New York: Macmillan, Inc., 1980.

Pilkis, S. J., and C. R. Park, "Mechanism of Action of Insulin," *Annual Review of Pharmacology* **14**: 365–88 (1974).

Podolsky, S., ed., "Symposium on Diabetes Mellitus," *Medical Clinics of North America* **62** (4): 625–869 (1978).

Seltzer, H. S., "Drug-Induced Hypoglycemia—A Review Based on 473 Cases," *Diabetes* **21**: 955–66 (1972).

Shen, S. W., and R. Bressler, "Clinical Pharmacology of Oral Antidiabetic Agents," *New England Journal of Medicine* **206**: 787–93 (1977).

Steiner, D. P., and N. Freinek, ed., "Endocrine Pancreas," *Endocrinology*, Vol. 1. Handbook of Physiology, Section 7. Washington, D.C.: American Physiological Society, 1972.

Unger, R. H., and L. Orci, "Role of Glucagon in Diabetes," *Archives of Internal Medicine* **137**: 482–91 (1977).

Walesky, M. E., "Common Problems in Managing Adult Diabetes Mellitus," *American Journal of Nursing* **78**: 871–90 (1978).

Williams, R. H., and D. Porte, Jr., "The Pancreas," in *Textbook of Endocrinology* (5th ed.), ed. R. H. Williams, pp. 502–626. Philadelphia: W. B. Saunders Company, 1974.

THE SEX HORMONES

Chapter 37

Female and male sex hormones are required for the normal development, function, and maintenance of the reproductive organs and secondary sex characteristics. In addition, the pregnant female requires hormones for the successful maintenance of pregnancy.

In this chapter we shall consider the normal physiological functions of the sex hormones and discuss their uses for the treatment of endocrine and nonendocrine disorders and as contraceptive agents. The use of drugs to increase the motility of the smooth muscle of the pregnant female uterus will be examined in the next chapter.

FEMALE SEX HORMONES

The *ovary*, the female gonad, is both the site of the formation of the ovum (egg) and the endocrine gland responsible for the synthesis and secretion of hormones that control the activity of the female reproductive system and determine secondary sex characteristics. Prior to the onset of puberty, the ovary is relatively dormant. At puberty ovarian function is initiated as is evidenced by the start of the menstrual cycle; this cycle continues for three or four decades and then ceases at menopause.

The Menstrual Cycle

The functional activity of the ovaries is under the control of two *gonadotropic hormones* namely, *follicle-stimulating hormone* (FSH) and *luteinizing hormone* (LH). The rate of secretion of FSH and LH is influenced by hypothalamic releasing factors. The following sequence of events occurs during the normal menstrual cycle (Figure 37-1).

FSH travels in the blood from the anterior pituitary to the ovary, where it stimulates the maturation of the Graffian follicles, from which the ovum will develop. This gonadotropin also activates the secretion of the female sex hormone *estrogen* from the maturing ovarian follicle. By 8 to 10 days after the start of menstruation and several days after the initiation of the release of estrogen, this hormone stimulates proliferation of the uterine mucosa (endometrium). The high blood levels of estrogen achieved by day 10 trigger two hypothalamically mediated effects on the release of gonadotropic hormones from the anterior pituitary: FSH release is markedly suppressed and LH secretion is activated.

On day 14 LH triggers the release of the ovum from the follicle. After *ovulation* has occurred, the ovum moves down the fallopian tube, where it becomes available for fertiliza-

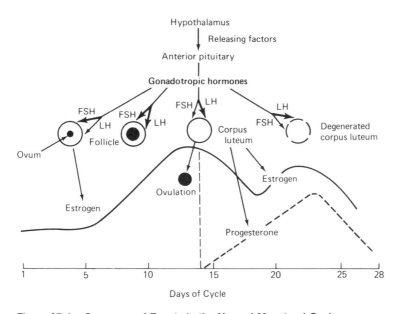

Figure 37-1. Sequence of Events in the Normal Menstrual Cycle.

tion by a sperm cell; the woman's most fertile period is between days 14 and 18. The remains of the ruptured follicle are converted to the *corpus luteum*, which is capable of secreting the sex hormones estrogen and progesterone.

During the second half of the menstrual cycle, *progesterone* initiates changes in the uterine mucosa that will provide a hospitable environment for implantation of a fertilized ovum. The cells of the uterus begin to stockpile fat and carbohydrate nutrient materials and the blood supply to the uterus is greatly enhanced. Progesterone also reduces the normal contractions of the smooth muscle of the uterus (myometrium).

Blood levels of estrogen and progesterone reach a post-ovulation peak on days 23 to 25. If the ovum has not been fertilized, several events occur, which culminate in *menstruation*. The high blood levels of progesterone initiate an inhibitory feedback mechanism, via the hypothalamus, which suppresses additional LH secretion from the pituitary. Reduced LH causes a degeneration of the corpus luteum, which in turn inhibits secretion of estrogen and progesterone. In the absence of hormonal support of the uterine mucosa, there is a breakdown and sloughing of its cells; menstruation begins and usually lasts for 3 to 5 days. Falling estrogen levels serve as a stimulus to the hypothalamus to activate the secretion of FSH by the pituitary, thus initiating the start of the next cycle.

If *fertilization* has occurred, generally between days 14 to 18 of the cycle, the implanted ovum in the uterine wall releases chorionic gonadotropin (HCG), which signals the corpus luteum to continue to secrete estrogen and progestrone for the first three months of pregnancy. Estrogen continues to maintain the proliferated uterine wall, while progesterone activates glandular secretions and reduces spontaneous contrac-

tions of the uterus. During the early weeks of gestation, the *placenta* begins to assume greater importance and begins releasing estrogen, progesterone, and *chorionic gonadotropin;* the presence of this last hormone, most active during the first trimester of pregnancy, is the basis for the pregnancy tests in current use. The high circulating levels of estrogen and progesterone during pregnancy inhibit the secretion of FSH, thus precluding the development of additional ova by the ovarian follicles. This last point is of fundamental importance for an understanding of the mechanism of action of the oral contraceptives. In the next chapter, we shall consider the effects of drugs on the motility of the pregnant uterus.

Gonadotropins

Gonadotropins found in the urine may be secreted by the anterior pituitary gland (FSH and LH) or by the placenta (HCG). *Human menopausal gonadotropin* (HMG) or *menotropins*, extracted from the urine of postmenopausal females, contains primarily FSH. Daily intramuscular injections of menotropins (Pergonal) for 9 to 12 days, followed by parenteral administration of chorionic gonadotropin, is clinically employed to induce ovulation in women who are infertile as the result of insufficient gonadotropins. The fertility-promoting effects of clomiphene, an antiestrogen, will be discussed in a later section of this chapter.

Human chorionic gonadotropin (HCG), extracted from the urine of pregnant females, possesses LH-like activity. In addition to the above described use, HCG is employed for the treatment of *cryptorchism*, the failure of one or both testes to descend from the abdominal cavity into the scrotum by puberty.

Estrogens

Of the three major estrogenic hormones secreted by the ovaries, namely, estradiol, estrone, and estriol, the first of these is released in the greatest quantities and is the most potent.

Effects Estradiol is required for the development of the female reproductive organs (vagina, uterus, and fallopian tubes) and secondary sex characteristics, including fullness of the breasts, appropriate distribution of body fat around the breasts and hips, soft skin texture, growth and distribution of body hair, and the nature of the female voice. Estrogens also play an essential role in the maintenance of the menstrual cycle and promote the growth of the ducts and nipples of the mammary glands. High doses of estrogen cause sodium retention, which may lead to fluid retention and edema.

Preparations and therapeutic uses

Natural and synthetic estrogenic hormones (Table 37-1) are available for the treatment of a wide range of endocrine disorders. After oral administration of the natural estrogens, they are rapidly metabolized and inactivated by the liver; they are, therefore, commonly given by subcutaneous or intramuscular injection. Semisynthetic and synthetic estrogens are suitable for oral use, vaginal administration, and topical application.

Menopausal symptoms A major therapeutic use of the estrogens is to alleviate the distressing symptoms associated with the menopause, "the change of life." With the onset of menopause, generally between 45 and 50 years of age, there is a gradual cessation of the ability of the ovaries to secrete estrogens. The absence of these hormones leads to characteristic symptoms of vasomotor instability including "hot flushes," fatigue, headache, muscle cramps, dizziness, nausea, anxiety, irritability, and vaginal atrophy. Estrogen therapy is highly specific and very effective in relieving these symptoms. Up to 25 percent of menopausal women will seek medical assistance and treatment.

Many physicians recommend that their patients take estrogens for 3 weeks of each month and continue therapy for several months up to a few years; long-term estrogen replacement therapy may increase the risk of endometrial cancer and cardiovascular disorders, as discussed shortly.

Estrogens are of proven value in the treatment of *atrophic vaginitis*. Their long-term benefits in the management of osteoporosis is questionable.

Menstrual disturbances Estrogens are reported to be helpful in relieving the pain and discomfort associated with *dysmenorrhea*, and replace the hormonal deficiency underlying *amenorrhea*. Abnormal uterine bleeding that is irregular, profuse, or prolonged and results from a hormonal imbalance can generally be controlled effectively with estrogens and progestins.

Miscellaneous uses Estrogens have been employed with reasonable success in the treatment of *prostate and female postmenopausal breast cancer* (Chapter 51) and are employed in combination with progestins as oral contraceptives (see page 327).

Adverse effects and precautions

The most common adverse effect associated with estrogen therapy is *nausea*, which usually dissipates with continued drug therapy. Large doses of this hormone or its synthetic derivatives may cause vomiting, loss of appetite, headache, salt and water retention, and breast tenderness.

Estrogen therapy is contraindicated during pregnancy because of potential risks to the fetus. Female offspring exposed to diethylstilbestrol *in utero* have been shown to have an increased risk of developing *vaginal or cervical cancer* or other nonmalignant changes to these structures later in life. Although such changes have not been clearly

Table 37-1 Representative Estrogenic Hormones

Generic name	Selected trade names	Usual adult dose	Distinguishing properties
Natural and Semisynthetic Estrogens			
Estrone	Theelin	IM: 0.1–0.5 mg 2–3 times weekly; vaginal suppositories (0.2 mg): 1 nightly	Aqueous suspensions have more prolonged actions than solutions in oil.
Estradiol	Progynon	IM: 0.22–1.5 mg 2–3 times weekly; SC pellet (25 mg): q. 3–4 months	Rapid metabolism and inactivation; esters preferred.
Estradiol cypionate	Depo-Estradiol	IM: 1–5 mg weekly	Very long duration of action.
Estradiol valerate	Delestrogen	IM: 20–30 mg q. 2–3 wks	Very long duration of action.
Ethinyl estradiol	Estinyl Feminone	PO: 0.02–0.05 mg o.d.	Highly active estrogen by mouth.
Estrogens conjugated	Premarin Menotab	PO: 0.3–1.25 mg o.d.; solutions for IM and IV injections and lotions and creams available.	Mixed estrogens extracted from urine of pregnant mares.
Esterified estrogens	Amnestrogen Femogen Menest	PO: 1.25 mg o.d.	Contains a mixture of sodium estrone sulfate and sodium equilin sulfate.
Piperazine estrone sulfate	Ogen	PO: 2.5 mg o.d.	When used for treatment of menopause, take for 3 weeks of each month.
Polyestradiol	Estradurin	IM: 40 mg q. 2–4 wks	Specifically intended for prostatic cancer; not recommended as replacement therapy.
Synthetic Estrogens			
Diethylstilbestrol (Stilbestrol)		PO: 0.2–0.5 mg o.d.; solution for injection and vaginal suppository available	DES was first synthetic estrogen; inexpensive; highly effective orally as substitute for natural estrogen. Effective but not recommended as postcoital contraceptive. Contraindicated during pregnancy. Nausea, vomiting and headache frequent after oral administration.
Chlorotrianisene	TACE	PO: 12–25 mg o.d.	Stored in body fat and slowly released, accounting for long duration of action.
Dienestrol		Vaginal cream	Treatment of atrophic vaginitis associated with menopause.

demonstrated with estrogens other than diethylstilbestrol, these drugs should also be avoided. Other studies suggest that estrogen therapy increases the risk of *congenital anomalies* (heart defects, limb reduction) in the offspring. In the past, estrogens were used to treat threatened or habitual abortion; considerable evidence is now available

documenting their ineffectiveness in preventing abortions.

The risk of *endometrial cancer* in postmenopausal women receiving estrogen therapy for prolonged periods is estimated to be 4.5 to 14 times greater than nonusers. Hence, when estrogens are to be employed for the management of menopausal symptoms, *the lowest effective dose should be used for the shortest period of time.* When prolonged estrogen therapy is required, women should be evaluated on at least a semiannual basis to determine whether a continued drug need exists.

The possible involvement of estrogens in causing *thromboembolic disorders* will be considered later. Potential drug interactions involving the estrogens are given in Table 37-5 (page 332) and nursing implications are summarized at the end of this chapter. The Food and Drug Administration requires that the patient be given a lay package insert (outlining the benefits and risks associated with estrogens) when the therapy is initiated.

Antiestrogens

Antiestrogens are drugs that suppress or antagonize the effects of estrogen. *Clomiphene* possesses such properties and has been used to successfully stimulate ovulation in many previously infertile women.

High blood levels of estrogens normally exert an inhibitory influence on the hypothalamus which, in turn, results in suppression of the release of gonadotropins from the anterior pituitary. Clomiphene is thought to act by blocking the inhibitory effects of estrogens on the hypothalamus, thus promoting the release of gonadotropins and stimulating ovulation.

Clomiphene (Clomid) is administered orally in doses of 50 to 100 mg for 5 days to several weeks. Ovulation occurs in 70 to 75 percent of appropriately selected patients, with pregnancy achieved in 25 to 30 percent.

The incidence of multiple births is considerably higher than normal in users of this drug. Frequently encountered adverse effects include cystic enlargement of the ovaries, breast enlargement, hot flushes, and nausea.

Progestins (Progestogens)

The most important natural progestin is *progesterone*, a hormone secreted by the corpus luteum and the placenta. This hormone induces changes in the uterine mucosa that provides nourishment and a more favorable environment for implantation of the fertilized ovum. During pregnancy, progesterone induces mammary gland duct development and reduces spontaneous contractions of the uterine smooth muscle by antagonizing the actions of estradiol and oxytocin.

High doses of progestins inhibit LH release, thus preventing ovulation. This effect may serve as the basis for the use of these hormones as contraceptive agents.

Preparations and therapeutic uses
Progesterone is poorly effective when taken by mouth. It is available for parenteral administration as an oily solution and as an aqueous suspension. Synthetic progestins are available that are active after oral administration (Table 37-2).

The ability of the progestins to suppress ovulation underlies their use for the treatment of dysmenorrhea and endometriosis.

Functional uterine bleeding is a common disorder, characterized by highly irregular menstrual cycles and periods of prolonged and excessive bleeding. This problem is most frequently observed in young girls prior to the onset of regular menstrual cycles and in mature women upon the approach of menopause. The immediate treatment objective is to terminate bleeding, and, thereafter, to regulate the cycle. Progestins are highly effective in achieving these goals.

While extensively used to prevent abortion, the therapeutic effectiveness of progestins has not been demonstrated. Moreover, use of these drugs during the first four months of pregnancy may result in the mas-

Table 37-2   Representative Progestogens

Generic name	Trade name	Usual adult dose	Distinguishing properties
Natural Progestogen			
Progesterone		IM: 5-10 mg o.d.	Ineffective orally; irritating at site of injection; very short duration of action.
Synthetic Progestogens			
Dydrogesterone	Duphaston Gynorest	PO: 10-20 mg o.d.	Unlike some other progestogens, lacks thermogenic, estrogenic, and androgenic activities; does not interfere with normal menstrual cycle.
Hydroxyprogesterone caproate	Delatutin	IM: 125-250 mg once per menstrual cycle	More potent and longer duration of action than progesterone.
Medroxyprogesterone acetate	Provera Depo-Provera	PO: 5-10 mg o.d. IM: 50-100 mg q. other week	Effective orally. Intramuscular product used for treatment of cancer.
Norethindrone	Norlutin	PO: 5-20 mg o.d.	Possesses estrogenic activity; can be used to delay menstruation.
Norethindrone acetate	Norlutate	½ that of norethindrone.	Same as norethindrone, but twice as potent.
Progestin Products for Contraceptive Use			
Medroxyprogesterone acetate	Depo-Provera C-150	IM: 150 mg q. 90 days	Long-acting contraceptive preparation; potential carcinogenic hazard and permanent infertility; withdrawn for use as contraceptive in U.S. Employed for treatment of uterine cancer.
Progesterone intrauterine device "Minipills" (Table 37-3, page 327)	Progestasert	Replace one year after insertion.	IUD with slowly released progesterone.

culinization of the external genitalia of the female fetus, as well as congenital heart and limb defects. Estrogens or progestins are effective in suppressing postpartum lactation.

Undesirable effects associated with progestin administration are generally mild and include nausea, headache, dizziness, edema, and weight gain, and such menstrual disturbances as spotting and breakthrough bleeding. Nursing precautions associated with progesterone administration appear at the end of the chapter.

Oral Contraceptives

Many methods are currently available to prevent pregnancy, including oral contraceptives, intrauterine devices (IUD), diaphragms, condoms, spermicidal foams, creams and jellies, and rhythm. The oral contraceptives are the most effective of these methods, and yet they are not without potential hazard to the ten million female American users.

Pharmacological actions and available products   The oral contraceptives act by one or more of the following mechanisms: (1) they prevent ovulation by blocking the release of FSH and LH from the anterior pituitary; (2) they increase the thickness of the cervical mucus, creating an unfavorable environment for sperm penetration and subsequent conception; or (3) they induce other changes in the cervical mucosa that prove

Table 37-3   Representative Oral Contraceptives

Trade name	Progestin (mg)	Estrogen (μg)	Relative dominance[c]
Combination Products[a]			
Demulen	Ethynodiol diacetate (1)	Ethinyl estradiol (50)	I
Ovulen	Ethynodiol diacetate (1)	Mestranol (100)	E
Ovcon-35	Norethindrone (0.4)	Ethinyl estradiol (35)	I
Brevicon, Modicon	Norethindrone (0.5)	Ethinyl estradiol (35)	I
Norinyl 1 + 50; Ortho-Novum 1/50	Norethindrone (1)	Mestranol (50)	I
Norinyl 1 + 80; Ortho-Novum 1/80	Norethindrone (1)	Mestranol (80)	I
Norinyl 2 mg; Ortho-Novum 2 mg	Norethindrone (2)	Mestranol (100)	E
Ortho-Novum 10 mg	Norethindrone (10)	Mestranol (60)	P
Loestrin 1/20	Norethindrone acetate (1)	Ethinyl estradiol (20)	P
Norlestrin 1/50; Ovcon 50	Norethindrone acetate (1)	Ethinyl estradiol (50)	I
Loestrin 1.5/30	Norethindrone acetate (1.5)	Ethinyl estradiol (30)	P
Norlestrin 2.5/50	Norethindrone acetate (2.5)	Ethinyl estradiol (50)	P
Enovid-E	Norethynodrel (2.5)	Mestranol (100)	E
Enovid 5 mg	Norethynodrel (5)	Mestranol (75)	E
Lo/Ovral	Norgestrel (0.3)	Ethinyl estradiol (30)	P
Ovral	Norgestrel (0.5)	Ethinyl estradiol (50)	P
Progestin-Only Products (Minipills)[b]			
Micronor; Nor-Q.D.	Norethindrone (0.35)	———	P
Ovrette	Norgestrel (0.075)	———	P

[a]Some of the combination products are taken once daily for 20 to 21 days, starting on day 5 of menstrual cycle; others, taken for the entire 28-day cycle, contain 21 tablets with estrogen and progestin and 7 inert tablets.
[b]The minipills are taken once daily, every day of the year.
[c]Key to abbreviations: E = estrogen dominant; P = progestin dominant; I = intermediate estrogen-progestin balance.

unfavorable for implantation of the fertilized ovum.

Oral contraceptives are classified as *combination products* and *progestin*-only minipills; they differ with respect to their composition, pharmacological actions, side effects, and schedule of administration (Table 37-3).*

The *combination products*, consisting

Sequential oral contraceptives were formerly available for use. Preparations of this type (Norquen, Oracon, Ortho-Novum SC) consisted of an estrogen (taken for 15 to 16 days) and an estrogen-progestin tablet (taken for the subsequent 5 to 6 days). These products were voluntarily withdrawn from the American market in 1976 because use of these products increased the risk of thromboembolic disorders and malignant tumors. The sequentials are less effective contraceptives than the combination products.

of both an *estrogen* and a *progestin*, are taken from the fifth day after the start of menstruation for the next 20 to 21 days, withdrawal bleeding occurs 2 to 4 days after the last dose. The next course of drug administration should be initiated 7 days after the last dose, whether or not bleeding has occurred. To eliminate the need for patients counting days between cycles, potentially resulting in the failure to take medication as directed, some products contain 7 tablets that are inert or contain iron to be taken during the hormone-free week; the suffix "28" generally appears in the trade name to designate such products.

The *minipills* contain only a *progestin* ingredient and are intended to be taken every day of the year regardless of whether bleeding occurs or not. The absence of estrogen in these products is intended to reduce the risk of thromboembolic disorders and carcinogenesis.

Effectiveness When all doses of these contraceptives are taken according to the prescribed schedule, the combination products represent the most effective method of contraception; their *theoretical effectiveness* is greater than 99 percent or, conversely, less than one pregnancy per 100 women-years.* With the minipill, approximately three pregnancies might be predicted per 100 women-years, with pregnancy risks highest during the first 6 months of use.

While pregnancies have been reported in women taking oral contraceptives as directed, in most cases failures result from *noncompliance* with the dosage regimen. See the nursing implications at the end of the chapter for how to advise patients who have omitted taking this medication as directed. The nurse should play an active role in the education of patients about the proper use of these drugs and stress the importance of their uninterrupted use.

Product selection Initial selection of the most appropriate oral contraceptive preparation should be based on a careful history and physical examination. Available combination products may have estrogen or progestin dominance or contain a balance of these hormonal activities (Table 37-3, page 327).

Products that are *estrogen-dominant* are preferred for patients exhibiting acne, hirsutism, depression, scanty menses, or small breasts, or when premenopausal estro-

*The rate of pregnancies during a given time period is a measure of the failure rate of that method. If we assume that ovulation occurs 13 times annually, for each woman there are 13 opportunities for conception to occur, or 1,300 per 100 women-years.

gen deficiency is evident. *Progestin-dominant* prepartions are useful for patients with mucorrhea, a history of nausea or bloating after previous use of oral contraceptives or during pregnancy, fibrocystic disease of the breasts, cyclic premenstrual weight gain, premenstrual tension, or dysmenorrhea. Progestin-only preparations may be preferred for contraceptive purposes to reduce the risk of thromboembolic disorders, such as thrombophlebitis, pulmonary embolism, and cerebral thrombosis.

Side effects and potential hazards

The most common side effects are similar to the early signs of pregnancy and include nausea, possible vomiting, breast fullness, weight gain, dizziness, fatigue, and depression. Irregular menstrual bleeding (breakthrough bleeding), scanty menstrual flow, or amenorrhea may also occur, particularly with progestin-dominant preparations.

Increased medical and public attention has been focused in recent years on the potential hazards associated with the use of oral contraceptives over extended periods of time. These possible dangers include increased risk of cardiovascular disorders, carcinogenesis, gall bladder disease, and diabetogenic effects. Since complications are also clearly associated with pregnancy, the high degree of contraceptive effectiveness of these drug must be weighed against their potential dangers.

Cardiovascular disorders Studies conducted in the last decade suggest that the risk of life-threatening *thromboembolic disorders* (thrombophlebitis, thrombotic stroke) is four to ten times greater in women using combination oral contraceptive preparations than in women of the same age who are not using these drugs. These blood clotting disorders are generally believed to be caused by the *estrogen* component; there is no evidence that the use of low doses of this hormone is free of the risk of abnormal clotting.

Oral contraceptives cause *essential hypertension* in a significant number of patients, particularly in those patients who have other risk factors for hypertensive disease. The incidence of hypertension appears to be correlated with the duration of oral contraceptive use and the dose of the progestin component; hypertension, usually mild to moderate in intensity, is generally reversible within 1 to 3 months after discontinuation of drug usage.

The risk of fatal and nonfatal *myocardial infarction* is increased by this drug class, particularly when used by women having other risk factors such as hypertension, cigarette smoking, diabetes mellitus, elevated cholesterol and triglyceride levels, and obesity. The risk of myocardial infarction in women with one risk factor increases fourfold above those with no risk factors and 10 and 78 times in women with two and three or more risk factors, respectively.

Carcinogenesis and tumors Considerable controversy exists in the literature about whether or not oral contraceptives and estrogens increase the risk of *cancer of the female breast and reproductive tract* (cervical and endometrial carcinoma). Strong evidence has been presented which indicates that the prolonged use of estrogens for the management of postmenopausal symptoms markedly increases the risk of endometrial cancer.

Many reports have documented an increase in *benign liver tumors* (hepatic adenomas), a previously rare disorder, in women using oral contraceptives; fatal intraperitoneal bleeding resulting from such tumors has been observed. Recent reports suggest that these drugs may transform benign adenomas into malignant tumors.

Other risks The increased incidence of gallstones and *gall bladder disease* (cholecystitis, cholangitis) is clearly associated with the use of oral contraceptives.

While there is no strong evidence suggesting that oral contraceptives cause diabetes mellitus, disturbances of *carbohydrate metabolism* and aggravation of diabetes may occur. These drugs should be used with great caution in women with carbohydrate metabolic abnormalities, latent diabetes, or a family history of this disease.

Precautions Oral contraceptives are contraindicated for use in women with thromboembolic disorders or a past history of these conditions, cerebral vascular or coronary artery disease, established or suspected carcinomas of the breast or reproductive tract, undiagnosed abnormal genital bleeding, or marked impairment of liver function.

Medication should be withdrawn upon the appearance of an unexplained sudden or gradual *reduction in vision* (possibly resulting from drug-induced ocular lesions) or the onset or worsening of migraine or other severe headaches. If pregnancy is suspected, these drugs should not be used because of possible progestin-induced masculinization of the female fetus and teratogenesis in fetuses of both sexes. Oral contraceptive use during the postpartum period interferes with lactation, decreasing both the quantity and quality of breast milk. Potential drug interactions involving the oral contraceptives are given in (Table 37-5, page 332), and nursing implications are summarized at the end of this chapter.

Other Hormonal Contraceptive Approaches

In this section, we shall briefly consider the use of the intrauterine administration of progestins as contraceptives and estrogens as "morning-after pills."

Progesterone intrauterine device

This T-shaped intrauterine device (IUD) contains a reservoir of progesterone; its trade name is Progestasert. The hormone is slowly released into the uterine cavity at a constant rate for at least one year. It is strongly recommended that a unit be replaced 1 year after insertion.

Progesterone exerts a local action to prevent pregnancy. This action may involve interference with sperm survival and alterations in the uterine environment rendering it hostile to implantation by the fertilized ovum. Progestasert is an effective contraceptive, although more expensive and not necessarily more effective in preventing pregnancy than IUD's that do not contain drugs. This product should not be used if pregnancy is suspected.

Morning-after pill

The estrogenic hormone *diethylstilbestrol* has been approved for postcoital use in emergency situations such as rape or incest or when pregnancy will threaten the woman's physical or mental well-being. The potential carcinogenic hazards of this drug preclude its use on a routine or frequent basis as a contraceptive agent. (See the adverse effects associated with estrogens given earlier.)

Since diethylstilbestrol acts by preventing implantation of the fertilized ovum, it should be taken within 72 hours after intercourse. Administration of this drug at a dose of 25 mg twice daily for 5 consecutive days is approximately 99 percent effective in preventing pregnancy. Nausea and vomiting frequently occur during this course of therapy.

MALE SEX HORMONES

The male sex hormones, referred to as *androgens*, have important effects on reproductive structures as well as on other body tissues. *Testosterone* is the most important androgen, and this steroid hormone is synthesized and secreted by the Leydig cells of the *testes.*

The androgens are responsible for the normal development and maintenance of the male secondary sex characteristics and male psyche, sex organs and related structures (testes, penis, prostate, seminal vesicles), and for the synthesis of sperm.

Among the major nonhormonal effects produced by androgens are those concerned with *protein anabolism.* Testosterone-induced stimulation of protein synthesis is associated with nitrogen retention, as well as retention of potassium, phosphorus, and sodium, leading to an increase in body weight and muscle mass. Research efforts have been directed toward developing synthetic testosterone-like compounds that possess minimal virilizing effects while retaining anabolic activity; these drugs are called *anabolic steroids.*

Preparations

Testosterone is readily absorbed after oral and parenteral administration but is rapidly metabolized and inactivated by the liver. Esters of this androgen (Table 37-4), administered as solutions in oil, have a considerably longer duration of action after intramuscular injection. Methyltestosterone is effective after oral and buccal administration. Synthetic anabolic steroids, highly active when taken by mouth, possess a more favorable anabolic/androgenic (virilizing) ratio than testosterone.

Therapeutic Uses

The primary clinical use of androgens is for the treatment of *hypogonadism* (eunuchism, cryptorchism, Klinefelter's syndrome) resulting from a failure of the testes to secrete testosterone. These drugs are also useful for

Table 37-4   Representative Androgens

Generic name	Selected trade names	Usual adult dose	Distinguishing properties
Androgen Replacement Therapy			
Testosterone		IM: 10-50 mg 2-6 times weekly SC: 450 mg (6 pellets) q. 4-6 mo	Ineffective orally; short duration of action. Relative androgenic: anabolic activity 1:1.
Testosterone cypionate	Depo-Testosterone	IM: 100-400 mg q. 1-4 wk	Long duration of action.
Testosterone enanthate	Delatestryl	IM: 100-400 mg q. 1-4 wk	Long duration of action.
Testosterone propionate		IM: 10-25 mg 2-4 times weekly; buccal tablets 5-20 mg o.d.	Short duration of action makes it unsuitable for long-term use.
Methyltestosterone	Metandren Oreton Methyl	PO: 10-50 mg o.d.; buccal dose: ½ oral	Effective orally, twice as potent as testosterone by buccal administration; liver toxicity.
Fluoxymesterone	Halotestin Ora-Testryl	PO: 2-20 mg o.d.	Five times more potent than testosterone and orally active.
Anabolic Steroids[a]			
Nandrolone phenpropionate	Durabolin	IM: 25-50 mg weekly	Less androgenic than testosterone; no liver toxicity or water retention.
Nandrolone decanoate	Deca-Durabolin	IM: 50-100 mg q. 3-4 wk	Long duration of action.
Oxymetholone	Adroyd Anadrol-50	PO: 5-10 mg o.d.	Orally active.
Stanozolol	Winstrol	PO: 2 mg t.i.d.	Strong anabolic and weak androgenic activity.
Oxandrolone	Anavar	PO: 5-20 mg o.d.	Same as stanozolol.
Methandrostenolone	Dianabol	PO: 2.5-5 mg o.d.	Same as stanozolol.
Ethylestrenol	Maxibolin	PO: 4-8 mg o.d.	Give for 6 weeks, 4-week rest period, resume drug for 6 weeks, if needed.

[a]These drugs have relatively greater anabolic activity than androgenic (virilizing) activity.

the treatment of male youths exhibiting delayed puberty.

Androgens are used in the palliative management of metastatic *breast cancer* in postmenopausal females and in premenopausal women after surgical removal of their ovaries (Chapter 51). Danazol (Danocrine), a synthetic androgen, is used for the treatment of *endometriosis* when other drugs cannot be tolerated. The usual dose is 400 mg twice daily for 3 to 6 months.

Anabolic steroids are used to increase body weight in patients with a negative nitrogen balance, such as after a severe debilitating illness or during convalescence after major surgery or severe injury. Employment of these drugs for the treatment of osteoporosis is predicated upon their ability to cause nitrogen and calcium retention.

Adverse Effects and Precautions

The use of androgens in females may result in signs of masculinization including growth

Table 37-5   Potential Drug Interactions Involving Sex Hormones

Sex hormone	Interacting drug/class	Possible consequences of interaction
Estrogens	Corticosteroids hydrocortisone	Estrogens may enhance the anti-inflammatory effects of hydrocortisone.
Estrogens Oral contraceptives	Oral anticoagulants (dicumarol)	Oral contraceptives increase the activity of clotting factors in the blood, thereby decreasing the anticoagulant response to dicumarol; increase in dose may be required.
Oral contraceptives	Barbiturates Rifampin (Rifadin, Rimactane)	These drugs may increase the rate of estrogen metabolism, thereby reducing the ability of the oral contraceptive to prevent pregnancy.
Anabolic steroids	Oral anticoagulants	Anabolic steroids (in particular methandrostenolone, norethandrolone, and oxymetholone) produce a well-documented increase in the tendency to hemorrhage. Prothrombin times should be monitored and a reduction in anticoagulant dosage may be required.
Anabolic steroids	Antidiabetic drugs	Anabolic steroids may decrease blood glucose levels in some diabetic patients, thereby enhancing the hypoglycemic effects of tolbutamide (Orinase) and decreasing insulin requirements.
Methandrostenolone (Dianabol)	Oxyphenbutazone (Tandearil)	This hormone increases plasma levels of oxyphenbutazone, potentially increasing toxicity.

of facial and body hair (hirsutism), acne, deepening of the voice, clitoral enlargement, menstrual irregularities, and regression of the breasts. All anabolic steroids produce some of these virilizing effects, but to a lesser extent than testosterone. Other adverse effects may include sodium and water retention resulting in edema, increased libido, jaundice and liver toxicity, and premature epiphyseal closure in prepubertal males, preventing further elongation of the long bones.

Anabolic steriods are employed by some athletes seeking to increase their muscle mass and body weight. Available evidence suggests that these drugs fail to increase muscle strength or physical performance; the apparent increase in muscle mass is attributed to fluid retention. In the absence of careful supervision by a medically trained individual, these drugs may be potentially dangerous, and, therefore, the nurse should strongly discourage indiscriminate use of them.

Androgens are contraindicated in male patients with known or suspected prostate or breast cancer and severe liver, kidney, or heart disease. Their use during pregnancy or lactation is contraindicated because of their masculinizing effects on the female fetus or breast-fed infant. Potential drug interactions involving androgenic compounds are summarized in Table 37-5.

Sex Hormones:
nursing implications

Estrogens

1. Use for symptoms of menopause is usually cyclic: 3 wk on drug, 1 wk off, or only for the first 25 days of each month. Dosing schedule employed to avoid continued stimulation of reproductive tissue, particularly the endometrium of uterus.
2. Prior to and periodically during estrogen therapy, physical examinations are recommended, with special attention to abdominal palpation of liver, breast examination, blood pressure (B.P.) and pelvic examination with Pap smear.
3. Instruct the patient to report any unusual vaginal bleeding. Withdrawal bleeding may occur in patients who have not had regular menstrual periods.
4. Nausea, a common side effect, may be relieved by taking the drug with meals; it usually disappears after 1-2 wk of therapy.
5. Instruct the patient to check for edema and monitor weight 2-3 times weekly and report sudden weight gain. Cyclic fluid retention may be managed with a low salt diet and a diuretic.
6. Teach patient to identify and report early signs of thromboembolic disorders: tenderness, pain, or swelling of legs; sudden severe headache or chest pain; unexplained visual disturbances.
7. Estrogen may alter glucose tolerance. Advise diabetic patients to report changes in sugar urine tests.
8. Have the patient report signs of liver damage: jaundice, pruritus, dark urine, light colored stools are all indications for liver function tests, which may require drug withdrawal.
9. Reassure male patients receiving estrogens that feminization and impotence are reversible and will disappear after termination of drug administration.
10. Be alert for behavioral changes or increased mental depression, which may be a symptom of a recurrent psychiatric disorder.

Progesterone

1. Instruct the patient to report unusual vaginal spotting or bleeding, signs of thromboembolic disorders.
2. Observe the patient for edema and report any sudden weight gain.
3. Instruct the patient to report symptoms of ophthalmic pathology: headache, dizziness, blurred vision or partial loss of vision, diplopia.
4. Inform the pathologist of progesterone therapy when relevant specimens are submitted.

Estrogen-Progestin Combination (Oral Contraceptives)

1. Patients receiving combination therapy are susceptible to the untoward effects produced by the individual ingredients as well as the following effects.

2. Prior to initiating therapy with oral contraceptives (the pill), the patient's weight and B.P. should be checked and recorded as a baseline. The patient should return in 3 mo for evaluation of: weight, B.P., fasting blood glucose or 2-h post-glucose levels, triglycerides, SGOT, and palpation of right upper quadrant of the abdomen to rule out early liver pathology.

3. To reduce the risk of later fertility and menstrual problems, the pill is not advised for the adolescent patient until after at least 2 yr of well-established menstrual cycles and until physiological maturity has occurred.

4. Teach patients to take pills exactly as prescribed to prevent pregnancy. They should be advised to take pills at a regular time each day, such as at bedtime. If 1 pill is missed, it should be taken as soon as possible. If 2 consecutive pills are missed, the patient should double the dosage for the next 2 days and then resume the regular schedule; it is advisable to use additional contraceptive measures for the remainder of the cycle. If 3 doses are missed, drug administration should be resumed 7 days after the last pill was taken; another method of contraception should be used when not taking the pill and for 7 days into the new cycle.

5. Withdrawal bleeding normally occurs 2–5 days after the last dose, but the regular pill dosage schedule should be followed regardless of when bleeding occurs.

6. Intramenstrual spotting may occur during the first through third cycles that the medication is taken. Persistent intramenstrual spotting may represent an indication for need to adjust dosage or oral contraceptive product and should be reported to physician.

7. If the prescribed regimen has been properly followed and 2 consecutive periods are missed, the patient should see the physician to rule out pregnancy. If dosage schedule has not been followed, the possibility of pregnancy should be considered at the time the first period is missed.

8. When pregnancy is desired, the pill should be discontinued, and the patient should be advised to use an alternative method of contraception for at least 3 months to reduce the risk of congenital defects in the fetus.

9. Anovulation or amenorrhea after termination of the pill may persist for 6 mo or longer.

10. Pills should not be taken by nursing mothers.

11. The heavy smoker has a higher risk of developing venous thrombosis than the nonsmoker.

12. Check B.P. periodically. Drug-induced hypertension is usually reversible with drug withdrawal.

13. Sudden abdominal pain should be reported immediately to rule out ectopic pregnancy or hepatic adenoma.

14. Inform the patient that pill administration increases cervical mucous and susceptibility to vaginal infections that are difficult to treat. Patient should report vaginal itching, burning, or malodorous discharges.

SUPPLEMENTARY READINGS

Bingel, A. S., and P. S. Benoit, "Oral Contraceptives: Therapeutic Versus Adverse Reactions, with an Out-

look for the Future," *Journal of Pharmaceutical Sciences* **62**: 179–200, 349–62 (1973).

Brotherton, J., *Sex Hormone Pharmacology*. New York: Academic Press, Inc., 1976.

Chan, L., and B. O'Malley, "Mechanism of Action of Sex Steroid Hormones," *New England Journal of Medicine* **294**: 1322–28, 1372–81, 1430–37 (1976).

Dickey, R., "Diagnosis and Management of Patients With Oral Contraceptive Side Effects," *Journal of Continuing Education in Obstetrics and Gynecology*, January 1978, pp. 19–39.

Drill, V. A., "Oral Contraceptives: Relation to Mammary Cancer, Benign Breast Lesions, and Cervical Cancer," *Annual Review of Pharmacology* **15**: 367–85 (1975).

Ewing, L. L., and B. Robaire, "Endogenous Antisperm Agents: Prospects for Male Contraception," *Annual Review of Pharmacology and Toxicology* **18**: 167–87 (1978).

Hafez, E. S. E., and T. M. Evans, eds., *Human Reproduction: Conception and Contraception*. New York: Harper & Row Publishers, Inc., 1973.

Hatcher, R. A., and others, *Contraceptive Technology 1978–1979*, 9th revised edition. New York: Irvington Publishers, 1978.

Huff, J. E., and L. Hernandez, "Contraceptive Methods and Products," in *Handbook of Nonprescription Drugs* (6th ed.), pp. 247–57. Washington, D.C.: American Pharmaceutical Association, 1979.

Kellie, A. E., "The Pharmacology of the Estrogens," *Annual Review of Pharmacology* **11**: 97–112 (1971).

Kochakian, C., "Definition of Androgens and Protein Anabolic Steroids," *Pharmacology and Therapeutics* **1**(B): 149–77 (1972).

Longson, D., "Androgen Therapy," *Practitioner*, **208**: 338–48 (1972).

Ory, H. W., "Association Between Oral Contraceptives and Myocardial Infarction—A Review," *Journal of the American Medical Association* **237**: 2619–22 (1977).

Rahwan, R. G., "Pharmacological Approaches to Birth Control: Contraceptives, Intraceptives, Abortifacients," *U.S. Pharmacist* **2**(9): 30-42, **2**(10): 56–72 (1977).

DRUGS AFFECTING UTERINE MOTILITY

Chapter 38

During a first pregnancy, the human female uterus increases twentyfold in weight and its smooth muscle fiber (*myometrium*) increases in length tenfold. Endogenously released progesterone (Chapter 37) depresses the normal rhythmic contractions of the pregnant uterus. Late in the third trimester of pregnancy, progesterone levels fall, and spontaneous and drug-induced uterine motility markedly increases.

There are three well-defined stages in normal labor. The *first stage* begins with the onset of labor pains and terminates when there is complete dilation of the cervix; contractions of the uterine muscle occur every 15 to 20 minutes. During the *second stage*, uterine contractions progressively increase in force, frequency, and duration. The end of this stage is marked by delivery of the baby. In the *third stage*, occurring after the birth of the baby, the uterus becomes smaller in size and there is complete expulsion of the placenta and membranes. Normal postpartum blood loss during this stage varies from 300 to 600 ml.

Oxytocics, drugs that stimulate the smooth muscle of the uterus, are used to induce labor at term and control postpartum hemorrhage. Routine use of oxytocics during the first two stages of labor is generally not recommended. Drugs in the oxytocic class include oxytocin, the ergot alkaloids, and the prostaglandins (Table 38-1). In this chapter, we shall discuss these drugs and also consider the use of ergot alkaloids for the treatment of migraine.

OXYTOCIN

Oxytocin is a natural protein hormone secreted by the posterior pituitary (Chapter 33). The capacity of the myometrium to contract in the presence of this hormone increases during pregnancy and becomes maximal at term. Synthetic preparations of oxytocin (Pitocin, Syntocinon) are available for therapeutic use.

Administration

In most cases, oxytocin is considered to be the drug of choice when *induction of labor at term* is therapeutically indicated. Ineffective when taken orally, oxytocin is usually administered by slow intravenous infusion (in 5 percent dextrose) at an initial rate of 5 milliunits per minute. If no response is obtained within 15 minutes, the infusion rate can be gradually increased, up to 20 milliunits per minute. An average dose of 4000 milliunits (4 units) is required to induce labor. After labor has been initiated, drug administration should be terminated.

Since patient sensitivity varies, uterine activity must be carefully monitored during oxytocin administration to prevent sustained tetanic uterine contractions resulting in uterine rupture, impairment of placental circulation, and fetal death. Contractions rapidly cease after termination of oxytocin infusion. After infusions of extended duration, the antidiuretic properties of oxytocin may cause maternal water intoxication with convulsions and coma; this risk is increased in patients with toxemia of pregnancy. The use of a saline solution rather than dextrose reduces this potential hazard. Nursing implications are summarized at the end of this chapter.

Oxytocin may be intramuscularly administered to control postpartum bleeding and promote uterine involution, but ergot alkaloids are generally preferred. A nasal spray containing synthetic oxytocin (Syntocinon) is employed to initiate milk let-down.

ERGOT ALKALOIDS

Ergot is a fungus (*Claviceps purpurea*) that grows on rye and other grains. This fungus, found in the grainfields of North America and Europe, has been shown to be responsible for various epidemics of gangrene of the extremities dating from ancient times to the present century; chronic ergot poisoning was referred to as St. Anthony's fire.

At least five alkaloids have been isolated from ergot; the two most important of these are *ergonovine*, employed as an oxytocic agent, and *ergotamine*, the drug of choice for the treatment of migraine. The general properties of selected natural and synthetic ergot alkaloids are summarized in Table 38-1.

Pharmacological Effects

The ergot alkaloids produce smooth muscle contraction and α-adrenergic blockade.

Smooth muscle contraction   Ergonovine causes direct stimulation of smooth

Table 38-1   Oxytocic and Ergot-Related Antimigraine Drugs

Generic name	Trade name	Usual dose	Distinguishing properties
Ocytocic drugs			
Oxytocin	Pitocin Syntocinon	Labor: 4,000 milliunits by IV infusion. Postpartum bleeding: 3-10 units, IM; repeat in 30 min, PRN.	Drug of choice for induction of labor. Not effective for midpregnancy abortion. Ergot alkaloids preferred for control of postpartum bleeding. Synthetic oxytocin is available as a nasal spray to promote initial milk let-down.
Ergonovine maleate	Ergotrate	IM: 0.2 mg q 6 h PO: 0.2 mg t.i.d.	Used in Stage 3 of labor and to control postpartum bleeding. Less effective than ergotamine for migraine.
Methylergonovine maleate	Methergine	PO: 0.2 mg q.i.d. for not more than 2 days postpartum. IM: 0.2 mg q. 2-4 h PRN.	Same as ergonovine, but more effective orally.
Dinoprost tromethamine (Prostaglandin $F_2\alpha$)	Prostin F2 alpha	40 mg by slow intra-amnionic injection; repeat in 24 h PRN.	Drug of choice for second-trimester therapeutic abortions. No major advantages over oxytocin for routine delivery at term.
Dinoprostone (Prostaglandin E_2)	Prostin E2	Insert 20-mg vaginal suppository every 3-5 h until abortion occurs.	Used for 12-week to second-trimester abortions, induction of labor after fetal death or missed abortion, and treatment of hydatidiform moles. Not lethal to fetus, so live birth is possible.
Carboprost (Synthetic PG $F_2\alpha$ derivative)	Prostin/15 M	IM: 250 μg q 1.5-3.5 h	High incidence of gastrointestinal side effects.
Antimigraine drugs			
Ergotamine tartrate	Gynergen Ergomar Ergostat	PO: 1 mg, repeated up to 6 mg daily or 12 mg weekly. IM or SC: 0.25-0.5 mg, up to 1 mg daily or 2 mg weekly.	Drug of choice for migraine and other vascular headaches. Gastrointestinal effects common. Excessive dosage may result in severe vasoconstriction and gangrene, numbness, and tingling of fingers and toes; changes heart rate.
Dihydroergotamine mesylate	D.H.E. 45	IM: 1 mg q. h up to 3 mg	Only active parenterally. Less effective drug but less nausea and vomiting than ergotamine.
Ergotamine tartrate and caffeine	Cafergot	PO: 1 tablet q. 30 min up to 3 daily or 6 weekly. 1 rectal suppository q. h up 5 weekly.	Tablets: 1 mg ergotamine + 100 mg caffeine. Suppositories: twice these concentrations. Caffeine enhances cerebral vasoconstrictor properties of ergotamine.
Methysergide maleate	Sansert	PO: 2 mg t.i.d.	Indicated for prevention of migraine; ineffective for acute attack. Gastrointestinal and behavioral side effects; many contraindications; patient should remain under close medical supervision (see text).

Table 38-1   Continued

Generic name	Trade name	Usual dose	Distinguishing properties
Propranolol	Inderal	PO: 160–240 mg daily.	β-adrenergic blocking agent used for the treatment of cardiovascular disorders. Indicated for prevention of migraine. Relatively low incidence of adverse side effects.
Miscellaneous ergot derivatives			
Dihydroergotoxine mesylate	Hydergine	IM or IV: 0.3–1 mg. Sublingual: 0.5 mg	Peripheral vasodilator.
Bromocriptine	Parlodel	PO: maximum 15 mg q. 6 h	Relief of amenorrhea and galactorrhea. Investigational drug for Parkinson's disease.
Lysergic acid diethylamide (LSD)			Psychotomimetic with no approved medical indications (Chapter 23).

muscle, effects most readily observed on the uterus and blood vessels. The ability of ergonovine and its semisynthetic derivative methylergonovine to cause myometrial contractions is greatest at term and during the postpartum period. Ergotamine and its derivative dihydroergotamine produce peripheral vasoconstriction and capillary endothelial damage. These effects are thought to be responsible for the gangrene observed in chronic ergot poisoning and, in lower doses, for its beneficial effects in the treatment of migraine headaches.

Adrenergic blockade   Ergot alkaloids of the ergotoxine type produce α-adrenergic blockade and were used in the past as peripheral vasodilators and as antihypertensive agents. Ergotamine and dihydroergotamine also produce adrenergic blockade, but ergonovine and methylergonovine do not.

Ergonovine

Ergonovine (Ergotrate) and methylergonovine (Methergine) possess potent oxytocic properties. These drugs are commonly administered during the third stage of labor to produce uterine contractions, thus controlling postpartum bleeding.

After intravenous or intramuscular administration of therapeutic doses (0.2 mg), these drugs have a rapid onset of action (less than 5 minutes) and a long duration of action (up to 6 hours). To promote uterine involution and reduce the risk of bleeding, these drugs are often given orally (0.2 mg, three times daily) for several days after delivery.

Adverse effects include nausea, vomiting, and more rarely, a rise in blood pressure. Since ergot alkaloids do not produce normal uterine contractions, they should not be employed during the first two stages of labor.

Ergonovine is only moderately effective in the treatment of migraine, but it is preferred by some patients because it produces less gastrointestinal side effects than ergotamine.

Ergotamine

Ergotamine (Gynergen) has remained the drug of choice for the treatment of migraine and other vascular headaches since its clinical introduction over 50 years ago.

The cause of *migraine* is poorly understood. The headache is usually unilateral in origin, is most common in the temple, and is associated with nausea and photophobia. An attack, which may be extremely disabling, varies in duration from a few minutes to several days. The early phases of the attack are believed to be associated with vasoconstriction of the cranial blood vessels followed by a pulsating vasodilation of these blood vessels. Ergotamine is thought to produce its beneficial effects by producing vasoconstriction and by reducing pulsations of these blood vessels.

Administration and precautions

Ergotamine is extremely effective in relieving migraine attacks in almost all patients; it is most effective when taken during the early stages of migraine. After subcutaneous or intramuscular administration (0.25 to 0.5 mg), the headache disappears within 15 minutes to 2 hours. Relief of headache requires an average of 5 hours after sublingual or oral administration of 4 to 5 mg, but these routes of administration may fail to be effective in severe attacks.

The nurse should caution the patient that the *smallest effective dose* of ergotamine should be used to manage migraine. During a 24-hour period, not more than 1 mg should be given parenterally or 10 mg by mouth. Excessive doses of this drug may produce severe vasoconstriction and gangrene of the extremities; early symptoms include a cold and numb feeling in the feet and legs and muscle pains. Other common symptoms associated with excessive ergotamine administration include headache, nausea, vomiting, diarrhea, and dizziness. Other nursing implications associated with the use of antimigraine agents are summarized at the end of this chapter.

Methysergide

Methysergide (Sansert) is ineffective for the relief of an acute attack of migraine. It and propranolol are the only drugs currently approved to *prevent* attacks. When a dose of 2 mg is taken orally three times daily, this synthetic ergot derivative has been found to be effective in preventing or reducing the intensity and frequency of migraine episodes.

The most common adverse effects include nausea, abdominal cramps, dizziness, insomnia, confusion, and depersonalization similar to that produced by LSD (Chapter 23). Long-term use of methysergide has been shown to produce *retroperitoneal fibrosis*, which may result in obstruction on the urinary tract. Fibrotic disorders of the heart and lungs have also been reported. This drug should be reserved for use in patients with headaches that are frequent or severe and uncontrollable and who are under close medical supervision.

Methysergide is contraindicated during pregnancy and in patients with peripheral vascular disorders, coronary artery disease, severe hypertension, kidney, liver or pulmonary disorders, rheumatoid arthritis, or other collagen diseases or disorders that may cause fibrosis. It is strongly recommended that the patient be examined at 6-month intervals and that a drug-free holiday of several weeks duration be maintained between courses of therapy.

PROSTAGLANDINS

The role of prostaglandins as possible mediators of the inflammatory response has been previously considered (Chapter 21). Natural prostaglandins and their synthetic derivatives are currently being evaluated for the treatment of many clinical disorders, including bronchial asthma, gastric ulcers, hypertension, and nasal congestion. In this chapter, we shall consider the obstetrical uses of these remarkable compounds.

Prostaglandins of the E and F class (PGE and PGF) have been shown to be involved in many phases of the endocrine regulation of reproductive function, including stimulation of gonadotropic hormone secretion by the anterior pituitary gland and ovulation. To date, greatest interest has focused upon the progressive increase in sensitivity of the pregnant uterus to the oxytocic actions of the prostaglandins, which reaches its peak at term. These compounds may play a physiological role in labor and parturition.

Therapeutic Uses

Prostaglandin $F_2\alpha$ (*dinoprost tromethamine, Prostin F2 alpha*) and E_2 (*dinoprostone, Prostin E2*) have been approved for use in the United States for induction of second-trimester abortion; dinoprost has also been used for induction of labor at term.

Induction of therapeutic abortion During the first trimester of pregnancy, the suction-curettage method of aborting fetuses is generally satisfactory. Prior to the introduction of the prostaglandins, intra-amnionic injection of 150 to 250 ml of a hypertonic (20 percent) solution of sodium chloride was the most widely used method for inducing a therapeutic abortion between the 14th and 24th week of gestation. This method did not always prove to be effective and was associated with inducing the sudden death of the mother as the result of rapid intravascular absorption.

Prostaglandins are the safest and most effective drugs available for terminating pregnancy during the second trimester of gestation. Drug-induced increase in uterine motility is thought to be responsible for these abortifacient effects.

To reduce the incidence of adverse systemic effects, intra-amnionic instillation of dinoprost (40 mg) is preferred rather than other routes of drug administration; if abortion is not complete within 24 hours, an additional 10 to 40 mg may be given. In one study, 80 percent of the patients aborted within 24 hours and 100 percent aborted within 48 hours.

Dinoprostone is available as a vaginal suppository (20 mg). It is recommended that a suppository be inserted high in the vagina every 3 to 5 hours until abortion occurs; the patient should be kept in a supine position for 10 minutes after insertion. The average time for abortion to occur is about 26 hours, but the time may range from 4 to 54 hours. This drug has been found to induce second-trimester abortions in 90 percent of all patients; of these, three-fourths are complete.

Carboprost (Prostin/15 M), indicated for inducing abortion between the 13th and 20th weeks of gestation, is administered by deep intramuscular injection. An initial 250 μg dose is recommended followed at 1.5 to 3.5-hour intervals by additional 250 to 500 μg doses. Carboprost also stimulates the smooth muscle of the gastrointestinal tract, an action that results in a higher incidence of nausea, vomiting, and diarrhea than with other prostaglandin derivatives.

The major side effects observed with these natural prostaglandins include a very high incidence of nausea, vomiting, and diarrhea; chills and fever have been reported with dinoprostone and carboprost. Nursing implications associated with the use of dinoprost appear at the end of this chapter.

Induction of labor at term While intravenous administration of the prostaglandins is effective in inducing labor at term, these drugs have a considerably longer onset of action than oxytocin and, in most cases, offer no clear advantages. You will recall that oxytocin can increase uterine contractions throughout pregnancy, but it produces its maximum effects at term. Prostaglandins, by contrast, are effective oxytocics throughout gestation and are, therefore, preferred when labor must be induced during an early stage of pregnancy for the management of missed abortion or in fetal death. Unlike intra-amnionic hypertonic saline solutions, prostaglandins do not kill the fetus, and some live births can occur when these drugs are used to induce abortions late in the second trimester.

Drugs Affecting Uterine Contractions and Antimigraine Agents: **nursing implications**

Oxytocics

1. Assess condition of the patient prior to initiating drug therapy. Monitor blood pressure (B.P.), fluid intake and output ratio, strength and duration of uterine contractions, and fetal heart tones and rate. A qualified physician should be immediately available to manage complications.
2. For inducement or enhancement of labor, oxytocin should be administered in a dilute solution employing a constant infusion pump; 5 units oxytocin per 1000 ml dextrose in water or normal saline administered initially at 5 milliunits/min (15 drops/min).
3. Overdosage may occur at very low infusion rates and produce uterine hypertonus and abnormally frequent contractions. Overstimulation usually subsides within a few minutes after stopping the infusion.
4. Closely monitor uterine contractions and fetal heart and vital signs at least every 15 min during drug administration.
5. During periods of prolonged IV infusions, watch for signs of water intoxication: drowsiness, listlessness, headache, confusion, anuria, and edema. Report changes in levels of alertness, fluid intake and output ratio, and edema.
6. If contractions are prolonged and if electric monitor records contractions above 50 mm Hg, stop infusion to prevent fetal anoxia and notify physician.

Dinoprost

1. The benefits and risks of dinoprost-induced abortion should be explained to the patient.
2. Monitor B.P., pulse, and uterine contractions after drug administration. Significant changes may indicate hemorrhage.
3. Gastrointestinal symptoms (nausea, vomiting, abdominal cramps, diarrhea) may indicate accidental administration of drug into maternal bloodstream.
4. The drug is administered via a transabdominal intra-amnionic catheter after checking that no blood is present in amnionic fluid.
5. The drug does not cause fetal death; live birth is possible if abortion is performed at end of second trimester.
6. If the drug fails to terminate pregnancy, another method is usually used because of teratogenic potential of prostaglandins.

Antimigraine Agents

1. Teach the patient the action of drug and timing for administration to obtain maximum relief of migraine symptoms. Drug therapy should be initiated as soon as possible after onset of prodromal symptoms: scintillating scotoma, visual field defects, paresthesia.
2. Instruct the patient to report side effects associated with excessive vasoconstriction: cold or numb digits, claudication.

3. Patients taking drugs prophylactically should be cautioned to discontinue drugs gradually to prevent migraine headache rebound.

4. Help the patient identify and learn to avoid physical or emotional stresses or dietary substances that precipitate attacks.

5. Drugs should not be given to patients with peripheral vascular disorders, coronary artery disease, severe hypertension, or collagen disease or during pregnancy (because of oxytocic effects).

SUPPLEMENTARY READINGS

Behrman, H. R., and G. G. Anderson, "Prostaglandins in Reproduction," *Archives of Internal Medicine* **133:** 77–84 (1974).

Caldeyro-Barcia, R., and H. Heller, *Oxytocin*. New York: Pergamon Press, Inc., 1961.

Dalessio, D. J., *Wolff's Headache and Other Head Pain* (3rd ed.). New York: Oxford University Press, Inc., 1972.

Goldberg, V. J., and P. W. Ramwell, "Role of Prostaglandins in Reproduction," *Physiological Reviews* **55:** 325–51 (1975).

Karim, S. M. M., ed., *Prostaglandins and Reproduction*. Baltimore: University Park Press, 1975.

Rall, T. W., and L. S. Schleifer, "Oxytocin, Prostaglandins, Ergot Alkaloids, and Other Agents," in *Goodman and Gilman's The Pharmacological Basis of Therapeutics* (6th ed.), ed. A. G. Gilman, L. S. Goodman, and A. Gilman, Chapter 39, pp. 935–50. New York: Macmillan, Inc., 1980.

Romney, S. L., and others, *Gynecology and Obstetrics: The Health Care of Women*. New York: McGraw-Hill Book Company, 1975.

Scheife, R. T., and J. R. Hills, "Migraine Headache: Signs and Symptoms, Biochemistry, and Current Therapy," *American Journal of Hospital Pharmacy* **37:** 365–74 (1980).

Wilson, D. E., ed., "Symposium on Prostaglandins," *Archives of Internal Medicine* **133:** 29–146 (1974).

Chapter 39

THE VITAMINS

Vitamins are substances required by the body for carrying out essential metabolic reactions. Although these substances are needed in relatively small amounts, vitamins must be supplied by the diet to maintain the health of the individual because they cannot be biosynthesized.

In this chapter, we shall examine the rational uses of vitamins. Because detailed considerations of the physiological effects of vitamins and the medical disorders resulting from their deficiency are presented in other courses in the nursing curriculum, these aspects will not be discussed in this text. The comparative properties of water-soluble and fat-soluble vitamins are summarized in Table 39-1 and 39-2, respectively.

RECOMMENDED DAILY ALLOWANCES

Since 1940, the Food and Nutrition Board of the National Research Council has published a set of *"Recommended Daily Allowances"* (RDA) for vitamins and other nutrients. The RDA (Tables 39-1 and 39-2) are recommendations for the amounts of vitamins that should be consumed daily to provide the known nutritional needs of most normal and healthy persons living in the United States under usual environmental conditions. These values should not be confused with *minimum daily requirements* (MDR), which differ for each individual; in most instances, the RDA is several times greater than the MDR.

A vast amount of confusion and misinformation exists about foods and the need for vitamin supplements. Notwithstanding many promotional claims to the contrary, most healthy Americans ingesting a well-balanced diet obtain a sufficient quantity of vitamins to adequately satisfy their bodies' needs. Reports appearing in lay publications describing the beneficial effects of large doses of vitamins in the treatment or cure of disorders related to nonvitamin disorders should be read with healthy skepticism by nurses.

EXCESSIVE VITAMIN INTAKE

The use of vitamin supplements in doses greatly in excess of the established RDA is at best economically wasteful and may be

Table 39-1　Water-Soluble Vitamins

Vitamin (synonyms)	Common dietary sources	Recommended daily allowance[a]			
		Unit	Infants	Children $<$ 4 yrs	Children $>$ 4 yrs and adults
B$_1$ (Thiamine, Thiamin)	Yeast, pork, wheat germ.	mg	0.3-0.5	0.7	1.1-1.5
B$_2$ (Riboflavin)	Yeast, eggs, green vegetables, meat.	mg	0.4-0.6	0.8	1.2-1.7
Niacin (Nicotinic acid)	Yeast, liver, meat.	mg	6-8	9	13-19
B$_6$ (Pyridoxine)	Yeast, liver, wheat germ.	mg	0.3-0.6	0.9	2
B$_{12}$ (Cyanocobalamin)	Liver	mg	0.5-1.5	2	3
Biotin	Eggs, meat, milk.	mg	——[b]	——[b]	——[b]
Pantothenic acid	Yeast, eggs, liver.	mg	——[b]	——[b]	——[b]
Folacin (Folic acid)	Liver, yeast, milk, green vegetables.	μg	30-45	100	400
C (Ascorbic acid)	Citrus fruits, green peppers, vegetables.	mg	35	45	60

[a] *Recommended Daily Allowances* (9th ed.), Washington, D.C.: National Academy of Sciences, 1979. (For healthy persons living in the United States)

[b] None established.

Physiological functions	Deficiency disorders	Daily adult therapeutic dose (mg)	Remarks
Carbohydrate metabolism; synthesis of acetylcholine.	Beri-beri peripheral neuritis, heart failure. Behavioral disorders. Muscle weakness.	25–50	Large intravenous doses may cause anaphylactic reactions.
Prosthetic group of enzyme systems involved in carbohydrate and amino acid metabolism and oxidation-reduction reactions.	Skin lesions, glossitis, visual disorders; possible skeletal deformities of fetus if deficiency during pregnancy.	5–15	No adverse effects with excessive doses.
Prosthetic group of NAD and NADP, coenzymes essential for life.	Pellagra (skin lesions, gastrointestinal disorders; behavorial aberrations).	20	Used with B_1 and B_2 for treatment of chronic alcoholism. May cause flushing, itching, nausea.
Acts as coenzyme pyridoxal phosphate in amino acid metabolism, for example, biosynthesis of neurotransmitters.	Skin disorders. Convulsions (infants).	5–150	Deficiency very rare in adults.
Normal function of bone marrow (erythrocyte maturation) and nervous system.	Pernicious anemia.	0.1 mg IM 1–2 times weekly.	Used for treatment of pernicious anemia and megaloblastic anemias.
Metabolic reactions involving transfer of carboxyl groups.	Skin disorders, loss of appetite.	0.3	Difficult to demonstrate biotin deficiency in humans.
Unit of coenzyme A required for acetylation reactions.	Neuromuscular disorders.	10	Same as biotin.
Required for synthesis of purines, pyrimidines and amino acids; formation of erythrocytes.	Megaloblastic anemias, glossitis, diarrhea, weight loss.	0.25–1	The daily requirements of this vitamin are 0.8 mg during the last trimester of pregnancy. Folic acid administration can mask pernicious anemia, which can lead to neurological damage.
Formation of intracellular collagen, bones and teeth; cellular oxidation-reduction reactions.	Scurvy (abnormalities of capillaries, bones, connective tissues).	500–1,000	Readily destroyed during cooking. High daily doses (1–4 g) recommended for treatment of common cold; effectiveness questionable. Possible gastrointestinal upset, kidney or bladder stone formation.

Table 39-2   Fat-Soluble Vitamins

Vitamin (synonyms)	Common dietary sources	Recommended Daily Allowances[a]			
		Unit	Infants	Children < 4 yr.	Children > 4 yr. and adults
A A_1 = retinol	Fish liver oils, eggs, milk, butter, green leafy and yellow vegetables.	I.U.	2,100	2,000	2500–5000
D D_2 = ergocalciferol D_3 = cholecalciferol	Fish, eggs, butter, milk (fortified).	I.U.	400	400	200–400
E (tocopherol)	Vegetable fats and oils, dairy products, meat, cereals, vegetables.	I.U.	4–6	7	10–15
K (menadione) K_1 = phytonadione	Leafy green vegetables, tomatoes, liver.	——[b]	——[b]	——[b]	

[a] *Recommended Daily Allowances* (9th ed.), National Academy of Sciences, 1979. (For healthy persons living in the United States)

[b] None established.

harmful. The *water-soluble vitamins* (B and C) generally possess low toxicity, and, when consumed orally in large amounts, are rapidly excreted in the urine. The potential adverse effects associated with these vitamins are summarized in Table 39-1, and drug interactions with these compounds appear in Table 39-3 (page 348); drug interactions with vitamin B_{12} and folic acid are summarized in Table 40-2 (page 353).

The *fat-soluble vitamins* (A, D, E, and K), by contrast, accumulate in fat when taken in excessive quantities. Ingestion of vitamins A and D in amounts greatly larger than their daily requirements results in toxic syndromes referred to as *hypervitaminosis* A and D (Table 39-2).

INSUFFICIENT VITAMIN INTAKE

When a vitamin deficiency is present or suspected, supplemental vitamin therapy is therapeutically indicated. *Vitamin deficiency* may result from inadequate intake, impaired gas-

Physiological functions	Deficiency disorders	Daily adult therapeutic dose	Consequences of overdosage	Remarks
Formation of rhodopsin-protein in retina for dark adaptation. Maintenance of epithelial cells.	Night blindness. Abnormalities of connective tissues, bones, nerves, skin infections, reproduction.	25,000 I.U.	Hypervitaminosis A: irritability, loss of appetite, skin and bone disorders, enlargement of spleen and liver, hard swelling of extremities.	Topical use of retinoic acid (tretinoin, Retin-A) for acne vulgaris.
Promotes intestinal absorption of calcium and phosphorus. Regulates movement of these minerals in bone. Required for normal growth of children.	Rickets (infants and children). Osteomalacia (adults).	1,000–50,000 I.U.	Hypercalcemia: weakness, headache, gastrointestinal, kidney, heart disorders.	Also used for treatment of hypoparathyroidism.
Antioxidant may be related to polyunsaturated fats in diet. May stabilize cell membranes, for example, erythrocytes.	Rarely observed in humans, usually associated with impaired fat absorption. Animals: abortions and muscle weakness.	30 I.U.	None known.	Only use is for vitamin deficiency with fat absorption impaired.
Formation of blood clotting factors in liver.	Hemorrhagic disorders in premature infants.	2–5 mg	Hemolysis of erythrocytes, kernicterus, liver jaundice.	Menadione used to treat coumarin anticoagulant overdosage.

trointestinal absorption, or increased tissue requirements.

Inadequate vitamin intake is very common in many parts of the world and exists in the United States most often as the result of poverty. Vitamin deficiencies may also be the consequence of ignorance, poor eating habits, emotional or physical illnesses, greatly restricted food intake by individuals on diets seeking to manage obesity, or food faddism (for example, among vegetarians). Inadequate vitamin intake is often observed in chronic alcoholics. Since single-vitamin deficiences are rare in such individuals, multiple-vitamin therapy is generally prescribed.

Impairment of vitamin absorption may result from a wide variety of malabsorption syndromes and other gastrointestinal disorders, including pernicious anemia, tropical sprue, prolonged diarrhea, and diseases of the liver and biliary tract. Some drugs have been found to impair vitamin absorption (Table 39-3).

Increased tissue requirements may result from conditions rendering a previously adequate diet no longer sufficient in supply-

Table 39-3   Drug Interactions Involving Vitamins

Vitamin	Interacting drug/class	Potential consequences
B_1	Alkaline solutions	Thiamine hydrochloride is unstable and breaks down in neutral or alkaline solutions (carbonates, citrates, barbiturates).
B_6	Levodopa	Pyridoxine at doses greater than 5 mg antagonize beneficial effects of levodopa in Parkinson's disease.
B_{12}	Table 40-2	
Folacin	Table 40-2	
C	Tricyclic antidepressants Amphetamine Quinidine	High daily doses of ascorbic acid (2 g) acidify the urine and may enhance the urinary excretion of basic drugs.
Calcium ascorbate	Digitalis glycosides	This vitamin preparation should not be used in patients receiving digitalis; calcium may precipitate cardiac arrhythmias.
D K	Mineral oil	Mineral oil interferes with absorption of fat-soluble vitamins; impairment of vitamin K absorption in pregnant females may cause hemorrhaging in newborn.
K (menadione)	Oral anticoagulants	Mutual antagonism between these drugs; menadione used to treat overdosage of coumarin derivatives.

ing the greater demands of the body. Vitamin requirements are increased during pregnancy, lactation, menstruation, and during periods of growth, wound healing, hard work, and stress. Disorders increasing the rate of body metabolism, such as hyperthyroidism, also increase the needs of tissues for vitamins.

The nurse possesses the professional training required to educate the lay public about the proper dietary intake and rational use of vitamin supplements to enable them to maintain good health. Nursing implications are summarized at the end of this chapter. Use of excessive quantities of vitamins is not without potential hazard and is frequently economically unjustified.

Vitamins:
nursing implications

1. Teach the patient and his or her family the requirements for adequate vitamin intake through diet. Individualize dietary planning, utilizing economic food products when appropriate and adapting the diet for specific cultural preferences and physiological needs.
2. Explain the meaning of minimum daily requirements and how to read labels of vitamin products to determine adequacy and avoid unnecessary excess and overdosage.
3. Observe patients for symptoms of vitamin deficiency, especially in children, the elderly, and those with chronic diseases.
4. Advise the patient not to take mineral oil with the fat-soluble vitamins (A, D, E, K) because they will not be absorbed normally.
5. Vitamain K is used for the treatment of primary and drug- (coumarin-) induced hypoprothrombinemia. It cannot reverse the anticoagulant effects of heparin.

SUPPLEMENTARY READINGS

Boehne, J. V., and M. R. Spivey Fox, "Vitamins and Other Nutients," in *Remington's Pharmaceutical Sciences*, ed. A. Osol and J. E. Hoover (15th ed.), Chapter 52, pp. 935–70. Easton, Pennsylvania: Mack Publishing Co., 1975.

DeLuca, H. F., and J. W. Suttie, eds., *The Fat Soluble Vitamins*. Madison: University of Wisconsin Press, 1970.

DiPalma, J. R. and D. M. Ritchie, "Vitamin Toxicity," *Annual Review of Pharmacology and Toxicology* 17: 133–48 (1977).

Dykes, M. H. M., and P. Meier, "Ascorbic Acid and the Common Cold. Evaluation of its Efficacy and Tox-

icity," *Journal of the American Medical Association* 231: 1073–79 (1975).

Food and Nutrition Board, National Research Council, *Recommended Daily Allowances* (9th ed.). Washington, D.C.: National Academy of Sciences, 1979.

Goodhart, R. S., and M. E. Shils, eds., *Modern Nutrition in Health and Disease* (5th ed.). Philadelphia: Lea & Febiger, 1973.

Ivey, M., "Nutritional Supplement, Mineral, and Vitamin Products," in *Handbook of Nonprescription Drugs* (6th ed.), pp. 141–74. Washington, D.C.: American Pharmaceutical Association, 1979.

Robinson, C. H., *Normal and Therapeutic Nutrition* (14th ed.). New York: Macmillan, Inc., 1972.

Poe, D. A., "Drug-Induced Deficiency of B Vitamins," *New York State Journal of Medicine* 71: 2770–77 (1971).

DRUG TREATMENT OF ANEMIAS

Chapter 40

The major function of *erythrocytes* (red blood cells) is to carry oxygen from the lungs to the tissues. Approximately 97 percent of the oxygen transported is carried in loose chemical combination with *hemoglobin*, the major component of erythrocytes. Conditions characterized by a reduction in the number of circulating erythrocytes or in the amount of hemoglobin are called *anemias*. In anemic disorders, the blood is unable to adequately satisfy the oxygen requirements of

tissues, especially during periods of exercise, thus reducing the endurance of patients with such diseases, causing them to fatigue readily.

There are many causes of anemia, some of which include: (1) excessive blood loss; (2) erythrocyte hemolysis, resulting from hereditary disorders (sickle-cell anemia), erythroblastosis fetalis (a disease of the newborn in which maternal antibodies destroy the erythrocytes of the baby), and drugs (primaquine and other antimalarial drugs, sulfonamides, nitrofurantoin, aspirin, acetanilid, and other analgesic-antipyretics); (3) bone marrow failure (the site of erythrocyte formation) caused by excessive exposure to radiation (nuclear bomb blast) or drugs (chloramphenicol, sulfonamides, certain anticancer drugs); and (4) defective formation of hemoglobin (iron deficiency anemia) or erythrocytes (megaloblastic anemias, including pernicious anemia).

This fourth group of anemias, the subject of this chapter, is very responsive to treatment with *hematinic* or *antianemic agents* such as iron, vitamin B₁₂, and folic acid. We shall begin our discussion with a brief consideration of the normal formation of erythrocytes and hemoglobin.

ERYTHROCYTES AND HEMOGLOBIN

Erythrocytes are produced in the bone marrow at a rate that is normally sufficient to replace aged cells that are constantly being removed from the circulation. It has been estimated that over 100 million erythrocytes are formed each hour and have an average life-span of 120 days. These cells are formed in several stages, progressing from large, immature cells containing a nucleus but not hemoglobin to small, non-nucleated biconcave disks containing hemoglobin (erythrocytes).

Erythrocytes are packed with 200 to 300 million molecules of *hemoglobulin*, with each molecule consisting of the protein globulin and heme, a pigment containing iron. Erythropoiesis (red-cell production) requires amino acids for the synthesis of globulin, iron, and minute amounts of vitamin B₁₂, folic acid, vitamin B₆, and copper.

The diet usually supplies an adequate amount of these essential substances. For the most part, anemias result when iron is removed from the body at a rate exceeding that

provided by the diet or when insufficient amounts of vitamin B₁₂ or folic acid are absorbed from dietary sources. We shall now consider iron deficiency and megaloblastic anemias, the types the nurse is most likely to encounter in practice.

IRON-DEFICIENCY ANEMIA

The most common form of anemia throughout the world and the most prevalant nutritional deficiency in the United States results from an iron deficiency. Early symptoms are generally vague and include feelings of weakness and fatigue, loss of appetite, dizziness, and skin pallor. Microscopic examination of blood samples from advanced cases reveals small and pale erythrocytes that are poorly filled with hemoglobin; hence, iron-deficiency anemia is referred to as *hypochromic microcytic anemia.*

Iron Metabolism

Of the total body stores of iron, approximately 60 percent circulate in the blood as hemoglobin. Twenty-six mg of iron are liberated each day as the result of normal red blood cell breakdown, and only 1 mg is lost in the urine and bile; this amount represents the normal daily adult requirement of this mineral, which increases to 4 mg during periods of growth, menstruation, and pregnancy. The iron retained by the body is employed for the synthesis of new molecules of hemoglobin.

The average daily North American or European diet contains 6 mg of iron per 1,000 kilocalories or about 15 to 20 mg. Good dietary sources of iron include green vegetables, eggs, beef, liver, and chocolate; milk is a poor source of this mineral.

Iron in foods or provided as a supplement is absorbed from the stomach and small intestines to the extent of 5 to 10 percent in normal individuals and about 10 to 30 percent in iron-deficient patients; hence the amount of iron ingested must be ten times as great as the daily body requirements. The extent to which iron is absorbed from the gastrointestinal tract depends upon the state of the body's iron reserves and not on the hemoglobin content of the blood. During pregnancy, iron utilization is greater than normal, causing a depletion of reserves; the pregnant woman, whether anemic or not, absorbs two to ten times as much iron as the nonpregnant female.

Control of iron absorption is mediated by *apoferritin*, a compound present in the mucosal cells of the small intestines. Gastric acid of the stomach increases the ionization of iron and the reduction of iron (ferric) salts to their ferrous state, which also facilitates absorption. Antacids (alkalinizing agents), used by patients for the treatment of peptic ulcer, and milk impair iron absorption.

After absorption has occurred, the glycoprotein *transferrin* transports iron to storage sites in the bone marrow, spleen, and liver for subsequent hemoglobin biosynthesis.

Iron Deficiency

The most common cause of iron deficiency is *excessive blood loss*, commonly produced by gastrointestinal bleeding resulting from disease (gastroduodenal ulcer or carcinoma, hemorrhoids), drugs (aspirin, phenylbutazone, reserpine, oral anticoagulants), or blood loss during delivery of a baby or menstruation. The average daily loss of iron during normal menstruation, spread evenly over the menstrual cycle, is 0.5 to 1 mg. Hookworm and other intestinal parasites are important causes of blood loss and iron deficiency in many countries.

Inadequate dietary intake is rarely a cause of iron deficiency in healthy men of any age and in postmenopausal women. Women who have borne several children in rapid succession often have an iron intake insufficient to meet the increased requirements associated with pregnancy. Since cow's milk is low in iron, extended periods of bottle feeding may result in a deficiency of this mineral; this problem is most common in immature infants or those born with insufficient iron reserves. A very high incidence of iron-deficiency anemia is observed between the ages of 6 months and 3 years, especially in 1- to 2-year-old children. One report found the incidence of anemia in 1-year-old children ranges from 25 to 75 percent in impoverished areas to 5 to 15 percent in middle class areas of the United States. Individuals restricting their diets because of weight control or lack of interest in eating (elderly persons) may also develop iron deficiency.

Malabsorption of iron from the diet may occur in prolonged cases of diarrhea and other intestinal disorders or in patients with partial gastrectomy.

Iron Supplementation

Adjustments in diet generally do not prove satisfactory in the management of iron deficiency anemia, and iron supplementation is usually required. Drugs containing iron are available for oral and parenteral administration (Table 40-1), with the former preferred in most cases. Nursing implications associated with iron preparations are summarized at the end of this chapter.

Oral iron preparations Oral *ferrous sulfate* is the least expensive iron preparation available and is the drug of choice for the treatment of iron deficiency anemia. The relatively high incidence of undesirable gastrointestinal side effects (which are dis-

Table 40-1   Iron Preparations

Generic name	Selected trade names	% Elemental iron	mg Elemental iron per 1 tablet/1 ml	Usual total daily adult dose
Oral Preparations				
Ferrous Sulfate (Heptahydrate)	_____ Mol-Iron	20	60 mg per 300 mg 39 mg per 195 mg; 10 mg/ml	600–1,200 mg
Ferrous Sulfate (dried)	Feosol Fer-In-Sol	30	65 mg per 200 mg; 9 mg/ml	600–800 mg
Ferrous Gluconate	Fergon	11.6	37 mg per 320 mg; 7 mg/ml	960–1,600 mg
Ferrous Fumarate	Feostat Ircon	33	66 mg per 200 mg	600–800 mg
Ferrocholinate	Chel-Iron	12	40 mg per 333 mg; 10 mg/ml	666–999 mg
Parenteral Preparation				
Iron Dextran injection	Imferon		50 mg/ml	A test dose of 25–50 mg IM on 1st day, 250 mg every day or every other day.

cussed shortly) has led to the introduction of many solid (pill) and liquid (drops) products containing iron (Table 40-1). The nurse should note, however, that the extent to which a preparation is absorbed is proportional to the amount of soluble elemental (free or ionic) iron present; the greater this amount, the greater will be the degree of gastrointestinal distress. Hence, ferrous sulfate and other iron salts that are well absorbed are those preparations which are most likely to produce distress; preparations containing slowly released iron (which are far more expensive) are less effectively absorbed and are less useful in the management of anemia. Some of the widely promoted iron products ("iron tonics for tired blood") are usually well tolerated, but the low iron content and high cost of these products fails to justify their use.

The largest effective dose of ferrous sulfate that can be taken in the absence of adverse side effects should be employed. Subjective feelings of well-being may be reported within several days after the initiation of therapy but these are probably psychological rather than pharmacological effects. Oral therapy should be continued for several weeks after hemoglobin levels have returned to normal; the normal duration of therapy is 4 to 6 months.

Adverse effects   Between 5 to 10 percent of patients receiving normal therapeutic doses of iron salts will experience such symptoms of *gastrointestinal distress* as constipation or diarrhea, nausea, and epigastric pain. Administration of these drugs after meals, three times daily, generally reduces these side effects. A number of drugs can reduce the absorption of iron salts; these interactions and others are summarized in Table 40-2.

The nurse should inform patients prior to the initiation of therapy that iron preparations will color the feces dark red or black and that this should not be interpreted as a sign of gastrointestinal bleeding. Patients tak-

Table 40-2   Potential Drug Interactions Involving Antianemic Drugs

Antianemic drug	Interacting drug/class	Potential consequences
Oral iron preparations	Antacids Calcium carbonate Aluminum hydroxide Magnesium hydroxide Magnesium trisilicate	Iron forms insoluble complexes with these compounds resulting in an impairment of iron absorption. Moreover, since acidity (from gastric juice) favors iron absorption, antacid neutralization of this acidity also impairs absorption.
	Tetracycline antibiotics Tetracycline (Achromycin, Panmycin, Steclin, Tetracyn, and others) Methacycline (Rondomycin) Doxycycline (Vibramycin)	Iron preparations bind tetracyclines in the gastrointestinal tract impairing the absorption of these antibiotics. Iron should be given 2 h before or after tetracycline derivatives.
Folic acid	Antiepileptics Phenytoin (Dilantin) Phenobarbital Primidone (Mysoline)	These drugs, phenytoin in particular, impair folic acid absorption and possibly its metabolism, causing megaloblastic anemia. Administration of folic acid may reduce seizure control.
	Chemotherapeutic agents Methotrexate (Amethopterin) Trimethoprim Pyrimethamine	These drugs antagonize folic acid potentially resulting in megaloblastic anemia.
	Oral contraceptives	Can impair folic acid absorption.

ing liquids containing soluble iron salts should be advised to place the drops or liquid well back on the tongue to avoid staining dental enamel; alternatively, the liquid should be taken in a small volume of water or fruit juice and administered through a straw.

Acute toxicity Patients should be warned to keep iron products out of the reach of children. Accidental poisoning with this drug class is a common occurrence in children, with 50 percent of these cases having a fatal outcome. Doses of 1 g of ferrous sulfate may be toxic, with lethal doses ranging from 3 to 18 g.

Symptoms of toxicity may occur within 30 minutes to several hours and include gastrointestinal signs (nausea, vomiting, often containing blood, and diarrhea) and shock. If death does not occur within 6 hours, there may be a transient period of apparent recovery followed by cardiovascular collapse and death within 12 to 48 hours.

Emergency treatment can be started in the home by inducing vomiting and by giving eggs or milk to form an insoluble iron-protein complex. *Deferoxamine mesylate* (Desferal), a specific iron chelating agent, has been used to successfully treat acute iron poisoning in children. A dose of 500 mg of this drug is administered intravenously or intramuscularly at 4-hour intervals; not more than 6 g should be given within a 24-hour period. Deferoxamine is contraindicated in patients with severe renal disease or anuria since the drug and the chelate it forms with iron are excreted primarily by the kidney.

Parenteral iron preparations   Parenteral iron should be employed only after oral therapy has proved to be ineffective because of the lack of a therapeutic response (resulting from failure to absorb adequate amounts of iron) or the inability or unwillingness of the patient to take iron by mouth.

While oral preparations are inexpensive, safe, and effective, parenteral iron is costly, painful, and sometimes dangerous. Moreover, similar therapeutic responses are achieved after the administration of equivalent doses of iron given by mouth and injection.

Iron complexed with dextran (Imferon) is a commonly used parenteral preparation. A test dose of 25 or 50 mg is administered on the first day, and, if no adverse reaction occurs, is followed by adult doses of up to 250 mg daily or every other day until normal levels of hemoglobin and body stores of iron are achieved. This drug is administered by deep intramuscular injection. A Z-tract injection technique into the upper outer quadrant of the buttock should be employed to avoid leakage back into subcutaneous tissues; brown discoloration occurs at the site of injection and may persist for 1 to 2 years or longer.

Allergic responses and even fatal anaphylactic reactions have occurred after administration of iron dextran. Relatively common side effects include soreness and inflammation at the site of injection, headache, fever, nausea, vomiting, and regional lymphadenopathy.

MEGALOBLASTIC ANEMIAS

Formation of erythrocytes requires vitamin B_{12} and folic acid. In the absence of these B-complex vitamins, the large, nucleated erythrocyte-precursor blood cells (megaloblasts) fail to mature. Examination of the bone marrow and blood of such patients reveals a marked decrease in the number of erythrocytes and a great number of macrocytes; the latter are large, misshapen, hemoglobin-packed cells with a life-span one-third that of normal erythrocytes. These hematological disorders, called *megaloblastic* or *macrocytic anemias*, include pernicious anemia, tropical sprue, celiac disease, and idiopathic steatorrhea.

Pernicious Anemia

Pernicious anemia, the most prevalent of the megaloblastic anemias, affects about 0.1 percent of the population and occurs during middle and late life. In addition to causing anemia, this once invariably fatal disorder affects all cells of the body, particularly those of the nervous system and gastrointestinal tract.

Causes and symptoms   The normal daily body requirements of vitamin B_{12} are extremely small, only 1 μg (1 millionth gram); a normal diet containing liver, meat, seafood, eggs, and milk more than adequately supplies these needs. The most common cause of pernicious anemia is the *failure to absorb* this vitamin from the intestinal tract. Absorption of this vitamin requires the presence of an *intrinsic factor*, a glycoprotein that is secreted by the parietal cells of the stomach and is present in normal gastric secretions. Pernicious anemia is associated with an atrophy of the gastric mucosa. This leads to an absence of the intrinsic factor, thus accounting for a failure to absorb the *extrinsic factor*, vitamin B_{12}.

The anemia associated with this disease causes the patient to be pale and experience shortness of breath (dyspnea), the latter resulting from the lack of adequate oxygen to the tissues. Levels of white blood cells and platelets are also low, and this accounts for increased susceptibility to infection and bleeding tendencies, respectively.

One of the most characteristic signs of this disease is *achlorhydria*, the absence of hydrochloric acid in gastric secretions. This lack of gastric acid is responsible for the marked loss of appetite and subsequent weight loss. Glossitis, an inflammation of the tongue, is commonly observed. A variety of *nervous system disorders* are seen, including numbness and tingling of the hands and feet, unsteadiness and difficulty in walking, progressive weakness, degeneration of the spinal cord, and adverse behavioral changes. Nursing implications associated with pernicious anemia, vitamin B_{12}, and folic acid are summarized at the end of this chapter.

Vitamin B_{12}

Vitamin B_{12} (cyanocobalamin), a compound containing cobalt, is essential for the normal functioning of all cells, especially those in the bone marrow, nervous system, and gastrointestinal tract. This vitamin participates in reduction reactions, those biochemical reactions involving the transfer of methyl groups, and in DNA synthesis.

Administration In the absence of the intrinsic factor, absorption of vitamin B_{12} is extremely modest (1 percent) and not reliable. Since high oral doses (100 to 1000 μg) are required and are quite expensive, therapy by mouth is generally reserved for patients refusing injections. Cyanocobalamin (Betalin 12, Redisol, Rubramin PC) is highly effective after intramuscular or subcutaneous injection. This drug is usually parenterally administered at a dose of 30 μg on a daily basis for 5 to 10 days, followed by maintenance doses of 100 μg at monthly intervals.

Hydroxocobalamin (alphaRedisol), a semisynthetic cyanocobalamin derivative, is more slowly absorbed from its intramuscular site of injection and is less rapidly excreted in the urine. This drug achieves higher and more prolonged blood levels than cyanocobalamin after the administration of equivalent doses.

Therapeutic aspects The therapeutic response to vitamin B_{12} in the treatment of pernicious anemia is usually dramatic. Elevations in mood and feelings of wellbeing are observed within 48 hours, followed soon thereafter by improved appetite and increased strength. After approximately 10 days, levels of white blood cells and platelets return to normal, while 4 to 8 weeks are required for erythrocyte levels to return to normal.

While administration of this vitamin arrests further neurological damage, the restoration of nervous system function depends largely on the duration of impairment rather than its severity. Greatest improvements can be observed in patients whose walking has been impaired for less than 3 months, with little benefit noted when impairment has persisted for several years. Vitamin therapy ameliorates many of the gastrointestinal disturbances but does not correct the basic defect underlying pernicious anemia; gastric mucosal atrophy persists, and there is no restoration of the deficient intrinsic factor. The nurse should explain to the patient that injections of cyanocobalamin do not cure this disease, and that therapy must continue for a lifetime. Injections of cyanocobalamin are relatively painless, and even high doses are devoid of toxicity.

The only established clinical indication for cyanocobalamin administration is for the management of a deficiency of this vitamin. There is no evidence justifying the use of this vitamin to stimulate growth, for the treatment of liver diseases or dermatological or behavioral disorders, or as a general tonic or appetite stimulant. The indiscriminate prescribing of "shotgun" antianemic preparations to all anemic patients, most of whom do not have pernicious anemia, at best represents an unnecessary expense for the patient. The use of such products, not uncommonly containing iron, vitamin B_{12}, liver, stomach, B-complex vitamins, vitamin C, and minerals, may mask the neurological complications of pernicious anemia or gastric carcinoma.

Folic Acid

Folic acid (Folacin, pteroylglutamic acid) serves as a coenzyme in intermediary metabolic reactions in which one-carbon units are transferred; such reactions are associated with amino acid and DNA synthesis.

Good dietary sources of folic acid include liver, kidney, dry beans, asparagus, broccoli, and mushrooms. The minimum daily adult requirement is 0.05 mg, with a recommended daily allowance of 0.4 mg.

Deficiency A deficiency of folic acid is primarily characterized by *megaloblastic anemia*, which cannot be differentiated from the same hematological disorder associated with a vitamin B_{12} deficiency. Other common symptoms associated with a folic acid deficiency include glossitis, diarrhea, and weight loss. You should note that the major clinical difference between these two B-vitamin deficiencies is the absence of neurological disorders in the case of folic acid.

Causes of folic acid deficiency include malnutrition, intestinal malabsorption disorders (tropical sprue, celiac disease, steatorrhea), gastroectomy, and pregnancy, when vitamin requirements are increased. Chronic alcoholics often have a deficiency of this vitamin. A number of drugs (antiepileptic, anticancer, and antimalarial) have been shown to produce varying degrees of folic acid de-

ficiency by inhibiting its absorption or by inhibiting its utilization in essential metabolic reactions (Table 40-2). These drug-induced deficiencies can often be managed by supplementing folic acid intake.

Administration and precautions
Folic acid is effectively absorbed after oral administration and is usually prescribed in daily doses of 0.1 to 1 mg; no adverse effects are associated with the administration of this vitamin.

Use of folic acid is indicated for the treatment of megaloblastic anemias resulting from a deficiency of this vitamin in adults and children and may be used during the third trimester of pregnancy. Parenteral administration of folic acid or leucovorin (folinic acid) should be reserved for patients with intestinal malabsorption disorders or when oral therapy is not possible. *Leucovorin* is also employed to diminish the toxicity and counteract the effects of an overdose of such folic acid antagonist anticancer drugs as methotrexate (Chapter 51).

Doses of 0.1 mg of folic acid may mask the megaloblastic anemia associated with pernicious anemia, while allowing the neurological defects to progress and even worsen. Hence, prior to the administration of folic acid, the possibility of pernicious anemia should be excluded. Folic acid should be co-administered only with vitamin B_{12} (in multivitamin preparations) when a deficiency of *both* vitamins is present. Food and Drug Administration regulations prohibit the inclusion of more than 0.1 mg of folic acid in nonprescription multivitamin preparations.

Drug Treatment of Anemias:
nursing implications

Oral Iron Preparations

1. Iron-deficiency anemia should be treated with oral iron preparations after other types of anemia are ruled out by examination.
2. The cause of iron deficiency must be identified and corrected as: inadequate dietary iron intake; impaired iron absorption; drug-induced causes such as high doses of aspirin; excessive blood loss, such as occult gastrointestinal bleeding, or excessive menstrual bleeding.
3. Iron therapy is generally continued for 2–3 mo after hemoglobin levels have returned to normal to allow replacement of the iron store of the body.
4. Oral iron preparations are best absorbed when taken between meals but are usually taken with food to decrease gastric upset. Administer liquid preparations well diluted with water or fruit juice through a straw to prevent staining of teeth.
5. Inform the patient that drug may cause dark red or black stools. Diarrhea or constipation should be reported and may be relieved by adjusting dosage or diet.
6. Caution the patient to keep oral preparations out of reach of children. Overdosage can be fatal. In case of accidental overdosage, emergency treatment can be initiated at home by inducing vomiting and by giving eggs or milk to form an insoluble iron-protein complex.
7. Teach the patient and his or her family principles of a balanced diet emphasizing iron-rich foods: dried fruit, green vegetables, dried beans, wheat germ, egg yolk.

Iron Dextran Injection

1. Recommended only for severe anemia with hemoglobin less than 7.5 g per 100 ml, or when patient cannot tolerate oral iron.
2. Should not be co-administered with oral iron. Discontinue use unless hemoglobin level increases by at least 2 g per 100 ml within 3 wk.
3. Patient should receive a small test dose prior to a full therapeutic dose; anaphylactic reactions have occurred with this drug.
4. Review specific Z-tract injection technique prior to administering this drug.
5. Exercise care when aspirating; dark color of medication can obscure blood in syringe if accidentally injecting into blood vessel.

Vitamin B_{12}

1. Emphasize to patients with pernicious anemia that parenteral vitamin therapy must continue throughout life to prevent irreversible neurological damage.
2. When oral preparations are used for B_{12} deficiency, the drug should be mixed with fruit juice and administered promptly with meals to enhance absorption.
3. Instruct the patient to report any illness which may increase need for B_{12}.

Folic Acid

1. Rule out pernicious anemia prior to administering folic acid for treatment of anemia. Folic acid administration can mask pernicious anemia, allowing irreversible neurological damage to occur.

2. Cause of deficiency should be identified and corrected, if possible, as: dietary deficiency or induced by drugs such as oral contraceptives, phenytoin (Dilantin), or barbiturates.

3. Folates are available in yeast, liver, fresh green vegetables, and fruit. Approximately 50-90% of folate content is destroyed by cooking or canning.

SUPPLEMENTARY READINGS

Chanarin, I., *The Megaloblastic Anemias.* Philadelphia: F. A. Davis Co., 1969.

Dreyfus, J. C., ed., *Hematopoietic Agents*, Vol. I, "Hematinic Agents." Oxford: Pergamon Press, Inc., 1971.

Hallberg, L., H. G. Harwerth, and A. Vannotti, eds., *Iron Deficiency.* New York: Academic Press, Inc., 1970.

Hardisty, R. M., and D. J. Westheral, eds., *Blood and Its Disorders.* Philadelphia: J. B. Lippincott Company, 1974.

Herbert, V., ed., "Nutritional Anemias," *Seminars in Hematology* **7**: 2–106 (1970).

Levin, R. H., "Iron Deficiency Anemia in the Pediatric Patient," in *Clinical Pharmacy and Therapeutics*, eds., E. T. Herfindal and J. L. Hirschman, Chapter 26, pp. 331–41. Baltimore: The Williams & Wilkins Company, 1975.

Stebbins, R., J. Scott, and V. Herbert, "Drug-Induced Megaloblastic Anemias," *Seminars in Hematology* **10**: 235–51 (1973).

Surgenor, D. M., ed., *The Red Blood Cells* (2nd ed.). New York: Academic Press, Inc., 1974.

VI Section

CHEMOTHERAPEUTIC AGENTS

Chapter 41

INTRODUCTION TO CHEMOTHERAPY

In 1900, 23 percent of all deaths in the United States were caused by influenza, pneumonia, and tuberculosis, with 2.3 percent of the population succumbing to diphtheria. At the turn of the century, there was little hope a nurse could offer the patient with such infectious diseases as cholera, meningitis, scarlet fever, and various streptococcal and staphylococcal infections. Viral pneumonia is the only infectious disease remaining on contemporary lists of the ten leading causes of death in the United States. The remainder of these infectious diseases have ceased to be major health problems in this country or are amenable to treatment.

Many factors have contributed to the reduction in morbidity and mortality associated with infectious diseases; these include advances in preventive medicine, more effective public health laws, improved tests for the early diagnosis of disease, and better training of physicians, nurses, and other members of the health care team. Undoubtedly, one of the most important factors has been the development of highly effective chemotherapeutic agents.

The objective of *chemotherapy* is to use a drug to kill or prevent the multiplication of an invading organism or cancer cell without causing harm to the patient. We shall consider such invading organisms or parasites to include bacteria, fungi, protozoa, worms, or viruses. Classically, *antibiotics* were defined as chemotherapeutic agents produced or derived from microorganisms; in recent years this definition has been expanded to include drugs that are synthetic or semisynthetic derivatives of natural products produced by living cells.

In this chapter, we shall discuss general principles of chemotherapy, including the mechanisms of action of these drugs, the development of microbial resistance, and therapeutic aspects and adverse effects associated with their use. Subsequent chapters in this section of the text will deal with specific chemotherapeutic agents employed for the management of bacterial, fungal, viral, protozoan, worm, and neoplastic disorders. Antiseptics and disinfectants, drugs used to destroy microorganisms on body surfaces or inanimate objects, will also be considered in this section.

MECHANISMS OF ACTION OF ANTIMICROBIAL AGENTS

Chemotherapy is predicated upon the fundamental principle that the drug is more toxic to the parasite than it is to the host (patient); this is referred to as *selective toxicity*. For some chemotherapeutic agents, such as penicillin, the drug is far more toxic to bacteria than it is to the patient; by contrast, we shall observe that many of the drugs employed for the treatment of cancers are only slightly more toxic to the malignant tumors than they are to the normal cells.

Some antimicrobial agents are able to kill bacteria, while others suppress only their growth and ability to reproduce; these drugs are referred to as *bactericidal* and *bacteriostatic* agents, respectively. This distinction is often concentration-dependent, that is, at low doses, a bactericidal antibiotic may exert a bacteriostatic effect. While bacteriostatic agents are able to inhibit the growth and reproduction of bacteria, *host defense mechanisms* (white blood cells and antibodies) must be operative to eradicate the disease-causing microbe. In the absence of such mechanisms, bacteriostatic drugs merely retard the spread of infection, with the patient often experiencing a relapse after the withdrawal of medication. To be most effective clinically, bactericidal agents also require the cooperation of functional host defenses.

Antimicrobial agents kill or inhibit the growth of microbes by one or more of the following mechanisms: competitive antagonism, inhibition of cell wall synthesis, impairment of cell membrane function, inhibition of protein synthesis, or inhibition of nucleic acid synthesis. Fundamental differences exist between the structure and/or function of the cells of the parasite and the host; these differences account for the selective toxicity of the antimicrobial agents.

Competitive Antagonism (Antimetabolites)

Some antibacterial agents act by interfering with the utilization of nutritional substances that are essential for the growth and reproduction of microbes. For many microorganisms, para-aminobenzoic acid (PABA) is an essential dietary requirement needed for the synthesis of folic acid, a building block in the manufacture of purines and eventually of nucleic acids. Whereas mammals are able to directly utilize dietary sources of folic acid, few bacteria are capable of employing this preformed vitamin provided by their environment.

It is generally believed that the antibacterial *sulfonamides*, which are similar to PABA chemically, act by interfering with the ability of microbes to synthesize folic acid from PABA. The latter nutrient and the antimetabolite sulfonamides both compete for the same enzyme that catalyzes the incorporation of PABA into the folic acid molecule. Animals and microbes that require preformed sources of folic acid and that, therefore, do not require PABA, are not susceptible to the growth-inhibiting effects of the sulfonamides. Other chemotherapeutic agents that act as competitive antagonists by mechanisms similar to the sulfonamides include drugs used for the treatment of tuberculosis (para-aminosalicylic acid), malaria (pyrimethamine), and leprosy (the sulfones).

Inhibition of Cell Wall Synthesis

One of the fundamental differences between bacterial and mammalian cells is the presence of a *rigid cell wall* in bacteria. In addition to providing the microbe with a definite shape, the cell wall enables the bacterium to maintain a much higher internal osmotic pressure than exists in the external environment. The cell wall is composed of polysaccharide (carbohydrate) chains that are cross-linked with amino acids; some of these individual carbohydrate and amino acid components are not found in mammalian cells.

Penicillin blocks cell wall synthesis of daughter cells of multiplying bacteria by preventing the cross-linking of amino acids on the polysaccharide chains. Other antibiotics that inhibit bacterial cell wall synthesis, although not necessarily by the same mechanism as penicillin, include the cephalosporins, bacitracin, vancomycin, and cycloserine. Drug-induced interference with cell wall synthesis may lead to lysis and death of the daughter microbial cell.

Inhibition of Cell Membrane Function

The *cell membranes* of microbial and mammalian cells serve as barriers to control the transfer of compounds between the external environment and the interior of the cell. Damage to the membrane results in a loss of essential intracellular constitutents (purines, pyrimidines, proteins) and the uncontrolled movement of other compounds into the cell; damage to or death of the parasite results.

Bacterial and fungal cell membranes are more readily disrupted by some chemotherapeutic agents than are the membranes of mammalian cells. *Polymyxin B* forms a complex with the phospholipid constituent of the cell membrane of gram-negative bacteria, causing a nonselective increase in membrane permeability. *Amphotericin B* also impairs cell membrane function, but unlike polymyxin B, acts only on the membranes of fungi.

Inhibition of Protein Synthesis

By a variety of different complex mechanisms, many of the most clinically useful antibiotics produce their antimicrobial effects by *inhibiting protein synthesis*. Chloramphenicol and erythromycin are thought to attach to one of the two subunits of the ribosome and block the formation of peptide bonds between amino acids; the former drug may also prevent the attachment of messenger ribonucleic acid (RNA) to the ribosome. Tetracyclines are believed to inhibit protein synthesis by blocking the binding of the amino acid-transfer RNA complex to ribosomes. Streptomycin binds to the ribosome in such a manner that incorrect amino acids are laid down, thus resulting in the formation of nonfunctional proteins.

Inhibition of Nucleic Acid Synthesis

Cell replication requires the continuous synthesis and normal functioning of deoxyribonucleic acid (DNA); once DNA is destroyed, the cell is incapable of replacing it and, as a consequence, is unable to form new RNA molecules. The anticancer agent dactinomycin and the antiviral drug idoxuridine block DNA synthesis, while the antitubercular drug rifampin inhibits RNA synthesis. In general, drugs that inhibit nucleic acid synthesis have a relatively low degree of selective toxicity (that is, they are relatively toxic to the host).

RESISTANCE TO ANTIMICROBIAL AGENTS

Resistance to an antimicrobial agent is said to exist when a strain of microrganisms becomes less sensitive or totally insensitive to drugs that ordinarily inhibit their growth or cause their deaths. The emergence of drug resistance should not be confused with the natural resistance of microorganisms to chemotherapeutic agents. The development of drug resistant bacterial strains is of obvious importance to the nurse when attempting to manage infectious diseases.

There are many different mechanisms that account for the emergence of bacterial resistance to antimicrobial agents. (1) Microbes can become resistant to certain antibiotics by producing enzymes that are capable of inactivating those chemotherapeutic agents. Staphylococci resistance to penicillin G has been attributed to the ability of these bacteria to form *penicillinase*, an enzyme capable of hydrolyzing and destroying the antimicrobial activity of penicillin. Synthetic penicillin derivatives have been developed that are not susceptible to penicillinase inactivation. (2) Resistance may result from an alteration in normal bacterial metabolism to overcome or circumvent the ability of antibacterial drugs to inhibit their growth. Some sulfonamide-resistant bacteria have acquired the ability to directly utilize preformed folic acid and do not require environmental PABA. (3) The microbial strain may lose the specific target structure attacked by the antibiotic or cause alterations in the drug resulting in the blockade of biologically active parts of the molecule. L forms of bacteria become resistant to penicillin because they can survive in the absence of a cell wall. R-factors, which can be transferred from one bacterial species to another, block the active site of antibiotics. (4) Changes may occur in the structure of the microbe that prevents the antimicrobial agent from entering the cell. Resistance to chloramphenicol, the tetracyclines, aminoglycosides, and the polymyxins have been associated with alterations in the permeability of the microbial cell to these drugs.

GENERAL CONSIDERATIONS IN ANTIMICROBIAL THERAPY

When employed judiciously, antibiotics are often capable of producing dramatic beneficial effects in the treatment of infectious disorders. By contrast, the improper use of these drugs has resulted in severe morbidity and mortality from drug-induced allergy and toxicity, as well as the development of infections far more severe than those originally present and the appearance of antibiotic-resistant strains of microorganisms. In an attempt to reduce such adverse drug reactions, many hospitals have instituted automatic *stop orders*, which limit the number of days a given antimicrobial agent can be administered; continued use of that drug requires a new prescription from the physician.

Since antimicrobial agents are not uniformly effective against all microbes, the selection of the most appropriate drug should be based upon the *identity of the offending microorganism(s)*. While it is ideally desirable to delay the initiation of antimicrobial therapy until after bacteriological laboratory reports are received that identify the microbe and indicate the sensitivity of the microorganism to different antibiotics (*disk test*), in life-threatening conditions it is often not possible to wait for such information. Broad-spectrum antibiotics (drugs effective against a wide range of microorganisms) or the simultaneous use of multiple antibiotics may have to be employed until the laboratory reports that indicate more specific drugs are received. Such laboratory results are not infallible and, in the final analysis, good clinical judgment must be exercised regarding the selection of the most appropriate therapy.

The *simultaneous administration of multiple antimicrobial agents* may be beneficial in some therapeutic situations, while detrimental to the patient's recovery in other cases. As a general rule, an additive antibacterial effect will be obtained when two bactericidal or two bacteriostatic drugs are used in combination. By contrast, the use of a bactericidal (penicillin) and a bacteriostatic (tetracycline) drug in combination may result in a diminished therapeutic advantage to the patient. Why should this be the case? Bactericidal drugs are most effective in killing bacteria during active phases of multiplication; if growth is suppressed by a bacteriostatic agent, the bactericidal drug is less effective in producing its lethal effects. It should be noted that exceptions have been observed clinically to these general rules.

Combination antimicrobial therapy is rationally indicated in four clinical situations: (1) for the treatment of infections caused by more than one bacterial species, such as peritonitis, wounds, and urinary tract disorders; (2) to delay the emergence of bacterial resistance, such as in the treatment of tuberculosis; (3) to increase the effectiveness of antimicrobial therapy in the management of such

specific diseases as tuberculosis, enterococci infections, brucellosis, and Haemophilus influenzae; and (4) for the treatment of severe infections in which the etiology has not been identified.

Once therapy is initiated with the most appropriate chemotherapeutic agent(s), in the absence of drug-induced toxicity, allergy, or superinfection (see the next section), it is essential that drug administration be *continued at optimal doses for a sufficient period of time* to completely eradicate the microorganism. An inadequate dosing schedule or premature termination of drug therapy may lead to the emergence of drug-resistant microbial strains and the possible relapse of the patient. In general, chemotherapy should be continued for at least several days after the patient becomes asymptomatic. An important nursing responsibility involves the education of non-hospitalized patients about the critical importance of taking their antimicrobial agents at the times of day and for the number of days prescribed by their physician. The patient should be advised about the potential dangers of discontinuing their medication without consulting their physicians when they "feel better."

ADVERSE EFFECTS TO ANTIMICROBIAL AGENTS

The nurse will observe three general types of adverse effects to antimicrobial agents, namely, toxicity, hypersensitivity reactions, and superinfections.

Toxicity

In the subsequent chapters in this section, we shall observe that each class of chemotherapeutic agents is capable of producing side effects and toxic effects; many of these adverse reactions are relatively specific for each drug class.

Prior to the selection of an antimicrobial agent and the dose of that drug and throughout the course of therapy, the patient's *renal function* should be assessed. Administration of "usual doses" of drugs that are eliminated largely by the kidney to patients with compromised renal function may cause severe or even lethal effects as the result of accumulation of the drug or its toxic metabolites. Many antimicrobial agents are themselves nephrotoxic and, therefore, may cause or aggravate renal failure. The kidney function of newborn or premature infants is often underdeveloped. Special dosage schedules must be employed in such infants to prevent toxicity resulting from toxic accumulation of drugs. Drugs that are eliminated almost entirely by the kidney include the penicillins, cephalosporins, aminoglycosides (gentamicin, kanamycin, streptomycin), some tetracyclines, vancomycin, and polymyxin.

Hypersensitivity Reactions

Hypersensitivity or *allergic reactions* to chemotherapeutic agents are most commonly encountered in patients with a history of allergic disorders or with allergies to other classes of drugs; many of these adverse effects have been attributed to antigen-antibody reactions (Chapter 53). These hypersensitivity reactions vary in clinical manifestations and in severity from a mild skin rash to a fatal anaphylactic reaction. It is obviously essential that the nurse obtain a careful and complete drug history from the patient prior to the initiation of antimicrobial therapy. Particular attention should be directed toward the patient's adverse response to drugs previously administered. Once a drug allergy has been identified, it is essential that this information be placed conspicuously in the patient's medical record or hospital chart; in addition, it is essential that patients be clearly informed of their allergies to such drugs.

Unless it is absolutely imperative to employ the offending antibiotic and no alternative chemotherapeutic agent is suitable for use, that drug should never be readministered once an allergic response has been identified. Patients with hypersensitivity reactions to one member of an antimicrobial class should not receive any other members of that same class; for example, an allergic reaction to any penicillin derivatives mandates that all penicillin derivatives should be avoided.

Superinfections

Superinfection (or *suprainfection*) is the development of a new infection, either bacterial or fungal in etiology, arising during antimicrobial management of the primary infection. While the risk of superinfection is low with narrow-spectrum antibiotics such as penicillin, it is a common occurrence when tetracycline and other broad-spectrum antibiotics are employed, especially during protracted courses of therapy and in children under 3 years of age. Broad-spectrum antibiotics suppress the growth of normal nonpathogenic inhabitants of the gastrointestinal, genitourinary, and respiratory tracts, disrupting the normal microbial balance, and permitting bacteria and fungi to freely proliferate. Disease-producing microbes may emerge that are highly resistant to available antimicrobial agents. The nurse should be vigilant for the appearance of common symptoms associated with superinfections, including diarrhea, fever, anal pruritus, and vaginal discharges.

NURSING RESPONSIBILITIES AND PRECAUTIONS

There are scores of antimicrobial agents available for clinical use, with many of these drugs marketed under a variety of trade names.

While it is not reasonable to expect that the nurse will become expert in the unique properties of each of these drugs, he or she should master the general pharmacological properties and adverse effects that distinguish each class of antimicrobial agents. Moreover, the nurse should be able to identify the antimicrobial class of commonly prescribed drugs. This information is of importance to prevent the inadvertent administration of an antimicrobial agent when the patient has a history of allergy to another member of that class.

To limit the emergence of bacterial resistance to antimicrobial agents, it is essential that the nurse administer these drugs according to the *prescribed dosing schedule* over the entire 24-hour period. The importance of taking these drugs at their prescribed times must be impressed upon patients or members of their families who are assuming responsibility for them at home. Moreover, nurses should not administer—nor should patients take—outdated antibiotics.

Antibiotics are administered intravenously for the management of life-threatening disorders or when it is necessary to maintain very high blood levels of the antimicrobial agent. These drugs should be dissolved in neutral solutions (pH 7.0–7.2) of isotonic saline (0.9 percent) or dextrose (5 percent) in water and, to avoid the frequent occurrence of chemical and physical incompatibilities, antibiotics should not be mixed with other drugs.

The *misuse* of antibiotics by patients is thought to be quite widespread. Antibiotics remaining from a previous illness are often used by the patient or members of the family or shared with neighbors to treat diseases with apparently similar symptoms. The nurse has an important responsibility in educating patients about the potential dangers of such self-medication.

Introduction to Chemotherapy:
nursing implications

1. The microorganism should be cultured and tested for sensitivity to antimicrobial agents prior to initiating therapy, if possible. If the microbe is subsequently determined to be resistant to the original drug ordered, a new antimicrobial agent can be substituted after the laboratory results are obtained.

2. A careful drug history should be obtained prior to antibiotic administration to determine whether the patient has experienced an allergic reaction to that drug or a member of the same antibiotic class.

3. When administering an antibiotic, carefully observe the patient for symptoms of an allergic reaction, for example, skin rash, urticaria, or anaphylactic shock; such reactions require emergency treatment with oxygen and epinephrine.

4. If the patient experiences an allergic reaction, make conspicuous note of this adverse reaction on the patient's chart. Instruct the patient to notify all physicians of this allergy, and advise the patient to avoid the use of this drug class in the future unless the physician specifically prescribes it after reviewing the patient's history of drug allergy.

5. Observe the patient for signs of superinfections (black, hairy tongue, nausea, diarrhea, anal pruritis, vaginitis) caused by overgrowth of nonsusceptible microorganisms.

6. Instruct the patient about the importance of taking the medication at the recommended intervals to maintain optimal blood levels and thereby maximize the benefits associated with drug administration.

7. Impress upon the patient the importance of completing the entire course of therapy even though the patient becomes asymptomatic before all the medication is taken. Unused medication should be discarded.

8. Withhold the newly prescribed drug and check with the physician when two or more drugs with a potential for causing a similar toxic reaction (neurotoxicity, ototoxicity, nephrotoxicity) are ordered.

9. To preclude the possibility of precipitation or other drug-drug interactions, do not mix antibiotics with other drugs when preparing IV solutions.

SUPPLEMENTARY READINGS

Albert, A., *Selective Toxicity* (6th ed.). New York: John Wiley & Sons, 1979.

Appel, G. B., and H. C. Neu, "The Nephrotoxicity of Antimicrobial Agents," *New England Journal of Medicine* 296: 663-70, 722-28, 784-87 (1977).

Conn, H. F., ed., "Efficacy of Antimicrobial and Antifungal Agents," *Medical Clinics of North America* 54: 1075-1354 (1970).

Garrod, L. P., H. P. Lambert, and F. O'Grady, *Antibiotic and Chemotherapy* (4th ed.). Baltimore: The Williams & Wilkins Company, 1973.

Handbook of Antimicrobial Therapy. New Rochelle, N.Y.: Medical Letter, Inc., 1976.

Jawetz, E., "The Use of Antimicrobial Combinations," *Annual Review of Pharmacology* 8: 151-70 (1968).

Kabins, S. A. "Interactions Among Antibiotics and Other Drugs," *Journal of the American Medical Association* 219: 206-12 (1972).

Kagan, B. M., ed., *Antimicrobial Therapy* (2nd ed.). Philadelphia: W. B. Saunders Company, 1974.

Klastersky, J., ed., *Clinical Use of Combinations of Antibiotics,* New York: John Wiley & Sons, Inc., 1975.

Lerner, P. I., M. C. McHenry, and E. Olinsky, eds., "Symposium on Infectious Diseases," *Medical Clinics of North America* 58: 463-708 (1974).

Lowbury, E. J. L., and G. A. J. Ayliffe, *Drug Resistance in Antimicrobial Therapy.* Springfield, Ill.: Charles C Thomas, Publisher, 1974.

McCracken, G. H., Jr., "Pharmacological Basis for Antimicrobial Therapy in Newborn Infants," *American Journal of Disease of Childhood* 128: 407-19 (1974).

Pratt, W. B., *Chemotherapy of Infection.* New York: Oxford University Press, 1977.

Sande, M. A., and G. L. Mandell, "Chemotherapy of Microbial Diseases," in *Goodman and Gilman's The Pharmacological Basis of Therapeutics* (6th ed.), eds. A. G. Gilman, L. S. Goodman, and A. Gilman, Section XII, Chapters 48-54, pp. 1080-1248. New York: Macmillan, Inc., 1980.

Sanders, W. E., Jr., and C. C. Sanders, "Toxicity of Antibacterial Agents: Mechanism of Action on Mammalian Cells," *Annual Review of Pharmacology and Toxicology* 19: 53-83 (1979).

Tobey, L. E., and T. R. Covington, "Antimicrobial Drug Interactions," *American Journal of Nursing* 75: 1470-73 (1975).

SULFONAMIDES AND URINARY TRACT ANTI-INFECTIVE DRUGS

Chapter 42

In this chapter we shall discuss the sulfonamides, antimicrobial agents that are primarily employed for the treatment of urinary tract infections and that are also useful for the treatment of systemic and topical infections. We shall also make brief reference to a group of drugs with clinical utility limited to infections of the urinary tract.

SULFONAMIDES

The sulfonamides (commonly referred to as *sulfa drugs*) are totally synthetic compounds, not derived from living cells, and, therefore, cannot be classified as antibiotics. At the time of their introduction in 1935, the sulfonamides were the first class of relatively nontoxic, clinically useful antibacterial agents. With the emergence of bacterial resistant strains and the development of much more effective antimicrobial agents, the relative importance of the sulfonamides in contemporary therapeutics has markedly diminished. Their major uses are for the treatment of urinary tract infections, where they continue to enjoy widespread popularity because

of their established effectiveness, low toxicity, and relatively low cost. They are also widely used in ocular infections.

Antimicrobial Activity

As discussed in Chapter 41, the sulfonamides block the utilization of para-aminobenzoic acid (PABA) in the synthesis of folic acid. As a consequence, these drugs are able to inhibit the growth and reproduction of microbes that must synthesize folic acid and that are incapable of utilizing the sources of this compound provided by their environment. Since human cells utilize dietary folic acid, the sulfonamides are not especially toxic to these host cells.

All sulfonamides possess essentially the same spectrum of antimicrobial activity. The sulfonamides exert their bacteriostatic effects against a wide range of gram-positive and gram-negative cocci and gram-negative bacilli, chlamydiae, actinomycetes, nocardia, and certain protozoa. However, with the development of resistant strains, their effective therapeutic antimicrobial utility is considerably reduced.

Administration and Fate

When used for the treatment of systemic infections, sulfonamides are most often administered orally. The sodium salts and acetyl and diethanolamine derivatives of several sulfonamides (sulfisoxazole, sulfadiazine) are available for intravenous use; the salts of most sulfonamides are too alkaline—and therefore, too irritating—to permit their subcutaneous or intramuscular injection. Insoluble derivatives (phthalylsulfathiazole) are not absorbed from the gastrointestinal tract after oral administration and are used for their antimicrobial effects in the gut. Sulfonamides may also be applied to the eyes (sodium sulfacetamide) or to the skin (mafenide). The properties of selected sulfonamides in common therapeutic use are summarized in Table 42-1.

After oral administration, most sulfonamides are rapidly absorbed from the gastrointestinal tract and are widely distributed to most body fluids and tissues, including the central nervous system and across the placental barrier to the fetus. Once in the blood, sulfonamides bind to plasma albumin to varying degrees, ranging from less than 10 percent to over 90 percent depending upon the particular drug; the extent of plasma protein binding is decreased in patients with severe renal failure.

The major products of sulfonamide metabolism, the acetylated metabolites, are formed to varying degrees with different sulfonamides; while they lack antibacterial activity, they retain the potential of the parent drug for causing toxic effects and allergic responses. Moreover, the acetylated derivatives of some of the older sulfonamides (sulfadiazine, sulfamerazine, sulfamethazine) are less soluble than the parent drug in the urine resulting in crystalluria and related kidney damage. The sulfonamides achieve high concentration in the urine and are primarily eliminated from the body by the *kidney*.

Classification of Sulfonamides

The American prefix for these drugs is *sulfa*, while the British prefix is *sulpha*. The sul-

Table 42-1 Representative Sulfonamides

Generic name (trade name)	Usual oral adult doses		Remarks
	Initial	Maintenance	
Short-acting systemic sulfonamides			
Sulfisoxazole (Gantrisin; Sulfalar; SK-Soxazole)	2–4 g	4–8 g in 4–6 doses per 24 h	Rapid onset and short (4 h) duration of action. Prototype sulfonamide for urinary tract infections; high solubility in urine, little kidney toxicity. Less useful for systemic infections. Administered orally, topically (ears, eyes, nose), and parenterally.
Sulfadiazine (Microsulfon)	2–4 g	4–8 g in 3–6 doses per 24 h; sodium salt used IV	Prototype sulfonamide for systemic infections because of good tissue penetrating properties. Potential danger of crystalluria minimized by administration of alkaline salts (sodium bicarbonate) and maintenance of high urinary output.
Trisulfapyrimidines (Neotrizine, Sulfose, Terfonyl, Triple Sulfa)	2–4 g	2–4 g in 3–6 doses per 24 h	Tablets or oral suspension containing equal amounts of sulfadiazine, sulfamerazine, and sulfamethazine at $\frac{1}{3}$ the normal full dose of each. Lower incidence of crystalluria and kidney damage.

Table 42-1   Continued

Generic name (trade name)	Usual oral adult doses		Remarks
	Initial	Maintenance	
Sulfachlorpyridazine (Nefrosul, Sonilyn)	2-4 g	2-4 g in 3-6 doses per 24 h	Similar to sulfisoxazole.
Sulfacytine (Renoquid)	0.5 g	250 mg q.i.d. for 10 days	More potent than most sulfonamides; lower dose required.
Intermediate-acting systemic sulfonamides			
Sulfamethoxazole (Gantanol)	2 g	1 g 2-3 times daily	Similar to sulfisoxazole, but more slowly absorbed and excreted; duration of action of 8-12 h.
Sulfamethoxazole/400 mg + trimethoprim/80 mg (Bactrim, Septra)		2 tablets b.i.d. for 12-14 days	Antimicrobial spectrum of combination greater than individual drugs; reduction in bacterial resistance. Useful in chronic urinary tract and systemic bacterial infections. To prevent recurrent urinary tract infections, give in small daily doses over extended periods of time.
Long-acting systemic sulfonamides			
Sulfamethoxypyridazine (Midicel)	1 g	1 g o.d. or q.o.d.	Rapid absorption, very long duration of action. Used for chronic therapy. Low drug levels in urine. Danger of severe and sometimes fatal skin rashes (Stevens-Johnson syndrome) limiting utility; characterized by high fever, headache, stomatitis, rhinitis, urethritis.
Sulfameter (Sulla)	1.5 g	0.5 g o.d.	Similar to sulfamethoxypyridazine; no advantages.
Insoluble, poorly absorbed sulfonamides			
Phthalylsulfathiazole (Sulfathalidine)		1 g q. 4 h	Action limited to gastrointestinal tract; treatment of ulcerative colitis; no proof of efficacy when used preoperatively to "sterilize" gut.
Sulfasalazine (Azulfidine, Sulcolon)		2-8 g per 24 h in 4-8 doses	Treatment of ulcerative colitis. Drug may interfere with synthesis of vitamin K by intestinal bacteria; instruct patient to report any bleeding.
Topical sulfonamides			
Mafenide (Sulfamylon)		8.5% cream applied 1-2 times	Prevention of infections of burns by gram-positive and gram-negative bacteria; risk of fungal superinfection. Causes pain on application. Inhibits enzyme carbonic anhydrase, potentially resulting in alkaline urine and metabolic acidosis.
Silver sulfadiazine (Silvadene)		1% cream	Same use as mafenide, but no pain nor risk of adverse systemic effects.
Sulfacetamide Sodium (Bleph; Sodium Sulamyd; Sulf-10)		10-30% ointment applied 2-8 times daily to eyes. 0.05-0.1 ml of 10-30% sol to eyes q. 2-3 during day, less often at night.	Treatment of ocular infections, including conjunctivitis, corneal ulcer, and trachoma (with systemic sulfonamides); ointment may impair healing; risk of fungal superinfection.

fonamides can be divided into four major groups: (1) short-to-intermediate-acting systemic sulfonamides; (2) long-acting systemic sulfonamides; (3) insoluble, poorly absorbed sulfonamides; and (4) topical sulfonamides. The properties of representative members of each of these classes are summarized in Table 42-1.

Short- and intermediate-acting sulfonamides

The *short-acting sulfonamides*, including sulfisoxazole, sulfadiazine, sulfacytine, and sulfachlorpyridazine, are rapidly absorbed after oral administration, achieving peak blood levels within 2 to 3 hours. Therapeutic blood levels may be maintained by administering these drugs at 4- to 8-hour intervals. The short-acting drugs produce high concentrations in the urine and are usually the sulfonamides of choice for the treatment of urinary tract infections. The newer members of this class are relatively safe, well tolerated, and have a low risk of crystalluria. Moreover, unlike the long-acting sulfonamides, exposure to these drugs can be rapidly terminated upon appearance of serious adverse reactions.

The *intermediate-acting sulfonamide*, sulfamethoxazole, is less rapidly absorbed than the short-acting drugs and is more slowly excreted. Sulfamethoxazole may be administered at 12-hour intervals and is useful in the treatment of infections requiring prolonged courses of therapy.

Long-acting sulfonamides

The long-acting sulfonamides, sulfameter and sulfamethoxypyridazine, are relatively rapidly absorbed but require several days for the elimination of a single dose. Although the administration of a single daily dose may prove to be more convenient for the patient, the low concentrations of these drugs in the urine and cerebrospinal fluid make them less effective than the short-acting sulfonamides

for the treatment of urinary tract infections and infections involving the central nervous system, respectively. Severe toxic effects have been associated with the use of the long-acting sulfonamides.

Insoluble, poorly absorbed sulfonamides

Phthalylsulfathiazole is poorly absorbed from the gastrointestinal tract after oral administration. In the gut, this inactive parent compound is hydrolyzed to the antimicrobial agent sulfathiazole. These drugs have been used for the treatment of intestinal infections and to reduce the microbial population prior to surgery.

Topical sulfonamides

Preparations containing topical sulfonamides are used on the skin and mucous membranes and in the eye. With the exception of mafenide, sulfonamides applied to the skin are ineffective because pus and cellular debris readily inhibit their action. The most important clinical uses of topical sulfonamides are for the treatment of mild ocular infections and to prevent sepsis in patients with severe burns. Sulfonamide preparations (for example, Sultrin) are also available for intravaginal insertion to treat infections of the mucous membrane surfaces.

Therapeutic Uses

Sulfonamides are among the most important antimicrobial drugs for the treatment of acute, uncomplicated *urinary tract infections*. They are also used for chronic suppressive therapy of urinary tract infections caused by *Escherichia*, *Proteus*, *Pseudomonas*, and the *Klebsiella-Enterobacter* groups. Since resistance rapidly develops during the course of suppressive therapy, the sulfonamides can be employed alternately with nitrofurantoin (Table 42-3, page 373) or other anti-infective agents. The short-acting sulfonamides are employed alone, or a combination of sulfamethoxazole and trimethoprim may be effectively used. Prompt reduction of the bacteriuria, as denoted by a negative urine culture within 4 days after the initiation of therapy, is a clinical indication of the effectiveness of the therapy selected. Nurses should stress to patients the importance of continuing drug therapy for 10 to 14 days, even after the patient feels asymptomatic, to reduce the danger of relapse and the emergence of resistant bacterial strains.

Respiratory infections (including bronchitis), otitis media, tonsillitis, and pharyngitis caused by susceptible strains of streptococci, pneumonococci, or *Haemophilus influenzae* may respond to sulfonamide administration, but antibiotics are superior and are generally preferred. Although not the drugs of first choice, sulfonamides are also used alone or in combination with other antimicrobial agents for the treatment of bacillary dysentery, nocardiosis, actinomycosis, and toxoplasmosis. Whether given orally or applied locally to the conjunctival sac, sulfonamides are among the most useful drugs for the treatment of trachoma, an ophthalmic disease.

Although extensively employed to reduce the microbial population of the gut prior to surgery, there is no clear evidence supporting their efficacy when compared with appropriate surgical technique and careful preoperative and postoperative care. Sulfasalazine is a poorly absorbed drug that is used for the treatment of ulcerative colitis; the beneficial effects of this drug are thought to be independent of its antibacterial actions.

Mafenide is an effective agent when topically applied for the prevention of infections of burns caused by a wide variety of gram-positive and gram-negative bacteria; superinfections by fungi may occur. Unlike mafenide, silver sulfadiazine causes no pain upon application and does not cause adverse systemic effects.

Trimethoprim-sulfamethoxazole

Clinical experience reveals that the antimicrobial spectrum of these two antimicrobial agents is wider than the spectrum of each individual drug. These two drugs act by inhibiting consecutive steps in the microbial synthesis and utilization of folic acid, resulting in a broader antimicrobial spectrum of activity and a marked reduction in the development of resistant bacterial strains.

Some clinicians view the trimethoprimsulamethoxazole combination (Bactrim, Septra) to be the treatment of choice for acute and chronic urinary tract infections. This combination has also proved useful in the treatment of typhoid and paratyphoid fevers and bacterial infections of the nose, throat, skin, ear, soft tissues, and bone, as well as septicemia, brucellosis, enteric fevers, uncomplicated gonorrhea, cholera, and malaria.

The combination is generally well tolerated, with the adverse effects primarily those attributed to the sulfonamide component. Blood dyscrasias and crystalluria have been reported. Since trimethoprim is a potential teratogenic agent, this combination should be avoided during pregnancy.

Adverse Effects and Precautions

The sulfonamides cause numerous and diverse side effects in about 5 percent of patients. These adverse effects include hypersensitivity reactions as well as toxic effects to the urinary tract and blood. Potential drug interactions involving the sulfonamides are summarized in Table 42-2. Nursing implications are summarized at the end of this chapter.

Table 42-2   Potential Drug Interactions Involving Sulfonamides and Urinary Tract Anti-Infectives

Interacting drug/class	Potential consequences
Sulfonamides	
Local anesthetics (benzocaine, procaine, tetracaine, buta-caine) Para-aminobenzoic acid (PABA)	PABA-derivative local anesthetics and PABA (a component in some non-prescription analgesics) may antagonize the antibacterial effects of sulfonamides.
Methenamine mandelate (Mandelamine)	Coadministration of less soluble sulfonamides (sulfadiazine) with methenamine and its salts (which form formaldehyde and acidify the urine) may result in sulfonamide precipitation (crystalluria).
Oral anticoagulant agents (coumarin-type) Oral hypoglycemic agents sulfonylureas (tolbutamide) Methotrexate	Sulfonamides can potentially displace these highly plasma protein bound drugs enhancing their pharmacological activity and toxicity; significance of interaction not clinically documented.
Nalidixic acid and oxolinic acid	
Oral anticoagulants	Displacement of anticoagulants from plasma protein binding sites increasing risk of bleeding.
Methenamine	
Acetazolamide (Diamox) Sodium bicarbonate	These drugs make the urine alkaline and impair conversion of methenamine to formaldehyde, thus interfering with the antimicrobial activity of methenamine.

Hypersensitivity reactions involving the skin and mucous membranes include urticaria and maculopapular rashes (often accompanied by itching and fever) as well contact dermatitis, photosensitivity, often severe skin reactions, and the potentially fatal Stevens-Johnson syndrome. If a rash develops after sulfonamide administration, therapy should be immediately terminated and the cause of the rash ascertained. Patients exhibiting a hypersensitivity reaction to one sulfonamide will generally show similar reactions to other sulfonamides; hence, this class of drugs is usually contraindicated in patients with a sensitivity to any sulfonamide.

Urinary tract toxicity, including crystalluria, hematuria, and partial or complete suppression of urine output, may occur after sulfonamide administration. Older drugs in this class may precipitate in the kidneys and other parts of the urinary tract in neutral or acidic urine; the risk of crystalluria is minimal with sulfisoxazole and other soluble sulfonamides. Nurses should impress upon their patients the importance of maintaining a *high fluid intake.* The adult daily urine output should be 1,200 to 1,500 ml. Alkali therapy with sodium bicarbonate may be required if the urine volume is low or if the urine is acidic. Sulfonamides may also cause toxic nephrosis or hypersensitivity reactions involving the urinary tract.

Blood disorders, while uncommon, may be sufficiently serious to warrant discontinuation of drug administration. These disorders of the hematopoietic system include acute hemolytic anemia (with blacks and individuals of Mediterranean origin at greater risk), aplastic anemia, agranulocytosis, thrombocytopenia, and eosinophilia. White blood cell counts and tests of hemoglobin levels should be performed every 3 to 5 days to permit drug withdrawal during an early and less severe stage of toxicity. Nurses should advise patients to report the appearance of rashes, sore throat, or purpurea to their physician. The use of these drugs near term increases the risk of kernicterus in the newborn and is contraindicated; they should not be given to nursing mothers for the same reason. Anorexia, nausea, vomiting, and diarrhea are not uncommon side effects with sulfonamide administration.

URINARY TRACT ANTI-INFECTIVE AGENTS

The urinary tract anti-infectives or antiseptics are a group of diverse drugs with minimal

Table 42-3   Urinary Tract Anti-Infective Drugs

Generic name (trade name)	Antimicrobial spectrum	Usual adult dose	Remarks
Sulfonamides	Gram-positive and gram-negative cocci and gram-negative bacilli. Resistant strains develop.	See Table 42-1; usually orally administered.	Short-acting sulfonamides preferred. Potentially cause allergic reactions, kidney toxicity, and blood disorders. Maintenance of adequate urine output essential.
Nitrofurantoin (Furadantin, Cyantin)	Gram-positive and gram-negative microbes except some *Proteus* and *Pseudomonas*. Resistance slowly develops.	PO: 50–100 mg q.i.d. Can be given for extended periods of time.	Important drug for urinary tract infections. No cross-resistance with other antimicrobial agents. Increased antibacterial activity in acidic urine. Anorexia, nausea, and vomiting common side effects; hypersensitivity reactions reported.
Nalidixic acid (NegGram)	Gram-negative bacteria except *Pseudomonas*. Rapid emergence of resistance strains.	PO: 1 g q.i.d. for 1–2 wk	Low incidence of toxicity; gastrointestinal disturbances, skin rashes, double vision. May give false-positive test for glucose in urine.
Oxolinic acid (Utibid)	Similar to nalidixic acid.	PO: 750 mg b.i.d.	Very similar to nalidixic acid; only difference is longer duration of action.
Methenamine hippurate (Hiprex, Urex) mandelate (Mandelamine)	Wide spectrum of gram-positive and gram-negative organisms.	PO: Mandelamine and mandelate salt; i g q.i.d., PC & HS. Hippurate salt: 1 g b.i.d.	Antibacterial effects attributed to release of formaldehyde in acid urine. Maintain urine below pH 5.5. Useful for chronic suppression of bacteriuria, since no bacterial resistance develops. Avoid use with sulfonamides. Most common side effect is gastrointestinal disturbance.
Dimethyl sulfoxide; DMSO (Rimso-50)	Symptomatic relief of interstitial cystitis.	Instillation of 50 ml directly into bladder and allow to remain for 15 min.	No proof of effectiveness for treatment of bacterial infections. Garlic-like taste or odor on breath may last for hours.

systemic antibacterial effects. The ability of these drugs to eliminate or suppress the bacterial count of the urine (bacteriuria) may be useful in the treatment of chronic urinary tract disorders such as pyelonephritis (inflammation of the renal pelvis) and cystitis (inflammation of the bladder). The properties of commonly used urinary tract anti-infective agents are summarized in Table 42-3; drug interactions involving these agents appear in Table 42-2 (page 372).

Sulfonamides and Urinary Tract Anti-Infective Drugs: nursing implications

1. Severe untoward reactions (such as blood dyscrasias) require immediate discontinuation of drug administration. Instruct the patient to report to the physician fever, sore throat or mouth, malaise, unusual fatigue, joint pain, pallor, bleeding tendencies, rash, or jaundice. Serum sickness, which may appear 7-10 days after the initiation of therapy, is characterized by eruption of purpuric spots and pains in the limbs and joints.

2. Advise the patient to avoid prolonged exposure to sunlight to reduce the risk of phototoxic sensitivity reactions.

3. Monitor fluid intake and output of the patient. Encourage adequate fluid intake to maintain a daily urinary output of 1500 ml to prevent crystalluria and calculi formation.

4. Daily check of urinary pH is recommended: an acidic urine decreases the solubility of sulfisoxazole; nitrofurantoin has greater antibacterial activity in acidic urine and methenamine is only active in acidic urine.

5. Advise the patient about dietary modifications that will alter the urinary pH to maximize the benefits of therapy: cranberry juice or vitamin C acidify the urine, while sodium bicarbonate may be ordered to alkalinize the urine.

6. Patients with recurrent urinary tract infections should be referred for a urological examination to rule out upper urinary tract disease.

7. Women with a first urinary tract infection usually require 10 days of drug therapy, while those with chronic infections may need 2-3 wk of drug administration. Low doses of antimicrobial agents may be prescribed for prolonged periods to prevent recurrent infections.

8. Instruct female patients with recurrent urinary tract infections on general measures to prevent re-infection: after intercourse empty bladder, drink 2 glasses of water, and take medication if it is ordered for this time of day; after a bowel movement wipe from front to back; wear cotton underwear and avoid tight fitting clothing which may increase perineal moisture; seek prompt treatment for vaginal discharge; if vaginal mucosa is dry, use a water-soluble lubricant such as KY jelly.

9. Diabetic patients receiving oral hypoglycemic agents (sulfonylureas such as tolbutamine or chlorpropamide) should be observed for hypoglycemic reactions and should have blood glucose levels checked prior to and during the course of sulfonamide therapy.

SUPPLEMENTARY READINGS

Anderson, E. R., "Women and Cystitis," *Nursing '77* **7**(4): 50–53 (1977).

Hirschman, J. L., and E. T. Herfindal, "Urinary Tract Infection," *Journal of the American Pharmaceutical Association* **NS 11:** 619–23 (1971).

Symposium. "Trimethoprim-Sulfamethoxazole," *Journal of Infectious Diseases* **128** Suppl.: 425–816 (1973).

Weinstein, L., M. A. Madoff, and C. A. Samet, "The Sulfonamides," *New England Journal of Medicine* **263:** 793–800, 842–49, 900–7 (1960).

PENICILLINS AND CEPHALOSPORINS

Chapter 43

In this chapter we shall consider the penicillins and cephalosporins. These antibiotics cause the death of susceptible bacteria by a common mechanism of action.

PENICILLINS

The penicillins were the first class of antibiotics to be discovered, and they continue to remain among the most important and widely prescribed antibacterial agents. The term *penicillins* is used to designate the natural products of the *Penicillium* molds or their semisynthetic derivatives. *Penicillin G* or benzylpenicillin is the most important of the naturally produced penicillins and is the most potent member of this antibiotic class.

Antimicrobial Activity

Penicillins are bactericidal at high concentrations and bacteriostatic at low concentrations. The bactericidal action of these drugs has been attributed to their ability to inhibit bacterial cell wall synthesis in daughter cells of multiplying bacteria, more specifically, by preventing the cross-linking of peptides on the mucopolysaccharide chains. This results in an increased movement of water into the bacterial cell and its bursting. These lethal effects are most pronounced when the bacteria are in a rapid growth phase; simultaneous administration of bacteriostatic agents such as the tetracyclines may reduce the bactericidal effectiveness of the penicillins.

Table 43-1 Comparative Properties of Penicillin Derivatives

Generic name (synonym)	Selected trade name	Penicillinase resistant	Gastric acid stable	Antibacterial spectrum	Usual adult dose range	Remarks
Penicillin G (Benzylpenicillin) potassium or sodium	Pentids Pfizerpen G	No	No	Particularly effective versus gram-positive bacteria (for example, staphylococci, streptococci); less active versus gram-negative bacteria (except gonococci, meningococci).	Very wide range.	Prototype and most potent, least toxic, penicillin. Absorption after oral administration undependable and should be avoided in severe infections. Give 1 h before or 2–3 h after meals. Oral dose 3–5 times higher than parenteral. Intramuscular route preferred.
Penicillin G benzathine	Bicillin Permapen	No	No	Same as penicillin G	IM: 300,000–3 million units 3 times weekly to once monthly.	Longest duration of action of penicillin preparations; sustained blood levels for 1–4 weeks. Useful prophylaxis of rheumatic fever. Orally active.
Penicillin G procaine	Crysticillin A.S., Duracillin A.S., Pfizerpen-AS, Wycillin	No	No	Same as penicillin G	IM: 300,00–1.2 million units 1–2 times daily.	Only administered intramuscularly. Local anesthetic effects of procaine make injections less painful than benzathine. Allergic reactions to procaine.
Penicillin V (phenoxymethyl penicillin)	Compocillin-V, Pen-Vee K, V-Cillin K	No	Yes	Same as penicillin G.	PO: 125–500 mg q. 6–8 h	Less potent and effective, but more acid stable than penicillin G and better absorbed from gastrointestinal tract. Employed only orally.
Methicillin	Azapen, Celbenin, Staphcillin	Yes	No	Gram-positive bacteria, especially penicillinase-resistant staphylococci.	IM or IV: 1–2 g q. 4–6 h	First penicillinase-resistant penicillin. Primary indication is for treatment of penicillinase-producing staphylococci. Less active than nafcillin and isoxazolyl penicillins. Unstable in acid, cannot be given orally. Intramuscular injections painful.
Oxacillin	Bactocill, Prostaphlin	Yes	Yes	Same as methicillin.	500 mg–2 g, PO, or 250 mg–2 g, IM or IV q. 4–6 h	Isoxazolyl penicillins (oxacillin, cloxacillin, and dicloxacillin) have similar antibacterial spectra; they are more potent than methicillin and less active than penicillin G against gram-positive cocci. Little or no activity against gram-negative bacteria.

Generic Name	Trade Names			Spectrum	Dosage	Remarks
Cloxacillin	Cloxapen, Tegopen	Yes	Yes	Same as methicillin.	PO: 250-500 mg q. 6 h	See oxacillin. Not all patients allergic to penicillin G may be sensitive to cloxacillin.
Dicloxacillin	Dycill, Dynapen, Pathocil, Veracillin	Yes	Yes	Same as methicillin.	PO: 125-500 mg q. 6 h	See cloxacillin. Best orally absorbed penicillinase-resistant penicillin.
Nafcillin	Nafcil, Unipen	Yes	Yes	Same as methicillin.	250 mg to 1 g, PO, or 500 mg IM or IV q. 4-6 h	Not absorbed as well orally as isoxazolyl penicillins. See Oxacillin.
Ampicillin	Amcill, Omnipen, Penbritin, Polycillin	No	Yes	Broad-spectrum: gram-positive bacteria (except penicillinase-forming) and gram-negative.	PO: 250 mg to 1 g q. 6 h; IM or IV: 200-500 mg q.i.d.	First broad-spectrum penicillin. Useful for treatment of gram-negative infections of gastrointestinal and urinary tracts. Well absorbed after oral administration.
Hetacillin	Versapen	No	Yes	Same as ampicillin.	PO: 225-900 mg q. 6 h	Hetacillin is metabolized in the body to ampicillin, its active metabolite.
Cyclacillin	Cyclapen	No	Yes	Similar to ampicillin but not as broad-spectrum.	PO: 250 mg q. 6 h	Reported lower incidence of gastrointestinal effects and skin rash than ampicillin.
Amoxicillin	Amoxil, Larotid, Polymox, Wymox	No	Yes	Same as ampicillin.	PO: 250-500 mg q. 8 h	Similar to ampicillin, but reported to produce higher blood levels and less diarrhea. Food has little effect on absorption of amoxicillin.
Carbenicillin	Geopen, Pyopen	No	Yes	Similar to ampicillin.	IV: 200-500 mg/kg/day; IM: 1-2 g q. 6 h	High activity against Proteus and moderate activity against Pseudomonas. Particularly useful for treatment of severe urinary tract infections. Intramuscular injections are painful. Large intravenous doses may be nephrotoxic.
Ticarcillin	Ticar	No	No	Gram-negative bacteria.	IV or IM: 1-3 g q. 4-6 h	New drug recommended for treatment of severe respiratory and genitourinary tract infections caused by gram-negative bacteria (susceptible strains of Pseudomonas, Proteus). Intramuscular injections should not exceed 2 g.

With several notable exceptions, most penicillins have a narrow spectrum of antibacterial activity (Table 43-1). They are considerably more active against gram-positive bacteria (for example, staphylococci, streptococci, pneumonococci, clostridia) than against gram-negative bacteria. Notable exceptions are the gram-negative gonococci and the spirochete responsible for causing syphilis (*Treponema pallidum*), which are susceptible to penicillins. Ampicillin and carbenicillin have a broad-spectrum of antimicrobial activity.

Resistance of many gram-positive and gram-negative bacteria to penicillin may be natural or acquired and has been attributed primarily to their ability to produce penicillinase, an enzyme capable of inactivating penicillin G. Semisynthetic penicillins such as methicillin, oxacillin, and the isoxazolyl derivatives are resistant to breakdown by bacterial penicillinase (Table 43-1). Other mechanisms of bacterial resistance to penicillin have been shown to exist.

Administration and Fate

Absorption Penicillin G is poorly and irregularly absorbed from the gastrointestinal tract after oral administration and is subject to chemical breakdown and biological inactivation by gastric acid. Oral administration of penicillin G should never be employed for the treatment of severe infections. To prevent its binding to foods, which reduces the rate and extent to which penicillin G is absorbed, this drug should be administered 1 hour before or 2 to 3 hours after meals. Milk, divalent and trivalent cation antacids, and oral ferrous salts also inhibit the absorption of penicillin (Table 43-3, pages 382–383).

Intramuscular injection is the preferred route of administration of penicillin G. The rate of absorption from these intramuscular sites may be slowed to produce a prolonged action by the use of relatively insoluble penicillin salts in a suitable vehicle. After a single injection, therapeutic blood levels persist for 12 to 24 hours after procaine penicillin and for 1 week or more after benzathine penicillin G. The intravenous route of administration by continuous infusion is used only when it is essential to maintain very high blood levels, such as in the treatment of subacute bacterial endocarditis.

Distribution Penicillins are widely distributed in the fluids and tissues of the body, including across the placental barrier. Under normal conditions, only low concentrations of the penicillins are found in the cerebrospinal fluid; these levels are reported to increase, but to an unreliable extent, when the meninges are inflamed. On rare occasions penicillin may be injected intrathecally, but this route of drug administration may cause severe adverse reactions.

The relative distribution of penicillins is influenced by their degree of plasma-protein binding. Penicillin G, penicillin V, methicillin, and ampicillin are protein-bound to a moderate extent (20 to 75 percent), while oxacillin and the other isoxazolyl derivatives are highly protein-bound (90 to 98 percent). With the latter drugs, lower levels of free drug are available for antibacterial action, thus potentially delaying the onset of the therapeutic response.

Excretion Penicillin is rapidly excreted by the kidneys into the urine, and this represents the major route of drug elimination. Probenecid (Benemid) inhibits the renal tubular excretion of penicillin, thus increasing and prolonging therapeutically effective blood levels. Newborns and individuals with impaired renal function tend to maintain higher drug levels for longer periods of time.

Therapeutic Uses

Notwithstanding the development of many new antibiotics, the penicillins remain the most widely used antibacterial agents. Their principal virtues include high potency, a bactericidal action, and low toxicity. Penicillin G is the drug of choice for the treatment of infections caused by pneumococci (pneumonia, empyema, meningitis, osteomyelitis, acute suppurative mastoiditis, endocarditis, peritonitis, and pericarditis); streptococci, particularly β-hemolytic streptococci, also referred to as *Group-A-Strep* pyogens (scarlet fever, pharyngitis, meningitis, pneumonia, endocarditis, otitis media, mastoiditis); meningococci (meningitis, meningococcemia, endocarditis); gonococci (gonorrhea); *Treponema pallidum* (syphilis); *Bacillus anthracis* (anthrax); and clostridia (gas gangrene; tetanus).

Ampicillin, a broad-spectrum penicillin derivative, is highly effective for the treatment of gram-negative bacillary infections caused by *Salmonella* (typhoid and paratyphoid fever, bacteremia, acute gastroenteritis); *Shigella* (acute gastroenteritis), and *Haemophilus influenzae*. Carbenicillin, a new broad-spectrum penicillin, has proven to be highly effective in the treatment of urinary tract and respiratory tract infections caused by *Proteus* and *Pseudomonas*. The prophylactic use of penicillin has been demonstrated to be effective in streptococcal infections, rheumatic fever, gonorrhea, and syphilis and in preventing bacterial endocarditis in patients with congenital or acquired heart disease of any kind who will be undergoing surgical or dental procedures.

Adverse Effects

While the penicillins possess a very low order of toxicity, their ability to cause hypersensitivity reactions is of great therapeutic significance. Nursing implications associated with penicillin administration are summarized at the end of this chapter.

Toxicity   Penicillin is the most selectively toxic chemotherapeutic agent currently available and is virtually nontoxic in human patients with normal kidney function. One patient was reported to have received 240 million units (144 g) of penicillin intravenously on a daily basis for 6 weeks without experiencing toxicity.

Most of the toxic effects of penicillin have been attributed to irritation, and include local pain and inflammation after the intramuscular injection of concentrated drug solutions; thrombophlebitis may occur after intravenous injection. Under certain circumstances, the central nervous system is particularly sensitive to the irritating effects of penicillin. Parenteral administration of large doses to patients with impaired renal function may cause twitching or localized or generalized seizures.

Most penicillin preparations are administered as the sodium or potassium salt; there are approximately 1.7 milliequivalents of potassium and sodium per million units (2.8 milliequivalents per gram) of their respective penicillin G salts. Hence the nurse should not overlook toxicity resulting from the cationic load, particularly in patients with impaired renal function.

Superinfection   Penicillin, like other antibiotics, can markedly alter the size and nature of the normal bacterial population of the gastrointestinal and upper respiratory tracts. The incidence of superinfection with penicillin G is considerably less than after the administration of such broad-spectrum antibiotics as the tetracyclines.

Hypersensitivity reactions   It has been estimated that from 5 to 10 percent of all American adults are hypersensitive to penicillin, and this probably represents the most common drug allergy. Hypersensitivity may occur after administration by any route, although the highest incidence is observed after its topical application.

The clinical manifestations of penicillin hypersensitivity may be of one of three types: (1) An *immediate anaphylactic reaction* characterized by circulatory collapse, edema of the larynx, and obstruction of respiration, which may rapidly be fatal. It is estimated that several hundred individuals die annually in the United States as the result of penicillin-induced anaphylaxis. (2) A reaction like *serum sickness*, less rapid in onset, with fever, urticaria, or other adverse skin reactions, and in severe cases, arthralgia and joint effusions and enlargement of the spleen and lymph nodes. (3) *Contact dermatitis* of delayed onset which may occur in nurses, physicians, and pharmacists who prepare penicillin solutions but who have never received this drug orally or by injection.

Prior to administration of penicillin to the patient, regardless of the route of administration, the nurse should ascertain whether the patient has experienced an adverse reaction to penicillin. Patients allergic to one penicillin derivative are generally allergic to all other penicillins and possibly to cephalosporin derivatives (see page 381). Hence these drugs should not be readministered to such patients. At present, diagnostic skin tests for penicillin have not proved to be completely reliable and may, themselves, be dangerous.

Penicillin Derivatives

Although penicillin G is the most potent and least expensive member of this antibiotic class and still remains the drug of choice for the vast majority of infections responsive to the penicillins, this natural derivative suffers from several major disadvantages.

Semisynthetic derivatives of penicillin G that overcome one or more of these shortcomings (Table 43-1) have been prepared.

Penicillin G is *unstable in the acidic environment of the stomach* and is irregularly absorbed after oral administration. Although less potent, penicillin V has an antimicrobial spectrum similar to penicillin G and is more stable and better absorbed from the gastrointestinal tract after oral administration. This drug is available only for oral use and is not intended to serve as a substitute for parenteral penicillin when it is indicated.

Many disease-causing staphylococci have been demonstrated to be penicillin resistant because of their ability to release *penicillinase* (β-lactamase), an enzyme that inactivates penicillin G. Penicillinase-resistant penicillins have been developed that are able to resist attack by this degradative enzyme; such drugs include methicillin and the isoxazolyl derivatives (Table 43-1). These drugs are considerably less active than penicillin G in the treatment of infections susceptible to therapy by the natural agent. These penicillinase-resistant drugs should be reserved for use only in the treatment of staphylococcal infections that are resistant to penicillin G.

The final inherent shortcoming of penicillin G is its rather *limited spectrum of antimicrobial activity*. Ampicillin, a very extensively prescribed drug, is somewhat less effective than penicillin G for the treatment of infections caused by gram-positive coccal bacteria. By contrast, ampicillin is very useful for the management of urinary and respiratory tract infections caused by gram-negative organisms. This drug is not penicillinase-resistant; it is available for oral and parenteral administration.

Nursing Precautions

Implicit nursing precautions have been indicated already. The most important of these involve hypersensitivity reactions. The nurse must determine whether the patient has previously experienced a hypersensitivity reaction to penicillin; if so, an alternative drug should be selected. After penicillin administration, the nurse should be vigilant for the appearance of immediate life-threatening hypersensitivity reactions, as well as those having a delayed onset.

Oral penicillins should be administered about 1 hour prior to or 2 to 3 hours after meals. Milk, oral iron supplements, and antacids containing divalent and trivalent cations bind most penicillins, interfering with the rate and extent to which these antibiotics are absorbed and substantially reducing their blood levels. Potential penicillin-drug interactions are summarized in Table 43-3, (pages 382–383).

CEPHALOSPORINS

The *Cephalosporium* fungus was first isoated in 1948 off the coast of Sardinia in the sea near a sewer outlet. The cephalosporin antibiotics closely resemble the penicillins in several respects. Both groups are chemically related and exert their bactericidal effects by inhibiting cell wall synthesis. In general, the cephalosporins are penicillinase-resistant. Although the reported incidence of cross-allergenicity between cephalosporins and penicillins is generally low, the nurse should exercise caution since hypersensitivity reactions to the former drugs occur more frequently in patients who have exhibited allergic reactions to penicillin.

Antimicrobial Activity

The antimicrobial activity of the cephalosporins is broader than penicillin G and more closely resembles ampicillin; the cephalosporins are less active than the penicillins against gram-positive bacteria, with the exception of penicillinase-producing staphylococci. In addition, these antibiotics are effective in the treatment of infections caused by some strains of such gram-negative bacteria as *Escherichia*, *Salmonella*, *Shigella*, *Proteus*, and *Klebsiella*.

While some cephalosporins are effective orally, others are not sufficiently well absorbed from the gastrointestinal tract and must be administered by intramuscular or intravenous injection (Table 43-2).

While the cephalosporins represent an effective class of chemotherapeutic agents, with the exception of *Klebsiella* infections, they are generally not recommended to be the primary drug of choice for any infectious disease. These drugs represent useful alternatives for the treatment of a variety of infectious disorders that are nonresponsive to the penicillins.

Adverse Effects

Approximately 5 percent of the patients receiving the cephalosporins develop *allergic reactions*, including fever, eosinophilia, skin rashes, serum sickness, or anaphylaxis.

Severe local pain may be experienced after intramuscular injection, while repeated intravenous injections may result in the development of phlebitis or thrombophlebitis; these adverse reactions, resulting from local irritation, are most common after cephalothin (Keflin) administration. While cephaloridine (Loridine) administration produces less irritation at the site of injection, the danger of nephrotoxicity producing tubular necrosis far overshadows this advantage. Cephaloridine is the only member of this antibiotic class causing kidney damage, and this drug is not recommended in patients with impaired renal function. Potential interactions involving the cephalosporins appear in Table 43-3. Nursing implications are summarized at the end of this chapter.

Table 43-2   Comparative Properties of Cephalosporin Derivatives

Generic name	Selected trade names	Usual adult dose	Remarks
Orally inactive			
Cephalothin Sodium	Keflin	IM (deep) or IV: 500 mg to 1 g q. 4-6 h	Antibacterial spectrum similar to penicillin, but penicillinase-resistant. Ineffective orally, intramuscular injection painful. Adjust dose in severe renal failure.
Cephaloridine	Loridine	IM or IV: 250 mg to 1 g 2-4 times daily	Penicillinase resistance. Cross-sensitivity in penicillin-allergic patients. Unlike other cephalosporins, possesses nephrotoxic potential. Drug interferes with tests for cross-matching of blood.
Cefazolin Sodium	Ancef, Kefzol	IM or IV: 750 mg to 4 g daily in 3-4 divided doses	Recommended for respiratory, urinary tract, skin, and soft tissue infections. Less pain than cephalothin after IM injection.
Cephapirin Sodium	Cefadyl	IM or IV: 500 mg to 2 g q. 4-6 h	Penicillinase-resistant. Nausea common.
Cefamandole Nafate	Mandol	IM or IV: 500 mg to 1 g q. 4-6 h	Wider spectrum of antibacterial activity against gram-positive and gram-negative bacteria. Penicillinase-resistant. Indications similar to cefazolin. Adjust dose in renal failure.
Orally active			
Cefaclor	Ceclor	PO: 250 to 500 mg q. 8 h.	Most useful oral cephalosporin for treatment of otitis media caused by *Haemophilus influenzae.*
Cefadroxil monohydrate	Duricef	PO: 1 g b.i.d.	Long duration of action. Not useful for treatment of respiratory tract infections.
Cephalexin	Keflex	PO: 250 mg to 1 g q. 6 h	Penicillinase-resistant. Food slows rate of absorption. Gastrointestinal side effects.
Cephaloglycin	Kafocin	PO: 250-500 mg q. 6 h for 10 days	Penicillinase-resistant. Most useful for severe urinary tract infections. Causes severe diarrhea. Poorest absorption after oral administration.
Cephradine	Anspor, Velosef	PO: 250-500 mg q. 6 h IM or IV: 500 mg-1 g q.i.d.	Same uses as cefazolin. Unlike other cephalosporins, active against enterococci. Excellent absorption orally; food slows, but does not decrease absorption. Only cephalosporin active by mouth and injection.

Table 43-3   Potential Drug Interactions Involving Penicillins and Cephalosporins

Antibiotic	Interacting drug/class	Potential consequences
Penicillins and cephalosporins	Bacteriostatic antibiotics for example, tetracyclines, erythromycin, chloramphenicol	Use of bacteriostatic antibiotics may theoretically reduce the antibacterial effects of bactericidal agents (penicillins, cephalosporins); this interaction has not been well documented clinically.
Penicillins and cephalosporins (cephalothin, cephapirin)	Probenecid (Benemid)	Probenecid inhibits the renal tubular excretion of these antibiotics, thus increasing and prolonging their blood levels.

Table 43-3   (Continued)

Antibiotic	Interacting drug/class	Potential consequences
Penicillin G	Divalent (calcium, magnesium), trivalent (aluminum) cation antacids. Oral iron preparations (for example, ferrous sulfate)	These metals inhibit the absorption of penicillin G after oral administration.
Cephaloridine	Colistin (Coly-Mycin) Aminoglycosides (Table 46-1) Furosemide (Lasix) Ethacrynic acid (Edecrin)	Use of these nephrotoxic or potentially nephrotoxic agents with cephaloridine increases the risk of kidney damage.

Penicillins and Cephalosporins: nursing implications

Penicillins

1. The incidence of penicillin hypersensitivity among American adults is estimated to be as high as 10%; therefore, a careful medication history should be taken prior to initiation of therapy.

2. If the patient is determined to be allergic to penicillin, this should be clearly noted on the chart. Instruct the patient to inform physicians of this allergy whenever medical treatment is rendered. Advise the patient to wear a tag or carry a card indicating this allergy.

3. After penicillin administration, observe the patient for possible allergic reaction and have epinephrine, corticosteroids, and oxygen available for emergency use. Allergic reactions most commonly occur in patients with a history of asthma, hay fever, or atopic dermatitis.

4. Allergic reactions may occur within 20 min or may appear days or weeks after therapy is initiated.

5. Instruct the patient to report skin rashes, fever, joint pains, or pruritis.

6. Oral penicillins should be taken 1 h before or 2–3 h after meals. Milk, antacids, and oral iron supplements can also interfere with penicillin absorption and should be avoided, if possible, during the course of antibiotic therapy.

7. When a patient is being treated for gonorrhea and primary syphilis is suspected, a dark field examination should be performed and monthly serological examinations performed for 4 mo after the completion of treatment.

Cephalosporins

1. Drug-induced severe diarrhea may require discontinuation of medication.

2. After chronic drug administration, observe the patient for superinfections caused by nonsensitive microorganisms, most commonly *Pseudomonas*, and vaginal monilial infections.

3. In diabetes use Tes-Tape to evaluate glycosuria since false positive tests may be obtained with Clinitest tablets or Benedict's solution.

SUPPLEMENTARY READINGS

Barza, M., "Antimicrobial Spectrum, Pharmacology and Therapeutic Use of Antibiotics, Part 2: Penicillins," *American Journal of Hospital Pharmacy* **34:** 57–67 (1977).

Barza, M., and P. V. M. Miao, "Antimicrobial Spectrum, Pharmacology and Therapeutic Use of Antibiotics, Part 3: Cephalosporins," *American Journal of Hospital Pharmacy* **34:** 621–29 (1977).

Bear, D. M., M. Turck, and R. G. Petersdorf, "Ampicillin," *Medical Clinics of North America* **54:** 1145–59 (1970).

Flynn, E. H., ed., *Cephalosporins and Penicillins: Chemistry and Biology.* New York: Academic Press, Inc., 1972.

Moellering, R. C., and M. N. Swartz, "The Newer Cephalosporins," *New England Journal of Medicine* **294:** 24–28 (1976).

Schwartz, M. A., Chemical Aspects of Penicillin Allergy," *Journal of Pharmaceutical Sciences* **58:** 643–61 (1969).

Thrupp, L. D., "Newer Cephalosporins and Expanded-Spectrum Penicillins," *Annual Review of Pharmacology* **14:** 435–67 (1974).

ERYTHROMYCIN AND OTHER ANTIBIOTICS EMPLOYED AGAINST GRAM-POSITIVE ORGANISMS

Chapter 44

In this chapter, we shall consider the pharmacology and therapeutics of drugs with antimicrobial activity limited primarily to gram-positive bacteria. These drugs, the most widely used of which is erythromycin, are employed primarily in patients who are intolerant to penicillin or in the treatment of penicillin-resistant bacterial infections.

ERYTHROMYCIN

Erythromycin possesses an antimicrobial spectrum similar to that of penicillin G. It is active against most gram-positive bacteria, in particular, streptococci, staphylococci, pneumonococci, and corynebacteria; neisseria, haemophilus, and mycoplasma are also susceptible. The bacteriostatic effects of erythromycin have been attributed to its ability to inhibit protein synthesis by binding to bacterial ribosomes.

The erythromycins are primarily employed as penicillin substitutes in patients who are allergic to the latter drug. They are useful for the treatment of mild to moderate infections when oral therapy is appropriate

(Table 44-1). The emergence of resistant strains in susceptible bacterial populations has markedly reduced the therapeutic utility of these antibiotics.

The incidence of adverse effects and allergic reactions to the erythromycins is generally low. When given in large oral doses, these antibiotics may cause loss of appetite, nausea, vomiting, or diarrhea. Tablets with acid-resistant (enteric) coating may be given with meals to reduce the incidence of these mild gastrointestinal disturbances. Erythromycin estolate (Ilosone) has been reported to be *hepatotoxic*, an effect that appears to be unique only to this ester of erythromycin. Cholestatic hepatitis, most commonly seen after 10 days of therapy, is characterized initially by nausea, vomiting, and abdominal cramps; these symptoms are followed by fever and jaundice or other signs of impairment of liver function. These symptoms generally disappear within days after the termination of drug therapy. Nursing implications appear at the end of this chapter.

LINCOMYCIN AND CLINDAMYCIN

The chemical derivatives lincomycin (Lincocin) and clindamycin (Cleocin) have antibacterial activity similar to that of erythromycin. Clindamycin is more potent, better absorbed, and reported to cause less diarrhea than lincomycin. The most important clinical indication for clindamycin is for the treatment of severe anaerobic infections caused by bacteroides not sensitive to penicillins, especially *Bacteroides fragilis.*

The incidence and severity of severe toxicity, most commonly involving the gastrointestinal tract, usually restrict the use of these drugs to the treatment of several specific infections in hospitalized patients only.

Table 44-1   Erythromycins and Other Antibiotics Used Against Gram-Positive Organisms

Generic name	Selected trade names	Usual adult dose	Remarks
Erythromycin	E-Mycin, Erythrocin, Ilotycin, Robimycin	PO: 250 mg q. 6 h	Prototype erythromycin derivative with antibacterial activity similar to penicillin G. Enteric coating on tablets required to prevent destruction by gastric acid. Up to 4 g daily may be given in divided doses. Available as tablets, rectal suppositories, ophthalmic ointment.
Erythromycin estolate	Ilosone	PO: 250 mg q. 6 h	More acid stable than erythromycin and absorption less affected by food in stomach. Cholestatic hepatitis seen only with this derivative.
Erythromycin ethylsuccinate	EES, Pediamycin	PO: 400 mg q. 6 h; IM: 100 mg q. 4-8 h	Relatively nonirritating, suitable for intramuscular injection. Used as pediatric oral suspension.
Erythromycin gluceptate	Ilotycin gluceptate	IV: 15-20 mg/kg daily. Continuous infusion preferred but may be given at 6-h intervals.	Used for treatment of severe infections; larger doses may be used. The infusion rate should be slow to avoid pain along vein.
Erythromycin lactobionate	Erythrocin lactobionate		
Erythromycin stearate	Bristamycin, Erythrocin Stearate, Erypar; Ethril, Wyamycin S	PO: 250 mg q. 6 h	Same as erythromycin. More stable in gastric acid. Hydrolyzed in small intestines to yield erythromycin.

Table 44-1   Continued

Generic name	Selected trade names	Usual adult dose	Remarks
Troleandomycin	Tao	PO: 250–500 mg q.i.d.	Antibacterial activity similar to erythromycin, but less active and no advantages. Gastrointestinal side effects.
Lincomycin	Lincocin	PO: 500 mg t.i.d., IM: 600 mg q. 24 h	Antibacterial activity similar to erythromycin. May be used to treat infections caused by microbes resistant to penicillin and erythromycin. Can cause severe diarrhea and potentially fatal colitis.
Clindamycin	Cleocin	PO: 150–300 mg q. 6 h; IM or IV:600–1200 mg daily in 2–4 equal doses.	Same antimicrobial activity as lincomycin, but better absorbed and less toxic; severe colitis reported. Most useful for treatment of anaerobic infections caused by bacteroides.
Vancomycin	Vancocin	IV: 500 mg q. 6 h or 1 g q. 12 h	Reserved for treatment of life-threatening infections caused by gram-positive cocci unresponsive to safer antibiotics. Can cause severe nephrotoxicity and permanent deafness.
Novobiocin	Albamycin	PO: 250 mg q. 6 h PO, IM, or IV: 500 mg q. 12 h	Narrow-spectrum antibiotic, primarily active against gram-positive cocci. High incidence of allergic reactions and rapid emergence of bacterial resistance suggest that this drug has rare therapeutic utility.
Spectinomycin	Trobicin	IM (deep): 2 single injections of 2–4 g	Used only for treatment of acute genital and rectal gonorrhea. Adverse effects: pain at site of injection; nausea, chills, and fever.
Bacitracin	———	IM: Infants under 2.5 kg: 900 units/kg/24 h. Over 2.5 kg: 1,000 units/kg/24 h	Use restricted to infants with staphylococcal pneumonia and emphysema. Severe risk of nephrotoxicity limits systemic usefulness.
Bacitracin	Baciguent	Skin and ophthalmic ointment.	Used for treatment of skin and eye infections alone or in combination with other drugs.

Table 44-2   Potential Drug Interactions Involving Lincomycin and Clindamycin

Antibiotic	Interacting drug/class	Potential consequences
Lincomycin	Cyclamates Kaolin-pectin (Kaopectate)	These drugs markedly inhibit lincomycin absorption after oral administration.
Lincomycin Clindamycin	Neuromuscular blocking agents.	These two antibiotics possess neuromuscular blocking activity, which may enhance the activity or prolong the duration of surgical neuromuscular blocking agents.

Severe and persistent diarrhea may be associated with pseudomembranous colitis and may lead to acute ulcerative colitis and death. If severe diarrhea occurs, antibiotic administration should be terminated and therapy initiated to control the diarrhea and restore the normal fluid and electrolyte balance. Since large amounts of these drugs are excreted in the urine unmetabolized, the doses employed must be reduced in patients with impaired renal function.

The available preparations, doses, and distinguishing characteristics of antibiotics employed primarily for the treatment of gram-positive infections are summarized in Table 44-1. Potential drug interactions involving these drugs are summarized in Table 44-2.

Erythromycin and Other Antibiotics Employed Against Gram-Positive Organisms:
nursing implications

Erythromycin

1. Antimicrobial activity may be reduced in acid medium and by presence of food in the stomach. Administer at least 1 h before or 2-3 after meals; avoid fruit juices.
2. During prolonged therapy periodic liver function tests and blood counts are recommended.
3. Observe the patient for overgrowth of nonsusceptible microorganisms. Appearance of resistant strains of staphylococci are common after prolonged therapy, causing fever, sore mouth, enteritis, perianal irritation, pruritis, or vaginitis.

Lincomycin

1. Twenty percent of patients receiving lincomycin experience diarrhea. Drug administration is usually restricted to hospitalized patients with specific indications.
2. Instruct the patient to report any change in bowel frequency or perianal irritation or blood or mucus in stools.
3. If severe diarrhea occurs, medication should be discontinued and treatment initiated to control diarrhea. Opiates or Lomotil may prolong and worsen the diarrhea. Appropriate medical treatment includes fluid and electrolyte replacement, protein supplementation, and possibly corticosteroids.

SUPPLEMENTARY READINGS

Braun, P., "Hepatoxicity of Erythromycin," *Journal of Infectious Diseases* **119**: 300–306 (1969).

Graham, R. C., Jr., "Antibiotics for Treatment of In-
fections Caused by Gram-Positive Cocci," *Medical Clinics of North America* **58**: 505–17 (1974).

Griffith, R. S., and H. R. Black, "Erythromycin," *Medical Clinics of North America* **54**: 1199–1215 (1970).

TETRACYCLINES AND CHLORAMPHENICOL

The tetracyclines and chloramphenicol are antibiotic agents possessing a broad-spectrum of antimicrobial activity. While the tetracyclines are used for the treatment of a wide range of microbial infections, the risk of severe toxicity has limited the safe and rational use of chloramphenicol to only a few highly selected diseases.

TETRACYCLINES

Tetracyclines are among the most widely employed antimicrobial agents, and of the antibiotics in common therapeutic usage, they have the broadest spectrum of antimicrobial activity. Drugs in this antibiotic class all have the same general antimicrobial spectrum, pharmacological effects, therapeutic uses, and adverse effects. Differences exist among the members of the tetracycline class with respect to their degrees of absorption after oral administration, durations of action, suitabilities for parenteral administration, and relative incidence of adverse effects (Table 45-1).

Antimicrobial Activity

The antimicrobial activity of the tetracyclines has been attributed to their inhibition of bacterial protein synthesis by blocking the binding of the amino acid-transfer RNA complex to ribosomes. Their relatively selective inhibitory effects on microbial growth rather than on host cells may be the result of differences in the permeability and concentration of the drug by the microbial cells.

The tetracyclines are broad-spectrum antibiotics, with activities against gram-positive and gram-negative bacteria, mycoplasma, *Treponema pallidum*, leptospira, rickettsia, chlamydia, and some protozoa, including amebas.

Administration and Fate

All tetracyclines are incompletely absorbed from the gastrointestinal tract after oral administration. Their absorption is greatly impaired by calcium, magnesium, antacids containing aluminum, and oral iron preparations. The calcium in milk and dairy products also reduces the absorption of tetra-

Table 45-1   Comparative Properties of Tetracycline Derivatives

Generic name	Selected trade names	Usual adult dose	Remarks
Tetracycline	Achromycin V, Panmycin, Sumycin, Tetracyn	PO: 250–500 mg q.i.d. IM: 250 mg q. 24 h IV: 250–500 mg q. 12 h	Prototype tetracycline; see text for general discussion. Drug is eliminated primarily in urine; dose must be adjusted in renal failure. Available for oral, parenteral, ophthalmic and otic use. Gastrointestinal side effects less than oxytetracycline but more than demeclocycline.
Oxytetracycline	Terramycin	PO: 250–500 mg q.i.d. IM: 250 mg q. 24 h	Same uses as tetracycline, in particular, intestinal amebiasis (Chapter 49). High incidence of gastrointestinal side effects.
Democlocycline	Declomycin	PO: 450–900 mg daily in 2–4 divided doses	More potent than tetracycline. Long biological half-life. Photosensitive reactions (extreme sunburn) most common with this tetracycline derivative.
Methacycline	Rondomycin	PO: 600 mg daily in 2–4 divided doses	Long biological half-life. Photosensitivity reactions more common than tetracycline. Avoid use in patients with impaired renal function.
Doxycycline	Doxychel, Vibramycin	PO: 100 mg b.i.d. on day 1, followed by 50–100 mg 1–2 times daily IV: 100–200 mg q. 24 h	Best absorbed tetracycline, not inhibited by foods but impaired by antacids. Greater potency than tetracycline, long half-life, low rate of urinary excretion; plasma levels and duration of action not greatly influenced by renal insufficiency. Photosensitivity reactions.
Minocycline	Minocin, Vectrin	PO or IV: 200 mg followed by 100 mg q. 12 h	More potent, longer half-life than tetracycline. Bacterial resistance, especially staphylococci, of low incidence. Photosensitivity reactions reported; vestibular toxicity (dizziness, nausea, vomiting). Antacids and iron, but not food and milk, markedly impair absorption.

cyclines lowering the blood concentration of these antibiotics. To prevent these problems, tetracyclines should be administered at least 1 hour prior to antacids or meals or 2 hours after.

All members of this class are bound to plasma proteins from 20 percent (tetracycline) to 90 percent (doxycycline, methacycline, demeclocycline); those drugs that are most protein-bound have the slowest rates of renal excretion and the longest biological half-lives. The tetracyclines are generally widely distributed throughout the tissues and fluids of the body. Penetration into the cerebrospinal fluid is generally quite low after oral drug administration.

Tetracyclines are specifically stored in growing bones and teeth. This may result in *brown discoloration of teeth*, an effect most prominent when tetracyclines are taken between the ages of 2 months and 2 years, when permanent teeth are being calcified. The intensity of discoloration is dependent upon the total dose of tetracycline administered to the child. Similarly, administration of tetracyclines to pregnant patients, especially during the second trimester of pregnancy, has been shown to cause discoloration of their children's teeth. It is generally recommended that, if possible, this class of antibiotics be avoided during pregnancy and by children under 8 years of age.

Therapeutic Uses

The tetracyclines are among the most widely used classes of anti-infective agents because of their effectiveness after oral administration, relatively low toxicity, and extensive spectrum of antimicrobial activity, making them useful for the management of infections of mixed microbial etiology.

A partial listing of major therapeutic uses includes treatment of infections caused by rickettsia (Rocky Mountain spotted fever, murine and endemic typhus, Q fever, and rickettsialpox, for all of which tetracyclines are the drug class of choice); chlamydia (psittacosis, *Lymphogranuloma venereum*, trachoma, and inclusion conjunctivitis, for all of which the tetracyclines are the drug class of choice or are considered highly effective); mycoplasma ("atypical" viral pneumonia); gram-positive and gram-negative bacteria (brucellosis, tularemia, cholera, gonorrhea, syphilis); and ameba (amebic dysentery). When susceptible bacteria are responsible for the infection, tetracyclines are commonly employed for the treatment of urinary, biliary, and respiratory tract infections and skin infections, particularly acne.

Adverse Effects and Precautions

Hypersensitivity reactions have been associated with tetracycline administration, although not commonly. Such reactions involve the skin (rashes, urticaria, fixed skin eruptions, generalized exfoliative dermatitis) and respiratory system (asthmatic-like responses, angioedema); anaphylactoid reactions can occur even after oral use. Cross-sensitization exists among the various tetracycline derivatives.

The most common adverse effects noted after oral administration of tetracyclines involve *gastrointestinal disturbances* and include anorexia, epigastric distress, nausea, vomiting, and diarrhea. These symptoms are generally not disabling but, when severe, medication must be discontinued or at least interrupted and reinitiated at a lower dosage level. These symptoms may be reduced by advising the patient to take the medication with food, *not* milk. It is essential that diarrhea resulting from gastrointestinal irritation be differentiated from the diarrhea associated with superinfection.

The broad antimicrobial spectrum of the tetracyclines commonly causes marked alterations in the normal floral population and balance, resulting in *superinfections* (suprainfections). This most commonly occurs in the intestinal tract, but may also involve the mouth, lungs, anus, and vagina and results from an overgrowth of the yeast monilia, or the bacteria staphylococci, enterococci, *Proteus*, or *Pseudomonas*. Staphylococcal enterocolitis, which may occur at any time during or shortly after tetracycline administration, must be rapidly diagnosed since it is frequently fatal. The nurse should be alert for the symptoms of superinfection, which include diarrhea, dryness of the mouth, oral lesions, hoarseness, glossitis, pharyngitis, and anal or vaginal pruritis.

The tetracyclines may cause liver and kidney injury. Most hepatotoxic reactions have been reported after the parenteral administration of large daily doses (1 to 2 g), although this effect may also occur after large oral doses. The risk of hepatotoxicity is increased in pregnant patients, those with pre-existing kidney or liver disorders, or those to whom the tetracyclines are administered with other drugs capable of causing liver injury. With the exception of doxycycline (Vibramycin) and minocycline (Minocin), drugs which are not eliminated to a large extent in the urine, the tetracyclines are not advised for use in patients with *renal impairment.* Tetracycline-induced injury to the kidney, which has been reported to produce fatalities, is directly related to the tetracycline employed, the dose and duration of therapy, and the degree of pre-existing renal insufficiency. Symptoms of kidney toxicity include azotemia, acidosis, weight loss, nausea, and vomiting.

Photosensitivity reactions have been noted after the administration of some tetracycline derivatives, in particular, demeclocycline (Declomycin); this adverse response is less frequent with tetracycline and has not been observed with minocycline. This reaction is generally manifested as an extreme sunburn upon exposure to sunlight in the ultraviolet range and is reversible over a period of days to weeks. Nurses should advise their patients, especially those with fair skin, to avoid direct exposure to the sun after receiving demeclocycline.

As we mentioned earlier, short- or long-term therapy with the tetracyclines may cause brown discoloration of the teeth of children and the offspring of pregnant women receiving these drugs. This risk of discoloration is greatest from midpregnancy to 2 years of age, but continues until the age of 7 years and possibly longer. The intensity of the discoloration of the teeth appears to be related more to the total dose of antibiotic received than to the duration of drug administration.

Tetracyclines have been shown to delay the rate of blood coagulation and may enhance the effects of the coumarin-type anticoagulants. This effect has been attributed to the ability of the tetracyclines to cause chelation of calcium and also to alter plasma lipoproteins (Chapter 31). The tetracyclines are irritating after intravenous administration and can cause thrombophlebitis.

Nurses should not administer and should advise their patients not to take *outdated* and degraded tetracycline. Patients ingesting such drugs have experienced a type of Fanconi syndrome characterized by

Table 45-2 Potential Drug Interactions Involving Tetracyclines and Chloramphenicol

Antibiotic	Interacting drug/class	Potential consequences
Tetracyclines	Divalent (calcium, magnesium) and trivalent (aluminum) cation antacids Milk and dairy products	Well documented that antacids reduce absorption of orally administered tetracyclines, thus decreasing blood levels of these antibiotics; the tetracyclines should not be administered within 1–2 h after antacids.
	Oral iron preparations, for example, ferrous sulfate	Iron impairs absorption of oral tetracycline; if not possible to avoid use of iron, give 3 h before or 2 h after tetracyclines.
	Methoxyflurane (Penthrane)	Enhanced risk of nephrotoxicity.
Doxycycline	Carbamazepine (Tegretol) Phenytoin (Dilantin) Barbiturates	Administration of these anticonvulsants enhances the rate of metabolism of doxycycline, lowering blood levels and potentially reducing its antimicrobial effects.
Chloramphenicol	Oral anticoagulants, coumarin-type	Chloramphenicol decreases vitamin K production by intestinal bacteria and inhibits coumarin metabolism; both result in potential enhancement of anticoagulation with increased risk of bleeding.
	Oral hypoglycemic agents, sulfonylureas	Chloramphenicol increases the plasma half-life of tolbutamide (possibly by inhibiting its metabolism), with strong risk of hypoglycemic reaction.
	Cyclophosphamide (Cytoxan) Phenytoin (Dilantin)	Chloramphenicol may inhibit metabolism of these drugs increasing the risk of toxicity.

nausea, vomiting, polyuria, polydipsia, proteinuria and glycosuria. Drug-interactions involving the tetracycline class of antibiotics are summarized in Table 45-2. Nursing implications appear at the end of the chapter.

CHLORAMPHENICOL

Chloramphenicol (Chloromycetin, Mychel) is a broad-spectrum antibiotic; its therapeutic uses should be restricted to the treatment of those serious infections that fail to respond to less dangerous drugs.

Antimicrobial Activity and Therapeutic Uses

The antimicrobial activity of chloramphenicol has been attributed to its ability to inhibit protein synthesis by attaching to the bacterial ribosome and interfering with the formation of peptide bonds between amino acids. It is also capable of inhibiting the protein synthesis of mammalian bone marrow cells.

Chloramphenicol is rapidly absorbed from the gastrointestinal tract. It is well distributed in body fluids and achieves therapeutic concentrations in the cerebrospinal fluid and the brain, making it useful for the treatment of infections of the central nervous system. After subconjunctival injection, it penetrates the aqueous humor of the eye. Chloramphenicol sodium succinate, a water-soluble derivative, is available for parenteral administration.

Chloramphenicol inhibits many strains of gram-positive and gram-negative bacteria, rickettsia, chlamydia, and the mycoplasmas. It is the drug of choice for the treatment of typhoid fever and other systemic *Salmonella* infections (osteitis, meningitis). While the tetracyclines are the treatment of choice in rickettsial diseases, chloramphenicol is indicated in patients allergic to the tetracyclines

and in those who are pregnant or who have impaired renal function. Chloramphenicol is also highly effective in the clinical treatment of meningitis caused by sensitive strains of *Haemophilus influenzae* and many strains of anaerobic bacteria. The usual oral adult dose is 2 to 3 g daily.

Adverse Effects

It is not uncommon for the irritating effects of chloramphenicol on the gastrointestinal tract to cause nausea, vomiting, and diarrhea within several days after the initiation of therapy. The cause of these symptoms should be differentiated from superinfections, which appear within 5 to 10 days.

The routine use of chloramphenicol as an antimicrobial agent has been and should continue to be sharply restricted because of its ability to cause *bone marrow depression*, resulting in severe and potentially fatal blood dyscrasia—including anemia, pancytopenia, thrombopenia, and *aplastic anemia*. The last mentioned is an irreversible and often fatal blood disorder characterized by a marked reduction in circulating red blood cells, leukocytes, and blood platelets. This condition is not dose-related nor is it seen in all patients; it is believed to be a genetically-determined idiosyncratic reaction to this antibiotic. In view of the potential risk of aplastic anemia, patients receiving chloramphenicol should be under very close medical supervision for periodic blood studies. Nurses should instruct patients to immediately report to their physicians the appearance of bleeding tendencies, sore throats, or other symptoms potentially indicative of a new infectious process.

In older children and in adults, chloramphenicol is readily inactivated by a glucuronic acid conjugation reaction. Newborns lack the enzyme required to catalyze this reaction during the early weeks of life and, moreover, do not have sufficiently well-developed renal function to excrete the drug; as a consequence, chloramphenicol levels become markedly elevated. The resulting "gray syndrome" in neonates is manifested by vomiting, abdominal distention, progressive pallid cyanosis (ashen-gray color), acute circulatory failure, and, in some instances, death. Only under highly unusual circum-stances should chloramphenicol be administered during the first 4 weeks of life, and then the daily dose should not exceed 25 mg/kg of body weight; after this age, the daily dosage of 50 mg/kg may be given.

Potential drug interactions involving chloramphenicol are summarized in Table 45-2. Nursing implications are summarized below.

Tetracyclines and Chloramphenicol: nursing implications

Tetracyclines

1. Administer the drug at least 1 h before or 2 h after meals. If nausea, vomiting, or diarrhea occur, administer with foods other than calcium-rich foods such as dairy products.
2. Tetracyclines should not be administered to pregnant patients or children up to 8 years of age to prevent brown discoloration of teeth.
3. Check expiration date before administering the drug, and instruct the patient to discard all unused tetracyclines. Ingestion of outdated and decomposed tetracycline may cause a Falconi-like syndrome.
4. Observe for overgrowth of nonsensitive microorganisms: black hairy tongue; monilial vaginitis; diarrhea may result from superinfection (requiring discontinuation of medication) or local irritation of tissues. Prevent or treat pruritus ani by cleansing the anal area with water several times each day and after each bowel movement.
5. Instruct the patient to avoid prolonged exposure to sunlight or ultraviolet light, since tetracyclines may increase sensitivity to severe sunburn resulting from a phototoxic reaction.
6. Observe patients on IV therapy for redness, swelling, and pain along the vein.
7. Check fluid intake and output because impaired renal function may result in extremely high drug levels, leading to toxicity. Observe patients with impaired kidney function for acidosis, anorexia, nausea, vomiting, and dehydration.

Chloramphenicol

1. Administration is usually restricted to hospitalized patients to permit observation for early signs of severe side effects.
2. Baseline complete blood counts and reticulocyte cell counts are recommended prior to the initiation of therapy, at 48-h intervals during the course of therapy, and periodically after its termination. Bone marrow depression may occur weeks or months after the end of drug administration.

3. Bone marrow depression may be dose-related and reversible or dose-unrelated and irreversible. Frequent laboratory tests and close observation are essential. Report immediately sore throat, fatigue, fever, or petechiae.

4. To reduce the risk of "gray syndrome" (manifested by vomiting, abdominal distention, progressive pallid cyanosis, and acute circulatory failure), chloramphenicol should not be administered to infants during the first 4 wk of life unless other effective drugs are not available.

SUPPLEMENTARY READINGS

Barza, M., and R. T. Schiefe, "Antimicrobial Spectrum, Pharmacology and Therapeutic Use of Antibiotics, Part 1: Tetracyclines," *American Journal of Hospital Pharmacy* **34:** 49–57 (1977).

Neuvonen, P. J., "Interactions with the Absorption of Tetracyclines," *Drugs* **11:** 45–54 (1976).

Ory, E. M., "The Tetracyclines," *Medical Clinics of North America* **54:** 1173–86 (1970).

Snyder, M. J., and T. E. Woodward, "The Clinical Use of Chloramphenicol," *Medical Clinics of North America* **54:** 1187–97 (1970).

Woodward, T. E., and C. L. Wisseman, Jr., *Chloromycetin (Chloramphenicol)*. New York: Medical Encyclopedia, Inc., 1958.

AMINOGLYCOSIDES AND POLYMYXINS

Chapter 46

The aminoglycosides and the polymyxins are two groups of antibiotics with antimicrobial activity limited primarily to the treatment of gram-negative infections.

AMINOGLYCOSIDES

The aminoglycosides share common chemical, antimicrobial, pharmacological, and toxicological characteristics. The members of this class include streptomycin (the oldest and best studied drug in this group), neomycin, gentamicin, kanamycin, tobramycin, amikacin, and paromomycin (Table 46-1).

Antimicrobial Activity

Streptomycin binds to bacterial ribosomes and is thought to inhibit protein synthesis by causing the misreading of the messenger

Table 46-1 Comparative Properties of Aminoglycoside Derivatives

Generic name	Selected trade names	Usual adult dose	Remarks
Streptomycin		IM: 1–4 gm o.d.	Used for treatment of gram-negative bacterial infections and tuberculosis (Chapter 47). Rapid development of bacterial resistance. Highly useful for tularemia and bubonic plague. Only administered intramuscularly. Potential renal impairment or ototoxicity with all aminoglycosides.
Neomycin	Mycifradin	IM: 15 mg/kg/day in 4 equally spaced doses.	Effective for gram-negative systemic infections, but, because of toxicity, reserved for hospitalized patients for whom no other drug is effective. Used topically for local infections; prolonged use may cause elevated systemic levels and ototoxicity.
Gentamicin	Garamycin	IM: 0.8–3 mg/kg/day in 3 equal doses q. 8 h for 7–10 days.	Treatment of gram-negative infections (especially *Pseudomonas*) of urinary tract, eye and skin. Narrower range of safety than kanamycin. Effective versus some gram-positive bacteria (staphylococci). Dose must be reduced in impaired renal function for systemic aminoglycosides.
Kanamycin	Kantrex Klebcil	IM: 7.5 mg/kg q. 12 h; IV: 15 mg/kg/day, in 2–3 divided doses. PO: 1–4 g t.i.d. for 5–7 days.	Not absorbed orally; used for intestinal infections. Useful for gram-negative septicemias. Bacterial resistance develops. Ototoxicity and reversible nephrotoxicity.
Tobramycin	Nebcin	IM or IV: 3 mg/kg q. 8 h	New drug similar to gentamicin, effective versus *Pseudomonas.*
Amikacin	Amikin	IM or IV: 15 mg/kg/day in 2–3 divided doses.	New drug similar to gentamicin.
Paromomycin	Humatin	PO: 25–35 mg/kg/day in 3 divided doses with meals for 5–10 days.	Major use is for the treatment of acute and chronic intestinal amebiasis (more effective drugs available); ineffective for extraintestinal amebiasis (Chapter 49).

RNA (mRNA) information. The ability of the other aminoglycosides to inhibit protein synthesis is probably accomplished by a mechanism that is similar to that produced by streptomycin.

The aminoglycosides are active against gram-negative rods, most notably, sensitive strains of *Enterobacter* (*Aerobacter*), *Proteus*, *Pseudomonas*, and *Serratia*. Gentamicin, tobramycin, and amikacin are particularly active against kanamycin-resistant strains. Some gram-positive organisms, in particular, staphylococci, are inhibited by the aminoglycoside antibiotics; in most instances, however, the serious toxicity associated with these drugs precludes their use alone for the treatment of infections caused by these organisms. Streptomycin and kanamycin possess activity against *Mycrobacterium tuberculosis* (Chapter 47). The aminoglycosides are generally inactive against streptococci, pneumonococci, clostridia, bacteriodes, rickettsia, fungi, and viruses.

Bacterial resistance to streptomycin is common and develops rapidly, thus limiting the utility of this drug for the long-term treatment of bacterial infections. The development of resistance to other aminoglycosides has been demonstrated but occurs at a much slower rate than to streptomycin.

Cross-resistance may develop between aminoglycosides and, when this occurs, it is generally complete.

Administration and Fate

The aminoglycosides are well absorbed after intramuscular injection, producing peak serum levels within approximately 1 hour. In patients with normal kidney function, minimal serum levels are achieved after oral administration, although repeated oral doses in patients with impaired renal function may result in toxicity. Similar adverse effects may occur when these drugs are applied topically to extensive denuded areas such as wounds or burns, or after irrigation of closed cavities or infected wounds. No absorption occurs through the intact skin.

Once entering the blood, the aminoglycosides are generally distributed throughout the body except to the central nervous system and the humors of the eye. The aminoglycosides have a marked affinity for the *kidney* and have a tendency to accumulate in this organ. They are not metabolized to an appreciable extent and are removed from the body in the urine. Considerable adjustments in dosage must be made in patients with renal impairment to prevent the appearance of serum levels capable of producing toxicity.

Therapeutic Uses

Gentamicin, kanamycin, tobramycin, and amikacin are parenterally administered to treat bacteremias and infections caused by a variety of aerobic gram-negative rods that are resistant to less toxic antibiotics such as the penicillins and cephalosporins. These infections may involve the respiratory system, soft tissues (including burn infections), bone, urinary tract, and the central nervous system (employing an intrathecal injection). In certain infectious disorders, the aminoglycosides are employed in combination with other anti-infective agents. Streptomycin and kanamycin are used in combination with other drugs for the treatment of such mycobacterial infections as tuberculosis or meningitis. Streptomycin and penicillin are used for the treatment of enterococcal endocarditis, while this aminoglycoside may be employed with tetracycline or chloramphenicol in tularemia and bubonic plague.

Kanamycin, neomycin, and paromomycin are employed orally to control diarrhea caused by enteropathogenic *Escherichia coli* and are also used postoperatively to suppress intestinal flora. These aminoglycosides reduce the population of ammonia-producing bacteria in the intestines and are used as adjuncts in the treatment of hepatic coma.

Gentamicin and neomycin are employed topically to treat serious infections of wounds and burns caused by gram-negative organisms. Neomycin is often included as an ingredient in nonprescription topical preparations for minor lacerations, abrasions, or burns.

Adverse Reactions

The use of the aminoglycosides may be associated with significant ototoxicity or renal impairment; patients with impaired kidney function are particularly at risk.

Ototoxicity, both auditory and vestibular, may occur in patients treated at doses that are higher or for periods that are longer than recommended. High frequency *deafness* usually occurs first, and notwithstanding drug withdrawal, may progress to total loss of hearing. Symptoms of *vestibular toxicity* include dizziness, vertigo, or ataxia, and are often signs of impending complete loss of hearing. Auditory toxicity is more common with kanamycin and neomycin, while vestibular toxicity is more frequently observed with gentamicin and streptomycin.

Nephrotoxicity is most frequently mani-

Table 46-2   Potential Drug Interactions Involving Aminoglycosides and Polymyxins

Antibiotic	Interacting drug/class	Potential consequences
Aminoglycosides	Ethacrynic acid (Edecrin) Furosemide (Lasix)	These diuretics are ototoxic in their own right; potentiation of aminoglycoside ototoxicity.
Aminoglycosides Polymyxins	Amphotericin B (Fungizone) Cephalosporins (for example, cephaloridine) Methoxyflurane (Penthrane)	These drugs are potentially nephrotoxic in their own right; potentiation of antibiotic nephrotoxicity.
Aminoglycosides Polymyxins	Skeletal muscle relaxants Ether	The antibiotics are capable of producing some neuromuscular blockade; may enhance and prolong blockade produced by skeletal muscle relaxants and ether, with potential respiratory failure. Well documented.
Neomycin	Penicillin V Digoxin	Orally administered neomycin inhibits intestinal absorption of these drugs.
Neomycin	Oral anticoagulants, coumarin-type	Orally administered neomycin may decrease vitamin K production by intestinal bacteria, thus potentially enhancing anticoagulation and the risk of bleeding.

fested by transient proteinuria or retention of nonprotein nitrogen; severe azotemia may occasionally occur. Nephrotoxic reactions are generally not serious, are usually reversible, and do not represent reasons to withhold the use of these drugs. The aminoglycosides should not be administered with other nephrotoxic agents (Table 46-2).

The aminoglycosides produce varying degrees of *neuromuscular blockade*, and apnea may occur if they are given by rapid intravenous injection or to patients with myasthenia gravis. Respiratory paralysis may occur if these antibiotics are administered soon after the use of general anesthetics or neuromuscular blocking agents (Table 46-2).

Various allergic reactions have been reported after the use of aminoglycosides, and cross-sensitization among the members of this class is common.

Nursing Precautions

All patients treated with aminoglycosides must be under close supervision. Monitoring of kidney and eighth cranial nerve (auditory and vestibular) function is essential in patients with known kidney impairment. Sim-

ilar testing should be instituted in patients with normal kidney function at the initiation of therapy who show signs of nitrogen retention. Evidence of ototoxicity or nephrotoxicity may require discontinuation of aminoglycoside administration or a reduction in dosage. The coadministration of other nephrotoxic or neurotoxic drugs should be avoided. Potential drug interactions are given in Table 46-2 and nursing implications involving the aminoglycosides are summarized at the end of this chapter.

POLYMYXINS

The polymyxins are peptide antibiotics with selective antibacterial activity against gram-negative bacilli. The only two members of this group employed clinically are polymyxin B (Aerosporin) and polymyxin E, more commonly known as colistin (Coly-Mycin S); colistimethate (Coly-Mycin M) is a derivative and parenteral form of colistin.

Antimicrobial Activity

The polymyxins are primarily active against gram-negative bacilli, in particular, *Pseudo-*

monas, *Escherichia, Haemophilus, Klebsiella, Enterobacter, Salmonella,* and *Shigella; Proteus* and gram-positive organisms are resistant.

The polymyxins exert their bactericidal effects by attaching to the cell membrane of bacteria, disrupting its function, causing a loss of essential intracellular materials, and resulting in the death of the bacterial cell.

Administration and Therapeutic Uses

The polymyxins are not absorbed from the gastrointestinal tract after oral administration. Colistin is used orally to treat diarrhea caused by enteropathic *Escherichia coli* in children with enteritis.

These antibiotics are primarily used for the treatment of urinary tract infections caused by gram-negative organisms (especially *Pseudomonas*) that are resistant to other antimicrobial agents. The introduction of gentamicin (Garamycin) and carbenicillin (Geopen, Pyopen) in recent years has markedly reduced the clinical use of the polymyxins. The polymyxins are also used to treat pulmonary infections and meningitis caused by *Pseudomonas*. Since the polymyxins do not enter the cerebrospinal fluid after systemic injection, intrathecal injection is required. The polymyxins may be administered

to adults with normal kidney function at doses of 2 to 5 mg/kg of body weight by intramuscular injection.

Polymyxin B is useful for the treatment of infections of the skin, mucous membranes, eye, and ear.

Adverse Effects

The nephrotoxic risk associated with systemic administration of polymyxin B, and to a lesser extent colistin and colistimethate, have limited the therapeutic utility of the polymyxin derivatives. These drugs are also capable of causing neuromuscular blockade. Polymyxin B and colistin cause irritation and severe pain after intramuscular injection, while colistimethate is practically non-irritating after intramuscular or intravenous injection. Normal systemically administered doses must be reduced in patients with renal impairment.

Transient neurological disturbances such as dizziness, ataxia, slurred speech, blurred vision, numbness of the extremities, and muscle weakness may occur after polymyxin administration, particularly in patients with impaired renal function.

Potential drug interactions involving the polymyxins are summarized in Table 46-2.

Aminoglycosides and Polymyxins: **nursing implications**

Aminoglycosides

1. Observe the patient for signs of ototoxicity, which are usually preceded by vestibular or auditory symptoms: nausea, vomiting, high-pitched tinnitus, impaired hearing, and feeling of fullness in the ears. Hearing damage may be reversible if the drug is withdrawn at the first sign of tinnitus or dizziness; residual impairment may be permanent in other patients. Take safety precautions with patients exhibiting vestibular dysfunction (for example, assist with ambulation, use side rails).

2. Audiometric tests should be performed before, during, and several months after the discontinuation of drug.

3. Ototoxicity is most likely in the elderly, in patients with impaired renal function, and in patients receiving high doses or the concurrent administration of other ototoxic drugs.

4. Monitor the patient's fluid intake and output. Encourage fluid intake to maintain a daily urinary output of 1500 ml.

5. Observe the patient for signs of nephrotoxicity: oliguria, casts in the urine, proteinuria and increased blood urea nitrogen, nonprotein nitrogen, and serum creatinine levels.

6. Administer deep IM to minimize pain and local irritation.

Polymyxins

1. Observe the patient for ototoxicity and nephrotoxicity as described above.

2. Transient neurological disturbances may occur; watch for changes in speech or drowsiness. Instruct the patient to report visual or ototoxic changes, weakness or paresthesias, such as a tingling sensation involving the mouth or tongue.

3. Warn the patient to avoid potentially hazardous activities requiring mental alertness and coordination while taking medication.

4. When these drugs are to be administered intramuscularly, have oxygen and IV calcium chloride available in case of apnea.

SUPPLEMENTARY READINGS

Barza, M., and R. T. Scheife, "Antimicrobial Spectrum, Pharmacology and Therapeutic Use of Antibiotics—Part 4: Aminoglycosides," *American Journal of Hospital Pharmacy* 34: 723–37 (1977).

Bunn, P. A., "Kanamycin," *Medical Clinics of North America* 54(5): 1245–56 (1970).

Cox, C. E., "Gentamicin," *Medical Clinics of North America* 54(5): 1305–15 (1970).

International Symposium on Gentamicin. "A New Aminoglycoside Antibiotic." *Journal of Infectious Diseases* 119: 341–540 (1969).

Jawetz, E. "Polymyxin, Colistin, and Bacitracin," *Pediatric Clinics of North America* 8: 1057–71 (1961).

Lorian, V., "The Mode of Action of Antibiotics on Gram-Negative Bacilli," *Archives of Internal Medicine* 128: 623–32 (1971).

Pittinger, C., and R. Adamson, "Antibiotic Blockade of Neuromuscular Function," *Annual Review of Pharmacology* 12: 169–84 (1972).

CHEMOTHERAPY OF TUBERCULOSIS AND LEPROSY

Chapter 47

Tuberculosis and leprosy are two chronic diseases caused by acid-fast mycobacteria. The treatment of these mycobacterial infections presents a number of therapeutic problems resulting from inadequacy of the normal human host defense mechanisms, the metabolic characteristics of the myobacteria, the lack of bactericidal effects of some of the available drugs, the development of bacterial resistance, and the appearance of adverse effects by the available chemotherapeutic agents which often limits the use of these drugs at optimal doses.

TUBERCULOSIS

Tuberculosis (TB) is a chronic, sometimes fatal, infection, potentially of lifelong duration, caused by *Mycobacterium tuberculosis*. The most common means of spreading this disease is by inhalation of coughed or sneezed infectious material; infection may also occur by ingestion. While pulmonary tuberculosis is the most prevalent type, infection may occur in any organ or organ lining of the body. Infection of the kidneys and central nervous system (tubercular meningitis) are not uncommon.

In 1900 tuberculosis was the leading cause of death in the United States. The reduction in the death rate observed in this century has been generally attributed to improved housing, nutrition, and social awareness. Since the discovery of the highly effective antitubercular drugs streptomycin (1945) and isoniazid (1951), the decline in mortality has been even more rapid. In spite of these advances, it has been estimated that as many as five million people die annually throughout the world as the result of this disease.

Prior to the development of effective antitubercular agents, treatment was designed to increase host resistance and involved prolonged periods of rest at sanitariums. Chemotherapy is the most effective modality now available for the management of tuberculosis. In contemporary practice, patients are generally hospitalized for that relatively short period of time required to initiate and stabilize chemotherapy; thereafter, patients are treated on an outpatient basis and are required, in general, to take their medications for 1 to 3 years. The nurse must advise the patient to take the prescribed medication as directed, without interruption. To prevent relapse, the patient should not discontinue taking the medication when "feeling better" without medical authorization.

The nurse will observe that a combination of two or more drugs are virtually always employed for the treatment of all active tuberculosis infections. Combined therapy delays the development of bacterial resistance (one of the most important problems encountered in the treatment of tuberculosis) and increases the antibacterial effects (therapeutic efficacy) of the medication. In addition to isoniazid, the mainstay of the chemotherapy of tuberculosis, other primary antitubercular drugs include streptomycin, ethambutol, and rifampin. Secondary agents, less useful because of reduced clinical efficacy, potential toxicity, or patient intolerance are summarized in Table 47-1. Nursing implications are summarized at the end of this chapter.

Streptomycin

The antibiotic streptomycin was the first chemotherapeutic agent found to be unequivocally effective for the treatment of tuberculosis. Streptomycin is only effective when administered intramuscularly, and, therefore, its usefulness in long-term therapy is limited since most patients are now treated as outpatients and orally effective drugs are currently available.

When employed in combination with other drugs—most commonly isoniazid—streptomycin remains an important drug in the chemotherapy of tuberculosis, especially during the early weeks or months of therapy of severe, potentially life-threatening forms. The use of other drugs in combination with streptomycin delays the appearance of streptomycin-resistant bacterial strains.

Although streptomycin is related to the potentially nephrotoxic aminoglycoside antibiotics (Chapter 46), it has been administered daily for up to 6 months with little or no evidence of kidney toxicity. Streptomycin causes selective toxicity to the *eighth cranial nerve* when given in high doses for a long period of time. The neurotoxic effects of this drug are manifested to a greater extent by vestibular deficits than deafness.

The pharmacology and toxicology of streptomycin and related aminoglycosides are considered in Chapter 46; potential drug interactions involving streptomycin are summarized in Table 46-2 (page 397).

Isoniazid

Isoniazid (Niconyl, Nydrazid), often referred to as INH and isonicotinic acid hydrazide, is the most useful antitubercular drug currently available because of its high tuberculostatic potency, therapeutic efficacy, low toxicity, inexpensiveness, ease of administration, and patient acceptance. The mechanism of action of this synthetic drug is unknown.

Administration and fate   After oral administration, isoniazid is readily absorbed from the gastrointestinal tract and is distributed to all tissues and body fluids, including the central nervous system and cerebrospinal fluid. Metabolism of isoniazid, by an *acetylation reaction* to form acetylisoniazid, is under *genetic* control. Two groups of individuals have been identified: those people that are "slow" metabolizers and those that are "rapid" metabolizers (and, hence, inactivators) of this drug. In the American population, there are approximately equal numbers of rapid and slow inactivators, while the percentage of slow inactivators is markedly different among other ethnic groups:

Table 47-1   Drugs Used for Treatment of Tuberculosis

Generic name (selected trade names)	Usual adult dose	Adverse effects	Remarks
Primary Drugs			
Isoniazid [INH] (Niconyl, Nydrazid)	PO or IM: 5 mg/kg or 300 mg o.d.	Peripheral neuropathy and other neurological effects; possible risk of hepatitis.	Most effective drug for treatment and prophylaxis of TB. Development of bacterial resistance less than streptomycin. Lower dose in slow acetylators. Prevent or treat peripheral neuritis with pyridoxine.
Streptomycin	IM: 1 g o.d. for 2–3 weeks, then 1 g 2–3 times weekly.	Vestibular disturbances (vertigo, dizziness, tinnitus), hearing losses, nephrotoxicity, allergic reactions.	Used in combination with other anti-TB drugs; most beneficial effects during early weeks or months of therapy; rapid development of bacterial resistance. Only active parenterally.
Ethambutol (Myambutol)	PO: 15–25 mg/kg o.d.	Ocular toxicity (decreased visual acuity, loss of color discrimination); peripheral neuritis.	Eye tests recommended prior to and at 1-mo intervals after onset of therapy. Terminate therapy upon loss of visual acuity.
Rifampin (Rifadin, Rimactane)	PO: 600 mg o.d.	Well tolerated; abdominal, muscle, joint pain; risk of liver dysfunction.	Highly effective semisynthetic antibiotic. Use in combination with other anti-TB drugs delays emergence of bacterial resistance. Harmlessly colors urine and other fluids orange-red.
Secondary drugs			
Aminosalicylic acid, para-aminosalicylic acid [PAS] (Teebacin)	PO: 12 g o.d., in 2–3 divided doses p.c.	Severe gastrointestinal disturbances (nausea, vomiting, diarrhea), allergic reactions (fever, joint pain, skin rashes).	Formerly widely used in combination with other drugs. Other orally active drugs better tolerated. Potential drug interactions in Table 47-2.
Cycloserine (Seromycin)	PO: 0.5–1 g daily, in 3 divided doses p.c.	Neurological disturbances (muscle twitching to convulsive seizures) and psychotic disorders.	Treatment must be initiated in a hospital to establish appropriate dose and patient response. Neurological side effects may be treated with pyridoxine.
Ethionamide (Trecator-SC)	PO: 0.5–1 g o.d. in 3 doses p.c.	Patient intolerance because of gastrointestinal disturbances; potential liver toxicity.	Daily doses of 0.5 g tolerated, but questionable therapeutic effectiveness. Poor patient acceptance at 1 g daily. Divided daily doses may reduce gastrointestinal side effects.
Capreomycin (Capastat)	IM (deep): 1 g o.d. for 60–120 days, then 2–3 times weekly for 18–24 mo.	Kidney toxicity most common and significant; potential for vestibular disturbances and deafness.	As effective as streptomycin, but nephrotoxicity limits clinical potential. Always administered with one or more anti-TB drugs.
Pyrazinamide [PZA]	PO: 20–35 mg/kg o.d. in 3–4 divided doses.	Liver toxicity; hyperuricemia (with or without gout symptoms)	Analog of nicotinamide. Toxicity may outweigh potential therapeutic benefit. Available in hospitals only.

American Indians (21 percent), Japanese (13 percent), and Eskimos (5 percent). Slow inactivators appear to have an autosomal homozygous recessive hereditary trait and are more likely to develop polyneuritis than rapid inactivators.

Isoniazid is the drug most commonly employed for the treatment of active tuberculosis; it is used in combination with ethambutol, rifampin, or streptomycin to enhance the clinical response and delay the emergence of resistant tubercle bacilli. It is used alone in prophylaxis.

Adverse effects   The most common and significant adverse effects associated with isoniazid administration are those affecting the peripheral and central nervous systems; they are thought to result from a drug-induced pyridoxine (vitamin B_6) deficiency. The prophylactic administration of pyridoxine, 100 mg daily, prevents the development of these nervous system dysfunctions. Among these adverse effects are peripheral neuritis, muscle twitching, dizziness, convulsions, and behavioral changes, including psychoses.

During the past decade it has been established that isoniazid can cause severe *hepatic necrosis*, potentially leading to death. Although the mechanism underlying this liver toxicity has not been established, its incidence has been demonstrated to increase with age; drug-induced hepatitis is rare in patients less than 20 years of age and rises to 2.3 percent in individuals over 50 years old. Alcohol consumption may also increase the risk of liver toxicity. Nurses should advise their patients to be alert for the early signs of liver toxicity, including fatigue, weakness, malaise, and anorexia. Other undesirable effects associated with isoniazid administration include gastrointestinal disturbances and allergic reactions. Potential drug interactions involving isoniazid are summarized in Table 47-2.

Table 47-2   Potential Drug Interactions Involving Antitubercular Drugs

Antitubercular drug	Interacting drug/class	Potential consequences
Isoniazid	Phenytoin (Dilantin)	Isoniazid inhibits phenytoin metabolism, increasing the risk of toxicity.
Isoniazid + Rifampin		Possible increased risk of isoniazid hepatotoxicity.
Isoniazid	Aluminum hydroxide gel (Amphogel)	Antacid inhibits intestinal absorption of isoniazid, reducing plasma levels; give isoniazid 30 min prior to antacid.
Rifampin + PAS		PAS inhibits intestinal absorption of rifampin; administration of drugs should be spaced 8–12 h apart.
Rifampin	Oral contraceptives	Rifampin increases the metabolism of estrogens, decreasing the effectiveness of oral contraceptives, increasing the risk of pregnancy; an increase in dosage or alternative methods of contraception may be required.
Rifampin	Corticosteroids Narcotics Oral anticoagulants Warfarin	Rifampin increases the metabolism of these drugs.
Rifampin PAS	Probenecid (Benemid)	Probenecid inhibits the renal excretion of these drugs potentially increasing their toxicity.
Streptomycin		See Aminoglycoside interactions, Table 46-2.
Aminosalicylic acid (PAS)	Oral anticoagulants, coumarin-type	Salicylates displace coumarins from plasma protein-binding sites and may increase their anticoagulant effects.

Rifampin

Rifampin (Rifadin, Rimactane), a semisynthetic antibiotic, is viewed by some experts as the greatest contribution to the chemotherapy of tuberculosis since the introduction of isoniazid. This drug inhibits the growth of most gram-positive and gram-negative bacteria, as well as *Mycobacterium tuberculosis* and *M. leprae*, by inhibiting microbial RNA synthesis. Many bacteria rapidly acquire resistance to rifampin; thus—in an attempt to reduce the emergence of resistant strains of mycobacteria—the clinical uses of this drug have been restricted primarily to the treatment of tuberculosis, always in combination with other antitubercular drugs. Rifampin is also employed prophylactically in asymptomatic carriers of *Neisseria meningitidis* to eliminate meningococci from the nasopharynx; this drug is not recommended for the treatment of active meningococcal infections.

After oral administration, rifampin is well absorbed from the gastrointestinal tract. Because food delays its absorption, rifampin should be given as a single daily dose 1 hour before or 2 hours after meals. This drug is widely distributed throughout the body and achieves effective concentrations in many tissues and body fluids, including the cerebrospinal fluid. Nurses should forewarn their patients that rifampin may impart an orange-red color to their urine, feces, saliva, tears, sputum, and sweat, and that this coloration is harmless.

Adverse effects The incidence of adverse effects to rifampin is low and seldom requires termination of drug administration. Abdominal distress, aching pain in the muscles and joints, or cramping pains in the legs occur occasionally, especially during the early weeks of therapy. During this time asymptomatic jaundice may be noted; it generally dissipates without the necessity of discontinuing therapy. Jaundice, accompanied by symptoms of hepatitis, is potentially life-threatening and represents an indication for discontinuation of medication. Gastrointestinal distress (nausea, vomiting, diarrhea, abdominal cramps) and nervous system disorders (fatigue, drowsiness, headache, dizziness, inability to concentrate, muscle weakness) may occur. Intermittent administration of large doses of rifampin or the resumption of treatment after a lapse of days or weeks may result in adverse effects thought to be the consequence of hypersensitivity reaction. This reaction is characterized by flu-like symptoms, respiratory distress, purpura, and blood disorders. The use of this drug during pregnancy and in young children is not recommended. Potential drug interactions involving rifampin are summarized in Table 47-2.

Ethambutol

Ethambutol (Myambutol) is a synthetic drug with specific antimycobacterial activity. This drug is highly effective after oral administration, possesses a relatively low order of toxicity, and is acceptable to patients; for these reasons ethambutol has replaced aminosalicylic acid (PAS) as a primary drug in the combined chemotherapy of tuberculosis. The antimycobacterial effects have been attributed to an inhibition of RNA synthesis.

The most significant adverse effect produced by ethambutol is *ocular toxicity*, an effect that is dose-related (at daily doses of 50 mg/kg) and reversible over a period of weeks or months. Symptoms of toxicity include decreased visual acuity, loss of discrimination of the color green, and optic neuritis. Nurses should question patients about their vision during each regularly scheduled visit and advise patients to promptly report any visual changes, such as blurring or fading of vision. Treatment with ethambutol should be terminated immediately if these symptoms continue or if a substantial reduction in visual acuity is demonstrated in a complete eye examination. Administration of ethambutol to pregnant patients has produced no demonstrable adverse effects on the fetus.

LEPROSY

Leprosy (Hansen's disease) is a chronic disease caused by *Mycobacterium leprae*. This disease is characterized by lesions of the skin, nose, pharynx, larynx, and superficial nerves, often resulting in disfigurement and deformity in untreated patients. Although the nature of the transmission of leprosy is not well understood, it is currently believed that this disease has an extremely long incubation period and is readily acquired by contact with lepromatous patients during transient periods of increased susceptibility. In the United States, leprosy is endemic in Hawaii and in those states bordering on the Gulf of Mexico.

The *sulfone* derivatives (dapsone) are the drugs of choice in the treatment of leprosy, with clinical improvement noted in almost all cases. Treatment is continued until the skin lesions and mucosal lesions are healed and devoid of acid-fast bacilli; this is generally accomplished in no less than 2 to 3 years and may require as long as 6 to 8 years of chronic therapy. To prevent relapses, it is common practice to maintain sulfone administration indefinitely at one-third the full therapeutic dose. Drugs used for the treatment of leprosy are summarized in Table 47-3.

Table 47-3   Drugs Used for Treatment of Leprosy

Generic name	Trade name	Adult dosage range	Remarks and adverse effects
Sulfones			
Dapsone (DDS)	Avlosulfon	PO: 25 mg weekly to 100 mg 4 times weekly	Drug of choice for leprosy. Hemolysis, methemoglobinemia are common adverse effects; anorexia, nausea, vomiting may also occur.
Sulfoxone sodium	Diasone sodium	PO: 330 mg twice weekly to 330 mg 6 days weekly	Similar to dapsone; absorption erratic, expensive, seldom used.
Nonsulfones			
Amithiozone	Panrone; Tibione	PO: 50–200 mg o.d.	Alternative to sulfones; bacterial resistance develops. Anorexia, nausea, vomiting; bone-marrow depression (anemia, leukopenia, agranulocytosis) may also occur. Not available in U.S.
Clofazimine	Lamprene	PO: 100 mg o.d.	Useful secondary drug when bacterial resistance to sulfones exists.
Rifampin	Rifadin; Rimactane	PO: 300–600 mg o.d.	Black and red pigmentation may occur. Antitubercular drug currently being evaluated for treatment of leprosy.

Chemotherapy of Tuberculosis:
nursing implications

1. Successful treatment requires long-term therapy; 1 yr for prophylactic therapy and 1.5-2 yr for the original treatment of the active disease. Stress the importance of uninterrupted therapy and continuous medical supervision.
2. Therapeutic effects may be noted within 2-3 wk, with feelings of euphoria experienced by some patients. Teach the patient the importance of regular rest periods during the early phases of treatment.
3. Observe the patient for signs of hepatoxicity, and instruct the patient to report loss of appetite, fatigue, malaise, dark urine, or jaundice. Daily alcohol ingestion increases the risk of isoniazid hepatitis.
4. Ophthalmoscopic examination and vision testing is recommended before initiating therapy and periodically during therapy.

Isoniazid

1. Instruct the patient to report any signs of neurotoxicity, such as peripheral neuritis, which is usually preceded by numbness and tingling or burning of the feet and hands. Patients most susceptible are malnourished individuals, diabetics, and slow inactivators of isoniazid. Periodic liver function tests are advised.
2. Withhold the drug and report to the physician in case of marked central stimulation. Have parenteral sodium phenobarbital available in the event of convulsions.
3. Warn diabetics to watch for changes because diabetes is more difficult to control when patients are receiving isoniazid. True glycosuria and false positive Benedict's tests may occur.
4. Instruct the patient to take pyridoxine (vitamin B_6) daily to prevent deficiencies and reduce risk of neurotoxicity.

Rifampin

1. Watch for and instruct patients to report any signs of liver dysfunction.
2. Patients taking oral contraceptives should be advised to use other methods of birth control.
3. Inform the patient that drug colors urine, feces, saliva, tears, and sputum orange.

Ethambutol

1. The patient should have an ophthalmoscopic examination and visual acuity test prior to the initiation of therapy and every 2-4 wk during therapy. Instruct the patient to report loss of color discrimination or reduced visual acuity. Adverse effects on the eyes disappear several weeks to several months after therapy has been discontinued.
2. The drug should not be taken during pregnancy.
3. Reduced doses should be given to patients with impaired kidney function or gout.

SUPPLEMENTARY READINGS

Cochrane, R. G., and T. F. Davey, *Leprosy in Theory and Practice.* Baltimore: The Williams & Wilkins Company, 1964.

Mitchell, R. S., "Control of Tuberculosis," *New England Journal of Medicine* **276**: 842–48, 905–11 (1967).

Pinsker, K. L., and S. K. Koerner, "Chemotherapy of Tuberculosis," *American Journal of Hospital Pharmacy* **33**: 275–83 (1976).

Pyle, M. M., "Ethambutol and Viomycin," *Medical Clinics of North America* **54**(5): 1,317–27 (1970).

Robson, J. M., and F. M. Sullivan, "Antituberculosis Drugs," *Pharmacological Reviews* **15**: 169–223 (1963).

Shepard, C. C., "Chemotherapy of Leprosy," *Annual Review of Pharmacology* **9**: 37–50, 1969.

Symposium, "Rifampin in the Treatment of Tuberculosis," *Chest* **61**: 517–98 (1972).

ANTIFUNGAL AND ANTIVIRAL DRUGS

Chapter 48

While the nurse will encounter scores of drugs employed for the treatment of bacterial infections, relatively few safe and effective agents are available for the management of fungal and viral infections. Development of clinically useful antifungal and antiviral drugs, particularly for the management of systemic infections, represents a major challenge for biomedical scientists.

ANTIFUNGAL DRUGS

Most fungi are totally resistant to the available antibacterial agents. Although there are many topically active antifungal agents, to date only a limited number are sufficiently nontoxic to the host to be clinically useful for the treatment of systemic fungal infections (Table 48-1). Prior to discussing these drugs, we shall first briefly examine the nature of fungal infections.

Fungal Infections

Fungal (mycotic) infections may be placed in three therapeutic categories, namely, systemic infections, dermatophytic (skin) infections, and candidiasis (mucous membrane infections).

Systemic fungal infections are often difficult to diagnose, are chronic in nature, and

Table 48-1   Selected Antifungal Drugs

Generic name	Selected trade names	Clinical uses	Remarks
Amphotericin B	Fungizone	Systemic fungal infections; slow intravenous infusion; intrathecal injection; topical for candidiasis.	Wide range of antifungal activity for treatment of systemic infections. Kidney and liver toxicity, allergic reactions. Drug unstable; prepare fresh solutions. Increase daily IV dosage from 0.25 to 1 mg/kg.
Flucytosine [5-FU, 5-Fluorocytosine]	Ancobon	Orally active. Systemic fungal infections caused by *Candida, Cryptococcus, Cladosporium*, and *Torulopsis*.	Less toxic than amphotericin B. Can be used in renal impairment. Daily doses of 150 mg/kg.
Miconazole	Micatin Monistat I.V.	Systemic fungal infections caused Coccidioides, Candida, Cryptococcus, and Paracoccidioides. Topical—similar to haloprogin.	Rapid injection of undiluted drug may cause tachycardia or arrhythmia. Only given by IV infusion of 200-1200 mg per infusion over 1-20 wk period.
Potassium iodide		Cutaneous lymphatic sporotrichosis (drug of choice).	Side effects include: iodism, metallic taste, rhinitis, lacrimation, and salivation; 1 ml of saturated solution (1 g/ml) 3 times daily up to 12-15 ml daily for at least 6-8 wks.
Hydroxystilbamidine isethionate		Slow intravenous infusion for blastomycosis.	Side effects include: anorexia, nausea, vomiting, and headache. Protect solution from light and heat. Total course of 8 g given in daily doses of 225 mg.
Griseofulvin	Fulvicin-U/F, Grifulvin V, Grisactin, Gris-PEG	Orally for dermatophytic (tinea) infections.	Headache may be severe, but dissipates with time. Dose of microcrystalline preparation smaller and less toxic than macrocrystalline; daily dose 0.25-1 g of microsize and 125-500 mg ultramicrosize products.
Nystatin	Candex, Mycostatin, Nilstat	Orally and topically for candidal infections of skin, mucous membranes, gastrointestinal tract and vagina.	Too toxic for systemic infections. Oral side effects are nausea, vomiting, and diarrhea; 0.5-1 million units (orally) 3 times daily.
Tolnaftate	Tinactin Aftate	Topical—dermatophytic (tinea) infections. Ineffective against *Candida*.	Most effective for fungal infections on skin. Poor response on scalp and nails.
Haloprogin	Halotex	Topical—dermatophytic (tinea) and candidal infections.	Higher cure rate, lower relapse rate than tolnaftate. Local irritation, burning.
Clotrimazole	Lotrimin Mycelex	Similar to haloprogin.	Clinical improvement, including relief from pruritus, usually occurs within one week. Side effects include redness, stinging, blistering, and skin peeling.
Iodochlorhydroxyquin (clioquinol)	Vioform	Dermatophytic infections.	Antifungal-antibacterial activity.

Table 48-1 Continued

Generic name	Selected trade names	Clinical uses	Remarks
Triacetin	Enzactin Fungacetin	Athlete's foot and other superficial fungal infections.	Prevent contact with rayon fabrics.
Acrisorcin	Akrinol	Tinea versicolor (only).	Relapses are common.
Selenium sulfide	Selsun	Tinea versicolor and seborrheic dermatitis of scalp.	Irritating—avoid contact with eyes and genital areas.
Undecylenic acid and zinc undecylenate	Desenex	Athlete's foot and ringworm (except nails and hairy areas).	Keep away from eyes and mucous membranes.
Calcium undecylenate	Caldesene Cruex	Prophylaxis and therapy of jock itch (tinea cruris).	Also used for diaper rash, chafing, prickly heat, minor skin irritation.

can present a serious medical problem. The most important of these infections include histoplasmosis, blastomycosis, coccidioidomycosis, paracoccidioidomycosis, sporotrichosis, and cryptococcosis (torulosis). It is essential that patients with systemic infections be treated for a sufficiently long period of time to minimize the possibility of relapse. Because relapses of blastomycosis have been seen several months to many years after the arrest of this disease, remissions cannot be interpreted as cures. Amphotericin B is the most important drug available for the treatment of almost all systemic fungal infections; flucytosine and hydroxystilbamidine are useful in the treatment of selected disorders.

Dermatophytic infections, caused by such fungi as *Epidermophyton, Trichophyton,* and *Microsporum,* are limited to the skin, hair, and nails, and include such familiar diseases as ringworm and athlete's foot. Griseofulvin is the most useful orally administered drug for infections caused by dermatophytic fungi, while tolnaftate and haloprogin are highly effective drugs for topical application; many nonprescription products are available for the treatment of these infections, especially tinea pedis (athlete's foot).

Candidiasis usually affects moist skin or mucous membranes, including the gastrointestinal tract, although systemic diseases may occur. *Candida albicans* is the most common species causing disease in humans. Amphotericin B and nystatin are effective topically in the treatment of candidal infections of the skin and mucous membranes.

Antifungal Agents

Amphotericin B Amphotericin B (Fungizone) is an antibiotic useful for the treatment of topical infections; it is also the only antifungal agent sufficiently safe and effective for the management of a wide spectrum of systemic mycotic infections.

The antifungal activity of this drug involves its binding to certain sterols of the cell membrane of the fungus, causing disruption of the selective permeability characteristics of the membrane. This produces a loss of essential intracellular compounds and results in the death of the cell. Bacteria are thought to be resistant to the effects of amphotericin B because they lack the sterol required for drug binding to the membrane.

Orally administered amphotericin B is not absorbed into the blood. For the treatment of systemic infections, this drug is administered in 5 percent dextrose solution in water by slow intravenous infusion over a period of 4 to 6 hours. Some clinicians administer 0.25 mg/kg the first day, followed by an incremental dosage increase of 0.25 mg/kg daily until a dose of 1 mg/kg is reached; in very severe infections, the maximum total daily dosage may be 1.5 mg/kg. Drug administration may be required for 6 to 12 weeks or longer. For the treatment of fungal meningitis, 0.5 mg may be administered three times daily for 10 weeks or longer. A cream, a lotion, and an ointment containing 3 percent amphotericin B are also available for topical application.

Adverse Effects and Nursing Precautions

Adverse effects commonly observed after intravenous administration include chills, fever, sweating, vomiting, headache, and muscle and joint pain. These effects may be minimized by reducing the rate of infusion, administering the drug on alternate days, or by giving corticosteroids or aspirin. Impairment of liver and kidney function, anemia, marked hypotension, electrolyte disturbances (hypokalemia), neurological disturbances, and anemia are not uncommon and may result from the administration of therapeutic doses.

Detailed instructions for the storage, preparation, and administration of amphotericin B must be closely followed. Since this drug may cause irreversible renal failure, kidney function should be regularly assessed; renal impairment is a relative contraindication to this agent's use. Potential drug interactions involving amphotericin B are summarized in Table 48-2; nursing implications appear at the end of this chapter.

Flucytosine (5-FU, 5-Fluorocytosine)   Flucytosine (Ancobon) is a synthetic, orally active antifungal agent employed only for the treatment of serious systemic infections caused by susceptible strains of *Candida, Cryptococcus, Cladosporium*, and *Torulopsis*. Resistant mutant strains of *Candida* and *Cryptococcus* regularly and rapidly develop to this antifungal agent. The usual daily dosage is 150 mg/kg in divided doses at 6-hour intervals.

Less toxic than amphotericin B, flucytosine may cause nausea, vomiting, diarrhea, skin rashes, and blood disorders. Flucytosine appears to cause no renal toxicity, and, therefore, can be used in patients with renal insufficiency if the dosage is appropriately modified.

Griseofulvin   Griseofulvin (Fulvicin-U/F, Grifulvin V, Grisactin, Gris-PEG) is a

Table 48-2   Potential Drug Interactions Involving Antifungal Drugs

Drug	Interacting drug/class	Potential consequences
Amphotericin B	Corticosteroids	Corticosteroids may enhance potassium depletion induced by amphotericin B, resulting in cardiac dysfunction.
	Digitalis glycosides	Hypokalemia following amphotericin B may increase the risk of digitalis toxicity.
	Aminoglycoside antibiotics	Additive risk of nephrotoxicity.
	Skeletal muscle relaxants, tubocurarine-like	Hypokalemia induced by amphotericin B may enhance and prolong muscle relaxation, with potential respiratory failure.
Griseofulvin	Barbiturates, phenobarbital	Barbiturates increase the rate of griseofulvin metabolism and impair griseofulvin absorption, resulting in decreased blood levels and a marked reduction in antifungal activity.
	Oral anticoagulants, coumarin-type	Griseofulvin increases coumarin metabolism, decreasing its anticoagulant effects.

fungistatic antibiotic derived from a species of *Penicillium*. It is the only orally effective drug against dermatophytoses that cause tinea (ringworm) infections. This drug is ineffective against other fungi—including *Candida*—and bacteria. It is most useful for the treatment of tinea infections of the scalp and glabrous (smooth and bare) skin and less active in the management of chronic infections of the feet, palms, and nails.

Divided oral daily doses of 0.25 to 1 g* are employed, with the duration of therapy ranging from several weeks to more than 6 months, depending upon the type of infection being treated. Nurses should advise their patients that successful treatment requires careful adherence to the dosage schedule for the prescribed period of time. Frequent shampooing and trimming the hair and nails may improve the condition.

Serious adverse reactions are rarely observed with griseofulvin. Minor side effects include headache (which occurs often but disappears with continued drug administration), dryness of the mouth, nausea, vomiting, and diarrhea; hepatotoxicity, photosensitivity, and neurological disturbances have been reported. Allergic reactions to this drug may be manifested by fever, skin rashes, leukopenia, and serum sickness-type reactions. Drug interactions involving griseofulvin are summarized in Table 48-2; nursing implications are presented at the end of this chapter.

Nystatin Nystatin (Mycostatin, Nilstat) is an antibiotic employed primarily for the treatment of candidal infections of the skin, mucous membranes, gastrointestinal tract, and vagina. This drug is not suitable for the treatment of systemic infections; it is not absorbed from the gastrointestinal tract after oral administration and is too toxic to be ad-

*Ultramicrosize griseofulvin is approximately twice as active as the microsize (regular) formulations; the daily dose of an ultramicrosize tablet is 125 to 500 mg.

ministered parenterally. Nystatin has been used in combination with the broad-spectrum antibiotic tetracycline to prevent fungal overgrowth in the gastrointestinal tract resulting from superinfection; however, there is no evidence that such mixtures are of clinical value.

The usual adult oral dose of nystatin is 500,000 to 1,000,000 units, three times daily. This drug is also available as a vaginal tablet and as an ointment, cream, and powder for topical application.

Tolnaftate Tolnaftate (Tinactin) is effective topically against dermatophytic tinea infections. The drug is ineffective against candidal or bacterial infections. It is useful for the treatment of tinea infections of the skin. Relapses may occur and a second course of therapy may be required. Infections of the scalp, nails, soles, or palms generally do not respond well to topical medication. No significant adverse reactions have been reported after the application of this drug as a solution, cream, or powder.

ANTIVIRAL AGENTS

In contrast to the remarkable advances that have been made in the treatment of most infectious diseases, few antiviral drugs have been developed. Unlike bacteria, viruses have no metabolic enzymes of their own nor do they possess any mechanisms for self-regulation. They are capable of replicating only within a living host cell, employing the metabolic processes provided by the host. It is obvious that drugs potentially capable of killing or inhibiting the growth of the virus are also likely to seriously interfere with the life processes of the host cell.

In most instances, the appearance of the clinical manifestations of viral infections occurs at a time when the phase of viral multiplication is ending and the subsequent course of the disease has been largely determined. Destruction of the virus at this time will have little or no affect on the prognosis of the patient. Hence, to be clinically beneficial, the drug would have to be administered prior to the appearance of the disease, as *chemoprophylaxis.*

Idoxuridine and vidarabine are used for the treatment of an established viral infection, while gamma globulin, amantadine, and methisazone are chemoprophylactic agents.

Treatment of Viral Infections

Idoxuridine (IDU) Idoxuridine (Dendrid, Herplex, Stoxil) inhibits the replication of DNA by herpes simplex virus in the cornea and is, therefore, of value in the treatment of herpes simplex keratitis, a common cause of blindness. For the treatment of this ophthalmic disorder, 1 drop of a 0.1 percent aqueous solution is instilled in the conjunctival sac every hour during the day and every 2 hours during the night until substantial improvement is evident; thereafter, the interval between doses is doubled. The 0.5 percent ointment is applied every 4 hours during the day and once at bedtime. In recurrent episodes, the acute disease is often controlled, but scarring resulting from a previous episode is not improved. Moreover, complete healing or improvement is not observed in all instances.

Adverse effects associated with conjunctival administration of idoxuridine include irritation, pain, itching, inflammation, and edema of the eyelids, damage to the cells of the cornea, and photophobia. Nursing implications are summarized at the end of the chapter.

Vidarabine Vidarabine (Vira-A) appears to act by interfering with the early steps in viral DNA synthesis. This recently introduced drug is effective in the treatment of acute keratoconjunctivitis and recurrent epithelial keratitis caused by herpes simplex virus types 1 and 2. It is also useful in the treatment of superficial keratitis caused by the herpes simplex virus, which does not respond to topical idoxuridine, or when this antiviral agent cannot be used because of toxicity or hypersensitivity reactions. Systemic administration of vidarabine is effective in the treatment of herpes simplex viral encephalitis.

One-half inch of the ointment should be placed in the lower conjunctival sac five times daily at 3-hour intervals. If no signs of improvement are noted after 7 days or complete reepithelialization has not occurred within 21 days, other forms of therapy should be considered. Since chronic administration of vidarabine has been shown to cause tumor production in animal studies, the recommended frequency and duration of drug administration should not be exceeded. Common adverse effects after conjunctival administration include tearing, burning, irritation, and pain.

Vidarabine has been shown to reduce the mortality caused by herpes simplex viral encephalitis from 70 percent to 28 percent. Early diagnosis and treatment should be initiated because it does not alter morbidity and the resulting severe neurological sequelae in the comatose patient. This drug is administered by slow intravenous infusion at a daily dose of 15 mg/kg for 10 days. The package inset should be consulted for directions regarding the preparation of the solution for intravenous administration.

Viral Chemoprophylactic Agents

Gamma globulin Immune human serum globulin (gamma globulin) contains antibodies against viral antigens. This product interferes with the ability of the virus to penetrate the host cell. Administration of gamma globulin during the early period of incubation may modify such viral infections as measles, hepatitis, poliomyelitis, and rabies. A single intramuscular dose of 0.02 to 0.1 ml/lb of body weight confers protection for 2 to 3 weeks. Repeated injections may be necessary for protection against viral infections with long incubation periods.

Amantadine Amantadine (Symmetrel) is an orally active synthetic drug that acts by preventing the penetration of the virus into the host cell. It has proven to be effective in prevention of Asian (A_2) influenza, with clinically beneficial effects observed even when the drug has been administered as long as 20 hours after the onset of the illness. Increases in the rates of overall clinical improvement and disappearance of the signs and symptoms of the illness have been established.

The chemoprophylactic activity of amantadine is limited to the A_2 virus, with the use of this drug recommended during a documented A_2 epidemic, especially to patients of all ages who are deemed to be at high risk. The usual daily oral dose for adults and children over 9 years of age is 200 mg, with therapy recommended for 10 to 30 days. Children less than 9 years of age are given daily doses of 4.4 to 8.8 mg/kg, not to exceed 150 mg daily. Amantadine is also used for the treatment of Parkinson's disease (Chapter 19).

Reported side effects include increased nervousness, inability to concentrate, tremors, insomnia, and behavioral disorders. The incidence of these effects is low and is dose- and probably age-related, with elderly individuals more susceptible. Caution should be exercised when administering this drug to patients with cerebral atherosclerosis, psychiatric disorders, or epilepsy. This drug should not be given to pregnant women.

Methisazone Methisazone (Marboran) is a highly significant drug that is of established value in the prevention of smallpox in contacts within 1 to 2 days after exposure; it does not appear to be useful for the treatment of this viral infection. The only significant side effect associated with methisazone is vomiting, which is severe in many patients. Methisazone is available in Europe but not in the United States.

Antifungal and Antiviral Drugs: nursing implications

Amphotericin B

1. Administered intravenously only to hospitalized patients or those under close clinical supervision who have a confirmed diagnosis of a potentially life-threatening infection caused by a fungus susceptible to this drug.

2. Since this drug is fungistatic rather than fungicidal, several months of therapy are required to assure adequate treatment and to prevent relapse.

3. Detailed instructions for storage, preparation, and administration of drug must be closely followed. Acidic solutions containing electrolytes or preservatives should not be used to prepare infusions because they cause antibiotic precipitation. Fresh solutions should be prepared for each injection. Solutions containing a precipitate or foreign matter must be discarded.

4. Observe the patient for untoward reactions that may require discontinuation of IV drug administration or the intermittent use of drug: fever, chills, tremors, anorexia, nausea, or vomiting. Administration of antipyretics, antihistamines, or corticosteroids may be ordered to treat these adverse effects.
5. Monitor the patient's fluid intake and output and report decreased urine output and sediment or cloudiness in the urine. Weekly tests recommended: complete blood count, potassium levels, and renal function tests (BUN, NPN, serum creatinine). Renal damage is usually reversible if drug is discontinued at early signs of renal impairment.
6. Observe the patient for early signs of hypokalemia, especially if the patient is also receiving digitalis glycosides or corticosteroids: anorexia, drowsiness, muscle weakness, hypoactive reflexes, paresthesias.
7. Instruct the patient to report signs of ototoxicity: hearing loss, tinnitus, vertigo.
8. For local drug application, instruct the patient to rub the medication into the lesion. Reassure the patient that the medication will not stain skin. Cream or lotion can be removed from clothing by washing with soap and water; ointment can be removed by standard cleaning fluids.

Griseofulvin

1. Explain to the patient that while symptomatic relief may be experienced within 48–96 hours, the total duration of treatment depends upon the time required for the replacement of infected tissues. Usual durations of ringworm treatment: scalp or body, 2–4 wks; feet, 4–8 wks; fingernails, 4 months; toenails, 6 months.
2. Teach the patient the importance of hygienic measures to prevent recurrent infections; for example, in tinea pedis, the feet should be kept clean and dry.
3. The drug can be taken with meals to decrease adverse gastrointestinal effects. A high-fat diet enhances drug absorption from the intestines.
4. A complete blood count is recommended at weekly intervals during the first month of therapy. Instruct the patient to report symptoms of leukopenia: fever, sore throat, malaise.
5. Instruct the patient to avoid prolonged exposure to the sun because of possible photosensitivity reaction.
6. Warn the patient that alcohol ingestion during therapy may possibly cause tachycardia and flushing.

Idoxuridine

1. While receiving therapy, the patient should be carefully supervised by an ophthalmologist.
2. Therapy for corneal epithelial infections is usually continued for at least 3–5 days after corneal healing is demonstrated by loss of staining with fluorescein.
3. Drug should not be mixed with other medications and should not be used with corticosteroids.

SUPPLEMENTARY READINGS

Bauer, D. J., *The Specific Treatment of Virus Diseases.* Baltimore: University Park Press, 1977.

Bennett, J. E., "Chemotherapy of Systemic Mycoses," *New England Journal of Medicine* **290:** 30–32, 320–23 (1974).

Goldman, L., "Griseofulvin," *Medical Clinics of North America* **54:** 1339–45 (1970).

Hoeprich, P. D., "Chemotherapy of Systemic Fungal Diseases," *Annual Review of Pharmacology and Toxicology* **18:** 205–31 (1978).

Luby, J. P., M. T. Johnson, and S. R. Jones, "Antiviral Chemotherapy," *Annual Review of Medicine* **25:** 251–67 (1974).

Tilles, J. G., "Antiviral Agents," *Annual Review of Pharmacology* **14:** 469–89 (1974).

Weinstein, L., and T. W. Chang, "The Chemotherapy of Viral Infections," *New England Journal of Medicine* **289:** 725–30 (1973).

CHEMOTHERAPY OF MALARIA AND AMEBIASIS

Chapter 49

In this chapter we shall discuss the treatment of two diseases caused by unicellular protozoa. These diseases are *malaria*, the second most common disease affecting the human inhabitants of the earth, and *amebiasis*, a disease with a worldwide distribution, including the United States.

ANTIMALARIAL AGENTS

There are almost 200 million cases of malaria throughout the world, with two million deaths annually. Malaria was once endemic throughout the continental United States. Virtually all the cases of malaria that the nurse will now see in the United States are carried from malarious regions of the world by travelers or immigrants. Cases arising in the United States are, in almost all cases, induced by unintentional blood inoculation among drug-dependent individuals or by blood transfusions.

Malaria has been almost completely eradicated from most parts of the United States and Europe, and recent decades have witnessed a reduction in its incidence in Africa, Asia, and South America. While drugs have played a significant role in reducing morbidity and mortality, the most effective contribution to the control of this parasitic disease has involved eradication of its mosquito vector with the insecticide chlorophenothane (DDT).

Prior to considering the antimalarial agents, we shall briefly discuss the nature of this disease and the life cycle of the parasite.

Malaria

Malaria is clinically characterized by paroxysms of severe chills, fever, and profuse sweating. These episodes occur at clearly defined intervals, which are based upon the life cycle of the invading parasite. In the absence of treatment, malaria becomes chronic after recovery from the acute attack, with the patient experiencing repeated relapses.

This disease results from infestation by protozoa of the genus *Plasmodium*, four species of which affect a human host: *P. vivax*, *P. falciparum*, *P. malariae*, and rarely *P. ovale*. The microbe is transmitted to its host in the saliva of the female *Anopheles* mosquito. The onset of clinical symptoms after infestation, the recurring frequency of febrile paroxysms, and their severity differ according to the species involved. Tertian malaria (caused by *P. vivax*), the most common type, has a 26-day latency before symptoms are manifested after infestation; fever spikes occur every other day, with a relatively mild intensity.

The emergence of drug-resistant strains of *P. falciparum*, which causes the most life-threatening form of malaria, constitutes a major public health problem. Potential complications from falciparum malaria include hemolytic anemia, encephalopathy with confusion or coma ("cerebral malaria"), renal failure, and noncardiac pulmonary edema.

Life Cycle of the Parasite

To appreciate the rationale underlying the chemotherapy of malaria, an understanding of the plasmodium life cycle is essential. This life cycle consists of a sexual cycle in the mosquito and an asexual cycle in the verte-brate host (Figure 49-1). The disease vector, the female *Anopheles* mosquito, becomes the carrier of the plasmodium by ingesting the blood of a host containing both male and female forms of the parasite. In the stomach of the mosquito, the male gametocyte fertilizes the female gametocyte which, after numerous cell divisions, give rise to sporozoites. The sporozoites migrate to the salivary gland of the mosquito and are transferred to another vertebrate host by the bite of the mosquito.

The asexual cycle in humans consists of exo-erythrocytic and erythrocytic phases. Shortly after their injection into the blood, the sporozoites travel to liver cells, where they divide to form a liver (exo-erythrocytic) schizont containing many merozoites. The different latency periods observed with the various species of plasmodia (12 to 40 days) are attributed to variations in the length of this liver phase; during this period the patient is asymptomatic.

At the termination of this period, the affected liver cells burst, releasing merozoites into the blood. While some reinvade other liver cells, most gain access to erythrocytes, where they again multiply asexually. After maturation of the erythrocytic schizont, it ruptures, releasing merozoites. Rupture of the parasitized red blood cell is associated with the release of pyrogenic substances, which cause a rapid rise in body temperature. The released merozoites can reinvade erythrocytes, giving rise to repeated cycles of division, rupture, and fever; this is acute malaria. The interval between fever spikes is dependent upon the rate of merozoite division and red cell rupture. Disappearance of the plasmodium from the body (spontaneously or drug-induced) is associated with the absence of fever; exo-erythrocytic forms may persist in tissues for extended periods of time. Reappearance of the parasite in the

Asexual cycle in human

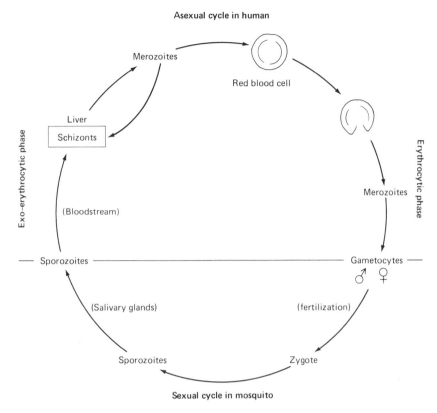

Figure 49-1. Life Cycle of the Plasmodium in the Mosquito and the Human Host.

blood after weeks or months produces a clinical relapse. A few of the merozoites released from the red blood cell undergo sexual division to form male and female gametocytes, these are ingested by the mosquito, starting the cycle anew.

Chemotherapy of Malaria

Treatment with antimalarial drugs has one of three primary objectives: prophylaxis, suppression of an acute attack, or the radical cure or complete elimination of the infection from the host. These aims are achieved by drug attack of the plasmodium at different stages in its life cycle. In this section we

shall discuss the major antimalarial drugs according to a classification based upon these major objectives. The nurse should bear in mind that this classification is not absolute; the use of some of these drugs for more than one treatment objective will be encountered. Representative antimalarial drugs appear in Table 49-1.

Prophylactic drugs   Prophylaxis involves the prevention of the malarial infection after the host is bitten by an infected mosquito. Such drugs are believed to act by eliminating the exo-erythrocytic forms of the parasite before they are able to invade red blood cells. The routine use of chemoprophylactic agents by residents of endemic

418

Table 49-1   Representative Antimalarial Agents

Generic name (trade name)	Usual adult dose	Adverse effects	Remarks
Quinine sulfate	PO: 300 mg to 1 g t.i.d. for 6-12 days. IV: 600 mg in 500 ml, diluent infused over 1 h; may be repeated twice at 8-h intervals.	"Cinchonism"-tinnitus, headache, nausea, visual and behavioral disturbances.	Has been generally replaced by less toxic, more effective drugs. Often used with pyrimethamine to treat chloroquine-resistant strains of *Plasmodium falciparum*. Also useful for nocturnal leg cramps. Give after meals.
Chloroquine (Aralen)	PO (phosphate): 600 mg initially, 300 mg 6 h later and on each of next 2 days. IM (hydrochloride): 200-500 mg, repeated in 6 h PRN.	Mild headache, visual disturbances, gastrointestinal upset.	Drug of choice in terminating acute attacks of vivax and faciparum malaria; cures latter. Suppresses vivax, relapses occur after drug withdrawal; not prophylactic. *P. falciparium* resistant strains emerging. Also used in extraintestinal amebiasis.
Hydroxychloroquine (Plaquenil)	PO: 620 mg initially, 310 mg 6 h later and on each of next 2 days.	Similar to chloroquine.	Similar to chloroquine with no advantages.
Amodiaquine (Camoquin)	PO: Same as chloroquine. Suppressive: 300-600 mg weekly.	Nausea, vomiting, diarrhea, dizziness.	Similar to chloroquine; less widely used.
Primaquine phosphate	PO: 15 mg o.d. for 14 days.	Abdominal distress; hemolytic anemia in patients with glucose-6-phosphate dehydrogenase deficiency.	Used for radical cure of relapsing vivax malaria; not useful for control of acute attack. Low incidence of side effects.
Quinacrine [Mepacrine] (Atabrine)	PO: 200 mg q. 6 h for 5 doses, then 100 mg t.i.d. for 6 days.	Yellow pigmentation of skin frequently occurs (apparently harmless); gastrointestinal upset.	Less effective and more toxic than chloroquine; rarely used.
Pyrimethamine (Daraprim)	PO: 25 mg once weekly	Anorexia and vomiting at high doses; occasional blood disorders.	Highly effective antifolate. Used primarily to prevent vivax and falciparum malaria. Used with quinine for chloroquine-resistant strains.
Trimethoprim	PO: 100 mg b.i.d.	Gastrointestinal effects, malaise, rarely blood disorders.	Used in combination with sulfonamides as antimalarial and antibacterial agent. See Chapter 42.
Tetracycline	PO: 250 mg q. 6 h for 7 days	Gastrointestinal effects.	Treatment of acute attack of chloroquine-resistant *P. falciparum*.

areas is not recommended because this practice favors the emergence of resistant strains of plasmodia; prophylaxis is suggested for use by people traveling to these areas. Primaquine, chloroguanide, and pyrimethamine are commonly employed chemoprophylactic agents.

Primaquine   While not useful for the suppression of an acute attack of malaria, primaquine is an effective prophylactic agent against all plasmodia and produces a radical cure of malaria caused by *P. vivax*, *P. ovale*, and *P. malariae*. It is also highly active against the gametocytes of all four malaria-causing species and is useful in preventing the transmission of this disease.

The most severe adverse effect associated with primaquine administration is acute hemolytic anemia, and this occurs in individuals with a glucose-6-phosphate deficiency. This genetically-linked disorder is observed most frequently in people whose ancestry originates in those areas in which malaria has been historically endemic, namely, the Mediterranean, Africa, and Southeast Asia. These individuals may also experience a similar adverse reaction with the sulfonamides, para-aminosalicylic acid, aspirin, certain vitamin K derivatives, and the antimicrobial nitrofurans (nitrofurantoin).

Other side effects include gastrointestinal distress, headache, disturbances of visual accommodation, and pruritis. Methemoglobinemia commonly occurs but rarely requires interruption of the usual 14-day course of therapy.

Pyrimethamine (Daraprim) is also used as a prophylactic agent, particularly against falciparum malaria. This drug should not be employed alone for the suppression of acute attacks because it has a slow onset of action in reducing fever and parasitemia. Pyrimethamine, in combination with quinine and a sulfonamide (sulfadiazine), has been used successfully to treat chloroquine-resistant strains of *P. falciparum*.

Suppressive drugs *Suppression* or a *clinical cure* involves the control of fever and other symptoms associated with an acute malarial attack. Suppressive drugs must be active against the asexual schizonts that multiply within the erythrocyte. These compounds, often referred to as *schizonticides*,

include quinine, chloroquine, and amodiaquine.

Quinine Quinine is the principal alkaloid obtained from the bark of the cinchona tree, which is indigenous to South America and also grows in Java. The use of this bark for the treatment of malaria originated in the seventeenth century, and quinine remained the primary antimalarial agent until World War II.

Effects. The primary action of quinine is on the asexual erythrocytic forms of the parasite. It has no effect on the exo-erythrocytic forms and, therefore, cannot be used as a prophylactic agent against any form of malaria, nor can it produce a radical cure of malaria caused by *P. vivax*, *P. malariae*, or *P. ovale*. Quinine can suppress the symptoms of malaria and is capable of producing rapid control of an acute attack. A major contemporary use of this drug is in combination with tetracycline or with pyrimethamine and a sulfonamide (sulfadiazine) for the control of chloroquine-resistant strains of *P. falciparum*. Quinine hydrochloride, administered intravenously, is also useful for the treatment of cerebral malaria.

Quinine possesses a wide spectrum of pharmacological effects that are unrelated to its antimalarial activity. While more toxic and no more effective than the salicylates, the analgesic and antipyretic actions of quinine have served as the basis for the use of this drug for the treatment of headache and muscle and joint aches and pains. Quinine has a curare-like effect on the motor end plate, thus decreasing its excitability. It is used to prevent nocturnal leg cramps and to alleviate muscle spasms and contractions that occur in myotonia congenita. It aggravates the muscle fatigue associated with myasthenia gravis and so has been employed as a diagnostic agent for this disorder.

The actions of quinine on the heart are

very similar to those produced by its isomer *quinidine* (Chapter 27), but the latter drug is preferred for the treatment of atrial fibrillation. Quinine causes a slight stimulant action on the uterus, while high doses are potentially capable of causing an abortion.

Adverse effects. Quinine salts are very *bitter* in taste, and when given orally in large doses may cause digestive disturbances. Because they are tissue (protoplasmic) poisons, these salts may cause pain, irritation, abscesses, and inflammation on injection.

The first signs of quinine overdosage are characterized by tinnitus (ringing in the ears), impaired hearing, blurred vision, dizziness, flushed and sweaty skin, and gastrointestinal disturbances; this toxic state is called *cinchonism*. Symptoms of toxicity involving the cardiovascular system include hypotension, widening of the QRS complex of the electrocardiogram, and, in more severe cases, ventricular tachycardia or ventricular fibrillation.

Quinine is capable of causing *blackwater fever* in patients being treated for falciparum malaria. Blackwater fever is a syndrome characterized by intravascular hemolysis, hemoglobinuria, azotemia, and renal failure; death may occur in 25 to 50 percent of these cases. The need to maintain the administration of quinine should be carefully re-examined at the first signs of hemolysis.

Chloroquine This compound is the drug of choice for the suppression of an acute malarial attack caused by *P. vivax*, *P. ovale*, *P. malariae*, and susceptible strains of *P. falciparum*.

Effects. The antimalarial effects of chloroquine (Aralen) have been attributed to its ability to block the synthesis of DNA and RNA. Chloroquine is highly active against the schizonts in the erythrocytes, thus ac-

counting for its ability to produce clinical cures. It is neither effective against the exoerythrocytic forms nor against the gametocytes of *P. falciparum* and cannot, therefore, be employed as a prophylactic agent. Plasmodial resistance to chloroquine may be the consequence of an impairment of drug transport across the cell wall of the parasite, resulting in inadequate drug concentrations available to inhibit nucleic acid synthesis.

Chloroquine is highly effective for the treatment of extraintestinal (hepatic) amebiasis, and is capable of producing complete and rapid cures (see the next section).

This drug has been found to produce beneficial therapeutic effects in the management of certain connective tissue diseases such as *rheumatoid arthritis* and *lupus erythematosus*. Successful treatment necessitates the use of high doses of chloroquine for long periods of time. The risk of toxic effects to the eye generally outweighs the benefits of such therapy.

Adverse effects. When used for the suppression of an acute malarial attack, chloroquine produces no toxic effects. Side effects may include occasional blurring of vision, headache, and dizziness. High doses may cause skin lesions, bleaching of the hair, behavioral aberrations (toxic psychosis with hallucinations and agitation), and electrocardiographic changes.

Chronic administration of high doses, such as for the treatment of rheumatoid arthritis, may cause severe and often permanent *ocular toxicity* involving the cornea and retina. Chloroquine is secreted in the tears, resulting in the formation of corneal deposits in 10 to 33 percent of those patients taking high doses. These deposits regress when drug administration is terminated. Early signs of retinal changes include halos around lights and blurring of vision. *Retinopathy* is progressive, often worsening after drug withdrawal; it may lead to blindness. Nurses should impress upon their patients the importance of having their vision tested and retinas examined every 3 months when receiving high-dose, long-term chloroquine administration. Nursing implications are summarized at the end of this chapter.

Curative drugs Radical cure of malaria denotes the complete elimination of all parasites from the body. This may involve the eradication of the reservoir of exo-erythrocytic parasites to prevent relapses and the destruction of gametocytes to prevent reinfection of mosquitoes. In falciparum malaria, no secondary exo-erythrocytic forms exist; hence elimination of the blood forms achieves both clinical and radical cure if there is no recurrence of parasitemia for 60 days after the termination of drug administration. Primaquine is the only widely used drug employed to accomplish radical cures.

AMEBICIDES

Amebiasis or amebic dysentary is a disease caused by *Entamoeba histolytica*. Infection by this protozoan may be restricted to the intestines, often causing ulceration of the mucosa; cases of intestinal amebiasis may be severe, mildly symptomatic, or even asymptomatic. This parasite may invade the liver, the primary site of extraintestinal amebiasis, where it may produce serious abscesses.

Amebicides are generally classified according to their primary site of action (Table 49-2). *Extraintestinal (tissue) amebicides*, drugs whose primary site of action is outside the intestinal lumen (including, but not limited to, the bowel wall and liver), include emetine and chloroquine. *Intestinal amebicides*, whose primary actions are restricted to the bowel lumen, include the organic ar-

senical carbasone, diiodohydroxyquin, and the antibiotic paromomycin. Metronidazole is the only effective drug for the management of intestinal and extraintestinal amebiasis. Successful treatment of amebiasis may require the concurrent or sequential use of more than one drug.

Metronidazole

Metronidazole (Flagyl) is the drug of choice for the treatment of both intestinal and extraintestinal amebiasis. It is favored because of its high degree of effectiveness after oral administration and relatively low toxicity. This compound is also the preferred drug for the treatment of infections of the vagina caused by the protozoan *Trichomonas vaginalis*. The dose employed in amebiasis (500 to 750 mg, three times daily for 5 to 10 days) is higher than the dose used in trichomoniasis (250 mg, three times daily, for 7 days).

Common side effects associated with metronidazole administration include nausea, anorexia, vomiting, diarrhea, abdominal cramping, headache, and an unpleasant, metallic taste. Nurses should advise patients to avoid the use of alcoholic beverages while taking this drug to preclude the risk of a disulfiram (Antabuse) reaction (Chapter 14). Metronidazole has been found to be carcinogenic in rodents but not, to date, in humans. This drug crosses the placenta and should not be administered during pregnancy. Nursing implications appear at the end of this chapter.

Emetine

Emetine, obtained from the South American ipecacuanha root, is capable of producing a rapid cure of an acute attack of extraintestinal amebiasis. It is considerably less effective for the management of chronic amebiasis.

When administered orally, emetine

Table 49-2   Representative Amebicidal and Antiprotozoal Agents

Generic name (other name) [trade name]	Usual adult dose	Principal therapeutic uses	Adverse effects	Remarks
Extraintestinal amebicides				
Emetine	SC or IM: 1 mg/kg (maximum 65 mg) o.d. for 3-10 days	Amebiasis, amebic hepatitis, balantidiasis, liver fluke infestations.	Frequent diarrhea, nausea, vomiting, skeletal muscle weakness.	High incidence of toxic effects, most dangerous of which are cardiovascular (changes blood pressure, heart rate, EKG).
Chloroquine [Aralen]	PO: 1 g o.d. for 2 days, then 500 mg o.d. for 2-3 wk IM: 200-500 mg o.d. for 10-12 days.	Malaria, amebiasis.	Mild headache, visual disturbances, gastrointestinal upset.	Less effective but less toxic than emetine. Chloroquine and emetine concurrently employed for hepatic amebiasis.
Intestinal amebicides				
Carbarsone	PO: 100-250 mg 2-3 times daily for 10 days	Intestinal amebiasis.	Gastrointestinal disorders, skin rashes, edema; danger hepatitis.	Organic arsenical, rarely used; less toxic drugs available; danger of cumulative toxicity.
Diiodohydroxyquin (iodoquinol) [Yodoxin]	PO: 650 mg t.i.d. for up to 3 wk	Intestinal amebiasis.	Rash, nausea, chills, abdominal cramps; danger of optic neuropathy.	Used, but not demonstrated effective, for traveler's diarrhea.
Paromomycin [Humatin]	PO: 25-35 mg/kg o.d. in 3 divided doses with meals for 5-10 days	Intestinal amebiasis. Also effective against gram-negative bacteria.	Gastrointestinal disturbances.	Antibiotic. Not systemically absorbed after oral administration.
Extraintestinal-intestinal amebicide				
Metronidazole [Flagyl]	PO: 750 mg t.i.d. for 10 days	Intestinal and extraintestinal amebiasis; infections by *Trichomonas vaginalis*.	Gastrointestinal disturbances, moniliasis.	Drug of choice in amebiasis. Shown to cause tumors in animals; human carcinogenic potential not established.
Miscellaneous antiprotozoan agent				
Suramin (Bayer 205)	IV: Prophylaxis: 1 g every 3 mo; Treatment: 1 g on days 1, 3, 7 and once weekly for 7 wk	Trypanosomiasis (except Chagas' disease); onchocerciasis; pemphigus. Also used as anthelmintic.	Early: nausea, vomiting, shock, loss of consciousness; later: sensory disturbances.	One of few drugs useful for trypanosomiasis. Intramuscular injection irritating. Available from the Center for Disease Control, Atlanta, Georgia.

causes irritation of the stomach and intestines and induces vomiting and diarrhea. The crude drug (syrup of ipecac) is employed as an emetic (Chapter 57) and expectorant. For the treatment of amebiasis, emetine is intramuscularly injected.

The therapeutic dose of emetine is close to one producing toxicity. This drug is slowly eliminated, creating the risk of cumulative toxicity, myocardial depression in particular. Nursing implications are summarized at the end of this chapter.

Diiodohydroxyquin (Iodoquinol)

Diiodohydroxyquin (Yodoxin) is an orally active drug useful for the treatment of mild or asymptomatic intestinal amebiasis. It is also employed prophylactically in "traveler's diarrhea," but evidence demonstrating its effectiveness is lacking.

The adverse effects of this drug are caused by the presence of *iodine* in the molecule and include skin rash, acne, enlargement of the thyroid gland, nausea, and abdominal cramps. Diiodohydroxyquin interferes with the results of thyroid function tests for several months after its administration. Its use is contraindicated in patients who are hypersensitive to iodine or who have liver disease.

Iodochlorhydroxyquin, an analog of diiodohydroxyquin, has been implicated in the development of *subacute myelo-optico-neuropathy* (SMON) when used on a daily basis for more than 14 days. The characteristics of this neurological disease include sensory impairment of the lower limbs, disturbances of gait, visual abnormalities, and behavioral disturbances. Iodochlorhydroxyquin is no longer marketed in the United States.

Paromomycin and Tetracyclines

Paromomycin (Humatin) is a broad-spectrum antibiotic that has direct activity against amebae in the intestinal lumen. It is effective for the treatment of acute and chronic intestinal amebiasis but ineffective in the management of extraintestinal amebiasis. The most frequently encountered side effects after oral administration are nausea and diarrhea.

The tetracycline antibiotics (Chapter 45) are active against amebae in the intestinal lumen and wall. Unlike paromomycin, which possesses direct amebicidal activity, the tetracyclines act indirectly by modifying the intestinal flora essential for the survival of the protozoa. The older tetracyclines, namely, tetracycline and oxytetracycline, are not as well absorbed from the bowel and are the most effective members of this antibiotic class. These drugs are used in combination with other amebicides for the treatment of intestinal and extraintestinal amebiasis.

Antimalarials and Amebicides: **nursing implications**

Chloroquine

1. Watch for side effects, especially in patients receiving high doses for prolonged periods; CNS disturbances: headache, fatigue, nervousness, irritability, emotional changes, hallucinations; skin: skin lesions, pruritis, dry skin, desquamation, changes in skin or

hair; muscular weakness or diminished deep tendon reflexes; blood dyscrasias; gastrointestinal disturbances.

2. Ophthalmoscopic and visual examinations should be performed prior to the initiation of therapy and periodically during prolonged therapy. Drug-induced corneal damage and retinopathy are often not reversible. Instruct patient to wear dark glasses in bright lights and report any changes in night vision or visual fields, scotomata, blurred vision, halos around lights, or difficulty focusing.

3. When chloroquine is administered for rheumatoid arthritis, improvements may not be noticed for 6–12 mo. Drug dosage will be adjusted depending upon therapeutic response and adverse effects.

4. Warn parents to keep this drug out of reach of children. Accidental overdose by children or in suicidal adults can cause acute toxicity in 30 min and death within 2 h. Acute toxic symptoms include headache, drowsiness, visual disturbances, cardiovascular collapse, convulsions, or cardiac arrest. Emergency treatment includes gastric lavage, barbiturates, vasopressors, oxygen; ammonium chloride and high fluid intake are employed to acidify the urine and promote renal excretion for several weeks to months until the drug is completely excreted.

5. Warn the patient that the drug may turn urine dark yellow-brown.

Metronidazole

1. Explain to the female patient that her sexual partner may be an asymptomatic carrier and may require drug therapy to prevent reinfection of female.

2. Women with trichomoniasis should be advised not to wear panty hose or tight underwear and to avoid bubble baths and commercial douche preparations. Review perineal hygiene with patient.

3. Warn the patient that ingestion of alcohol when receiving metronidazole therapy can result in a disulfiram-like reaction: sweating, nausea, vomiting, headache, flushing, palpitations.

4. Instruct the patient to report CNS toxicity, which requires drug discontinuation: tremor, ataxia, incoordination, paresthesias, numbness, impairment of pain or touch sensations.

5. Warn the patient that the drug may turn urine brown.

Emetine and Other Amebicides

1. Provide supportive care during periods of acute dysentary or extraintestinal amebiasis, including procedures to control diarrhea, maintain electrolyte balance, and prevent malnutrition.

2. Teach the patient and his or her family the necessity for thorough hand washing. This is especially important for food handlers and individuals working in schools and other institutions where the disease is likely to spread.

3. Patients treated with emetine should be hospitalized on absolute bed rest during therapy and for several days after treatment.

4. Observe the patient for and immediately report any increase in pulse or a decrease in blood pressure during the course of drug therapy; such cardiovascular changes may necessitate discontinuation of drug.

SUPPLEMENTARY READINGS

Hill, J., "Chemotherapy of Malaria. Part 2. The Antimalarial Drugs," in *Experimental Chemotherapy*, eds. R. J. Schnitzer and F. Hawking, Vol. 1, pp. 513–601. New York: Academic Press, Inc., 1963.

Powell, R. D., and W. D. Tigertt, "Drug Resistance of Parasites Causing Human Malaria," *Annual Review of Medicine* **19**: 81–102 (1968).

Powell, S. J., "Therapy of Amebiasis," *Bulletin of the New York Academy of Medicine* **47**: 469–77 (1971).

Rollo, I. M., "Drugs Used in the Chemotherapy of Malaria," in *Goodman and Gilman's The Pharmacological Basis of Therapeutics* (6th ed.), eds. A. G. Gilman, L. S. Goodman, and A. Gilman, Chapter 4–5, pp. 38–60, New York: Macmillan, Inc., 1980.

Thompson, P. E., and L. M. Werbel, *Antimalarial Agents: Chemistry and Pharmacology*. New York: Academic Press, Inc., 1972.

Woolfe, G., "The Chemotherapy of Amoebiasis," in *Progress in Drug Research*, ed. E. Jucker, Vol. 8, pp. 11–52. Basel: Birkhäuser Verlag, 1965.

Chapter 50

ANTHELMINTICS

Approximately one-third of the world's population is infested with *parasitic worms* or *helminths*. While the North American nurse will most commonly encounter intestinal nematode (roundworm) infestations, particularly pinworm in children, it should be noted that schistosomiasis (caused by blood flukes) is a chronic, serious infection afflicting 180 to 200 million people in Asia, Africa, the Caribbean, and South America. In many patients, multiple infestations may be present. In this chapter we shall discuss anthelmintics, chemotherapeutic agents used for the treatment and often cure of parasitic worm infestations in humans.

HELMINTHIASIS

Helminthiasis do not always cause clinical symptoms and, in some cases, do not represent severe health hazards to the host. By contrast, worm infestations may cause blood loss and anemia, mechanical injury to body organs, malnutrition (by appropriating the host's food), and general feelings of weakness and malaise. In large numbers, worms can cause mechanical obstruction of the intestines, bile duct, and lymphatics.

With few exceptions, most of the anthelmintics in contemporary practice are relatively specific in their spectrum of action (Table 50-1, pages 427–29). Prior to initiating therapy, therefore, an accurate diagnosis of the infesting worm(s) should be made. On occasion the parasitic worm can be identified by gross examination of the stool, although more often, an appropriate sample (stool, blood, urine, sputum, or body tissue) must be submitted to a parasitology laboratory for accurate diagnosis.

Worms that are parasitic to humans are classified as *nematodes*, *cestodes*, and *trematodes*.

Nematodes

Nematodes, commonly referred to as *roundworms*, are cylindrical, unsegmented worms varying in length from $\frac{1}{12}$ inch to over 1 foot. The *intestinal nematodes* include: *Ascaris lumbricoides* (roundworm), *Necator americanus* and *Ancyclostoma duodenale* (two species of hookworms), *Trichuris trichiura* (whipworm), *Strongyloides stercoralis* (threadworm), *Enterobius* (Oxyuris) *vermicularis* (pinworm), and *Trichinella spiralis* (pork roundworm).

Infestations of these parasites are caused by the ingestion of food or water polluted with the ova of the worms or by eating with hands contaminated with the ova. Nematode infestations are encountered throughout the world, with infestations caused by roundworms (ascariasis, estimated to have infected one billion persons), pinworms (enterobiasis), and pork roundworms (trichi-

nosis), most prevalent in the United States. Drugs of choice (*in italics*) and other effective agents for the treatment of infestations caused by intestinal nematodes include the following compounds: roundworms, *piperazine*, pyrantel pamoate; hookworm, *bephenium*, *pyrantel pamoate;* whipworm, *mebendazole;* threadworm, *thiabendazole*, pyrvinium pamoate; pinworm, *pyrantel pamoate*, piperazine; pork roundworm, corticosteroids (for the control of acute systematic manifestations), *thiabendazole*.

The primary tissue nematodes or *filiarial worms* include *Wuchereria bancrofti* (Central Africa, West Indies, South America) and *Wuchereria malayi* (Indonesia, Southeast Asia). These worms, transmitted by mosquitoes, live in and obstruct the lymphatic vessels, causing hyperplasia of lymphatic tissues (elephantiasis). The primary drug for the treatment of filariasis is diethylcarbamazine. It has been estimated that over 300 million persons are infected with filariasis.

Cestodes

Cestodes or *tapeworms* are flattened, segmented worms, with a head (scolex) and a variable number of segments; they vary in length from 1.5 inches to up to 30 feet. The four species of cestodes include *Taenia saginata* (beef tapeworm), *Taenia solium* (pork tapeworm), *Diphyllobothrium latum* (fish tapeworm), and *Hymenolepsis nana* (dwarf tapeworm).

Tapeworm infestations result from eating improperly (undercooked) meat or fish infested with larvae. While beef tapeworm is relatively harmless, pork tapeworm can be carried to the muscles and brain, resulting in potential adverse neurological and behavioral changes in the host. Niclosamide is the drug of choice for the treatment of tapeworm infestations; dichlorophen and paro-

Table 50-1 Representative Anthelmintics

Generic name (trade name)	Usual adult dose	Principal therapeutic uses	Adverse effects	Remarks
Antimony potassium tartrate; tarter emetic	Slow IV injection of 8 ml of 0.5% sol. on day 1, increased by 4 ml daily until 11th day, when 28 ml given; continue on alternate days until 500 ml (2.5 g) given.	Blood fluke (*Schistosoma japonicum*[a], *S. mansoni*; *S. haematobium*)	Rapid injection causes coughing, vomiting, dyspnea, bradycardia, hypotension. Long-term adverse effects on hert and liver.	Most active and toxic antimony compound. Use freshly prepared solutions. Extravasation causes severe tissue necrosis. Sudden death, particularly in malnourished patients, from ventricular abnormalities, and cardiovascular collapse. Contraindicated: cardiac or kidney disease and hepatic disorders not caused by schistosomiasis.
Bephenium hydroxynaphthoate (Alcopara)	PO: 5 g b.i.d. for 1–3 days	*Hookworm (Ancylosoma duodenale*[a], *Necator americanus*[a]), mixed hookworm-round worm (*Ascaris*) infections	Nausea and vomiting (bitter taste); especially in children.	Safe, well-tolerated drug. Correct diarrhea, dehydration, electrolyte imbalance prior to administration. No longer marketed in the United States.
Dichlorophen (Antiphen)	PO: 2–3 g q. 8 h for 3 doses	Tapeworms	Gastrointestinal distress, lassitude.	Useful for treatment of beef and pork tapeworms in humans and domestic animals. Use cautiously in patients with liver disease. Not marketed in the United States.
Diethylcarbamazine citrate (Hetrazan)	PO: 2–4 mg/kg t.i.d. for 1–4 wk	Filarial worms[a] (*Wuchereria bancrofti*[a]; *Brugia malayi*[a], *Loa loa*[a]; *Onchocerca volvulus*[a])	Headache, malaise, anorexia, nausea, vomiting. Allergic reactions (fever, itching, tachycardia, tachypnea, rash, lymphatic swellings).	Safe, effective drug for filariasis. Allergic reactions result from release of foreign protein from dying microfilariae or adult worms; symptoms persist for 3–7 days.
Hexylresorcinol	PO: 1 g at weekly intervals PRN	Whipworm; roundworm; hookworm; dwarf tapeworm	Painful ulceration of oral mucosa if capsules not swallowed intact. Occasional gastrointestinal distress.	Broad-spectrum anthelmintic activity with low toxicity; may be useful in mixed infections. More effective specific drugs available.
Mebendazole (Vermox)	PO: 100 mg A.M. and P.M. for 3 consecutive days	Whipworm[a] (*Trichuris trichiura*), roundworm, hookworm, pinworm	Transient abdominal pain and diarrhea.	Broad-spectrum anthelmintic useful for trichuriasis and mixed infections. Contraindicated during pregnancy.

427

Table 50-1 Continued

Generic name (trade name)	Usual adult dose	Principal therapeutic uses	Adverse effects	Remarks
Niclosamide (Yomesan)	PO: 2 doses of 1 g each at 1 h intervals	Tapeworms[a] (Taenia saginata (beef); T. solium (pork); Diphyllobothrium latum (fish); Hymenolepis nana (dwarf)	Nausea, vomiting, and intestinal colic infrequently observed.	Safe and highly effective in tapeworm infections. Patient should omit breakfast, eat 2 hr after last dose. Chew tablets, swallow with water. Not generally available in U.S.; obtained from Center for Disease Control, Atlanta, Ga.
Niridazole (Ambilhar)	PO: 25 mg/kg daily in 2 divided doses for 5-10 days	Blood fluke (S. haematobium[a]; S. mansoni; S. japonicum); Guineaworm (Dracunulus medinensis)	Weakness, anorexia, nausea, vomiting, diarrhea, abdominal cramps, headache, dizziness, muscle and joint pain, EKG changes, mood changes.	Should not be given to patients with history of liver disease, neuropsychiatric or convulsive disorders or during pregnancy. Not generally available in U.S; obtained from Center for Disease Control, Atlanta, Ga.
Paromomycin (Humatin)	PO: 25 mg/kg daily, in divided doses at mealtimes, for 5 days	Tapeworms	Gastrointestinal upset.	Aminoglycoside antibiotic (Chapter 46) used for treatment of tapeworm infestations and acute and chronic intestinal amebiasis (Chapter 49).
Piperazine: citrate (Antepar, Multifuge); phosphate (Piperaval)	PO: 3.5 g o.d. for 2 consecutive days	Roundworm[a] (Ascaris lumbricoides); pinworm	Nausea, vomiting, mild diarrhea, abdominal pain, headache.	Safe and widely used. All piperazine salts possess equivalent effectiveness. Available as tablets, syrups, wafers. Contraindications: impaired renal or liver function, convulsive disorders.
Pyrantel pamoate (Antiminth)	PO: 11 mg/kg (maximum 1 g) 1-3 days	Pinworm[a] (Enterobius vermicularis); round worm[a]	Gastrointestinal upset, headache, drowsiness, rashes, elevated SGOT values.	Highly effective drug. Use with caution in patients with liver dysfunctions.

Drug	Indication	Dose	Side effects	Comments
Pyrvinium pamoate (Povan)	Pinworm, threadworm	PO: 5 mg/kg (maximum 350 mg) in single dose, repeat in 2 weeks for pinworm; 5 mg/kg daily for 5-7 days for threadworm.	Nausea, vomiting, abdominal cramps, and rarely, photosensitivity.	Highly effective for pinworm and threadworm. Patients should be forewarned that drug stains stools bright red and will stain clothing if vomiting. Tablets should be swallowed immediately, not chewed, to avoid oral staining.
Quinacrine (Atabrine)	Alternative drug for treatment of beef and fish tapeworm.	PO: duodenal tube: 4 doses of 200 mg 10 min apart	Nausea and vomiting common at doses employed for tapeworm therapy.	Administer no food after the evening meal and an enema. Prior to treatment an antiemetic and sodium bicarbonate may be given; 2 h after last dose a saline laxative is administered to remove the worm and unabsorbed drug.
Stibophen (Fuadin)	Blood fluke (Schistosoma mansoni[a], S. japonicum; S. haematobium)	IM: 100 mg on day 1, then 300 mg on alternate days up to 2.5-4.6 g	Similar to antimony potassium tartrate.	Less toxic than antimony potassium tartrate. Contraindicated in severe liver, kidney or cardiac insufficiency.
Tetrachloroethylene	Hookworm	PO: 3-5 ml as single dose	Nausea, vomiting, dizziness, inebriation occur occasionally.	Low-bulk, low-fat meal on evening before drug; avoid use of alcohol before and 24 h after treatment; 2 h after drug, administer saline laxative. Patient should remain recumbent for 4 h after treatment.
Thiabendazole (Mintezol)	Threadworm[a] (Strongyloides stercoralis), cutaneous larva migrans[a] (creeping eruption)	PO: 25 mg/kg (maximum 3 g) b.i.d. for 1-4 days	Side effects common but mild and transient—dizziness, anorexia, nausea and vomiting; loss of mental alertness; rare severe toxicity.	Broad-spectrum antihelmintic; drug of choice in strongyloidiasis and first effective drug in creeping eruption. Effective in pinworm but less toxic drugs (pyrantel, pyrvinium, piperazine) are preferred.

[a] Drug of choice for these worms.

momycin are also considered to be effective agents. Approximately 2 hours after the administration of the anthelmintic, a laxative such as magnesium or sodium sulfate (15 to 30 g for adults) should be given to expel the worm and eliminate the unabsorbed drug. It is essential that the head of the worm be passed in the stool to prevent regrowth of the tapeworm.

Trematodes

The most important of the trematodes are the blood flukes *Schistosoma haematobium* (Africa, Middle East), *S. mansoni* (Africa, Caribbean), and *S. japonicum* (East Asia). These three species are responsible for the very extensive and dangerous infection *schistosomiasis* (or bilharziasis).

Humans are infected by bathing in fresh water contaminated by the larvae, which are harbored by the snails that act as intermediate hosts. Symptoms of schistosomiasis include urinary tract disorders, hepatosplenomegaly (enlargement of the liver and spleen), portal hypertension, and pulmonary involvement. The drugs of choice for the treatment of schistosomiasis are niridazole (*S. haematobium*), stibophen (*S. mansoni*), and antimony potassium tartrate (*S. japonicum*).

Other trematodes causing diseases in humans include *Paragonimus westermani* (lung fluke) in the Far East and South America, treated with bithionol; *Clonorchis sinensis* (Chinese liver fluke) in the Far East and in Chinese immigrants, treated with chloroquine; and *Fascidopsis buski* (intestinal fluke) in the Far East, treated with hexylresorcinol. These diseases result from the ingestion of undercooked infested crabs, snails (lung fluke), fish (Chinese liver fluke), or infested water nuts (intestinal fluke).

ANTHELMINTICS

Anthelmintics are drugs used for the treatment of helminthiasis and include drugs that act locally to expel worms from the gastrointestinal tract, as well as those compounds employed to treat systemic parasitic worm infestations.

The comparative characteristics of contemporary anthelmintics are given in Table 50-1. The mechanisms of action of these drugs are highly diverse and include: (1) induction of temporary or permanent muscle paralysis or narcosis in worms, leading to their expulsion from the gastrointestinal tract by peristalsis (hexylresorcinol, piperazine, pyrantel); (2) inhibition of the uptake of essential nutrients, such as glucose, or by interfering with biochemical reactions that are necessary for the survival of the parasitic worm (niclosamine, niridazole, pyrvinium, thiabendazole); and (3) sensitization of the helminth to phagocytosis by normal host defense mechanisms (diethylcarbamazine).

Cure rates of 80 to almost 100 percent have been reported after the use of primary anthelmintics for the treatment of roundworm, hookworm, whipworm, pinworm, threadworm, and tapeworm infestations. By contrast, there is an urgent need for the development of safer, more effective, easily administered, and inexpensive drugs for the prevention, treatment, and cure of schistosomiasis and filariasis.

The nurse should bear in mind that the successful prevention and cure of helminthiasis cannot be accomplished solely with drugs and should play an active role in educating patients about good hygienic practices and other appropriate measures to avoid infestation or reduce the incidence of helminthiasis.

Anthelmintics:
nursing implications

1. Instruct the patient and family members about diet, laxative enemas, and follow-up tests when treatment is to be administered in the home. Supplement with written instructions.

2. When treating a patient for pinworms, the entire family is usually treated. To prevent reinfestation, instructions should include: wash hands after elimination and prior to preparing food or eating; keep finger nails short; bathe daily and change bed linen and underwear daily. Eggs are destroyed by household washing solutions.

3. Several (2–3) weeks after treatment for roundworms, daily microscopic stool examinations should be performed until no further roundworm ova are found.

4. After the administration of laxatives or enemas in conjunction with anthelmintic therapy for hookworm or tapeworm, examine the fecal material for the head of the worm, which will be bright yellow.

SUPPLEMENTARY READINGS

Botero, D., "Chemotherapy of Human Intestinal Parasitic Diseases," *Annual Review of Pharmacology and Toxicology* **18**: 1–15 (1978).

Desowitz, R. S., "Antiparasite Chemotherapy," *Annual Review of Pharmacology* **11**: 351–68 (1971).

Goldsmith, R. S., "Anthelmintic Drugs," in *Review of Medical Pharmacology* (5th ed.), eds. F. H. Meyers, E. Jawetz and A. Goldfein. Chapter 63, pp. 634–63. Los Altos, California: Lange Medical Publications, 1976.

Marois, M., ed., *Development of Chemotherapeutic Agents for Parasitic Diseases*. Amsterdam: North-Holland Publishing Co., 1975.

Most, H., "Treatment of Common Parasitic Infections of Man Encountered in the United States," *New England Journal of Medicine* **287**: 495–98, 698–702 (1972).

Saz, H. J., and E. Bueding, "Relationships Between Anthelmintic Effects and Biochemical and Physiological Mechanisms," *Pharmacological Reviews* **18**: 871–94 (1966).

Standen, O. D., "Chemotherapy of Helminthic Infections," in *Experimental Chemotherapy*, eds. R. J. Schnitzer and F. Hawkins, Vol. 1, pp. 701–892. New York: Academic Press, 1963.

CANCER CHEMOTHERAPY

Second only to cardiovascular disease, cancer is the leading cause of death in the United States, claiming in excess of 350,000 victims annually. Each year almost twice this number of patients are diagnosed as having cancer, with the eight most common types of cancer accounting for over seven out of every ten cases; of these, approximately 70 percent will have a fatal outcome. These eight cancer types and the annual incidence of each in the United States are colon and rectal cancer (100,000), lung carcinoma (91,000), female breast cancer (88,000), prostrate cancer (56,000), uterine carcinoma (46,000), bladder and kidney cancer (43,000), lymphoma (29,000), and leukemia (21,000).

Although there are rare instances of spontaneous tumor regressions in the absence of treatment, death is almost always the inevitable result of cancer that has not been diagnosed and treated during the early stages. Early surgery and radiation still remain the most effective treatments of cancer, although chemotherapeutic agents, employed alone or in conjunction with other treatment modalities, are now capable of curing or markedly increasing the life expectancy of patients with a number of different types of cancer. Before discussing the chemotherapy of cancer, we shall briefly examine its general characteristics and possible causes.

CANCER

A *tumor* or *neoplasm* is a mass of new cells, where the growth is not under the control of the host. Tumors may be benign or malignant. *Benign tumors* (such as warts or moles) grow relatively slowly and remain at their site of origin. *Malignant tumors*, collectively referred to as *cancer*, have the following common characteristics: (1) Malignant cells undergo excessive and *uncontrolled growth*, usually manifested as a tumor. (2) Malignant tumors have lost the distinguishing morphological characteristics of their cells of origin and have reverted to a more primitive, embryonic-like, *undifferentiated cell type*. Moreover, not only do the cells of a malignant tumor differ in size and shape from normal cells, they also differ from each other. (3) Unlike normal cells and benign tumors which respect the borders of neighboring cells, malignant tumors actively *invade* and *penetrate* surrounding tissues, usurping their nutrients and vascular supply and utilizing these resources to support their growth and cell division. This ultimately results in the destruction and death of normal cells. (4) Malignant cells may set up secondary growths or *metastases* in parts of the body that may be far removed from their sites of origin. The cancer cell reaches these sites via the blood and lymphatic vessels. (5) A type of "acquired heredity" is observed in which the progeny of the malignant tumor cells retain the same carcinogenic potential.

General symptoms of cancer include pain, fever, weakness, and extreme weight loss. These symptoms result in part from compression pressure exerted by the tumor on surrounding tissues or organs, causing pain, impairment of function, and the ultimate destruction of these tissues or organs. The feelings of weakness and loss of weight may be attributed to the rapidly growing malignant cells nourishing themselves at the expense of normal cells.

Etiological Factors

The exact cause of cancer is unknown, and it appears unlikely that a single cause will be discovered that is responsible for this widely diverse group of diseases that we collectively call cancer. Among the factors thought to contribute to the development of cancer are the following: (1) *Chemicals*, particularly a large number of environmental compounds, have attracted widespread attention in recent years. The "tars" inhaled in cigarette smoke are undoubtedly responsible for the higher incidence of cancer of the lungs, larnyx, oral cavity, bladder, and pancreas observed among cigarette smokers when compared to nonsmokers. (2) *Viruses* have been implicated as a cause of cancer in many animal species and might also be involved in the etiology of human malignant tumors. (3) *Radiation*, whether natural (sunlight) or artificaly gen-

erated (atomic bombs or radiation employed for biomedical purposes), has been shown to increase the risk of various types of cancer. (4) Multiple influences, including sex, age, race, and genetic predisposition, affect the development of cancer.

CANCER CHEMOTHERAPY

The use of chemotherapeutic agents for the management of microbial infections has been far more successful than the drug treatment of cancers. The reasons for the different success rates between these chemotherapies becomes evident when we examine the fundamental differences between microbes and malignant cells.

Microbial cells have metabolic and nutritional requirements and a cellular morphology that are markedly different from their mammalian hosts (Chapter 41). Malignant cells, by contrast, are derived from the cells of their hosts, to which they retain close similarity. While the selective toxicity of antimicrobial agents is relatively high, this is not the case for most anticancer drugs. Preferential (but not selective) tumor toxicity may result from greater accumulation of the antineoplastic drug by the cancer cell than by the normal cell; this may be the result of greater cellular permeability.

Therapeutically effective doses of antineoplastic agents are toxic to both malignant and normal cells, with rapidly proliferating host cells most susceptible. These cells include the epithelial cells of the gastrointestinal tract (from mouth to anus), the hematopoietic (blood-cell forming) and germ cells, and hair follicles. With the exception of the steroid hormones, common adverse effects the nurse will observe after anticancer drugs include loss of appetite resulting in undernutrition, ulceration and bleeding of the gastrointestinal tract, severe diarrhea, nausea and vomiting,* alopecia (hair loss), and a marked reduction in one or more types of blood cells. With the reduction in white blood cells (leukopenia) is a resulting decrease in the effectiveness of the patient's immune response and defense mechanisms, leading to greater vulnerability to microbial infections. Subnormal platelet levels (thrombocytopenia) may potentially result in severe bleeding episodes. General nursing implications associated with the administration of anticancer drugs appear at the end of this chapter.

Evaluation of Therapeutic Response

The nurse should note that, in the context of cancer chemotherapy, the terms *effective* or *useful* do not necessarily denote a cure, a significant prolongation of the patient's life, or even the elimination of pain and suffering. These terms are used to denote one or more of the following drug-induced effects, which all represent signs of clinical improvement: (1) a reduction in tumor size, which may be detected by physical or radiological examination or other screening procedures; (2) a significant reduction in the amount of a tumor-released product or marker substance, which provides an indication of the amount of tumor present in the body; (3) a return to normal or an improvement in the function of an organ that was previously impaired as the result of the tumor; or (4) general signs of well-being, such as improved appetite, weight gain, or ambulation after a bedridden period.

Cancer chemotherapeutic agents are generally classified into the following categories: alkylating agents, antimetabolites, antibiotics, steroid hormones, plant alkaloids, and miscellaneous agents.

*Marihuana (Chapter 23) is being used on an experimental basis as an antiemetic agent in patients receiving cancer chemotherapy.

Alkylating Agents

Alkylating agents are *cytotoxic*, that is, they are general cell poisons that adversely affect the survival of both malignant and rapidly growing normal cells. In the interstitial water of the body, these drugs are converted to highly reactive, positively charged (cationic) intermediate compounds that are capable of chemically interacting with negatively charged (anionic) cellular groups in a nonspecific manner. In this way, alkylating agents interfere with the activity of enzymes and other endogenous compounds required for the regulation of essential cellular functions. Among the most important of these interactions are those involving the alkylation of the guanine molecule of chromosomal DNA. This chemical attachment produces cross-linking of DNA strands, which inhibits normal cellular mitosis and replication. These effects bear great similarity to those produced by ionizing radiation (x-ray), and, therefore, alkylating agents are sometimes referred to as *radiomimetic agents.*

This class of anticancer drugs is used for the treatment of malignancies of the hematopoietic system, neuroblastoma, and carcinoma of the breast and ovary; they are also employed for carcinoma of the lung, head and neck, and gastrointestinal tract. These drugs are capable of curing only Burkitt's lymphoma (a tumor of the face). The distinguishing properties of commonly employed alkylating agents are summarized in Table 51-1.

The most common adverse reactions of the alkylating agents involve the gastrointestinal tract, in particular, nausea and vomiting. These drugs often produce bone marrow depression, which may be irreversible. During the early course of therapy, blood cell counts should be made weekly; after a maintenance dose has been established, blood counts can be made at 2 to 3 week intervals. Nursing implications appear at the end of this chapter.

Table 51-1 Alkylating Agents Used as Anticancer Drugs

Generic name (other names) [trade name]	Usual adult dose	Principal therapeutic uses	Remarks
Nitrogen mustards			
Mechlorethamine (nitrogen mustard) [Mustargen]	IV: 0.4 mg/kg as single dose or in 2 divided doses on separate days. Intracavity: 10–20 mg; turn patient's position every 60 sec to 5 different positions	Hodgkin's disease, lymphosarcoma; mycosis fungoides; pulmonary carcinoma; malignant effusions of pericardial or peritoneal spaces.	Prototype nitrogen mustard derivative and most rapidly acting member of class. Nausea and vomiting 1–3 h after administration, vomiting persisting for 8 h. Bone marrow depression (leukopenia and thrombocytopenia) limits dosage. Extravasation into subcutaneous tissues causes painful inflammation and sloughing.
Cyclophosphamide [Cytoxan]	PO: 1–5 mg/kg o.d. IV: 10–20 mg/kg/ day (2–5 days), then 10–15 mg/ kg every 7–10 days or 3–5 mg/kg twice weekly.	Hodgkin's disease; acute lymphoblastic leukemia; neuroblastoma; follicular lymphoma, Burkitt's lymphoma; lymphosarcoma; multiple myeloma.	Clinical spectrum similar to mechlorethamine. Active orally. Alopecia common; thrombocytopenia less frequent; acute CNS abnormalities seen with other nitrogen mustards not observed. Maintain ample fluid intake and frequent voiding to prevent cystitis, dysuria, or hematuria.
Melphalan [Alkeran]	PO: 0.1–0.2 mg/kg/day for 7 days; drug-free period 2–4 weeks; then 2–4 mg/day	Multiple myeloma.	Bone marrow depression, nausea and vomiting infrequent; alopecia and renal changes not observed.
Uracil mustard	PO: 0.15 mg/kg once weekly for 4 weeks; if favorable response, continue until relapse.	Similar to mechlorethamine: Hodgkin's disease; chronic lymphocytic leukemia; malignant lymphoma.	Gastrointestinal and skin reactions, bone marrow depression.
Chlorambucil [Leukeran]	PO: 0.1–0.2 mg/kg/day (4–10 mg) in a single dose for 3–6 weeks.	Chronic lymphocytic leukemia; Hodgkin's disease; lymphosarcoma; giant follicular lymphoma.	Slowest acting and least toxic nitrogen mustard. Less bone marrow depression, nausea and vomiting than mechlorethamine. Drug is very poisonous—avoid inhaling particles or skin exposure.
Ethylenimine derivatives			
Triethylenemelamine (TEM)	PO: 2.5 mg o.d. for 3 days	Retinoblastoma.	Seldom used. Orally active, eratic absorption. Slow onset of action.

Table 51-1   **Continued**

Generic name (other names) [trade name]	Usual adult dose	Principal therapeutic uses	Remarks
Thiotepa (Triethylenethiophosphoramide) [Thiotepa]	IV: 0.4 mg/kg at 2-wk intervals	Breast and ovary carcinoma.	Bone marrow depression unpredictable, with onset of 5 to 30 days. Anorexia, nausea, vomiting, fever.
Alkylsulfonate			
Busulfan [Myleran]	PO: 4-8 mg o.d.	Chronic myelocytic leukemia; polycythemia vera.	Bone marrow depression, which may cause thrombocytopenia and bleeding; possible hyperpigmentation. Drug is very poisonous— avoid inhaling particles or skin exposure.
Nitrosoureas			
Carmustine (BCNU) [BiCNU]	IV: 100-200 mg/M^2 at 6-wk intervals	Hodgkin's disease (advanced, refractory); malignant and multiple melanoma; CNS tumors.	Bone marrow depression, observed 3-4 weeks after drug; hepatotoxicity infrequent but severe; pain along vein during infusion; nausea and vomiting.
Lomustine (CCNU) [CeeNU]	PO: 130 mg/M^2 as a single dose every 6 weeks	Brain tumors; Hodgkin's disease.	Similar to carmustine, but orally active.
Streptozocin (Streptozotocin) [Zanosar]	IV: 0.5-2 g/M^2 1-5 times weekly every 3 weeks.	Pancreatic islet cell; carcinoma (insulinoma).	Nausea and vomiting are common. Nephrotoxicity is not infrequent. Investigational drug.
Estramustine [Estracyt]	PO: 600 mg/M^2 o.d.	Prostate cancer.	Nausea, vomiting and mild gynecomastia. No bone marrow depression. Investigational drug.

Antimetabolites

The antimetabolites employed as antineoplastic agents chemically resemble endogenous compounds utilized in the biosynthesis of the nucleic acids DNA and RNA. These drugs inhibit nucleic acid synthesis by one of the following general mechanisms: by attaching to an enzyme and thereby preventing that enzyme from catalyzing an essential biochemical reaction; or by entering a biosynthetic pathway and being incorporated into the formation of a fraudulent end product that cannot be utilized by the cell for growth and multiplication.

Antimetabolites may interfere with the normal metabolism of folic acid, purines, or pyrimidines, all of which ultimately play an essential role in the biosynthesis of nucleic acids. The properties of antimetabolite antineoplastic agents are summarized in Table 51-2.

The entire spectrum of cancers are treated with the antimetabolites, although

Table 51-2   Antimetabolites Used as Anticancer Drugs

Generic name (other names) [trade name]	Dose	Principal therapeutic uses	Remarks
Folic acid analogs			
Methotrexate (amethopterin) [Mexate]	PO or IM: 15 mg/M^2 o.d. for 5 days. Other dosing schedules are used.	Acute lymphoblastic leukemia; choriocarcinoma; hydatidiform mole; lymphosarcoma; breast cancer.	Bone marrow depression with leukopenia, thrombocytopenia, bleeding, anemia; oral and gastrointestinal ulceration and bleeding; hepatotoxicity, worsened by alcohol ingestion. Leucovorin (citrovorum factor) useful antagonist in methotrexate toxicity.
Pyrimidine analogs			
Fluorouracil (5-fluorouracil; 5-FU) [Adrucil] Floxuridine [FUDR]	FU—IV: 12 mg/kg o.d. for 4 consecutive days, then 6 mg/kg every other day until day 12. FUDR-intra-arterial: 0.1-0.6 mg/kg/24 h by by constant infusion.	Gastrointestinal (colon, rectum, stomach, pancreas) and breast cancers. 5-FU used topically (Efudex, Fluoroplex) as cream or solution for actinic keratosis.	FUDR is rapidly metabolized to FU. Highly toxic drugs with low margins of safety; hospitalize patient during first course of therapy. Leukopenia primary adverse effect. Temporarily suspend therapy if aphthous stomatitis develops. Apply to skin lesion for 2-6 wks until ulcerative stage occurs.
Cytarabine (cytosine arabinoside, ARA-C) [Cytosar-U]	Rapid IV injection: 2mg/kg for 10 days. Continuous IV infusion: 0.5-1 mg/kg/day for 1-24 hr. SC: 1 mg/kg 1-2 times weekly.	Acute myeloblastic leukemia (adults); acute leukemias.	Side effects similar to methotrexate.
Purine analogs			
Mercaptopurine (6-mercaptopurine; 6-MP) [Purinethol]	PO: 2.5 mg/kg o.d.	Acute lymphoblastic leukemia; chronic myelocytic leukemia. Also immunosuppressant and treatment of ulcerative colitis.	Bone marrow depression; less gastrointestinal ulceration than folic acid antagonists. When allopurinol (Zyloprim) used to reduce hyperuricemia, reduce dose of mercaptopurine.
Thioguanine (6-thioguanine; TG)	PO: 2 mg/kg o.d.	Same leukemias as mercaptopurine.	Same adverse effects as mercaptopurine but fewer gastrointestinal reactions.

some of these drugs are more effective against specific types of neoplastic disorders. Acute leukemias respond favorably to mercaptopurine, thioguanine, methotrexate, and cytarabine, while the first two of these drugs may also be useful in the treatment of chronic myelocytic leukemia. Fluorouracil produces greater beneficial effects in carcinoma of the colon, breast, and ovary than of the stomach and pancreas. Methotrexate, employed alone or in combination with other drugs, has proved useful for the treatment of trophoblastic tumors (choriocarcinoma, chorioadenoma destruens, hydatidiform mole).

Bone marrow depression is observed with all antimetabolites; thrombocytopenia with bleeding can be managed with platelet transfusions, but it may be difficult to control when an infection is present. To reduce the severity of methotrexate toxicity, leucovorin (citrovorum factor, folinic acid) may be administered to "rescue" the patient several hours after this neoplastic agent. By contrast, considerable variation is observed among these drugs with respect to their relative toxicity on the gastrointestinal mucosa. Ulceration and bleeding of the gastrointestinal tract and diarrhea are commonly observed after methotrexate and fluorouracil administration, while mercaptopurine and thioguanine rarely cause these adverse effects. High doses of cytarabine cause nausea and vomiting in most patients but rarely cause mucosal damage. Methotrexate is reported to be an abortifacient and should not be administered during the first trimester of pregnancy.

Antibiotics

A number of antibiotics are currently being employed as antineoplastic agents; their principal uses and distinguishing adverse effects are given in Table 51-3. Most of these drugs exert their anticancer effects by interfering with the synthesis of DNA or RNA. With the exception of bleomycin, all other members of this class cause bone marow depression. Doxorubicin (Adriamycin) has been found to possess a relatively broad spectrum of antineoplastic action. The potential usefulness of this drug is limited by its cardiotoxic potential and irreversible congestive heart failure which is manifested when the total dosage administered exceeds $500 \text{ mg}/\text{M}^2$.

Steroid Hormones

The adrenocortical hormones and the sex hormones (analogs of testosterone, progesterone, and estrogen) are used for the treatment of neoplastic disorders (Table 51-4); the pharmacology of these steroid hormones has been considered previously (Chapters 34 and 37).

In contrast with other drugs used for the treatment of cancer that act nonselectively on rapidly multiplying cells, the steroid hormones possess a relatively high degree of selective toxicity; each hormone acts on specific tissues. The basis for the use of steroid hormones in the management of cancer is predicated upon the fact that cancers arising from tissues that are responsive to the effects of hormones retain the hormonal responsiveness of their tissues of origin. Depending upon the properties of the tissue of origin, alterations in the concentration of the hormones present may cause the cancer to increase or regress in size.

The sex hormones are employed for the treatment of cancers of the male and female breast, the prostrate, and the endometrium of the uterus. The beneficial effects of the sex hormones are generally temporary. The *adrenocortical hormones* possess antineoplastic activity against malignancies of the lymphatic system, particularly acute and chronic lymphatic leukemia and lymphomas. Resistance to the beneficial effects of the latter hormones develops rapidly in patients with acute lym-

Table 51-3 Antibiotics Used as Anticancer Drugs

Generic name (other names) [trade name]	Usual adult dose	Principal therapeutic uses	Remarks
Dactinomycin (actinomycin D) [Cosmegen]	IV: 0.5 mg o.d. for maximum of 5 days	Wilms' tumor; rhabdomyosarcoma; choriocarcinoma; carcinoma of the testes. Useful in patients with impaired renal or liver function in whom methotrexate is contraindicated.	Irritation or phlebitis at site of injection. Gastrointestinal, skin, and blood reactions occur frequently and may be serious; disappear upon drug withdrawal.
Doxorubicin [Adriamycin]	IV: 60–75 mg/M^2 as single injection at 21–day intervals	Acute lymphoblastic and myeloblastic leukemia; Wilms' tumor; neuroblastoma; soft tissue and bone sarcoma; breast, bladder, bronchogenic, metastatic thyroid cancers.	Highly impressive new anticancer drug. Serious irreversible cardiotoxicity (tachycardia, arrhythmias, EKG changes, progressive congestive heart failure) at total doses of 550 mg/M^2. High incidence of bone marrow depression.
Daunorubicin (daunomycin) [Cerubidine]	IV: 30–60 mg/M^2 o.d. for 3 days.	Acute leukemia.	Irreversible cardiotoxicity (see Doxorubicin), bone marrow depression.
Bleomycin [Blenoxane]	IV or IM: 10–20 units/M^2 1–2 times weekly	Squamous cell carcinoma of head, neck, penis, cervix, vulva; lymphomas; testicular carcinoma.	Danger of anaphylactoid reaction; patients with lymphomas should be given 2 units or less for first 2 doses. Pulmonary toxicity with risk of pulmonary fibrosis especially when total dose exceeds 400 units. Adverse reactions to skin and mucous membranes.
Mitomycin [Mutamycin]	IV—use either regimen at 6–8 week intervals: 20 mg/M^2 as single dose or 2 mg/M^2/day for 5 days, 2 drug-free days, 2 mg/M^2/day for 5 days.	In combination with other drugs for disseminated stomach or pancreas cancer. Does not replace surgery or radiation.	Toxic drug with low margin of safety. Bone marrow depression common. Extravasation may result in ulceration and sloughing.
Mithramycin [Mithracin]	IV: 25 mcg/kg for 8–10 days	Testicular carcinoma.	Therapeutic utility limited by severe toxicity to bone marrow, liver, kidneys. Bleeding syndrome, potentially fatal, usually begins with nosebleed.

Table 51-4   Steroid Hormones Used as Anticancer Drugs

Generic name (trade name)	Usual adult dose	Principal therapeutic use(s)	Remarks
Testosterone analogs			
Dromostanolone propionate (Drolban)	IM: 100 mg 3 times weekly for 8-12 wks	Female metastatic breast cancer (postmenopausal).	Less virilizing than testosterone; fluid retention. Contraindicated: male breast cancer and premenopausal women.
Testolactone (Teslac)	IM (deep): 100 mg, 3 times weekly. PO: 250 mg q.i.d.	Same use and contraindications as dromostanolone.	Essentially devoid of virilizing effects at therapeutic doses. Side effects: hypercalcemia; mild pain, irritation, and inflammation at site of injection.
Calusterone (Methosarb)	PO: 50 mg q.i.d.	Same use and contraindications as dromostanolone.	Virilizing effects in 20-25% of users; hypercalcemia.
Fluoxymesterone (Halotestin, Ora-Testryl)	PO: 15-30 mg o.d. in divided doses.	Inoperable female breast cancer.	Cholestatic jaundice in some patients.
Progesterone analogs			
Megestrol acetate (Megace)	PO: 40-320 mg in divided doses for at least 2 months	Advanced carcinoma of breast or endometrium.	No major adverse effects.
Medroxyprogesterone acetate (Depo-Provera)	IM: 400-1,000 mg per wk	Inoperable, recurrent, and metastatic endometrial carcinoma.	Contraindications: thrombophlebitis, stroke, carcinoma of breast, undiagnosed vaginal bleeding.
Estrogen analogs			
Diethylstilbestrol diphosphate (Stilphostrol)	PO: 150-600 mg/day in divided doses IV: 250-500 mg 1-2 times weekly	Prostate cancer.	Increased risk of thromboembolic disease (thrombophlebitis, pulmonary embolism, cerebral thrombosis) associated with estrogen use now conclusively established. Side effects: salt and water retention, behavioral and gastrointestinal disturbances.
Polyestradiol phosphate (Estradurin)	IM (deep): 40 mg every 2-4 wks or less frequently	Prostate cancer.	Continuous gradual release of estradiol. See cautions for diethylstilbestrol.
Tamoxifen (Nolvadex)	PO: 10 or 20 mg b.i.d.	Advanced breast cancer in postmenopausal women.	Antiestrogen effects; competes with estrogen for binding sites in breast. Common adverse effects: hot flashes, nausea, vomiting.

Table 51-4   Continued

Generic name (Trade name)	Usual adult dose	Principal therapeutic use(s)	Remarks
Adrenocorticosteroids			
Prednisone (Deltasone, Meticorten, Orasone)	PO: 60–100 mg o.d.	In combination with other drugs for acute leukemias, Hodgkin's disease, lymphomas, multiple myeloma, breast cancer.	Minimizes bleeding (acute leukemia), reduces hemolysis (lymphocytic leukemia), hypercalcemia, edema, and inflammation (CNS tumors). Gradually reduce dose. See Chapter 34 for side effects.

phatic leukemia. Hence, these hormones are administered in large doses for the shortest period of time required to achieve remission, with the dosage reduced as rapidly as possible. The hazards associated with the long-term use of high doses of the adrenocortical hormones have been previously discussed (Chapter 34).

Plant Alkaloids

Vinblastine and vincristine are two alkaloids possessing antineoplastic activity that have been isolated from the periwinkle plant (*Vinca rosea*). Although these compounds bear close chemical similarity, considerable differences exist with respect to their antineoplastic activity and adverse side effects (Table 51-5). Vincristine is primarily effective in the treatment of acute lymphatic leukemia, lymphomas, and certain solid tumors (particularly in children), while vinblastine is most useful for the treatment of Hodgkin's disease and choriocarcinoma. These drugs appear to act by arresting the mitotic cycle.

The most common adverse effects caused by vinblastine are nausea, vomiting, and leukopenia, the last of which limits the dosage that can be safely administered. Since alopecia may occur in 30 to 60 percent of patients, they should be advised of this adverse effect prior to the initiation of therapy. These alkaloids, in particular vincristine, cause a slowly developing neuropathy which is often manifested by a loss of deep tendon reflexes, paresthesia of the fingers and toes, and varying degrees of muscle weakness and paralysis; adverse behavioral changes may be noted in some patients. These neurological effects may persist for many months after the termination of drug administation. Nursing implications for vincristine appear at the end of this chapter.

Miscellaneous Agents

With the exception of the plant alkaloids discussed above, the drugs summarized in Table 51-5 lack a common chemistry, source from which they are derived, and mechanism of action and have different adverse side effects and therapeutic indications.

Combination Chemotherapy

The nurse will frequently observe that more than one drug is employed for the treatment of neoplastic diseases. In such instances, an attempt is made to use a combination of drugs with different mechanisms of action that act at different phases of the cell cycle and cause nonoverlapping toxicities so that maximum tolerated doses of each agent can be used. Ideally, such combination chemotherapy will enhance the antineoplastic effects without in-

Table 51-5   Plant Alkaloids and Miscellaneous Anticancer Drugs

Generic name (other name) [trade name]	Usual adult dose	Principal therapeutic uses	Remarks
Vinblastine (VLB) [Velban]	IV: 0.1 mg/kg/wk; increase by 0.05 mg/kg increments at 7-day intervals up to 0.5 mg/kg	Hodgkin's disease no longer responding to radiation or alkylating agents. With bleomycin for testicular cancer.	Extravasation causes severe irritation and pain which may result in phlebitis. Leukopenia common; nausea and vomiting less than alkalating agents; alopecia (30-60% of patients) may be reversible.
Vincristine (VCR) [Oncovin]	IV: 1.4 mg/M² per wk	Acute leukemia. Also Hodgkin's disease, lymphosarcoma, neuroblastoma, Wilms' tumor.	Extreme care in calculating and administering dose—overdosage may have serious or fatal outcome. Neurotoxicity (muscle weakness, paralysis cranial nerves) limits dosage; may cause behavioral depression; alopecia common.
Hydroxyurea [Hydrea]	PO: 20-30 mg/kg o.d. as single dose	Melanoma; chronic myelocytic leukemia; inoperable ovary cancer.	Bone marrow depression; leukopenia rapid and dose-dependent.
Procarbazine (MIH) [Matulane]	PO: 100-200 mg o.d. for one week, then 300 mg o.d.	Generalized Hodgkin's disease.	Gastrointestinal, blood, skin, CNS disorders.
Dacarbazine (DTIC) [DTIC-Dome]	IV: 2-4.5 mg/kg for 10 days repeated at 28-day intervals or 250 mg/M² daily for 5 days repeated at 21-day intervals.	Metastatic malignant melanoma.	Gastrointestinal and blood disorders most common. Extravasation may result in tissue damage and severe pain.
Mitotane (o,p'-DDD) [Lysodren]	PO: 9-10 g o.d. in divided doses	Inoperable adrenal cortex carcinoma (very rare disease).	High incidence of adverse effects affecting gastrointestinal tract, CNS, and skin.
Quinacrine (Atabrine)	Intracavity (intrapleural, intraperitoneal): 50-200 mg	Recurring pleural and peritoneal neoplastic effusions secondary to carcinomas. (Primary use of quinacrine in malaria.)	Adverse effects: fever, regional pain, dyspnea, nausea, vomiting, hallucinations.
Asparaginase (Elspar)	IV: 200 units/kg o.d. for 28 days.	Lymphocytic leukemia; malignant melanomas; lymphomas.	Rationale for use based upon qualitative difference between tumor and normal cell; gastrointestinal, liver, CNS disturbances, hypersensitivity reactions. Lack of bone marrow depression. Tumor resistance.

Table 51-5   Continued

Generic name (other name) [Trade name]	Usual adult dose	Principal therapeutic uses	Remarks
Gold Au-198 [Aureotope]	Intrapleural, intraperitoneal: 25-100 mCi	Pleural effusions and ascites.	Should not be administered during pregnancy, lactation, or in patients under 18 years.
Sodium Phosphate P-32 [Phosphotope]	PO: 6 mCi (polycythemia) IV: 3-5 mCi	Polycythemia vera; chronic myelocytic leukemia.	As effective as alkylating agents for myelocytic leukemia.
Cisplatin (cis-platinum) [Platinol]	IV: 100 mg/M^2 q. 4 wks	Genitourinary cancers (testicular, bladder, ovarian).	Nausea, vomiting, anorexia are common. Potential nephrotoxicity and ototoxicity (tinnitus or hearing loss).

creasing the rate or severity of toxicity; moreover, the appearance of drug resistance by the tumor may be delayed or even prevented.

While it is beyond the scope of this text to present a detailed discussion of combination chemotherapy, it should be noted that this approach has enhanced the therapeutic response in the following neoplastic diseases: acute leukemia; Hodgkin's disease; lymphomas; testicular, ovarian, and gastrointestinal carcinomas; childhood neuroblastoma; Wilms' tumor; and osteogenic sarcoma.

Cancer Chemotherapy: nursing implications

1. Utilize a holistic approach for the patient and family, considering possible changes in the patient's physical appearance and physical, social, and spiritual needs. Formulate realistic goals involving the nurse, physician, social worker, and other personnel in order to provide supportive and nonconflicting interventions for patient and family.

2. Prevent exposure of the patient to communicable diseases.

3. Prior to initiating therapy, establish a baseline for the patient including fluid intake and output patterns; bowel habits; and condition of blood picture and mouth. Determine the patient's psychological status and family relationships.

4. Teach the patient and his or her family about expected effects of drug and toxic effects which should be reported: bleeding in any part of the body, fever, jaundice, skin eruptions, bruising, and weight loss or gain. Early symptoms of toxicity may be manifested in the gastrointestinal tract and include oral ulcers, intestinal bleeding, or diarrhea. Prolonged vomiting or diarrhea can reduce blood volume, which may be manifested by decreased skin turgor, shrunken and dry tongue, postural hypotension, weakness, and confusion.

5. Bone marrow depression (sometimes reversible) is the major danger associated with cancer chemotherapy. The patient must have frequent blood counts and periodic bone marrow examination depending upon the drug type used. A sudden drop in white blood cell count below 2000/mm^3 or a platelet count below 100,000/mm^3 may indicate the need for a reduction in dosage or drug withdrawal.

6. Identify the nadir (the time at which bone marrow depression is most pronounced). The nadir varies with different drugs and may occur at different times for white cells and platelets. Knowledge of the nadir will permit the nurse to anticipate complications (such as infections or bleeding) and permit their early treatment.

7. Utilize nursing measures to counteract nausea: provide small servings of food liked by the patient; wait for nausea to pass prior to serving food; obtain an order for antiemetic medication, if needed; move patient slowly; keep environment well ventilated and free of odors.

8. Careful mouth care reduces nausea and prevents or treats stomatitis (manifested by dryness, erythema, or ulceration of mouth). Mild mouth washes and soft, bland diet may reduce discomfort. Apply lubricant to lips.

9. Temporary or permanent alopecia may result from treatment with some anticancer agents. Discuss this with the patient and facilitate cosmetic substitute if desired by the patient.

10. Extensive destruction of neoplastic cells releases large amounts of purines, which are metabolized to uric acid. Allopurinol (Zyloprim) may be ordered to prevent urate formation and decrease the risk of urate deposition, gouty arthritis, or renal calculi.

11. Drug solutions should be prepared according to the specific directions provided with the medication. Avoid contact with skin or inhalation of vapors. Check specific procedures to be employed in the event of drug contact with the skin or extravasation of drug into local tissues during parenteral administration.

Alkylating Agents

1. Immediately after intracavity administration, the patient should be repositioned every 60 sec for 5 min to assure full contact of drug with all parts of the cavity; patient positions include: prone, supine, right side, left side, knee-chest. Paracentesis may be performed 24–36 h later to remove any remaining fluid.

2. Monitor urinary output. Keep the patient well hydrated to help prevent hemorrhagic cystitis resulting from excessive drug concentrations in the urine. Instruct patient to report dysuria or hematuria.

3. Amenorrhea, resulting from the lack of follicular maturation after a course of therapy, is usually temporary but may persist for several months.

4. Instruct the patient to report ototoxic symptoms. High doses may cause tinnitus and deafness.

5. Therapy may precipitate herpes zoster, which usually necessitates interrupting medication.

Methotrexate

1. Warn the patient not to self-medicate with vitamins. Folic acid or its derivatives can alter the response to methotrexate.

2. Diabetes may be precipitated. Check for glycosuria periodically and instruct patient to report polyuria or polydipsia.

Dactinomycin

1. Observed the patient for signs of agranulocytosis, which may develop abruptly especially when drug is administered concurrently with radiation. Report weakness, fatigue, sore throat, chills, and stomatitis.

Vincristine

1. Gastrointestinal tract toxicity may result in severe constipation, which may require a high fiber diet, stool softeners, and suppositories to prevent impaction.

2. It may be possible to minimize hair loss by applying a scalp torniquet (to limit the concentrations of drug reaching the scalp) during and for 10–15 min after IV drug administration.

SUPPLEMENTARY READINGS

Bertino, J. R., and W. M. Hryniuk, "Disorders of Cell Growth," in *Clinical Pharmacology* (2nd ed.), eds. K. L. Melmon and H. F. Morrelli, Chapter 15, pp. 802–41. New York: Macmillan, Inc., 1978.

Bingham, C. A., "The Cell Cycle and Cancer Chemotherapy," *American Journal of Nursing* **78**: 1201–05 (1978).

Brodsky, I., and S. B. Kahn, ed., *Cancer Chemotherapy II.* New York: Grune & Stratton, Inc., 1972.

Chabner, B. A., and others, "The Clinical Pharmacology of Antineoplastic Agents," *New England Journal of Medicine*, **292**: 1107–13, 1159–68 (1975).

Cline, M. J., and C. M. Haskell, *Cancer Chemotherapy* (2nd ed.). Philadelphia: W. B. Saunders Company, 1975.

DeVita, V. T., and P. S. Schein, "The Use of Drugs in Combination for the Treatment of Cancer," *New England Journal of Medicine* **288**: 998–1006 (1973).

Hickey, R. C., ed., *Pharmacological Basis of Cancer Chemotherapy.* Baltimore: The Williams & Wilkins Company, 1975.

Holland, J. F., and E. Frei, III, ed., *Cancer Medicine.* Philadelphia: Lea & Febinger, 1973.

Levine, M. E., "Cancer Chemotherapy—A Nursing Module," *Nursing Clinics of North America* **13**: 271–280 (1978).

Miller, S. A., "Oncology Nurse and Chemotherapy," *American Journal of Nursing* **77**: 989–92 (1977).

Oberfield, R. A., ed., "Symposium on Malignant Disease," *Medical Clinics of North America* **59**(2): 237–504 (1975).

Pratt, W. B., and R. W. Ruddon, *The Anticancer Drugs.* New York: Oxford University Press, 1979.

Salmon, S. E., "Cancer Chemotherapy," in *Review of Medical Pharmacology* (6th ed.), eds. F. H. Meyers, E. Jawetz, and A. Goldfien, Chapter 45, pp. 480–516. Los Altos, California: Lange Medical Publications, 1978.

Sartorelli, A. C., and D. J. Johns, ed., *Antineoplastic and Immunosuppressive Agents.* Berlin: Springer-Verlag, 1975.

Stoll, B. A., ed., *Endocrine Therapy in Malignant Disease.* Philadelphia: W. B. Saunders Company, 1972.

ANTISEPTICS AND DISINFECTANTS

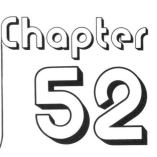

Chapter 52

Thousands of years before the nineteenth-century demonstration that bacteria were the primary cause of infectious diseases, embalmers in ancient Egypt had perfected the art of preserving mummies, which have been maintained to this day. Local antimicrobial agents are widely employed in clinics and hospitals, the household, in water purification, and for the preservation of foods and injectable drugs.

Considerable confusion exists about the precise meaning of the terms used to denote these drugs, and the nurse will note that these terms are sometimes used interchangeably. *Antiseptics* are chemicals, applied to living tissues, that are used to kill or prevent the growth of microorganisms. *Disinfectants* are chemicals, applied to inanimate objects, that destroy microorganisms by rapidly killing them. The term *germicide* is used to denote chemicals that destroy (kill) microorganisms.

ACTIONS AND USES

Unlike chemotherapeutic agents employed for systemic use, antiseptics and disinfectants possess little or no selective toxicity; that is, they are as toxic to the host cells as they are to the microbial parasite. Hence, although these drugs can be used to eliminate the microbial population on inanimate objects and can be applied to topical surfaces of the body, they lack the safety to be administered systemically.

Antiseptics and disinfectants kill or inhibit microbial growth by one of three primary mechanisms of action: (1) by *protein denaturation,* the drug produces a change in the structure of the microbial cell protein, which leads to its coagulation and destruction (phenols, alcohols, aldehydes); (2) by *surface tension reduction,* there is an increase in the permeability of the microbial cell membrane leading to the lysis and destruction of the cell (surface active agents); and (3) by *biochemical interference*, the drug may interfere with essential metabolic processes of the microbial cell resulting in inhibition of the ability of the cell to survive or multiply (compounds containing mercury).

Antiseptics are applied to living tissues to sterilize intact cutaneous and mucous surfaces and contaminated or infected wounds. These drugs should not be used on clean

446

wounds, since they inhibit tissue healing. Many authorities consider the washing of contaminated wounds with antiseptic solutions to be of questionable value and even possibly harmful. Careful washing or irrigation of the wound with soap and water or with an isotonic saline solution and removal of any foreign matter by mechanical means are considered to be more effective and less likely to injure the tissue. In addition, some antiseptics are inactivated by blood, pus, and the tissue proteins.

Tables 52-1 and 52-2 summarize the comparative properties of commonly used antiseptics and disinfectants, which have been classified according to their chemistry.

Table 52-1 Representative Antiseptics and Disinfectants

Generic name (other names) [trade name]	Method of application	Remarks
Alcohols		
Ethyl alcohol (alcohol; rubbing alcohol)	Topical (70%)	One of the widely used skin disinfectants; optimal concentration 70% (by volume). Effective bactericide; unreliable fungicide, virucide; inactive against dried spores.
Isopropyl alcohol (isopropanol)	Topical (70% undiluted)	Slightly greater bactericidal activity than ethyl alcohol.
Aldehydes		
Formaldehyde sol. (formol; formalin)	Disinfection of inanimate objects, (10–37%)	Effective but slow-acting disinfectant against bacteria, fungi, spores, viruses; highly disagreeable odor.
Acids		
Acetic acid	Topical: surgical dressings (1%); burn therapy sol. (5%); dermatological lotion (0.1%); bladder irrigation (0.25%).	Suppresses *Pseudomonas aeruginosa* in burns; suppresses vaginal infections; spermatocide. Can cause irritation and inflammation, especially in the vagina.
Boric acid [Borofax]	Ointment (5 and 10%); sol. (5%)	Little value as disinfectant but used as nonirritating antiseptic eye wash and ointment. Potentially toxic—containers should be labeled *Poison.* Symptoms: nausea, vomiting, diarrhea, headache, kidney damage, acute circulatory failure. Systemic absorption: after ingestion, serous cavities, abraded or inflamed skin. Medical use obsolete.
Halogen compounds		
Sodium hypochlorite sol. (bleach)	Disinfect instruments, root canal therapy (5%); skin germicide (0.5%), diluted 1:3	Diluted sodium hypochlorite sol. (0.5%) called *modified Dakin's solution;* disadvantages: dissolves blood clots and delays clotting. 5% sol. used as household bleach; ingestion by children causes irritation of mucous membranes.
Oxychlorosene sodium [Chlorpactin]	Topical (0.1–0.4% sol.)	Organic derivative of hypochlorous acid. Active against bacteria, fungi, viruses, molds, yeasts, and spores. Useful for treating localized infections particularly when resistant microorganisms are present.

Table 52-1   Continued

Generic name (other names) [trade name]	Method of application	Remarks
Iodine solution	Topical (2% aqueous sol.)	Effective nonirritating bactericide, fungicide applied to superficial lacerations. Preferred iodine preparation for use on skin and wounds.
Iodine tincture	Mild tincture (2% in alcohol); strong tincture (7% in alcohol)	Highly effective, but alcohol is irritating to wounds and does not contribute to antibacterial action. Addition of 3 drops of iodine tincture per quart of water kills bacteria and amebae in 15 min.
Povidone-iodine [Betadine, Frepp, Isodine, Povadyne]	Topical (1%); sol., spray, gargle, shampoo, surgical scrub, vaginal douche	Nonstinging organic iodine preparation with a broad spectrum of microcidal effects. Unlike iodine tincture, treated area may be bandaged or taped. Antiseptic on skin, mucous membranes; preoperative patient skin preparation and for washing and scrubbing of personnel. Discontinue if irritation, redness, or swelling develops. Prior to administering, ask patient about possible iodine allergy.
Mercury compounds		
Merbromin [Mercurochrome]	Topical (2% aqueous sol.)	Oldest organic mercurial antiseptic, commonly used in first-aid kits. Least effective commercial product.
Nitromersol [Metaphen]	Topical (0.2% sol. and 0.5% tincture)	Among best organic mercurials; tincture more germicidal than sol. Antistaph effects inferior to iodines and hexachlorophene.
Phenylmercuric acetate nitrate [Phe-Mer-Nite]	Topical (0.1–0.2%), disinfection of instruments (0.001–0.1%)	Inhibits bacteria and fungi, questionable sporicidal activity. Acetate used to treat vaginal infections and as preservative in ophthalmic sols. Nitrate is topical anesthetic.
Thimerosal [Merthiolate]	Topical as aerosol, sol., tincture (0.1%)	Although widely used, thimerosal has weak antibacterial and antifungal activity and is ineffective against spores; inferior to iodines and alcohol.
Silver compounds		
Silver nitrate	Ophthalmic sol. (1%)	Antiseptic, disinfectant, astringent, caustic. Effective bactericidal; used in newborns to prevent gonococcal infection ophthalmia neonatorum (wash immediately with water); sol. (0.5%) applied on dressings to prevent gram-negative burn infections.
Toughened silver nitrate (lunar caustic)	Pencil	For wound or mucous membrane cauterization and for removing granulation tissue. Moisten pencil in water and apply. Treated area will appear grayish-black.

Table 52-2 Representative Antiseptics and Disinfectants

Generic name (other name) [trade name]	Method of application	Remarks
Surface-active agents		
Benzalkonium chloride [Zephiran, Bactine, Germicin]	Topical: preoperative unbroken skin disinfection or treatment of superficial injuries (0.1% tincture); mucous membranes, broken skin (0.01–0.05% sol.) Disinfection: sterilization of surgical instruments (0.1%), with sodium nitrite (0.5%) to prevent rust of instruments.	Widely used all-purpose local antibacterial agent for application to skin and mucous membranes; ingredient in ophthalmic solutions and to disinfect contact lenses and surgical instruments. Low systemic toxicity if ingested; concentrated solution can produce corrosive skin lesions with deep necrosis and scarring. Diluted solution not generally irritating or sensitizing. Inactivated by soap.
Cetylpyridinium chloride [Cepacol]	Topical: sol. (1:2000) Lozenges: (1:500)	Local anti-infective agent used in a mouthwash and in throat lozenges.
Methylbenzethonium chloride (Diaparene)	Topical, in ointments, powders, creams, lotions	Local antiseptic used to treat ammonia dermatitis by application to skin and to diapers or underclothes.
Oxidizing agents		
Hydrogen peroxide (peroxide)	Topical (1.5–3%)	Short-acting, weak germicide with poor penetrability. Liberated oxygen mechanically removes tissue debris. Mouthwash (treat Vincent's stomatitis), vaginal douche.
Potassium permanganate	Topical (1:1000 to 1:10,000 sol.)	Useful anti-infective commonly employed for urethritis and as astringent in poison ivy.
Phenols and related compounds		
Phenol (carbolic acid)	Topical (1–2%)	Disinfectant of instruments; germicide at 1%. Ingredient in nonprescription mouthwashes, hemorrhoidal preparations, burn remedies, antipruritic (phenolated calamine lotion). Solutions stronger than 2% irritating to skin. Oral ingestion corrosive, painful; shock and death possible. Treat with gastric lavage with olive oil.
Resorcinol (resorcin)	Topical (1–20%) in lotions, gels, ointments.	Antifungal, antibacterial, local irritant used for treatment of ringworm, eczema, psoriasis, athlete's foot, seborrheic dermatitis; keratolytic for removal of corns, warts, calluses. May cause skin irritation or sensitization.
Hexachlorophene [pHisoHex, WescoHEX]	Topical (0.1–3%)	Strong bacteriostatic activity, particularly against gram-positive bacteria (staphylococci); little activity against spores; antifungal on inanimate objects. Used as antiseptic scrub by hospital personnel and dentists. Absorbed from intact skin, particularly after repeated applications; neurotoxic potential to infants. May cause erythema, dryness, and scaling in patients with sensitive skin.

Table 52-2   Continued

Generic name (other name) [trade name]	Method of application	Remarks
Chlorhexidine gluconate [Hibiclens, Hibitane]	Topical in liquid (4%), tincture (0.5%) for surgical hand scrub, hand wash, skin wound cleaner.	Rapid bactericidal activity against wide range of microorganisms. Active in presence of blood; does not delay wound healing. Keep out of eyes and ears.

SUPPLEMENTARY READINGS

Conference, "Hexachlorophene—Its Usage in the Nursery," *Pediatrics* **51**: Part II, 329–434 (1973).

Harmen, V. M., and S. M. Steele, *Nursing Care of the Skin: A Development Approach.* New York: Appleton-Century-Crofts, 1975.

Lawrence, C. A., and S. S. Block, ed., *Disinfection, Sterilization, and Preservation.* Philadelphia: Lea & Febiger, 1968.

Perkins, J. J., *Principles and Methods of Sterilization in the Health Sciences* (2nd ed.), Springfield, Ill.: Charles C Thomas, Publishers, 1969.

Reddish, G. F., ed., *Antiseptics, Disinfectants, Fungicides, and Chemical and Physical Sterilization.* Philadelphia: Lea & Febiger, 1957.

Zanowiak, P., "Topical Anti-Infective Products," in *Handbook of Nonprescription Drugs* (6th ed.), pp. 361–82. Washington, D.C.: American Pharmaceutical Association, 1979.

HISTAMINE AND ANTIHISTAMINES

Chapter 53

In this chapter we shall discuss the pharmacology of histamine, the role of this naturally occurring substance in allergies, and the therapeutic use of antihistamines for the symptomatic management of allergies and a variety of other medical disorders.

HISTAMINE

For approximately 70 years, histamine has been known to be present in both plants and animals, although to date, its precise role in normal physiology has yet to be defined. Histamine is found in most mammalian tissues and body fluids, with high concentrations in the skin, lungs, and stomach. A large percentage of total body histamine is present in the granules of *mast cells*, where it is bound to heparin. In these granules, histamine is not subject to enzymatic inactivation nor is it capable of producing its profound biologic effects.

Histamine Release

With the realization that histamine is at least partially responsible for mediating allergic reactions, considerable attention has been devoted toward learning more about those factors that cause its release from mast cells. In addition, chemical compounds (some of which the nurse will encounter as drugs) are able to cause the direct release of histamine by mechanisms that do not involve allergy.

Allergic disorders   An *allergy* is an exaggerated susceptibility to a substance that is attributable to an underlying *antigen-antibody reaction*. Substances that provoke the allergic response, the *allergens* (antigens), come from a myriad of sources and may include inhalants (which affect the respiratory tract), contactants (skin), and foods and drugs (skin, mucous membrane, blood, respiratory tract or digestive system). Representative drugs with high allergic potential include penicillin, aspirin, and the sulfonamides.

An *antigen* is a large molecule, usually a protein, that is capable of stimulating the formation of specific IgE *antibodies* (Figure 53-1). Most drug molecules are too small to be antigenic and must first combine with an endogenous carrier protein to form a drug-(hapten-) protein complex that is antigenic. When the body is first exposed to an antigen, antibody synthesis is stimulated and the body becomes sensitized to the presence of the antigen. Antibodies may circulate freely in the plasma or may be fixed in tissues. Upon re-exposure to that antigen or a very closely related substance, an antigen-antibody reaction occurs, resulting in the release of mediator

substances; these substances are directly responsible for the allergic symptoms. In humans, histamine and slow-reacting substances of anaphylaxis (SRS-A) are thought to be the primary mediators of the allergic response. At present, since only specific antagonists to histamine are clinically available (antihistamines), we shall restrict our subsequent discussion to the pharmacology of histamine.

Allergic reactions are often categorized as being immediate or delayed. *Immediate reactions* are generally observed after the antigenic substance has been rapidly absorbed, for example, after injection (foreign serums or a bee sting), ingestion (foods or drugs), or inhalation (pollens). By contrast, contactant allergens or those injected into the skin are more slowly absorbed and cause a *delayed reaction*.

In an immediate reaction, such as an anaphylactic shock, within minutes after re-exposure to the antigen the patient may complain of feelings of anxiety and a headache; these feelings are followed by circulatory and respiratory failure and shock. Unless prompt medical treatment (such as an injection of epinephrine) is initiated, death may result. It is, therefore, essential for the nurse to determine whether the patient has ever experienced an adverse drug reaction *prior* to administra-

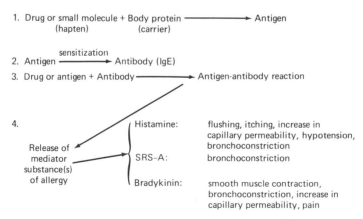

Figure 53-1.   Mechanisms of Allergic Reactions.

tion of a potential drug allergen or a chemically-related drug; for example, patients exhibiting an allergic response to one penicillin or sulfonamide will probably be allergic to all other members of these respective drug classes.

Nonallergic histamine release   A variety of drugs and other chemicals have been shown to stimulate the release of bound histamine from mast cells by mechanisms that do not appear to involve antigen-antibody reactions. Among the many *drugs* reported to cause histamine release include preoperative skeletal muscle relaxants (tubocurarine, dimethyltubocurarine, succinylcholine), narcotic analgesics (morphine, codeine, meperidine), organic compounds containing iodine that are employed exclusively as contrast media in diagnostic procedures (roentgenography), drugs used for the treatment of trypanosomiasis (stilbamidine), and the plasma substitutes dextran and polyvinylpyrrolidone (PVP).

Snake and insect *venoms* and *toxins* often contain enzymes and other proteins that are capable of causing the breakdown of mast cells, resulting in the release of histamine. After an insect sting, susceptible individuals—particularly those with a history of heart disease or asthma—may experience profuse sweating, marked hypotension, circulatory failure, and bronchoconstriction. In a very high percentage of cases, death occurs in less than one hour. Among these insects include bees, wasps, and hornets, stings from which resulted in over 200 deaths in the United States from 1949 to 1959.

Pharmacological Effects of Histamine

In humans, histamine causes contraction of the nonvascular smooth muscle of the bronchi and gastrointestinal tract, while causing relaxation of the vascular smooth muscle of minute blood vessels (capillaries). It is a potent stimulant of gastric acid production.

These effects have been attributed to the actions of this compound on *histamine receptors*, which have been subdivided into two types.* Contraction of nonvascular smooth muscles is mediated by activation of H_1-receptors, while enhanced gastric acid secretion involves H_2-receptors; relaxation of vascular smooth muscle and capillary vasodilation appears to be mediated by both H_1- and H_2-receptors. The actions of histamine on nonvascular smooth muscle and exocrine glands can be antagonized by specific blockers of each of these types of receptors, while a combination of both receptor-blocking drugs is required to antagonize the actions of histamine on capillaries.

Until relatively recently only antagonists of the H_1-receptors were available; these drugs are commonly referred to as *antihistamines* (Table 53-1, pages 454–455). While cimetidine (Tagamet) is the only H_2-antagonist now clinically available in the United States, the nurse should anticipate the appearance of pharmacologically similar drugs in the near future.

Cardiovascular system   Most of the major cardiovascular effects of histamine can be attributed, either directly or indirectly, to *vasodilation* of capillaries, arterioles, and venules. In addition, the permeability of the capillary membranes is increased, thus permitting the movement of plasma proteins and fluids into the extracellular spaces; this fluid accumulation results in edema. After sufficient amounts of plasma have escaped from the blood vessels, there is a reduction in the

---

*We have previously discussed several well-established precedents for the concept of multiple receptor types activated by a common chemical: epinephrine activates α-, β_1-, and β_2-adrenergic receptors, while acetylcholine activates muscarinic and nicotinic cholinergic receptor types.

Table 53-1   Representative H$_1$-Antagonist Antihistamines

Class and generic name	Selected trade names	Usual single oral adult dose (mg)	Properties of class or drugs
Ethanolamines			Class: High incidence of drowsiness and atropine-like (anticholinergic) side effects. Relatively low incidence of gastrointestinal upset.
Diphenhydramine[a]	Benadryl	25-50	Diphenhydramine: most widely used parenterally administered antihistamine for anaphylactic and other allergic reactions.
Dimenhydrinate[a]	Dramamine	50	Dimenhydrinate: motion sickness only.
Bromodiphenhydramine	Ambodryl	25	
Carbinoxamine	Clistin	4-8	
Doxylamine	Decapryn	12.5-25	
Ethylenediamines			Class: Lower incidence of drowsiness than ethanolamines; some dizziness. Mild gastrointestinal upset common.
Tripelennamine[a]	PBZ	50	Pyrilamine: Most common ingredient in nonprescription (OTC) sleep-aid preparations (Chapter 13).
Pyrilamine[a] (Neo-Antergan)		50	
Alkylamines			Class: Most potent class of H$_1$-antagonists (effective at lowest doses). Lowest incidence of drowsiness, making them most suitable for daytime use.
Chlorpheniramine[a]	Chlor-Trimeton, Histapan, Teldrin	2-4	Chlorpheniramine: Most widely used antihistamine.
Brompheniramine	Dimetane	4-8	
Dexchlorpheniramine	Polaramine	2	
Dimethindene	Forhistal	2.5	
Triprolidine[a]	Actidil	2.5	
Piperazines			Class: Relatively low incidence of drowsiness. Used primarily for prevention or treatment of motion sickness and postoperative nausea and vomiting. Duration of cyclizine and meclizine are 4-6 and 12-24 hours, respectively. Contraindicated during pregnancy.
Cyclizine	Marezine	50	
Meclizine[a]	Antivert		
	Bonine	25-50	
Phenothiazines			
Promethazine[a]	Phenergan	25	Promethazine: effective in motion sickness but high incidence of sedation.
Methdilazine	Tacaryl	8	Methdilazine and trimeprazine: used primarily as antipruritic (relieve itching); mild to moderate sedation.
Trimeprazine	Temaril	2.5	

Table 53-1   Continued

Class and generic name	Selected trade names	Usual single oral adult dose (mg)	Properties of class or drugs
Miscellaneous			
Azatadine	Optimine	1–2	Azatadine and cyproheptadine: histamine (H_1) and serotonin antagonists; antipruritic; moderate sedation. Cyproheptadine is contraindicated in glaucoma and urinary retention.
Cyproheptadine[a]	Periactin	4	
Diphenylpyraline	Diaphen, Hispril	2	

[a] Drug also marked under generic name.

circulating volume of blood, a decrease in blood pressure, and eventually shock. Hypotension activates a compensatory stimulation in heart rate in an attempt to restore circulation of an adequate amount of blood to maintain homeostasis. Profound histamine-induced vasodilation is also manifested by flushing of the face and upper trunk, a rise in skin temperature, and a throbbing vascular headache.

Intradermal injection of histamine produces a characteristic "triple response" consisting of (1) a rapidly appearing red spot at the site of injection resulting from dilation of small blood vessels; (2) a wheal consisting of localized edema and caused by increased capillary permeability; and (3) a bright red flare surrounding the wheal, a response mediated by an axon reflex involving peripheral sensory nerves.

Smooth muscles and exocrine glands Histamine stimulates nonvascular smooth muscles. In humans, particularly those suffering from such respiratory disorders as asthma, marked *bronchoconstriction* results from exposure to or marked release of histamine.

While capable of stimulating most exocrine glands, the most pronounced effects of histamine are noted on the *gastric glands* and manifested by an enhanced secretion of gastric acid (hydrochloric acid) and pepsin.

Clinical Uses

The contemporary clinical uses of histamine are very limited. Since it is rapidly inactivated by intestinal bacteria, it possesses little activity after oral administration and must be given parenterally. Histamine is employed as a diagnostic agent to assess gastric acid secretion. In this test, histamine (2.75 mg) is administered subcutaneously; in normal individuals, marked gastric acid secretion is noted. The absence of acid (achlorhydria) is caused by a loss of parietal cell function and is associated with pernicious anemia and some forms of stomach cancer.

The dose of histamine required to produce stimulation of gastric acid secretion often also causes flushing, sweating, tachycardia, hypotension, and a throbbing headache. *Betazole* (Histalog), a synthetic analog of histamine, is a potent stimulant of gastric acid secretion, although it causes a lower incidence of histamine-like adverse effects. This drug should, however, be used with great caution in patients with bronchial asthma. The usual adult dose is 50 mg administered subcutaneously.

Histamine is sometimes employed for

the diagnosis of *pheochromocytoma* (Chapter 6). Small doses of histamine (0.275 mg) stimulate the release of catecholamines from the adrenal medulla. In normal individuals, little change in blood pressure is observed, while in patients with pheochromocytoma, the massive release of catecholamines from the tumor results in a striking hypertensive response. The measurement of 24-hour urinary catecholamine excretion presents less potential risk to the patient than histamine administration and is currently the preferred procedure for the diagnosis of this disorder.

Repeated injections of histamine may reduce the sensitivity of patients with allergic disorders in which histamine is though to play a significant role as a mediator. This *desensitization* procedure has not been demonstrated to be generally effective.

H₁-ANTAGONISTS (ANTIHISTAMINES)

Two primary approaches are currently employed to prevent or antagonize the actions of histamine and thereby treat allergic disorders. These involve the use of physiological antagonists of histamine, such as the adrenergic (sympathomimetic) agents (Chapter 5) and the use of pharmacological antagonists such as blockers of H₁-receptors.

Physiological antagonists exert biological effects that are diametrically opposed to those produced by histamine. Whereas histamine causes bronchoconstriction, the adrenergic agents epinephrine and isoproterenol actively relax bronchial smooth muscle, producing bronchodilation, reopening airways that are essential for free and unobstructed breathing. *Pharmacological antagonists* compete with histamine for common cellular receptor sites. Unlike the physiological antagonists, antihistamines do not exert a positive

action themselves but rather restore normal function without improving upon it.

Actions

Antihistamines do not inhibit the synthesis or release of histamine, nor do they chemically or physically inactivate histamine. The H₁-antagonists are able to block histamine-induced contraction of the smooth muscles of the bronchioles and gastrointestinal tract; a combination of H₁- and H₂-antagonists is required to maximally inhibit capillary vasodilation. Histamine-induced stimulation of gastric acid secretion is unaffected by H₁-antagonists.

In addition to their ability to block the actions of histamine, antihistamines have a myriad of other actions, most of which cannot be explained on the basis of histamine antagonism. Some of these include effects on the central nervous system and antimotion sickness, antiparkinsonism, anticholinergic, and local anesthetic activities.

Adverse Effects and Toxicity

Although undesirable side effects are encountered when even therapeutic doses of H₁-antagonists are employed, severe adverse effects rarely occur. When we consider the very extensive use of these drugs, both alone and in combination with other compounds, the number of fatalities resulting from overdosage are extremely low. The undesirable effects caused by the antihistamines primarily involve the central nervous system, the autonomic nervous system, and the gastrointestinal tract. As you will note in Table 53-1, the relative incidence of these adverse effects differs among the five major classes of antihistamines. General nursing implications are summarized at the end of this chapter.

Central nervous system The most common undesirable effects associated with the use of the antihistamines, at both therapeutic and toxic doses, involve the central nervous system. In this regard, infants and very young children are particularly sensitive. In *young children*, toxic doses cause stimulation, which may be manifested as excitement, hallucinations, muscle tremors, and convulsions. Fixed, dilated pupils with a flushed face and fever are common at high doses. Convulsions may be controlled by the administration of thiopental sodium (Pentothal) or diazepam (Valium).

While some older children and adults may become restless, nervous, and unable to sleep, central nervous system *depression* is much more frequently encountered, resulting in impairment of both physical and mental performance. These effects vary in intensity from slight drowsiness to an inability to concentrate, dizziness with muscle weakness, deep sleep, and even coma. Tolerance develops to the drowsiness caused by therapeutic doses after several consecutive days of drug administration. The degree of depression produced is dependent upon the specific antihistamine, the dosage employed, and the susceptibility of the patient. There are no specific antidotes for antihistamine poisoning, with the treatment symptomatic and supportive in nature.

Nurses should strongly urge their patients to exercise extreme caution when operating motor vehicles or heavy machinery when taking antihistamines and avoid taking these drugs with alcohol, barbiturates, and other central nervous system depressants (Table 53-2).

Other adverse effects Since many antihistamines possess rather potent anticholinergic effects (in particular, the ethanolamine derivatives), it is not surprising that such drugs may cause dry mouth, blurred vision, and urinary retention. Gastrointestinal side effects may include loss of appetite, nausea, vomiting, gastric upset, and diarrhea. These unpleasantries can often be minimized by taking these drugs with meals.

Many of the H_1-antagonists are relatively powerful local anesthetics, and it is this action which serves as the basis for their topical use for the relief of itching or painful conditions of the skin and mucous membranes. Topical application of these drugs should be discouraged, because this route of administration is associated with a relatively high potential risk of allergic dermatitis.

The piperazine derivatives (cyclizine, meclizine) have been shown to produce fetal abnormalities in laboratory animals. Although similar teratogenic effects have not been demonstrated in humans, their use is

Table 53-2   Potential Drug Interactions Involving H_1-Antagonist Antihistamines

Interacting drug/class	Potential consequences

Central nervous system depressants
    alcohol
    antianxiety agents
    antipsychotic agents
    narcotic analgesics
    sedative-hypnotics
	Additive impairment of mental and physical function.

Anticholinergic agents (Table 8-2) Tricyclic antidepressants (Table 17-1)	Increased risk of atropine-like side effects, particularly in elderly patients when ethanolamine (diphenhydramine-type) antihistamines are employed.
Monoamine oxidase inhibitor antidepressants (Table 17-1)	MAO inhibitors may reduce rate of antihistamine metabolism, thus increasing the risk of adverse effects.

contraindicated in women who are pregnant or who may become pregnant.

Potential drug interactions involving the antihistamines are summarized in Table 53-2.

Therapeutic Considerations

There are approximately 30 chemically distinct H_1-antagonist antihistamines currently available. None of these drugs is completely effective for all patients or devoid of undesirable side effects. The major differences among the five major classes of antihistamines are not so much based upon differences in clinical effectiveness as upon the relative incidence of undesirable side effects (Table 53-1).

Antihistamines are among the most widely used classes of drugs. When appropriately employed, they are capable of providing the patient with a significant degree of symptomatic relief; unfortunately, these drugs are never capable of curing the underlying disease.

Allergic disorders Because of their diverse natures, sweeping generalizations cannot be made regarding the effectiveness of antihistamines in treating the many allergic disorders. Moreover, the relative effectiveness of a given drug for the management of a specific disorder may vary at different times during the year.

Antihistamines are highly effective (80 percent) for the symptomatic relief of *allergic rhinitis* (hay fever) early in the season, relieving sneezing, running nose, and itching of the eyes, nose, and throat. Later in the season, as the pollen (allergen) count rises, the degree of symptomatic relief provided by these drugs decreases proportionately. In vasomotor or *perennial rhinitis*, antihistamines may only provide partial relief to 50 percent of all patients.

The antihistamines are probably most effective in the management of acute and chronic *urticaria* (hives), with the itching and wheals rapidly relieved in 70 to 80 percent of all patients.

In acute life-threatening allergic disorders, such as *angioneurotic edema* or *anaphylactic shock*, the physiological antagonists (adrenergic agents, theophylline) are employed to actively reverse the respiratory distress provoked by bronchoconstriction. In such cases, it is imperative to provide the patient with rapid and positive bronchodilation. After such emergency therapy has produced its beneficial effects, antihistamines may be useful as adjunctive agents.

Antihistamines are generally ineffective for the management of *bronchial asthma*. As will be noted in Chapter 54, the bronchoconstriction associated with this respiratory disorder results from the release of multiple mediator substances, only one of which is histamine. Antihistamines are ineffective in blocking the adverse effects of SRS-A and other endogenous chemical mediators.

The nurse will observe the inclusion of an antihistamine in virtually all multiple ingredient preparations marketed for the treatment of the *common cold*. Notwithstanding early promotional claims and current misconceptions harbored by the general public, antihistamines are neither capable of curing the common cold nor shortening its duration. The symptomatic reduction in rhinorrhea (runny nose) often noted during the early phases of the cold may result from the anticholinergic effects of these drugs. The patient experiencing chronic allergic rhinitis superimposed upon a cold will probably benefit from antihistamine administration.

Motion sickness Among the most important uses of selected antihistamines is for the prevention and treatment of motion sickness associated with travel by land, air, or sea. In general, two major classes of centrally acting drugs are used for this disorder, namely, anticholinergic agents (scopolamine) and certain H_1-antagonists. Clinical studies have demonstrated that scopolamine is the most effective single drug for the prevention and relief of motion sickness. Of the antihistamines, promethazine (Phenergan) is most useful, with dimenhydrinate (Dramamine), cyclizine (Marezine), and meclizine (Antivert, Bonine) less effective. Since is is far easier to prevent motion sickness than to effect a cure, the nurse should recommend that patients take their medication approximately 30 minutes prior to starting the offending motion.

Parkinson's disease The use of selected H_1-antagonists for the treatment of Parkinson's disease has been discussed previously (Chapter 19). Among the antihistamines found to be useful are those possessing central anticholinergic (antimuscarinic) actions and include chlorphenoxamine (Phenoxene), orphenadrine (Disipal), and benztropine (Cogentin). Benztropine has pharmacological properties similar to diphenhydramine (Benadryl) and atropine.

While the antihistamines cause fewer side effects than levodopa (Bendopa, Dopar, Larodopa) or the anticholinergic-antiparkinson agents (Table 19-1, page 156), the antihistamines provide little benefit for the relief of tremors and salivation. The antihistamines are most commonly employed as adjuncts to levodopa therapy, particularly in the elderly, since their sedative properties may reduce the anxiety and insomnia associated with levodopa.

Insomnia The antihistamine pyrilamine is the most common ingredient contained in nonprescription medications intended for use as nighttime sleep-aids. Some clinical evidence suggests that pyrilamine (at single bedtime doses of 25 mg to a maximum of 100 mg) may be effective for the treatment of insomnia; the evidence supporting this conclusion is by no means overwhelming. This compound is considered relatively safe and possesses no abuse potential.

H_2-Antagonists

Prior to 1972 the only histamine antagonists developed were those capable of blocking the effects of histamine at its H_1 receptor. Histamine-mediated increase in gastric secretion was conspicuously refractory to blockade by these classical histamine antagonists.

In 1977 *cimetidine* (Tagamet) became the first H_2-antagonist approved for general clinical use in the United States. This orally active drug inhibits both histamine- and pentagastrin-induced secretion of gastric acid and pepsin, as well as the basal secretion of acid. Many experts believe that H_2-antagonists will revolutionize the management of *peptic ulcer disease*. Cimetidine has been found to be useful for the treatment of duodenal ulcers, Zollinger-Ellison syndrome, and gastric ulceration. The pharmacology and therapeutic uses of this drug will be considered in Chapter 55, when we discuss drugs employed for the treatment of peptic ulcer disease.

Antihistamines:
nursing implications

1. An attempt should be made to identify the allergen. If a severe allergic reaction to a drug has been experienced, the patient should be advised to wear identification indicating this fact.

2. Antihistamines may cause CNS depression, resulting in sedation, dizziness, impaired coordination or muscle weakness. This depression can be enhanced by the co-administration of other CNS depressants. Caution patients against driving or engaging in other activities requiring mental alertness and motor coordination until the effect of the antihistamine has been evaluated. Drowsiness may disappear spontaneously with continued use as tolerance develops.

3. Advise the patient to report side effects to physician. A reduction in the drug dosage may be indicated or a different drug may be preferable. The relative incidence of side effects varies among classes of antihistamines (Table 53-1, pages 454-455) and specific members of a class, as well as among patients.

4. Paradoxical CNS stimulation may occur, particularly in children, causing restlessness, insomnia, excitement, euphoria, palpitations, and tremors. Caution patient to store this drug out of the reach of children.

5. Overdose can cause CNS stimulation or depression, with the latter usually observed in adults. Stimulation is manifested by incoordination, hallucinations, and convulsions. Treatment is symptomatic and supportive.

6. When taken to prevent motion sickness, administer 30 min prior to motion.

7. Topical application of antihistamines should be limited to a short period. Prolonged use can result in rebound sensitization.

SUPPLEMENTARY READINGS

Beaven, M. A., "Histamine," *New England Journal of Medicine* **294**: 30–36, 320–25 (1976).

Bellanti, J. A., *Immunology* (2nd ed.). Philadelphia: W. B. Saunders Company, 1978.

Brand, J. J., and W. L. M. Perry, "Drugs Used in Motion Sickness," *Pharmacological Reviews* **18**: 895–924 (1966).

Douglas, W. D., "Histamine and 5-Hydroxytryptamine (Serotonin) and Their Antagonists," in *Goodman and Gilman's The Pharmacological Basis of Therapeutics* (6th ed.), eds. A. G. Gilman, L. S. Goodman, and A. Gilman, Chapter 26, pp. 609–46. New York: Macmillan, Inc., 1980.

Grillo, V. J., and K. F. Tempers, "Pharmacology and Therapeutic Use of Antihistamines," *American Journal of Hospital Pharmacy* **33**: 1200–07 (1976).

Kaliner, M., and K. F. Austen, "Immunologic Release of Chemical Mediators From Human Tissue," *Annual Review of Pharmacology* **15**: 177–89 (1975).

Parker, C. W., "Drug Allergy," *New England Journal of Medicine* **292**: 511–14, 732–36, 957–60 (1975).

Roth, F. E., and I. I. A. Tabachnick, "Histamine and Antihistamines," in *Drill's Pharmacology in Medicine* (4th ed.), ed. J. R. DiPalma, Chapter 48, pp. 995–1020. New York: McGraw-Hill Book Company, Inc., 1971.

Schacter, M., ed., *"Histamine and Antihistamines,"* Vol. 1. *International Encyclopedia of Pharmacology and Therapeutics*, Sec. 74. Oxford: Pergamon Press, Inc., 1973.

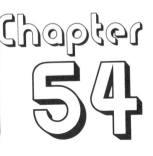

ANTIASTHMATIC AGENTS

Chapter 54

Bronchial asthma is a chronic disease characterized by respiratory distress resulting from episodic obstruction of airflow. This disease, affecting 1 to 2 percent of the population, is clinically manifested by wheezing, dyspnea, and coughing. In this chapter, we shall briefly review the physiology of the respiratory system, examine the types and causes of bronchial asthma, and then consider the use of drugs to treat this disease.

PHYSIOLOGY AND PATHOPHYSIOLOGY OF RESPIRATION

The *respiratory system* consists of a series of airways ultimately terminating in air sacs. The mouth and nasal passages lead to the pharynx and then to the trachea. The trachea divides into two large bronchi, each of which supplies air to one lung. Each bronchus subdivides into progressively smaller branches, namely, the bronchioles, alveolar ducts, alveolar sacs, and alveoli. There is a progressive thinning of the walls of each of these airways; at the level of the alveoli, the wall consists of a single cell.

The process of *internal respiration* involves the exchange of gases across the 150 million alveoli in each lung. Oxygen passes across the alveolar walls into the pulmonary capillaries surrounding the alveoli and is distributed throughout the body, while carbon dioxide moves in the opposite direction for ultimate elimination from the body. In patients with bronchial asthma, there is an interference with this free exchange of gases.

Sympathetic-Parasympathetic Influences

Bronchial smooth muscle tone, which determines the diameter of the bronchioles and their resistance to airflow, is under neural and humoral control. Normal tone is determined by a balance between sympathetic (adrenergic) and parasympathetic (cholinergic) influences. Activation of β-adrenergic receptors in the bronchioles, in particular the β_2-receptors (Chapter 5), causes bronchodilation (Figure 54-1), while stimulation of α-adrenergic receptors or cholinergic receptors cause bronchoconstriction (Figure 54-2). The catecholamines and acetylcholine re-

461

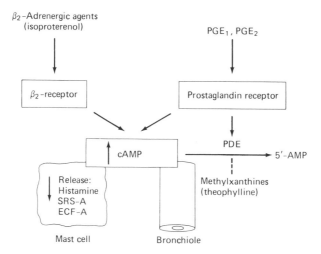

Figure 54-1. Pharmacological Basis for Antiasthmatic Agents. Beta-adrenergic agents and certain prostaglandins (PGE), via activation of their respective receptors, increase cyclic adenosine monophosphate (cAMP) levels in both mast cells and bronchial smooth muscle. Increased cAMP inhibits antigen-induced release of the chemical mediators of allergic asthma and bronchoconstriction (histamine, SRS-A, ECF-A) from mast cells and causes relaxation of smooth muscles (bronchodilation). Methylxanthines inhibit phosphodiesterase (PDE)-mediated inactivation of cAMP at both sites. The corticosteroids may act at both sites by multiple actions that may involve sensitization of the β_2-receptors to endogenous catecholamines, Cromolyn stabilizes the mast cell membrane preventing the release of the chemical mediators.

leased after the activation of adrenergic and cholinergic nerves, respectively, act indirectly on bronchial smooth muscle via the "second messengers," cyclic adenosine-3′,5′-monophosphate (cAMP) and cyclic guanosine monophosphate (cGMP), which have antagonistic actions.

Activation of the β_2-receptor stimulates the activity of the enzyme adenyl cyclase, which increases the conversion of adenosine triphosphate (ATP) to cAMP (Chapter 33); elevated levels of cAMP cause relaxation of smooth muscle, which results in bronchodilation. Beta-adrenergic stimulation can result from the release of endogenous cate-

cholamines or via the administration of drugs with sympathomimetic activity. Cyclic AMP is inactivated by the enzyme phosphodiesterase, and this enzyme can be inhibited by theophylline and related methylxanthines. Hence, the sympathomimetics and methylxanthines can increase cAMP concentrations by different mechanisms, both of which result in bronchodilation (Figure 54-1).

Cyclic GMP is under the control of the parasympathetic nervous system. Its concentration is increased by stimulation of the cholinergic vagus nerve (and the release of acetylcholine) or by the administration of

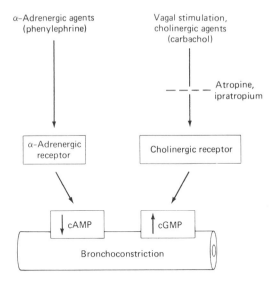

Figure 54-2.   Alpha-Adrenergic and Cholinergic Pathways Mediating Bronchoconstriction. Activation of the α-adrenergic receptor decreases cAMP; stimulation of the vagus nerve or administration of cholinergic agents increases levels of cyclic guanosine monophosphate (cGMP). Decreased levels of cAMP or increased levels of cGMP cause contraction of bronchial smooth muscle resulting in bronchoconstriction. Administration of atropine and related anticholinergic agents (ipratropium) produces bronchodilation by preventing activation of the cholinergic receptor.

cholinergic agents (Chapter 7). Increased concentrations of cGMP produce bronchoconstriction and a resulting increase in airway resistance, effects which can be antagonized by atropine and other anticholinergic agents (Figure 54-2).

Bronchial Asthma

Asthma usually occurs in episodes which vary in duration from a few minutes to several hours. Between attacks, respiratory function is essentially normal, and the patient is asymptomatic. An *asthmatic attack* usually begins with tightness in the chest, followed by coughing, wheezing, and dyspnea, which becomes progressively worse with time; expiration is more difficult than inspiration. These symptoms result from bronchial hypersecretion, bronchial mucosal edema which reduces the diameter of the lumen, and bronchial smooth muscle constriction. The sputum is thick and difficult to expectorate. Physical examination of the patient experiencing moderately severe symptoms reveals the use of accessory respiratory muscles with intercostal retraction; bilateral coarse breath sounds and wheezes are present, especially upon expiration, but no rales.

Status asthmaticus is an unrelenting attack lasting more than 24 hours. This condition is a medical emergency requiring hospitalization and may result in severe impairment of pulmonary function, cyanosis, and death.

Asthmatic patients are generally classified as having either extrinsic or intrinsic asthma, although many individuals have characteristics of both types. *Extrinsic (atopic, allergic) asthma* has an allergic basis and is generally characterized by its appearance in children and young adults; a family history of allergy; seasonal variation in the symptoms; positive skin tests and elevated circulating levels of immunoglobulin E (IgE); good responses to bronchodilators and cromolyn (Intal). By contrast, *intrinsic asthma* occurs later in life (over 35 years of age) and is characterized by a negative family history of allergy, negative skin tests, normal serum levels of IgE, the development of nasal polyps, and aspirin intolerance.

In patients with extrinsic (allergic) asthma, serum levels of IgE are generally elevated. Interaction of an allergen (antigen) with the IgE antibody bound to the membrane of a sensitized mast cell reduces intracellular levels of cAMP and results in the release of chemical mediators (Chapter 53); among the most important of these chemicals are histamine, slow-reacting substance of anaphylaxis (SRS-A), and eosinophil chemotactic factor of anaphylaxis (ECF-A). These chemicals, and perhaps others, cause contraction of bronchial smooth muscle, which is clinically manifested as bronchospasm. By contrast, increased intracellular levels of cAMP prevent the release of these chemical mediators from the sensitized mast cell (Figure 54-1).

As noted above, the normal control of bronchial smooth muscle occurs through a balance between opposing adrenergic and cholinergic influences. Intrinsic asthma may result from an imbalance in autonomic function. More specifically, it has been suggested that asthmatic bronchoconstriction may be caused by overactive cholinergic stimuli or inadequate β-adrenergic activation.

Factors precipitating asthmatic attacks Many factors have been shown to be capable of precipitating asthmatic attacks in susceptible individuals. These include psychological stimuli, pulmonary infections (increasing levels of antibodies in the lungs and stimulating mucus accumulation), physical exertion, atmospheric pollutants (including tobacco smoke), and drugs. Common examples of such drugs include compounds that block the β-adrenergic receptor (propranolol (Inderal)); increase the levels of cGMP (cholinergic agents); decrease intracellular cAMP levels by inhibiting prostaglandin synthesis (aspirin, indomethacin (Indocin), mefenamic acid (Ponstel)) or by activating the α-adrenergic receptor (phenylephrine (Neo-Synephrine)); stimulate the release of histamine from mast cells (d-tubocurarine, morphine, radiopaque organic iodides used as diagnostic agents). All these drugs should be administered with extreme caution to known or suspected asthmatic patients, if given at all.

DRUG TREATMENT OF BRONCHIAL ASTHMA

At present, no drug or other therapeutic procedure is capable of curing asthma or permanently correcting the fundamental aberration responsible for its origin. The available drugs are employed to prevent or manage acute attacks or exacerbations to permit the patient to carry out normal or near-normal activities. Nursing implications associated with the treatment of asthma are summarized at the end of this chapter.

Drugs used to manage asthma include the bronchodilator sympathomimetics and methylxanthines (theophylline derivatives), corticosteroids, cromolyn, and the expectorant-mucolytics; selected anticholinergic agents are currently being assessed for potential clinical use. Bronchodilator agents are the mainstay of asthma therapy and are employed to both prevent and terminate acute attacks.

Sympathomimetics

It will be recalled from Chapter 5 that the β-adrenergic receptors have been subdivided into two types: β_1-activation causes an increase in the force and rate of cardiac contraction, while β_2-stimulation leads to relaxation of the bronchial smooth muscle (bronchodilation) and muscle tremors. Alpha-adrenergic receptor activation causes contraction of vascular smooth muscle and may also give rise to bronchoconstriction. Recent years have witnessed the development and clinical introduction of more selective β_2-agonists for the treatment of asthma that have little or no α- and β_1-activities (Table 54-1).

Epinephrine and ephedrine *Epinephrine* has α- and β- (β_1- and β_2-) adrener-

Table 54-1   Comparative Properties of Sympathomimetic Bronchodilators

Generic name	Selected trade names	Usual adult dose	Adrenergic receptor	Remarks
Epinephrine	Adrenalin, Asmolin, Sus-Phrine Adrenalin chloride Bronitin Mist, Medihaler-Epi, Primatene Mist, Vaponefrin	SC: 0.2–0.5 mg (0.2–0.5 ml of 1:1,000 sol.) q. 2 h PRN Oral inhalation: least needed to obtain relief.	$\alpha_1, \beta_1, \beta_2$	Subcutaneous: arrest of acute asthmatic attack. Short duration of action. Adverse effects, α- and β-stimulation: anxiety, tremors, tachycardia, arrhythmias, hypertension. Avoid excessive inhalation: adverse effects (above), irritation bronchial mucosa, mucus accumulation.
Ephedrine		PO: 25–50 mg q. 3–4 h	α, β_1, β_2	Actions similar to epinephrine. Orally active, longer duration of action. Used to prevent asthmatic attacks. Adverse effects: central stimulation (nervousness, excitability, insomnia), cardiac palpitations, hypertension.
Pseudoephedrine	Novafed, Sudafed	PO: 60 mg 3–4 times daily	α, β_1, β_2	Similar to ephedrine with reportedly less central stimulation and hypertension. Useful nasal decongestant but antiasthmatic effects not clearly demonstrated.
Methoxyphenamine	Orthoxine	PO: 50–100 mg q.i.d.	β_1, β_2	Similar to ephedrine, with more selective β-effects and fewer cardiovascular effects.
Isoproterenol	Isuprel, Medihaler-Iso, Norisodrine	Oral inhalation, inhaler: 1–2 puffs up to 5 times daily Solution: 5–15 and 3–7 inhalations of 1:200 and 1:100 sol., respectively, up to 5 times daily Sublingual: 10–15 mg, 3–4 times daily	β_1, β_2	Potent β-stimulant. Effective in preventing and relieving bronchoconstriction. Short duration of action (1–3 h). Oral inhalation most effective route of administration. Overuse may cause palpitations, tachycardia, arrhythmias, hypotension, tremors, headache, nervousness; tolerance to bronchodilatory effects may occur or precipitate paradoxical severe asthmatic attack.
Isoetharine	Bronkosol, Bronkometer	Oral inhalation: q. 4–6 h	β_2 (some β_1)	Preferential β_2. Relatively short duration of action; comparable to isoproterenol, but fewer side effects.
Metaproterenol	Alupent, Metaprel	Oral inhalation: 2–3 puffs q. 4 h; not over 12 puffs per day PO: 20 mg q. 6–8 h	β_2 (some β_1)	Similar to isoproterenol but greater β_2-specificity (lower incidence of adverse cardiovascular effects) and longer duration of action. Oral preparation more effective, fewer adverse effects than ephedrine.

Table 54-1   Continued

Generic name	Selected trade names	Usual adult dose	Adrenergic receptor	Remarks
Protokylol	Ventaire	PO: 2–4 mg q.i.d.	β_1, β_2	Similar to isoproterenol, but effective orally and longer duration of action. Cardiac side effects. Not widely used.
Ethylnorepinephrine	Bronkephrine	SC or IM: 0.6–2 mg (0.3–1 ml)	β_1, β_2	Similar to isoproterenol but less active. May be useful in diabetic and hypertensive patients since it has little hyperglycemic or pressor effects.
Terbutaline	Brethine, Bricanyl	SC: 0.25 mg, repeated in 15–30 min PRN; dose not to exceed 0.5 mg in any 4-h period PO: 5 mg q 6 h	β_2	β_2-specific with little or no adverse effects on cardiovascular system; loses β_2-specificity when given by injection. Long duration of action. Muscle tremors common at 5-mg dose.
Albuterol (Salbutamol)		Oral inhalation: q. 4–6 h PO: 2–4 mg q. 4–6 h	β_2	Similar to terbutaline. Not approved for use in U.S.; widely used in Canada and Europe.

gic activities. The actions of this drug on the α-receptor produce vasoconstriction of the bronchial mucosal vessels, which causes a reduction in congestion and edema; this action is particularly prominent when epinephrine is inhaled. When these secretions are reduced, the mucous plugs become more viscid and tenacious and may occasionally be responsible for bronchoconstriction.

In normal clinical use the β_2-actions are far more pronounced, making epinephrine a highly useful bronchodilator agent for the management of an acute asthmatic attack; it has an onset of action of several minutes and a relatively short duration of action (2 to 3 hours). Oral epinephrine is rapidly inactivated by enzymes in the gastrointestinal tract, and so this drug is effective only when administered parenterally or by inhalation.

Frequent use of sympathomimetics, particularly epinephrine inhalation, can lead to *tolerance* is its bronchodilating effects, resulting in its relative or absolute ineffectiveness in managing an acute asthmatic attack. Withdrawal of the drug for several days may restore responsiveness of the bronchioles.

Ephedrine is among the most widely used bronchodilators in nonprescription antiasthmatic preparations. This sympathomimetic agent has both α- and β-activities but differs from epinephrine in several major respects. It is orally active, has a long onset of action (about 30 to 60 minutes), and a relatively long duration of action (3 to 5 hours). Ephedrine is clinically employed to *prevent* attacks in patients with mild asthma, while epinephrine is used to *terminate* acute attacks of moderate to severe intensity.

Isoproterenol   Isoproterenol (Isuprel), the most potent β-adrenergic stimulant, is a powerful relaxant of bronchial smooth muscle with minimal hypertensive effects. Since this sympathomimetic agent has equal activity on β_1- and β_2-receptors, the main adverse effects are on the heart (arrhythmias, anginal pain); tremors and headache may also occur.

This drug is well absorbed by inhalation but is unreliable after sublingual and oral administration. The usual dose is 0.1 mg (0.05 to 0.25 mg) by aerosol, which is generally provided by 1 to 2 puffs from metered dose inhalers. The nurse should instruct the patient to wait 1 to 2 minutes after the first dose before administering the second and not to use the inhaler more than three times during a single attack nor more frequently than every 3 hours. If these doses do not provide adequate bronchodilation in the absence of tachycardia or if respiratory symptoms seem worse after drug administration, the patient should be advised to consult the physician for additional drugs.

Selective beta₂ agents Selective β_2-agonists have preferential but not absolute activity on this receptor type. These drugs are preferred over epinephrine and isoproterenol for use in older patients, those with coronary artery disease, or those who are susceptible to arrhythmias. A side effect common to these drugs is β_2-mediated muscle tremors.

There are few outstanding differences among these drugs (Table 54-1). Oral administration of *metaproterenol* (Alupent, Metaprel) causes a higher incidence of side effects than when this drug is inhaled, although still fewer than ephedrine; by mouth this drug produces good but inconsistent bronchodilation. *Terbutaline* (Brethine, Bricanyl) has a long duration of action (at least 4 to 6 hours) after oral administration; the incidence of muscle tremors increase substantially when the dose is increased from 2.5 to 5 mg. The β_2-selectivity is markedly reduced after terbutaline injection and, when so administered, offers few advantages over epinephrine.

Adverse side effects and precautions The most frequently encountered adverse effects that are common to all β-adrenergic agents include cardiovascular effects (tachycardia, palpitations, dizziness, arrhythmias, hypertension), cerebral effects (anxiety, headache, nausea), and muscle tremors.

Contraindications to use, both relative and absolute, include acute coronary artery disease, cardiac disease, hyperthyroidism, cerebral arteriosclerosis, and hypertension; epinephrine should not be used in diabetic patients or those with narrow-angle glaucoma. Drugs with relatively potent α-activity (epinephrine, ephedrine) should be employed with caution in older men with prostatic hypertrophy, in whom these drugs can precipitate acute urinary retention. Other precautions appear in Chapter 6 and potential drug interactions involving sympathomimetic agents are summarized in Table 6-2 (page 61) and Table 54-3 (page 469).

Methylxanthines

Methylxanthines represent the other major class of bronchodilators commonly employed in the management of bronchial asthma (Table 54-2). The primary pharmacological effects of *theophylline*, the prototype drug in this class, are on the bronchi and cardiovascular system. These effects include relaxation of smooth muscle and bronchiolar tone, coronary artery dilation, reduction in peripheral vascular resistance, and a transient increase in cardiac output that results in diuresis of short duration; stimulation of skeletal muscle also occurs.

Since wide variation in the plasma half-life or theophylline is observed among patients (2.5 to 9.5 hours), individualized daily doses ranging from 400 to 3200 mg may be

Table 54-2 Comparative Properties of Methylxanthines

Generic name	Theophylline (%)	Equivalent dose, mg	Selected trade names	Usual adult doses	Remarks
Theophylline anhydrous	100	100	Aerolate, Bronkodyl, Elixophyllin, Matax[a] Quibron[a] Slo-Phyllin, Tedral[a] Theophyl, Theolair	PO: 200–250 mg q. 6 h Rectal: 250–500 mg q. 8–12 h	Plasma theophylline levels can be determined to increase therapeutic response and reduce toxicity; optimal plasma levels 1–2 mg/dl. Oral theophylline useful in mild to moderate asthma, given every 4–6 h on 24-h schedule to maintain blood levels; long-acting preparations less reliably absorbed than dyphylline or oxtriphylline. Liver disease increases plasma half-life; decrease dose 25–50%.
Theophylline monoethanolamine	75	133	Fleed Brand Theophyllin	Rectal: 250–500 mg q. 12 h	
Theophylline sodium glycinate	50	200	Gyhazan, Synophylate, Theofort	PO: 330–660 mg q. 6–8 h	
Theophylline calcium salicylate	48	208	Quadrinal[a]	PO: In mixtures only	
Aminophylline (theophylline ethylenediamine) anhydrous dihydrate	86 79	116 127	Somophyllin	PO: 200–300 mg q. 6–8 h Rectal: 250–500 mg b.i.d. IV (slowly in 10–20 ml diluent): 500 mg o.d.	Absorption from GI tract after oral or rectal administration is incomplete, slow, variable. Used IV to relieve acute bronchospasm or status asmaticus. Bronchodilator increases cardiac output, reduces venous pressure. Used with congestive heart failure, Cheyne-Stokes respiration, relief of pulmonary edema, paroxysmal noctural dyspnea. Relatively nontoxic; side effects are headache, dizziness, nervousness, nausea, vomiting, and epigastric pain.
Dyphylline (dihydroxypropyl theophylline)	70	143	Airet, Dilor, Lufyllin, Neothylline	PO: 300 mg q. 6–8 h IM: 250–500 mg several times daily	May be more consistently absorbed and less irritating orally than theophylline and aminophylline. Not recommended in angina pectoris or coronary disease. Is chemically related to theophylline, but unlike other drugs, is not a theophylline salt.
Oxtriphylline (choline theophyllinate)	64	156	Brondecon[a] Choledyl	PO: 200 mg q.i.d.	Better absorbed, less irritation orally than aminophylline. Development of tolerance infrequent.

[a]Selected antiasthmatic mixtures containing a methylxanthine.

required. Clinical studies reveal that the optimal therapeutic range of plasma theophylline is from 1 to 2 mg/dl (10 to 20 μg/ml). Lower levels are often ineffective, while at higher levels side effects are common and potentially very dangerous. When using theophylline derivatives, the dosage should be calculated on the basis of the amount of theophylline base present (Table 54-2). Intravenous aminophylline is the treatment of choice for severe acute asthmatic attacks.

Adverse effects The major adverse effects of theophylline result from local irritation of the stomach (anorexia, nausea, vomiting, abdominal distress) and stimulation of the central nervous system (irritability, agitation, insomnia, and, in overdosage, convulsions). Serious toxicity and death may occur at theophylline levels over 4 mg/ml without earlier signs of lesser toxicity.

Since the methylxanthines have fewer pronounced effects on the heart than epinephrine or isoproterenol, they are preferred to all but the most selective β_2-agents for use in patients with heart disease. Nevertheless, because the methylxanthines do increase the rate and force of contractions of the heart and cause tachyarrhythmias, particularly at high plasma levels, caution must be exercised. Potential drug interactions involving theophylline are summarized in Table 54-3.

Corticosteroids

For patients failing to respond to standard antiasthmatic agents, it may be necessary to initiate corticosteroid (adrenocortical steroid, glucocorticoid) administration. These drugs often provide dramatic therapeutic benefit and may even be life-saving. Their potential usefulness is limited by the adverse effects associated with long-term oral adminintration (Chapter 34). Potential drug interactions are summarized in Table 34-5.

The mechanism by which corticosteroids produce their antiasthmatic effects is not well understood; it is thought to involve multiple actions. Such actions may include reduction in the permeability of capillaries, vasoconstriction of these vessels, relaxation of bronchial smooth muscle, reduction in bronchial edema, and inhibition of antibody

Table 54-3   Potential Drug Interactions Involving Antiasthmatic Agents

Antiasthmatic agent/class	Interacting drug/class	Potential consequences
Sympathomimetics Theophylline	β-adrenergic blockers Propranolol (Inderal)	This β-adrenergic blocker has been demonstrated to antagonize the bronchodilatory effects of sympathomimetics (and may also possibly antagonize similar effects by theophylline and derivatives), potentially causing bronchospasm and inducing an asthmatic attack.
Ephedrine Pseudoephedrine	Monoamine oxidase inhibitor antidepressants Isocarboxazid (Marplan) Phenelzine (Nardil) Tranylcypromine (Parnate)	These drugs increase the amount of norepinephrine in storage sites of adrenergic neurons. Ephedrine (and other indirect-acting sympathomimetics, Chapter 5) can cause excessive catecholamine release resulting in severe hypertension.
Theophylline	Troleandomycin (TAO)	This antibiotic, which may be useful in the treatment of severe chronic asthma, inhibits the metabolism of theophylline, thus potentially increasing the risk of toxicity.

formation; they may also help restore the responsiveness of the bronchial smooth muscle of asthmatic patients to β-activation.

Aerosol administration: beclomethasone Corticosteroids can be administered orally (Table 34-2, page 289) or by inhaled aerosols for the management of chronic asthma. Intravenous injection of hydrocortisone (Solu-Cortef) controls status asthmaticus. The recent introduction of the synthetic corticosteroid beclomethasone dipropionate (Vanceril) represents an effective method of topical steroid administration (by inhalation) with very limited systemic absorption and few adverse effects.

Inhaled beclomethasone has been found to be as effective as orally administered glucocorticoids (prednisone) in controlling symptoms in patients with mild to moderate asthma requiring long-term corticosteroid therapy. The usual daily dose of beclomethasone is 400 μg, administered as 2 puffs from the aerosol four times daily. The most common side effect is oropharyngeal candidiasis. Nurses should recommend that their patients rinse their mouths and gargle with water after each inhalation to reduce the colonization by the fungus *Candida*. Beclomethasone is contraindicated in status asthmaticus and other acute asthmatic episodes requiring intensive measures.

The dosage requirements of orally administered corticosteroids can be reduced by 50 to 100 percent with the use of inhaled topical corticosteroids. To prevent the adverse effects associated with acute adrenal insufficiency (Chapter 34), the dose of the oral steroid must be slowly and cautiously reduced over a period of many weeks.

Cromolyn (Disodium Cromoglycate)

Cromolyn sodium (Intal) is not a bronchodilator and has no anti-inflammatory or anti-mediator (antihistaminic) activities. The antiasthmatic effects of this drug have been attributed to its ability to stabilize the membrane of the sensitized mast cell and thereby prevent the release of chemical mediators after an antigen-IgE interaction.

The patient must clearly understand that cromolyn is a *prophylactic* drug that must be taken on a daily basis for at least 3 to 5 days and often up to 1 month to become effective. It should not be used for the management of an acute asthmatic attack. Although most effective in young patients with extrinsic asthma, it is also useful in many adult patients with intrinsic asthma and in exercise-induced bronchospasm. Cromolyn may be used to help reduce or discontinue long-term corticosteroid therapy for asthma. It is particularly useful in children since it causes few acute or long-term side effects.

Patients should be advised that cromolyn capsules are inactive if swallowed. The fine, dry powder, contained in 20-mg capsules, is inhaled by the patient four times daily from a special hand-held, patient-activated Spinhaler. The use of a sympathomimetic bronchodilator aerosol 10 to 15 minues prior to cromolyn inhalation prevents episodes of bronchospasms that are often associated with the inhalation of this drug.

Mucolytics and Expectorants

In addition to bronchoconstriction, hypersecretion of mucus, which interferes with free breathing, is a common problem of asthma. Mucous plugs also increase the risk of pulmonary infections. The use of *expectorants* such as guaifenesin (glyceryl guaiacolate), potassium iodide, and ammonium chloride or *mucolytic agents* such as acetylcysteine (Mucomyst) and tyloxapol (Alevair) have not been demonstrated to be of definite clinical value in the removal of bronchial secretions and mucous plugs.

Water, by contrast, has been found to be most useful in liquifying mucus secretions, facilitating their removal and decreasing the formation of mucous plugs. In addition to suggesting increases in fluid intake, nurses should recommend that patients use vaporizers or cool-mist humidifiers.

Anticholinergic Agents

While atropine and most other anticholinergic agents cause relaxation of bronchial smooth muscle (Figure 54-2), they also produce a drying of the mucous membranes with the retention of sputum. The investigational drug ipratropium bromide (Sch 1000), an analogue of atropine, is an effective bronchodilator which may prove to be useful in selected patients with chronic asthma and bronchitis. When inhaled, this drug is effective in low doses that do not cause drying of the mucous membranes, dry mouth, blurred vision, or changes in heart rate.

Antiasthmatic Agents: nursing implications:

Assist the patient and family in planning long-term care to minimize asthmatic episodes. Include the following in the teaching plan: instructions on drug action, dosage schedule, side effects to report; need for adequate fluid intake to help liquify bronchial secretions; humidification of the environment, when needed; ways to avoid exposure to infection or irritants; and caution against taking nonprescription or prescription drugs without consulting the physician. Advise the patient not to smoke.

Ephedrine-Epinephrine

1. Before initiating therapy and after drug administration, record blood pressure and pulse rate; monitor these cardiovascular parameters frequently until they have stabilized.
2. Provide support and reassurance if the patient experiences nervousness and excitement after parenteral epinephrine administration.
3. Teach the patient how to monitor radial pulse and to report rapid or irregular pulse.
4. After prolonged periods of ephedrine use, observe for and instruct the patient to report decreased drug effectiveness. A drug-free period of 3-4 days may be required for restoration of responsiveness to drug.

Isoproterenol

1. Instruct the patient in proper use of nebulizer, and caution the patient to use the lowest effective dose required to relieve symptoms.
2. Tolerance to bronchodilating effects may develop after prolonged use. Instruct the patient to report to the physician if the usual dose does not produce the expected relief of symptoms.
3. Teach the patient expected effects and symptoms to report that require discontinuation of drug administration: increase in respiratory distress after drug administration; parotid gland swelling.

Methylxanthines

Individual patients metabolize methylxanthines at different rates; therefore dosage is determined by close monitoring of therapeutic response, development of tolerance, pulmonary function tests, and serum theophylline levels.

SUPPLEMENTARY READINGS

Austen, K. F., and L. M. Lichtenstein, ed., *Asthma: Physiology, Immunopharmacology, and Treatment.* New York: Academic Press, Inc., 1973.

Brown, M. S., and M. Collar, "Over the Counter Drugs for Upper Respiratory Symptoms," *Nurse Practitioner* 2(3): 18–20, 34–42 (1977).

Ellis, E. F., ed., "Symposium on Pediatric Allergy," *Pediatric Clinics of North America* 22(1): 1–266 (1975).

Fuhs, M., and A. M. Stein, "Better Ways to Cope with COPD," *Nursing '76* 6(2): 28–38 (1976).

Webb-Johnson, D. C., and J. L. Andrews, Jr., "Bronchodilator Therapy," *New England Journal of Medicine* 297: 476–82, 758–64 (1977).

Weinberger, M., and L. Hendels, "Pharmacotherapy of Asthma," *American Journal of Hospital Pharmacy* 33: 1071–80 (1976).

Weiss, E. B., and M. S. Segal, ed., *Bronchial Asthma—Mechanisms and Therapeutics.* Boston: Little, Brown & Company, 1976.

Wilson, A. F., and J. J. McPhillips, "Pharmacological Control of Asthma," *Annual Review of Pharmacology and Toxicology* 18: 541–61 (1978).

Ziment, I., *Respiratory Pharmacology and Therapeutics.* Philadelphia: W. B. Saunders Company, 1978.

Section VIII

DRUGS AFFECTING THE GASTROINTESTINAL TRACT

DRUG TREATMENT OF PEPTIC ULCER DISEASE

Chapter 55

Peptic ulcer, an acute or chronic lesion in the mucosa of the gastrointestinal tract, is a common disorder affecting 10 to 15 percent of the general population. In this chapter we shall briefly review the physiology of gastric secretion and the nature of peptic ulcer disease and then consider the management of this disease with antacids, anticholinergic agents, and H_2-receptor antagonists.

PHYSIOLOGY OF GASTRIC SECRETION

The secretory activity of the gastric (stomach) mucosa is influenced by central input transmitted via the cholinergic vagus nerve, local neural reflexes, and various gastrointestinal hormones. Gastric secretion in response to a meal can be divided into the cephalic, gastric, and intestinal phases, all of which proceed simultaneously.

The *cephalic phase*, resulting from parasympathetic (cholinergic) stimulation, is induced by the thought, sight, smell, or taste of food. Vagal stimulation increases the release of gastric juice, which consists of a mixture of hydrochloric acid (from parietal cells), pepsinogen (from chief cells), and gastrin (from mucosal cells). The presence of food in the stomach initiates the *gastric phase*. Dietary proteins simultaneously stimulate the release of *gastrin*, a hormone which activates further secretion of acid, and pepsinogen. The acidic (low pH) environment of the stomach favors the conversion of pepsinogen to *pepsin*, an enzyme which participates in the breakdown of proteins. The *intestinal phase* begins as the food enters the duodenum and is characterized by modest stimulatory and more pronounced inhibitory influences on gastric secretion; the latter influences are mediated by hormones secreted by the duodenum.

Experimental evidence suggests (but does not conclusively establish) that hista-mine may be a physiological mediator of acid secretion. Intravenously injected histamine causes a marked increase in the volume of gastric juice containing hydrochloric acid and pepsin. Upon activation by acetylcholine (released from the vagus nerve) or gastrin, histamine is released from cells in the gastric mucosa and stimulates the H_2-receptors of parietal cells, causing the release of acid (Figure 55-1).

PEPTIC ULCER DISEASE

The acid-peptic gastric juice digestion of sharply circumscribed areas of the mucosa is responsible for ulcer formation. The proteolytic enzyme *pepsin* acts with *gastric acid* to cause these mucosal erosions in the esophagus, stomach, or small intestines. The most common type, duodenal ulcers, occurs ten times as frequently as gastric ulcers.

Associated Factors

While acid and pepsin play a clear role in ulcers and ulcers do not form in the absence of acid, the etiology of peptic ulcer disease is not clearly understood. It remains a mystery why the normal resistance of the mucosa to acid and pepsin digestion is lost. A number of factors appear to contribute to the development of gastric or duodenal ulcer formation: (1) hormonal factors, since the incidence is higher in males than in females; (2) prolonged gastric hyperacidity; (3) rapid gastric emptying time, resulting in larger than normal amounts of unbuffered stomach acid spilling into the duodenum; (4) emotional factors, such as stress, anger, and hostility; and (5) genetic factors, as suggested by the higher incidence of duodenal ulcers in patients with a positive family history or blood type O.

Drugs have been identified as being potentially ulcerogenic. Such drugs include aspirin and related salicylates, phenylbutazone

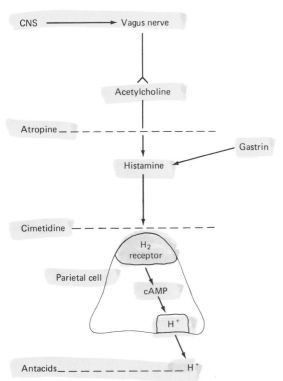

Figure 55-1 Diagrammatic Representation of Acid Secretion and Mechanisms of Antiulcer Drugs. Acetylcholine or gastrin can stimulate the release of histamine which activates the H_2-receptor resulting in acid (H^+) secretion; cyclic adenosine monophosphate (cAMP) is involved in acid secretion. Antiulcer drugs may act by (1) inhibiting the action of acetylcholine at the cholinergic receptor responsible for histamine release (atropine); (2) antagonizing the action of histamine at its H_2-receptor (cimetidine); and (3) neutralizing the acid released into the stomach (antacids).

(Butazolidin), oxyphenbutazone (Tandearil), indomethacin (Indocin), reserpine (Serpasil), many anticancer drugs (such as methotrexate), ethyl alcohol, caffeine, and nicotine. Corticosteroids were formerly believed to be ulcerogenic, but this concept has been challenged in recent years (Chapter 34). The nurse should note that these drugs are rarely the sole cause of peptic ulcer disease and more often aggravate or precipitate a preexisting condition.

Symptoms and Complications

Symptoms of "heartburn," nausea, and substernal pain are the most common complaints of patients with chronic gastric ulcers. This pain in the pit of the stomach may occur about one hour after meals and is usually relieved by eating or taking antacids. Nocturnal pain is more commonly associated with duodenal ulcers than those affecting the esophagus or stomach; patients typically awaken in pain during the early morning after sleeping many hours. The pain caused by a duodenal ulcer is variously described as gnawing, burning, cramp-like, or as a "heartburn." Some patients are asymptomatic. Not infrequently there is a remission of symptoms followed by their recurrence in a cyclic manner.

Nurses should educate patients about the potential *complications* of untreated peptic ulcer disease, the most important of which include: hemorrhage, manifested by black, tarry stools; acute perforation into the peritoneal cavity, the most serious complication and most common cause of death; penetration into adjacent organs; and pyloric obstruction, which interferes with the passage of food into the duodenum. A number of more serious disorders, including gastrointestinal carcinomas, cause ulcer-like pain; gastric ulcers are more likely to develop a malignancy than duodenal ulcers. Hence, it is essential that patients be accurately diagnosed and effectively treated. Extended periods of self-medication

with proprietary antacids can be hazardous and should be discouraged. Other nursing implications associated with peptic ulcer disease are summarized at the end of this chapter.

Antiulcer drugs   In our discussion of the management of peptic ulcer disease with drugs, we shall note that ulcer healing is promoted by reducing the amount of acid present. Examination of Figure 55-1 reveals that there are several potential mechanisms by which drugs might act: (1) The effects of acetylcholine can be antagonized at the cholinergic receptor responsible for histamine release. Atropine and a large number of synthetic anticholinergic (antimuscarinic) agents act by this mechanism. (2) The action of histamine at its H_2-receptor* on parietal cells can be blocked with specific antagonists such as cimetidine (Tagamet). (3) Antacids are used to neutralize the gastric acid released from parietal cells. Attempts have been made to reduce acid secretion by inhibiting the ability of gastrin to stimulate histamine release; at present, no clinically available drugs act by this mechanism. Synthetic prostaglandin (PGE_2) derivatives are currently being evaluated as potential antiulcer agents.

Antacids

Antacids, the mainstay of contemporary peptic ulcer disease therapy, are used to relieve ulcer pain and promote healing; these drugs will not necessarily prevent recurrences.

Two primary mechanisms are responsible for the beneficial effects of antacids: neutralization of gastric acid and reduction of the proteolytic activity of pepsin. Elevation of

---

*You will recall from Chapter 54 that histamine receptor sites are of two types: H_1-receptor activation increases contraction of intestinal and bronchial smooth muscle and is readily antagonized by classical antihistamines (H_1-receptor antagonists). H_2-receptor activation results in enhanced gastric acid secretion that is not modified by H_1-antagonists.

the pH of the gastric contents to more than 4 to 5 results in the virtually total inactivation of pepsin, and, at this pH, the damaging effects to the mucosa resulting from acidity are minimal.

To be maximally effective, the antacid must remain in the stomach for a sufficiently long period of time to neutralize the gastric acid. When administered to fasting patients, most antacids are effective only for 20 to 30 minutes before being emptied into the duodenum; this period is too short to produce a significant reduction in gastric acidity. Since maximum secretion of acid occurs about 1 hour after a meal, this is the most rational time for antacid administration. Antacids are usually given 3 to 4 times daily 1 hour after meals and at bedtime.

Choice of antacids Antacids have been classically classified as being systemic (absorbable) or nonsystemic (nonabsorbable). The former have systemic activity and may modify the electrolyte balance or change the pH of the extracellular fluid resulting in systemic (metabolic) alkalosis. Nonabsorbable antacids act exclusively in the gastrointestinal tract, and their adverse effects are generally limited to diarrhea or constipation. Sodium bicarbonate has long been known to have systemic activity after oral administration. It is now recognized that many antacids previously classified as nonabsorbable, while not capable of significantly altering the acid-base balance of the blood, have the potential for causing systemic toxicity.

Liquid preparations of antacids are generally more effective than tablets because they have a greater surface area available for interaction with and neutralization of acid. Nurses should encourage their patients to thoroughly chew tablets before swallowing them. In addition to considering the relative capacity of an antacid to chemically neutralize gastric acid, other factors to be taken into consideration when selecting a drug include palatability,

speed of onset and duration of action, side effects, and the patient's medical history (Table 55-1).

The potential of a *drug interaction* exists when antacids are being administered. The best-documented and most clinically relevant of these interactions involves the *tetracyclines*. Antacids containing calcium, magnesium, or aluminum form a nonabsorbable chelate with this antibiotic class, resulting in a significant reduction in blood levels. Other interactions result from the ability of antacids to alter the pH of the stomach and urine, thereby altering the normal absorption and urinary excretion of a number of drugs (Table 55-2, page 478). In some cases, antacids reduce the absorption of drugs by physically interacting with them by the process of adsorption. The clinical significance of these interactions has not been established. In general, it is best not to administer other oral drugs within 1 to 2 hours of antacids.

Sodium bicarbonate This drug has long been recognized as an inexpensive, effective, and rapid-acting household remedy for the treatment of "sour stomach." Unfortunately, sodium bicarbonate elevates the pH of the gastric contents more than the optimal 4 to 5; this results in a rapid increase in acid secretion or "acid rebound" and a short duration of relief.

Chronic administration leads to significant absorption, potentially resulting in *systemic alkalosis* and *sodium loading*; the latter should be avoided by patients on a low-sodium diet. Regular use of this drug with milk (intended to soothe ulcer pain) leads to an increase in calcium absorption and may precipitate the *milk-alkali syndrome*. This syndrome is characterized by hypercalcemia, renal insufficiency, and systemic alkalosis, causing such symptoms as nausea, vomiting, headache, anorexia, and mental confusion. These symptoms disappear after the discontinuation of the antacid and calcium.

Table 55-1   Comparative Properties of Representative Antacids

Generic name (synonyms)	Selected trade names (mls to neutralize 80 mEq of acid)[a]	Usual adult oral dose	Remarks
Sodium Bicarbonate (Baking Soda)	Alka-Seltzer	0.3-2 g 1-4 times daily	Widely used, potent, effective, rapid-acting. Disadvantages: "acid rebound," risk of systemic alkalosis, sodium overloading. Not recommended for chronic use.
Calcium Carbonate (Precipitated Chalk)	Chooz Titralac (20.7) Tums	0.5-2 g q. h	Rapid, prolonged, effective neutralization of gastric acid. In chronic use, risk of hypercalcemia with kidney impairment. Milk-alkali syndrome. Acid rebound. Tendency to constipate. Chalky taste.
Aluminum Compounds			Relatively low neutralizing capacity. Constipation common. Some systemic absorption.
Aluminum Hydroxide Gel	Amphojel (41.5) Alu-Cap	Suspension: 15 ml 4-6 times daily. Tablets: 600 mg 3-4 times daily	Tablets less effective than liquid. Used as antacid and for hyperphosphatemia in chronic renal failure.
Aluminum Carbonate Gel, Basic	Basaljel	10 ml q. 2-4 h	Useful for treatment of phosphatic renal calculi and for hyperphosphatemia in chronic renal failure.
Dihydroxyaluminum Aminoacetate	Robalate (70.8)	1-2 q.i.d.	Less effective than aluminum hydroxide gel.
Dihydroxyaluminum Sodium Carbonate	Rolaids	0.3-0.6 g PRN	Rapid action. Not recommended for patients on sodium-restricted diet.
Magnesium Compounds			Magnesium salts are slightly absorbable and have tendency to cause diarrhea. Should not be used in patients with renal insufficiency.
Magnesium Hydroxide (Milk of Magnesia) Magnesium Oxide	Mint-o-Mag	0.3-0.6 g q.i.d. 5 ml q.i.d. 0.25 g q.i.d.	All have the same properties, since magnesium oxide is converted to magnesium hydroxide in stomach, and milk of magnesia is a suspension of magnesium hydroxide. All are also used as mild laxatives (Chapter 56). Milk of magnesia is widely used.
Magnesium Carbonate (Carbonate of Magnesia)		0.5-2 g q.i.d.	Unlike magnesium oxide and hydroxide, carbon dioxide is liberated during acid neutralization. Common ingredient in nonprescription laxatives.
Magnesium Trisilicate		1 g q.i.d.	Slow onset, weak neutralizing action. Silicon dioxide formed in neutralization reaction may form protective coat over ulcer (significance ?) and adsorbs pepsin. Long-term use leads to development of silicate renal stones. Used in combination with other antacids.

477

Table 55-1   Continued

Generic name (synonyms)	Selected trade names (mls to neutralize 80 mEq of acid)[a]	Usual adult oral dose	Remarks
Aluminum/Magnesium Combinations			More palatable products with greater neutralizing capacity than aluminum hydroxide. Aluminum-induced constipation and magnesium-induced diarrhea balanced. Varying combinations of aluminum and magnesium salts. Most have relatively high sodium content.
Aludrox (28.5), A.M.T. (44.7), Creamalin (31.1), DiGel (32.7), Gelusil (60.2), Kolantyl Gel (47.3), Maalox (31.0), Mylanta (33.6), Trisogel (48.5), WinGel (35.6)			
Magaldrate	Riopan (36.2)	0.4–0.8 g q.i.d.	Aluminum magnesium hydroxide. Low sodium content but poor neutralizing capacity.

[a] Volume of antacid (ml) required to neutralize an equivalent amount of acid in vitro. The lower the volume of antacid, the higher its neutralizing capacity. To determine the in vitro neutralizing capacity of an antacid, divide 80 mEq by the ml of antacid noted in the table. For example, Titralac: (80 mEq)/(20.7 ml) = 3.86 mEq/ml. Data from Fordtran *et al.*, *N. Engl. J. Med.*, **288**, 923 (1973).

Table 55-2   Potential Drug Interactions Involving Antacids

Inhibition of Drug Absorption

Tetracyclines[a]
Chlorpromazine (Thorazine)
Digoxin (Lanoxin)
Isoniazid (INH)
Phenytoin (Dilantin)
Quinidine
Warfarin

Enhancement of Drug Absorption

Dicumarol

Increased Urinary Excretion

Aspirin and Salicylates
Quinidine

[a] Well-documented, clinically significant interaction resulting in a reduction in blood levels of these antibiotics.

Calcium Carbonate   This potent and effective antacid has a rapid onset and long duration of action. Although only a limited amount of calcium is absorbed when used infrequently, chronic drug administration may result in hypercalcemia, which in turn may lead to neurological disorders, renal calculi, and impaired kidney function. The milk-alkali syndrome has been reported in some patients.

Antacids containing aluminum   Aluminum salts, most often administered as the hydroxide, do not cause systemic alkalosis or acid rebound. The most common side effect associated with their use is *constipation*, which may lead to intestinal obstruction and fecal concretions in the elderly or in patients with decreased bowel motility. Phosphate depletion (*hypophosphatemia*) can result from aluminum binding and inhibition of the absorption of dietary phosphates. Common symptoms of acute hypophosphatemia include muscle weakness, anorexia, and malaise; chronic phosphate depletion may cause demineralization of bone and hypercalcemia, leading to kidney stone formation.

Results of recent clinical studies reject the long-held belief that insoluble aluminum salts are not absorbed and are nontoxic. Patients with chronic renal insufficiency (uremia) chronically receiving aluminum hydroxide for the management of hyperphosphatemia have been found to accumulate aluminum in the brain and develop a progressive neurological syndrome (*dialysis encephalopathy*) associated with a high incidence of mortality. These results suggest the need for extreme caution when aluminum-containing antacids are to be administered over extended periods of time.

Antacids containing magnesium Magnesium salts are more potent antacids than aluminum hydroxide gel and do not cause systemic alkalosis. The major side effect of these salts is *diarrhea*. Approximately 15 percent of an administered dose of magnesium is absorbed, and in normal individuals this is readily excreted in the urine. In patients with renal insufficiency, magnesium accumulates (hypermagnesemia) which may result in nausea, vomiting, hypotension, depressed reflexes, respiratory depression, and coma. Hence, magnesium salts should not be used in patients with impaired kidney function. Chronic use of magnesium trisilicate can lead to the development of renal stones.

Aluminum-magnesium combination antacids A large number of antacids available commercially contain a mixture of the salts of aluminum and magnesium (Table 55-1). Such preparations are more palatable and provide more effective neutralization of gastric acid than aluminum hydroxide. These mixtures, however, are unlike magnesium hydroxide when it is employed alone as they are unable to maintain the gastric pH above 4. The use of these salts in combination is intended to balance the diarrhea and constipation normally caused by each.

Most aluminum-magnesium combination products contain, as a contaminant, *sodium* in concentrations that might be excessive for individuals on a sodium-restricted diet. Magaldrate (Riopan), which is aluminum magnesium hydroxide, has a very low sodium content (0.7 mg per tablet or 5 ml).

This advantage may be offset by its low acid-neturalizing capacity.

Anticholinergic Agents

You will recall from Chapter 8 that atropine and related anticholinergic (antimuscarinic) agents reduce gastric acid secretion, decrease smooth muscle motility, and delay gastric emptying time. Since an ulcer does not form in the absence of acid and part of the pain associated with this disorder is caused by smooth muscle contractions, anticholinergic agents should, at least in theory, be ideally suited for the management of peptic ulcer disease. In practice, however, this has not been the case. It is the feeling of many clinicians that while these drugs may be of benefit for the management of peptic ulcer when employed in conjunction with dietary modifications and antacid administration, their ability to prevent ulcer recurrences over extended periods of time has not been well established.

The high doses of atropine-like drugs required to substantially reduce *gastric acid secretion* are almost always accompanied by such side effects as dry mouth, blurred vision, tachycardia, and difficulty in urination. Their ability to slow *gastric emptying time* prolongs the time available for antacids to neutralize gastric acid. However, this advantageous effect may be offset by the fact that the continued presence of food in the stomach provides a stimulus for the prolonged secretion of acid. These drugs are contraindicated in gastric ulcers because the delay of emptying time prolongs the duration of contact between the ulcer and the gastric contents. Atropine antagonizes acetylcholine-induced motility by blocking muscarinic receptor sites on smooth muscle; this is the basis for its antispasmodic effects.

Choice of drugs The naturally occurring belladonna alkaloids (atropine, scopolamine) are highly effective in reducing the motility and secretory activity of the gastro-intestinal tract. These drugs readily cross the blood-brain barrier and produce signs of central nervous system stimulation (restlessness, tremor, irritability, delirium, hallucinations).

Synthetic quaternary ammonium compounds have been developed (Table 55-3) that possess anticholinergic activity. When given orally, these drugs are less readily or reliably absorbed than are the natural or synthetic tertiary derivatives; this accounts for the considerable variation in response observed among patients. These drugs cause minimal central side effects.

Other chemical derivatives have been introduced that possess primarily antispas-modic activity, with little anticholingeric activity (Table 55-3). These drugs are used to relieve a wide variety of conditions characterized by spasms and hypermotility of the small intestines and colon. They are also employed as adjuncts in the management of functional bowel disorders, mild diarrhea, and nonobstructive cramping.

Administration and precautions Anticholinergic agents should be administered at least 1 hour prior to meals and at bedtime. The daytime dosage should be high enough to produce occasional side effects because it is generally assumed that if no side effects (such as dry mouth) are produced at a given dosage

Table 55-3   Antimuscarinic Antispasmodic Agents

Generic name	Selected trade names	Average adult oral dose
Belladonna Alkaloids		
Atropine sulfate	——	0.5 mg q.i.d.
Belladonna tincture	——	10–15 drops q.i.d.
Scopolamine (hyoscine) hydrobromide	——	0.5 mg q.i.d.
Belladonna alkaloids and phenobarbital	Belladenal, Bellergal, Butibel, Donnatal	
Belladonna Alkaloids, Quaternay Ammonium Derivative		
Methscopolamine bromide	Pamine	2.5 mg q.i.d.
Synthetic Quaternary Ammonium Compounds		
Anisotropine methylbromide	Valpin	50 mg t.i.d.
Diphemanil methylsulfate	Prantal	100–200 mg q.i.d.
Glycopyrrolate	Robinul	1 mg t.i.d.
Hexocyclium methylsulfate	Tral	25 mg q.i.d.
Isopropamide iodide	Darbid	5 mg b.i.d.
Mepenzolate bromide	Cantil	25–50 mg q.i.d.
Methantheline bromide	Banthine	50 mg q.i.d.
Oxyphenonium bromide	Antrenyl	5–10 mg q.i.d.
Propantheline bromide	Pro-Banthine	15 mg q.i.d.
Tridihexethyl chloride	Pathilon	25–50 mg q.i.d.
Synthetic Antispasmodic Agents[a]		
Dicyclomine hydrochloride	Bentyl, Di-Spaz	10 mg q.i.d.
Methixene hydrochloride	Trest	1 mg t.i.d.
Oxyphencyclimine hydrochloride	Daricon	10 mg b.i.d.

[a] Antispasmodic activity with little or no antimuscarinic activity and little effect on gastric secretion.

level, no therapeutic benefits are being obtained. Higher doses may be given at bedtime to inhibit nocturnal acid secretion; the side effects will not disturb the patient while sleeping.

In Chapter 8 we discussed the general adverse effects, precautions, and contraindications associated with the use of anticholinergic agents. In addition to being contraindicated in gastric ulcer, they should not be used in patients with reflux esophagitis. By decreasing the motility of both the esophagus and stomach and paralyzing the sphincter between them, they promote the reflux of gastric contents into the esophagus. Potential drug interactions involving anticholinergic agents are summarized in Table 8-2 (page 76).

H₂-Receptor Antagonists: Cimetidine

The first H₂-receptor antagonist became clinically available in the United States in 1977. This orally active drug, *cimetidine* (Tagamet) has been shown to antagonize gastric fluid (acid and, to a lesser extent, pepsin) secretion stimulated by histamine, insulin, food, physiological vagal stimulation, or pentagastrin (Pentavlon), a drug used to assess gastric secretory activity. Clinical tests performed in normal subjects and in patients with peptic ulcer disease reveal that cimetidine causes a marked reduction in both basal nocturnal and stimulated acid release and increases the gastric pH to 5 or more in most patients for 3 to 4 hours. The serum half-life of this drug is about 120 minutes.

Clinical uses and side effects Cimetidine causes a reduction in epigastric pain and subjective proof of ulcer healing or a reduction in ulcer size in patients with *duodenal ulcer disease*. Preliminary studies suggest that

this drug may also be of value for the management of gastric ulcers. Although many clinicians believe that the H₂-receptor antagonists will play a major role in the future treatment of peptic ulcer disease, a relatively high relapse rate occurs after the discontinuation of therapy.

The *Zollinger-Ellison syndrome* is characterized by a tumor of the exocrine pancreas, enormous secretions of gastric acid and pepsin, and severe ulceration of the stomach, duodenum, esophagus, and jejunum. This disorder is generally treated by performing a total gastrectomy; the pancreatic tumor is often removed because, not uncommonly, it is malignant. Cimetidine appears to be the first drug that effectively manages this disease, and its use may eliminate the need for the removal of the stomach.

The usual adult dose is 300 mg four times daily with meals and at bedtime. Antacids may be used as needed for the relief of pain. While ulcer healing generally occurs within the first 2 weeks, drug administration should be continued for 4 to 6 weeks, but not over 8 weeks. Cimetidine may be administered intravenously for hospitalized patients with pathological hypersecretory disorders. Since this drug is primarily eliminated by the kidney, doses should be reduced in patients with severely impaired renal function.

To date most of the side effects observed have been minor; they include headache, diarrhea, rash, pruritis, dizziness, and muscle pain. Mild gynecomastia (excessive development of male mammary glands) and neutropenia have been reported in a few patients. Elevations of serum creatinine and transaminase (SGOT/SGPT) occur in 5 to 25 percent of patients. The clinical significance of these findings is not clear; transaminase elevations have not been accompanied by liver damage.

Drug Treatment of Peptic Ulcer Disease:
nursing implications

1. Advise the patient to avoid self-medication with antacids and explain possible harmful effects. Sodium bicarbonate: acid rebound, excessive sodium intake, metabolic alkalosis; calcium carbonate: prolonged use with milk can cause milk-alkali syndrome or hypercalcemia in patients with kidney disease; antacids containing aluminum or magnesium or both: often contain high sodium content and are contraindicated in renal or cardiac disease.

2. Self-medication may mask underlying gastrointestinal pathology and delay medical treatment for serious disorders (for example, stomach cancer).

3. Teach the patient the expected effects of antacids and provide suggestions for maintaining normal bowel function. Products containing calcium or aluminum may cause constipation, while those containing magnesium tend to cause diarrhea.

4. Instruct patients with peptic ulcer disease about dietary modifications; for example, they should avoid irritating substances as coffee, black pepper, and alcohol.

SUPPLEMENTARY READINGS

Bass, P., "Gastric Antisecretory and Antiulcer Agents," *Advances in Drug Research* **8**: 205–328 (1974).

Burland, W. L., and M. A. Simkins, eds., "Cimetidine," *Proceedings of the Second International Symposium on Histamine H_2-Receptor Antagonists.* Amsterdam: Excerpta Medica, 1977.

Fordtran, J. S., S. G. Morawski, and C. T. Richardson, "In Vivo and In Vitro Evaluation of Liquid Antacids," *New England Journal of Medicine* **288**: 923–28 (1973).

Garnett, W. R., "Antacid Products," in *Handbook of Nonprescription Drugs* (6th ed.), pp. 1–18. Washington, D.C.: American Pharmaceutical Association, 1979.

Given, B. A., and S. J. Simmons, *Gastroenterology in Clinical Nursing.* St. Louis: C. V. Mosby Company, 1975.

Morrissey, J. F., and R. F. Barreras, "Antacid Therapy," *New England Journal of Medicine* **290**: 550–54 (1974).

Siepler, J. K., and others, "H_2-Receptor Antagonists," *American Journal of Hospital Pharmacy* **35**: 141–45 (1978).

LAXATIVES AND ANTIDIARRHEAL DRUGS

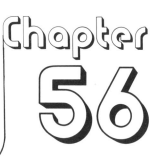

Chapter 56

Disorders of bowel function are common medical problems. In this chapter we shall briefly discuss the physiology of the digestive system and then consider constipation and diarrhea and the drugs used to manage these disorders.

PHYSIOLOGY OF THE DIGESTIVE SYSTEM

The alimentary tract is essentially a long, hollow tube surrounded by layers of smooth muscle. Coordination between adjacent layers of circular and longitudinal types of smooth muscle controls the movement of the intestinal contents. When circular muscle activity (tone) is increased, the lumen of the intestine becomes occluded and there is resistance to flow, resulting in constipation; the opiates produce constipation by this action. Alternatively, when the activity of circular muscle is decreased and more flaccid, such as may be caused by castor oil, the intestinal lumen opens more widely, offering little or no resistance to the flow of the intestinal contents; diarrhea may be the result.

Normal intestinal motility and peristalsis are maintained by the smooth muscles and the intrinsic nerves (Auerbach's and Meissner's plexuses). Activation of cholinergic nerves (the vagus and parasympathetic pelvic nerves) stimulates intestinal motility; blockade of cholinergic activity with atropine and related antimuscarinic agents reduces intestinal motility. Stimulation of the stretch receptors or sensory receptors of the intestinal mucosa by an increase in the bulk of the intestinal contents can also promote the propulsive peristaltic activity of the intestines.

Physiology of Defecation

After arriving in the cecum, the chyme (undigested and unabsorbed food residue) moves slowly in the lumen of the colon, where it is mixed by churning, nonpropulsive movements. These movements assist in the absorption of water and electrolytes and result in the solidification of the stool. Several times daily, generally after meals, the stool is propelled into the descending colon and sigmoid colon by a massive contraction. Subsequent movement of the stool into the rectum triggers the *defecation reflex*, which can be facilitated or inhibited by higher centers in the brain. If this reflex is inhibited, the rectum slowly relaxes and the defecation stimulus dissipates.

CONSTIPATION AND ITS TREATMENT

Constipation may be defined as an infrequent or difficult passage of feces; more precisely, it is a decrease in the frequency of bowel movements, accompanied by a prolonged and difficult passage of stool, followed by a sensation of incomplete evacuation. The normal frequency of bowel movements may vary from several times daily to once or twice per week.

Causes of Constipation

There are many widely diverse causes of constipation. The following are common. (1) *Psychological factors:* failure to respond to the defecation urge or to acquire the habit of regular defecation; emotional stress; depression. (2) *Nutritional factors:* starvation or dehydration; a diet containing insufficient bulk or foods that harden stools. (3) *Diseases:* paraplegia; multiple sclerosis; hypothyroidism; atony or spasm of the colon; hypertonicity of the ileocecal valve; benign or malignant tumors obstructing the intestinal lumen; hemorrhoids; anal fissures; hyperparathyroidism or other hypercalcemic states. (4) *Drugs:* antacids containing aluminum; calcium carbonate; anticholinergic agents; phenothiazine antipsychotic agents; tricyclic antidepressants; ganglionic blocking agents; salts containing iron; opiates; laxatives, when used at frequent intervals. (5) *Miscellaneous factors:* pregnancy; postpartum; decreased physical activity; old age.

Nursing Responsibilities

The nurse should actively participate in the education of patients about normal bowel function to prevent constipation whenever possible, precluding the unnecessary use of laxatives. A medical evaluation is fully justified and should be encouraged to determine the cause of constipation that persists for a period of several weeks. Temporary constipation, frequently associated with stressful situations or change in diet, is self-limiting. Several doses of a laxative may be beneficial in such situations.

The patient should be advised that the consistency, frequency, and quantity of the stool can normally be controlled by eating sufficient amounts of high-residue foods that are natural laxatives. Daily ingestion of 5 to 10 glassfuls of liquid or the equivalent in liquid foods (soups) and regular exercise are also beneficial in preventing constipation.

A frequent cause of constipation results from irregular bowel habits that have developed over long periods of inhibition of normal defecation reflexes. Clinical experience reveals that if defecation is not permitted to occur when these reflexes become excited, these reflexes become progressively weaker with time. The defecation reflex can also be inhibited by the pain of hemorrhoids or an anal fissure. The importance of initiating and maintaining good habits should be taught by the nurse using a vocabulary that is fully comprehensible to the patient.

Patients should be clearly warned not to take laxatives when experiencing undiagnosed abdominal pain. If the pain results from an inflamed appendix, the laxative may cause rupture of the appendix by increasing peristalsis. In addition, laxatives should not be administered to patients with an intestinal obstruction or fecal impaction. Nursing implications associated with the use of laxatives are summarized at the end of this chapter.

Laxative Misuse

The excessive use of laxatives by large segments of the population arises primarily from erroneous concepts about the normal physiology and pathophysiology of the body. Many individuals use laxatives to rid the body of toxic substances they believe will be absorbed into the blood in the absence of a daily bowel movement. While some people think that weakness and headaches result from constipation, others use laxatives for the treatment of the common cold, anger, and depression.

Although the occasional use of laxatives for the relief of constipation is relatively safe, regular use of these drugs can cause fluid and electrolyte (potassium) depletion and vitamin deficiency and often results in the development of a habit that is difficult to break. After a complete laxative effect has occurred, the bowel is devoid of food residues, and 2 to 3 days may be required prior to the next bowel movement. Many people fail to appreciate that this delay is normal and is to be anticipated. In the absence of a natural bowel movement, an additional dose of laxative is often taken or a stronger drug is used, leading to a vicious cycle. With repeated use of laxatives, normal defecation reflex mechanisms become blunted, eventually leading to total reliance upon these drugs for defecation. Treatment of the "laxative habit" often involves the temporary use of bulk-forming agents to increase the contents of the intestines in conjunction with professional training to establish regular bowel habits.

Drug Treatment of Constipation

Until recently, drugs used for the treatment of constipation were classified on the basis of their intensity of effect. The terms *laxative* or *aperient* refer to a "mild" drug that produces a formed stool in the absence of griping or abdominal cramps, while the terms *cathartic* or *purgative* are used to denote "harsh" drugs that produce loose watery feces, usually accompanied by abdominal cramping. This distinction, now falling into disfavor, is basically unsound because differences in the magnitude of the effect produced can be controlled by the dose administered. It should be noted that many authors use the terms *laxative* and *cathartic* interchangeably.

Laxatives are commonly classified on the basis of their presumed mechanism of action. The nurse should bear in mind, however, that this classification is not absolute because the mechanisms underlying the laxative effects of some drugs are not well understood, while others produce their effects by more than one mechanism. With these limitations in mind, we shall classify laxatives using the following categories: stimulants, saline laxatives, bulk-forming laxatives, emollients (lubricants), and fecal-softeners (wetting agents).

Stimulant laxatives Drugs in this class (Table 56-1) increase the propulsive peristaltic activity of the intestine by one or more of the following mechanisms: stimulation of the colonic intramural mysenteric plexuses; stimulation of the sensory nerves in the intestinal mucosa; direct stimulation of intestinal smooth muscle; and inhibition of water and electrolyte reabsorption from the intestinal lumen or enhancement of secretion of water into the lumen, increasing intraluminal pressure and stimulating peristalsis. The primary site of action of castor oil is the small intestine, while most other stimulant laxatives act in the colon.

Stimulant laxatives are useful for the treatment of acute constipation that does not respond to milder drugs. Other clinical indications include the management of consti-

Table 56-1   Representative Stimulant Laxatives

Generic name	Selected trade names	Usual adult dose	Onset of action	Remarks
Castor oil	Neoloid (mint-flavored castor oil emulsion)	PO: 15–30 ml	2 h	Complete emptying GI tract of gas and feces prior to proctoscopy or radiologic exam. Not for common constipation. Take chilled followed by fruit juice or carbonated beverages. Contraindicated during pregnancy.
Glycerin suppositories		Rectal: 3 g; children under 6 years, 1–1.5 g	15–30 min	Acts by stimulating rectal mucosa and by lubricating fecal matter. Can cause rectal irritation.
Bisacodyl	Dulcolax Theralax	PO and rectal: 10 mg	Oral: 6–8 h Rectal: 15–60 min	Suppositories may cause rectal irritation. Swallow tablets whole. Co-administration with antacids causes dissolution of enteric tablet coating, causing abdominal cramping and vomiting.
Phenolphthalein	Alophen Ex-Lax Feen-a-Mint Phenolax	PO: 60 mg	4–8 h	Very widely used. Colors alkaline urine pink. May cause a persistent skin rash (pink to purple) in hypersensitive individuals. Prolonged use may cause dehydration and electrolyte disturbances.
Anthraquinone derivatives				Color alkaline urine pink-red. Prolonged use causes pigmentation of colonic mucosa; harmless and slowly reversible. Excreted into breast milk; contraindicated in nursing mothers.
Cascara sagrada fluidextract	Cas-Evac	PO: 1 ml	8 h	Widely used. Mild, no cramping. May discolor urine.
Senna	Black-Draught Fletcher's Castoria Senokot X-Prep	PO: 1 t Rectal: 1 suppository	6 h 6 h	Purified preparation reported to produce colic and loose stools less than senna; little support of claim.
Sennosides A and B	Glysennid	PO: 12–24 mg		
Danthron	Dorbane Modane	PO: 75–150 mg	6–8 h	Colors urine pink-red.

pation caused by prolonged bedrest, hospitalization, or poor dietary habits or induced by other drugs. They are also employed to prepare the bowel prior to surgical and radiologic, proctoscopic, or colonoscopic procedures or prior to radiologic examination of the abdomen, especially barium enema examinations.

Precautions In general, the use of stimulant laxatives is not recommended in children. The intensity of action of these drugs is dose-dependent and varies from a mild laxative effect to severe griping and catharsis with resulting electrolyte imbalance (hypokalemia) and excessive fluid loss. This group of laxatives is most widely misused. Castor oil is contraindicated during pregnancy to preclude the potential risk of an abortion.

Stimulant laxatives containing anthraquinones (cascara, senna, danthron) color alkaline urine pink, and after periods of prolonged use cause a darkened pigmentation of the colonic mucosa (melanosis coli); this latter effect is generally considered to be harmless and is reversible 4 to 12 months after the drug is discontinued. These laxatives are excreted into the milk of lactating mothers at levels that may cause a laxative effect in the infant. It is generally recommended, therefore, that anthraquinone laxatives not be administered to lactating mothers. These precautions apply only to the anthraquinones and do not apply to castor oil, glycerin suppositories, or the diphenylmethane derivatives (bisacodyl, phenolphthalein). Glycerin suppositories also have lubricating properties and are, therefore, sometimes classified as emollients.

Saline laxatives Saline laxatives (Table 56-2) consist of nonabsorbable or poorly absorbable cations (magnesium, sodium, potassium) and anions (citrate, phosphate, sulfate, tartrate). A hypertonic solution of these salts causes the osmotic retention of a significant volume of water in the intestinal lumen. The resulting increase in intraluminal pressure mechanically stimulates stretch receptors, which increases peristalsis. In addition, magnesium ions may activate the release of the enteric hormone cholecystokinin (CCK), and this hormone stimulates intestinal motility and inhibits fluid absorption from the intestine. Both actions are thought to be responsible for the laxative effects.

Saline laxatives are administered to empty the bowel prior to surgery and radiologic, proctoscopic, or colonoscopic procedures. They are also used to hasten the elimination of orally ingested poisons present in the gastrointestinal tract and to remove parasites (worms) and toxic vermifuges after anthelmintic drug administration.

The relative palatability of the saline laxatives differs, and this serves as one consideration for selection of the most appropriate drug. Magnesium citrate solution, milk of magnesia, and sodium phosphate all have relatively pleasant tastes, while sodium sulfate has a bitter taste and, notwithstanding its effectiveness, is not widely used.

Precautions Saline laxatives must be carefully selected for patients with renal impairment and congestive heart failure. As much as 20 percent of the *magnesium* in saline laxatives containing magnesium is absorbed. This magnesium load is rapidly removed by the kidneys in normal individuals, while in patients with *impaired kidney function*, toxic levels of this cation may accumulate in the serum resulting in central nervous system depression, hypotension, muscle weakness, and electrocardiographic abnormalities. Laxatives containing magnesium or potassium are contraindicated in patients with renal insufficiency. Laxatives containing sodium are contraindicated in cardiac patients with edema, in those with evidence of congestive heart failure, or in those individuals maintained on a low-sodium diet.

Bulk-forming laxatives After the oral ingestion of these nondigestible polysaccharide and cellulose derivatives (Table 56-3), they absorb and retain very large

Table 56-2   Representative Saline Laxatives[a]

Generic name (trade name)	Synonyms	Usual adult dose	Remarks
Magnesium Carbonate	Carbonate of Magnesia	PO: 8 g	Also used as an antacid at lower doses. All magnesium-containing laxatives are contraindicated in renal insufficiency.
Magnesium Citrate Solution	Citrate of Magnesia; Citrate	PO: 200 ml	Pleasant tasting; keep refrigerated.
Magnesium Oxide		PO: 4 g	Also used as an antacid at lower doses.
Magnesium Sulfate	Epsom Salts	PO: 15 g	Effective and widely used. Administer dissolved in iced water or orange juice to mask nauseating taste. Effective in eliminating oral poisons.
Milk of Magnesia	MOM; Magnesium Hydroxide Mixture; Cream of Magnesia; Magnesia Magma	PO: 15 ml	Widely used mild laxative and, at lower doses, antacid. Is a suspension of magnesium hydroxide and volatile oil(s) for flavoring.
Potassium Sodium Tartrate	Rochelle Salt; Seignette Salt	PO: 10 g	Laxative properties of Seidlitz Powders result from inclusion of this compound.
Sodium Phosphate (Sal Hepatica)	Dibasic Sodium Phosphate; Disodium Orthophosphate; Disodium Hydrogen Phosphate	PO: 4 g	Highly palatable. Should not be confused with tribasic sodium phosphate, which is very alkaline and caustic.
Sodium Phosphate and Sodium Biphosphate Oral Sol. (Fleet Phospho-Soda) Enema (Fleet Enema)		PO: 20 ml Rectal: 120 ml	Oral solutions, mix with $\frac{1}{2}$ glass water, follow with full glass. Onset of action of enema 5 min. Pediatric doses of both preparations: $\frac{1}{4}$–$\frac{1}{2}$ adult dose.
Sodium Sulfate	Glauber's Salt	PO: 15 g	An effective, time-honored laxative with bitter taste.

[a]Onset of action 2–6 h. Most effective when taken with large volumes of fluid (240 ml) on an empty stomach.

volumes of water in the gut, causing hydration of the stool. By increasing the bulk of the intestinal contents and thereby increasing intraluminal pressure, they stimulate peristalsis, which facilitates the passage of the stool down the alimentary canal. A laxative effect is often obtained in 12 to 24 hours, but up to 3 days may be required to achieve a complete effect.

The nonabsorbed bulk-forming agents are relatively safe and represent a good initial class of drugs to employ for the treatment of constipation. This class of laxatives is the least subject to misuse. They have been shown to be effective in constipated postpartum or elderly patients, those with irritable bowel syndrome and diverticulosis, and chronic laxative misusers; they are also

Table 56-3 Representative Bulk-Forming and Emollient Laxatives and Fecal Softeners

Generic name (synonym)	Selected trade names	Usual adult dose	Onset of action	Remarks
Bulk-forming laxatives				Must be taken with water. Full laxative effect may require 3 days. Low misuse potential. Also used to increase bulk of stools when watery.
Carboxymethylcellulose		PO: 4-6 g	12-24 h	Commonly but unwisely used with dioctylsodium sulfosuccinate. Possible fluid retention in overweight patients.
Plantago Seed (Psyllium Seed)	Mucilose Siblin	PO: 7.5 g	12-24 h	Does not interfere with essential nutrient absorption, but may bind bile salts.
Psyllium Hydrophilic Colloid	Effersyllium Konsyl Metamucil	PO: 7 g	12-24 h	Widely used, effective, and safe laxative.
Bran (unrefined)		PO: 1-2 tbsp daily to start, doubling dose weekly to 6-8 tbsp.		Often contained in cereals.
Emollient laxatives (lubricants)				
Mineral Oil (Liquid Petrolatum)	Agoral Plain Kondremul Petrogalar	PO: 15-45 ml Rectal: 120 ml	6-8 h	Prolonged use of high doses may reduce fat-soluble vitamin absorption. Contraindicated during pregnancy. Potential danger of lipoid pneumonia.
Glycerin suppositories (Table 56-1)				
Fecal softeners (wetting agents)				
Dioctyl Calcium Sulfosuccinate	Surfak Colace	PO: 240 mg PO: 100 mg	1-2 days	Use in combination with other laxatives potentially dangerous; contraindicated in combination with
Dioctyl Sodium Sulfosuccinate (DSS)	Comfolax Disonate Doxinate Softon	2-3 times daily	1-2 days	mineral oil. May enhance absorption of other drugs (digitalis glycosides) with potential increased toxicity.

used to prepare patients prior to barium enema examinations. Drugs in this class are sometimes used to increase the bulk of stools in patients with chronic watery diarrhea; the number of evacuations is reduced and anal discomfort is relieved.

Precautions Because of the potential danger of fecal impaction or intestinal obstruction, the bulk-forming agents should not be taken by patients with intestinal ulcerations, stenosis, disabling adhesions, or difficulty in swallowing. Nurses should carefully instruct their patients to mix these laxatives with water or drink at least one glassful of liquid. To preclude the potential danger of their becoming lodged in the throat, these drugs should never be chewed or swallowed without water. Allergic reactions (urticaria, dermatitis, bronchial asthma) have been reported after their use. These drugs may bind salicylates, digitalis glycosides, and nitrofurantoin, thus impairing their absorption.

Emollient laxatives (Lubricants)

Mineral oil is the most important member of this class that is used as a laxative (Table 56-3); glycerin suppositories are sometimes classified as emollients. It has been suggested that mineral oil acts by softening the fecal material by retarding the absorption of water from the intestinal lumen. It may also act by coating the mucosal lining and fecal material, thus facilitating the "smooth" movement of the latter down the bowel.

This drug is recommended for use in those conditions in which straining during defecation is to be avoided, for example, after abdominal surgery, hernia, aneurysm, stroke, and myocardial infarction, and to prevent tearing of hemorrhoids or further laceration of fissures.

Precautions   In most patients, pruritis ani and anal leakage of oil are annoying side effects that cause discomfort and delay healing after rectal or anal surgery; granulomas may form at the site of healing wounds. Chronic administration of mineral oil (more than 2 weeks) may *decrease the absorption of food and fat-soluble vitamins* (A, D, E, and K), potentially resulting in a nutritional deficiency. Administration with meals should be avoided. Mineral oil is contraindicated during pregnancy because it can reduce the availability of vitamin K to the fetus; moreover, studies conducted in rodents suggest that this drug is carcinogenic. Severely debilitated patients and those receiving anticoagulants should not be given mineral oil. This emollient should not be co-administered with the dioctyl sulfosuccinates because of the danger of enhanced toxicity of the oil.

Lipoid pneumonia, caused by the use of nose drops with an oil base, may also result from the oral ingestion and subsequent aspiration of mineral oil. The elderly, infants, and debilitated patients are particularly at risk, especially when the oil is taken at bedtime. Chronic aspiration of even small amounts of mineral oil may cause tissue reactions.

Fecal softeners (Wetting agents)

The *dioctyl sulfosuccinates* (Table 56-3) soften the stool by lowering the surface tension, thus permitting the fecal mass to be penetrated by intestinal fluids. In addition to this surfactant effect, these drugs are thought to produce their laxative effects by inhibiting fluid and electrolyte absorption by the intestines. In recent studies they have been found to produce mucosal injury and epithelial cell toxicity.

The surfactant laxatives are employed for conditions in which straining at defecation is to be avoided, for example, after myocardial infarction or surgery of the rectum or anus or in postpartum patients. These drugs require 1 to 2 days to exert their full effects.

Precautions   Diarrhea is the only reported adverse effect associated with the use of these drugs. Dioctyl sulfosuccinates are often combined in commercial preparations with other laxatives, a practice that has little therapeutic justification and is potentially dangerous. The surfactant properties tend to enhance the systemic absorption of other drugs (such as mineral oil), which may lead to an exaggerated laxative effect and greater toxicity, to the liver in particular. Their use with mineral oil is contraindicated.

DIARRHEA

Diarrhea is the abnormally frequent passage of watery stools. Acute episodes of diarrhea are generally self-limiting and require little, if any, therapeutic intervention. In other situations, such as cholera or infantile diarrhea, immediate diagnosis and effective treatment are essential to avoid excessive electrolyte losses and dehydration. Chronic diarrhea is associated with certain inflammatory bowel diseases, radiation therapy to the abdominal area, and surgical removal of various segments of the bowel.

Causes of Diarrhea

Acute diarrhea may arise from many causes, including infectious organisms (usually bacterial in adults and viral in infants and young children); traveler's diarrhea, resulting from exposure (usually in foods and drinks) to a markedly different population of microbes; and foods that are excessively spicy or fatty or that contain a high percentage of roughage.

Diarrhea is a side effect that commonly occurs after drug administration. *Antibiotic-induced* diarrhea, the severity of which varies with the specific antibiotic used, is relatively common. Diarrhea caused by the first few doses of a drug can generally be attributed to the mild irritating properties of the drug, while diarrhea appearing days after the initiation of therapy usually results from antibiotic disruption of the normal intestinal flora. Alterations in the microbial population of the gut, with the development of *superinfections*, most commonly occurs after the administration of ampicillin, the tetracyclines, and other broad-spectrum antibiotics (Chapter 41).

Drugs that alter the autonomic control of intestinal motility, such as cholinergic agents and antihypertensive drugs (reserpine, guanethidine, methyldopa), may induce diarrhea. Diarrhea is also commonly associated with the use of colchicine, para-aminosalicylic acid, neomycin, lincomycin, clindamycin, and antacids containing magnesium.

Drug Treatment of Diarrhea

Diarrhea is a symptom, and its management should not be interpreted as a cure for its underlying cause. Antidiarrheal agents may provide only nonspecific symptomatic relief, while others (for example, drugs with antimicrobial or antiparasitic activity) act against its cause. In this chapter, we shall consider the three most commonly used classes of nonspecific antidiarrheal agents, namely, the opiates, anticholinergics, and adsorbents (Table 56-4); serotonin antagonists are used for the treatment of carcinoid. Nursing implications associated with the treatment of diarrhea are summarized at the end of this chapter.

Opiates Opium has been used for many centuries for the treatment of diarrhea and dysentery (Chapter 20). *Paregoric* (camphorated opium tincture) and other antidiarrheal products containing opium are generally considered to be safe and highly effective at the normally prescribed doses.

The abuse potential of the natural opiates is low when they are used for the treatment of acute diarrhea; the doses employed are low (and considerably less than analgesic doses) and not sufficiently well-absorbed after oral administration to cause alterations in mood. Chronic use of such drugs, such as for the management of ulcerative colitis, increases the risk of development of an opiate-dependent state.

Morphine, the active antidiarrheal ingredient in opium, reduces the rate of transit of chyme through the small intestines and colon. This effect has been attributed to the ability of morphine to inhibit effective peristaltic movements or to an increase in the circular smooth muscle tone of the intestines.

Diphenoxylate, a compound chemically related to meperidine (Demerol), is a highly effective antidiarrheal drug. The combina-

Table 56-4   Representative Antidiarrheal Agents

Generic name (synonym)	Selected trade names	Usual adult oral dose	Remarks
Opiates			Opium products are safe and effective; low abuse liability in antidiarrheal doses. Chronic use should be avoided.
Paregoric (Camphorated opium tincture)		5-10 ml, 1-4 times daily	Contains equivalent of 2 mg morphine per 5 ml and 45% alcohol.
Diphenoxylate (2.5 mg) with Atropine (0.025 mg)	Lomotil	5 mg q.i.d.	Very effective. Atropine added to prevent abuse. May cause respiratory depression in young children; reverse with narcotic antagonist.
Loperamide	Imodium	4 mg stat, then 2 mg after each unformed stool; daily dose not over 16 mg	Similar to diphenoxylate but few CNS effects; more potent, rapid onset, and longer duration of action. Improvement usually within 48 h.
Anticholinergics			Effective only at doses equivalent to 0.6-1 mg atropine sulfate. Narrow margin of safety.
Homatropine methylbromide		5 mg q.i.d.	More selective on gastrointestinal tract than atropine. Few CNS effects.
Adsorbents			
Kaolin and Pectin	*Kaopectate, Pargel*		Safe but not demonstrated effective antidiarrheal agent.
Polycarbophil		1 g q.i.d.	Safe and effective antidiarrheal.
Bismuth salts	Pepto-Bismol		Proof of effectiveness is lacking.
Lactobacillus organisms	Bacid, Lactinex		Proof of effectiveness is lacking.

tion of diphenoxylate and atropine is marketed as Lomotil. Atropine has been included at low doses to discourage diphenoxylate abuse; use of excessive doses of Lomotil will cause atropine-like side effects. This product has a low abuse potential and is preferred for the management of chronic diarrhea. High doses may cause respiratory depression and enhancement of other central depressants.

Loperamide (Imodium) is a recently introduced drug with diphenoxylate-like properties. It is more potent, has a longer duration of action, and causes less central depression than diphenoxylate.

Anticholinergic agents The use of anticholinergic agents for the treatment of diarrhea is based upon their ability to reduce intestinal smooth muscle tone and decrease the motility of the intestinal tract. The use of effective doses of these drugs, equivalent to 0.6 mg to 1 mg of atropine, is associated with a high incidence of side effects. Anticholinergic agents have a narrow margin of safety, especially in young children.

Adsorbents The adsorbents are the most commonly used class of antidiarrheal agents in nonprescription products. Adsorption is not specific. Drugs possessing this action not only adsorb toxins, bacteria, and other noxious materials that are responsible for causing diarrhea, but also nutrients, digestive enzymes, and orally administered drugs (lincomycin, cardiac glycosides, alkaloids, certain vitamins).

Generally taken as liquid suspensions, a dose is taken after each loose bowel movement until the diarrhea is controlled; large doses must be administered over short periods of time. The most widely employed adsorbents (kaolin, pectin, attapulgite, bismuth salts) are generally considered to be safe when used as directed; however, proof of their clinical effectiveness has not been established.

Serotonin antagonists Serotonin (5-hydroxytryptamine) is present in high concentrations in the gastrointestinal tract, mainly in enterochromaffin cells. It has been suggested, but not established, that serotonin is involved in the regulation of peristalsis. Tumors of the enterochromaffin cells (*carcinoid tumor*) release large amounts of serotonin and cause severe colic and diarrhea. The diarrhea associated with the carcinoid syndrome is well controlled with serotonin antagonists such as methysergide (Sansert) and cyproheptadine (Periactin); these drugs are more commonly employed for the management of migrane (Chapter 38) and itching (Chapter 53), respectively.

Laxatives and Antidiarrheal Drugs
nursing implications

Laxatives

1. Difficult or infrequent passage of stools is a very common symptom with many possible causes. Treatment must be determined by its etiology and individualized according to the age, physical condition, and preference of the patient.

2. Explain to patients the normal physiology of elimination and clarify any misconceptions. Advise the patient that a daily bowel movement is not essential for good health, and that normal frequency may vary among individuals from 2-3 times daily to 2-3 times per week.

3. When no organic pathology is present, dietary measures should be employed as the initial approach in the treatment of constipation. Encourage the patient to increase intake of bulk-forming foods such as fruits, vegetables, and whole grain cereals. Advise the patient to increase physical activity within the limits imposed by his or her physical condition. An upright position and mild to moderate exercise enhances peristalsis. Encourage the patient to reactivate awareness of distension of the colon and attempt to defecate in response to the defecation reflex; this reflex is most active after meals, especially breakfast.

4. Advise patients who experience a sudden change in bowel patterns or abdominal pain to contact their physician rather than self-medicate.

5. When a laxative is required, administer medication at a time when it will not interfere with the patient's digestion or absorption of nutrients.

6. Plan medication administration to allow the drug's effects to occur at a time that will not interfere with the patient's rest.

7. Administer castor oil in a palatable vehicle such as orange juice.

8. Encourage fluid intake when this enhances drug effectiveness, such as with bulk-forming laxatives.

9. Prior to drug administration inform the patient that drugs such as anthraquinones may change the color of urine.

Antidiarrheal Agents

1. Diarrhea may be a minor problem which is appropriately self-medicated. It may also be a symptom of a serious disease; self-medication, in this case, may mask the problem delaying diagnosis and effective treatment. Diarrhea is always a potentially serious problem in infants and young children and should not be self-medicated; severe dehydration may develop in the young patient in a short period of time.

2. Diarrhea accompanies many medical disorders and is treated according to the underlying etiology. Diarrhea may be a self-limiting natural defense mechanism by which the drug rids itself of a toxic or irritating substance.

3. Prolonged diarrhea can result in dehydration and electrolyte imbalance. Symptomatic treatment with antidiarrheal agents may prevent these complications.

4. Observe patients receiving Lomotil and other narcotics or barbiturates for additive CNS depression. Have naloxone (Narcan) available in the event of overdosage.

5. Opium tincture and paregoric are included in the Controlled Substances Act and must, therefore, be recorded in the narcotics book. Measure the dose accurately and administer in water. Opium tincture contains 25 times more morphine than paregoric. Observe patients receiving these drugs for prolonged periods for signs of physical dependence.

6. Teach the patient the expected effects of these drugs; when drug should be taken and when discontinued to avoid constipation; and to keep these drugs out of reach of children.

7. Instruct the patient about dietary modifications. Food is usually withheld or restricted to clear liquids such as broth, bouillon, weak tea, ginger ale, or gelatin for 24 h to reduce bowel stimulation. Bland diet is then added with progression to regular diet as tolerated.

SUPPLEMENTARY READINGS

Binder, H. J., "Pharmacology of Laxatives," *Annual Review of Pharmacology and Toxicology* 17: 355–67 (1977).

Black, C. D., N. G. Popovich, and M. C. Black, "Drug Interactions in the GI Tract," *American Journal of Nursing* 77: 1426–29 (1977).

Darlington, R. C., "Laxative Products," in *Handbook of Nonprescription Drugs* (6th ed.), pp. 37–54. Washington, D.C.: American Pharmaceutical Association, 1979.

Gaginella, T. S., "Management of Gastrointestinal Disorders. Part II. Use and Misuse of Laxatives," *Journal of Continuing Education in Pharmacy* 2(2): 19–28, 53–54 (1978).

Gaginella, T. S., "Management of Gastrointestinal Disease. Part III. Diarrheal Disease and Antidiarrheal Therapy," *Journal of Continuing Education in Pharmacy* **2**(3): 41–51 (1978).

Gaginella, T. S., and P. Bass, "Laxatives: an Update on Mechanism of Action," *Life Sciences* **23**: 1001–10 (1978).

Longe, R. L., "Antidiarrheal and Other Gastrointestinal Products," in *Handbook of Nonprescription Drugs* (6th ed.), pp. 25–36. Washington, D.C.: American Pharmaceutical Association, 1979.

Pietrusko, R. G., "Use and Abuse of Laxatives," *American Journal of Hospital Pharmacy* **34**: 291–300 (1977).

Section IX

TOXICOLOGY

Chapter 57

TREATMENT OF ACUTE POISONING

Toxicology is the study of poisons and includes consideration of their biological actions and effects, procedures for detecting their presence, and treatment of the poisoned patient. Poisons can be therapeutic agents, compounds employed in the household or industrial setting, or chemicals present in the air, water, or food.

Acute poisoning, whether accidental, suicidal, or criminal in nature represents a major problem in the United States. In 1976 the National Clearinghouse for Poison Control Centers processed 147,277 reports of poisoning throughout the United States. Reliable estimates suggest that there are actually ten times this number of poisonings

each year and, of these, over 3,000 result in fatalities; one-fourth to one-third of these deaths occur in children under 5 years of age.

ROLE OF THE NURSE

By virtue of their unique training and experience, nurses can play a significant role in the prevention of accidental poisonings and the administration of immediate assistance until the patient is treated by experts in this area.

Nurses should actively educate the parents of young children to lock up all potentially toxic chemicals or, if this is not possible, keep such materials out of the reach of their children. Outdated or unused medications and household products should be discarded. The five most common categories of products ingested in 1976 by children under 5 years of age, in descending order of frequency, were: plants (excluding mushrooms and toadstools); soaps, detergents, and cleaners; vitamins and minerals; aspirin; and antihistamines and cold medicines. It is significant to note that most of the accidental ingestions and fatalities in young children do not involve substances that their parents would traditionally classify as poisons.

Parents should not be misled by using adult standards of palatability to predict the types of materials that their children will ingest. Young children will eat almost anything, regardless of its taste or caustic nature. By contrast, when administering medication to children, parents should be admonished not to call it "candy" in an attempt to encourage an unwilling child to ingest it.

When poisoning is suspected, the nurse should immediately contact a physician or the local poison control center to obtain expert advise on treatment procedures that are advised or contraindicated. Steps should be initiated promptly thereafter to remove the poison from contact with the patient. The nurse should attempt to determine the identity of the poison (usually found on the label of the container), the quantity ingested, and the estimated period of time that has elapsed between the suspected poisoning and notification of the nurse or other health professional.

In the absence of observing the patient ingest the poison or finding an empty container nearby, poison identification may largely depend upon the signs or symptoms manifested by the patient. The nurse should look for burns about the mouth, injection marks, skin rashes, or alterations in the normal function of the respiratory, cardiovascular, or nervous systems. Since chemical analysis of vomitus, urine, or stools may be of subsequent diagnostic or medicolegal significance, the nurse should safeguard such specimens.

TREATMENT OF ACUTE POISONING

The primary rule for the first-aid treatment of acute poisoning is to *remove the poison from contact with the patient* (unless this is contraindicated) and to *secure expert medical assistance at the earliest possible moment.* Supportive measures such as maintenance of breathing by instituting artificial respiration, are often essential for the survival of the comatose patient. Poisoning commonly results from local exposure to or ingestion of the toxic substance.

Local Exposure

Various chemicals, in particular acids and alkalis, are toxic to the skin, eyes, and mucous membranes. In most instances injury results from direct irritation of the affected area, although some chemicals are capable of producing systemic toxicity after transcutaneous absorption (for example, chlorinated or organophosphate (anticholinesterase) insecticides or those insecticides containing nicotine (Black Leaf 40)).

Materials spilled on the *skin* are best removed by washing with large volumes of water, using soap if available. Vinegar (acetic acid) or baking soda (sodium bicarbonate) can be used to neutralize alkalis (lye) and acids, respectively.

Exposure of the *eye* to caustic chemicals can cause chemical burns to the cornea and conjunctiva. The eye should be gently washed with very large volumes of water for at least 5 minutes, with the eyelids held open during this time. Contact lenses, if worn, should be removed. The patient should not be permitted to rub the eyes. In all cases, an ophthalmologist should be contacted without delay.

Oral Ingestion

Oral ingestion of poison may result in injury to the mucous membranes of the gastrointestinal tract or systemic toxicity after absorption. Treatment approaches include removal of the poison from the stomach (by inducing emesis or employing gastric lavage), inactivation of the poison (using local or systemic antidotes), or by hastening its elimination from the body.

Emptying the stomach

Emesis Removal of poisons from the stomach can be most effectively carried out by inducing emesis, and this is often the treatment of choice. Compared with gastric lavage, emesis is more rapid, less traumatic to the patient, more efficient in emptying the stomach and duodenum, and more convenient to perform.

Induction of emesis and gastric lavage are *contraindicated* in patients experiencing seizures or after ingestion of a strong acid or alkali (risk of further corrosive damage to the esophagus with possible perforation) or petroleum distillates such as gasoline, kerosene, and cleaning fluids (risk of aspiration of the vomitus). In addition, emesis should not be attempted in patients who are comatose or unconscious (risk of aspiration of vomitus), who are in late pregnancy (risk of inducing a spontaneous abortion), or who have a history of cardiac disease.

Vomiting can be induced by mechanical stimulation or with emetic agents. These processes will not be effective if the stomach is empty and, therefore, the patient should be given 1 or 2 glassfuls of water prior to induction of emesis. Gagging may be accomplished by tickling the back of the throat with a finger or a spoon handle. Unfortunately, mechanical stimulation induces vomiting in only a relatively small percentage of patients, and the volume of vomitus is low when compared to that induced by chemical methods.

Syrup of ipecac is a highly effective emetic; it can be obtained at pharmacies at low cost, without a prescription, and in 1-ounce quantities. Nurses should encourage all families with young children to have this drug readily available in their homes in the event of an emergency. This *syrup* should never be confused with ipecac *fluidextract* which is fourteen times as strong and potentially toxic.

The syrup is about 90 percent effective in inducing emesis within 30 minutes, with an average induction time of 20 minutes. In children over one year of age, the recommended dose is 15 ml (1 tablespoon) followed by a glassful of water. This dose may be repeated in 15 to 20 minutes if emesis has not occurred. Since physical activity enhances drug effectiveness, the patient should be encouraged to move around until emesis occurs.

Apomorphine, a direct stimulant of the chemoreceptor trigger zone in the medulla, usually acts within 3 to 5 minutes after its subcutaneous injection. The emesis induced by this drug is more violent and complete than with ipecac syrup. Since this drug is only effective after parenteral administration, it is not suitable for inclusion in a first-aid kit in the home.

This morphine derivative is a depressant of the central nervous system that should be used with extreme caution when the ingested poison is also a central depressant. Narcotic antagonists, such as naloxone (Narcan), at a dose of 0.01 mg/kg, may be used to terminate the protracted emesis often induced by apomorphine, as well as to reverse its depression of the central nervous system. The usual subcutaneous dose of apomorphine is 5 mg in adults and 0.066 mg/kg in children. If two doses fail to induce vomiting, no additional doses should be given. This drug is unstable at room temperature and must be refrigerated; a green or brown colored solution indicates that the drug has decomposed and should not be used.

Substances such as copper sulfate, zinc sulfate, and antimony potassium tartrate (tarter emetic) are inherently toxic compounds and are not recommended for use as emetic agents. Mustard water (prepared from dry mustard powder) is relatively ineffective and unpalatable but may be used in an emergency if ipecac syrup is unavailable.

Gastric lavage This procedure is employed to remove unabsorbed poisons from the upper gastrointestinal tract and is most useful in comatose, hysterical, or otherwise uncooperative patients. Lavage may be lifesaving and is indicated within 2 to 4 hours after the ingestion of most poisons, except as noted above; its effectiveness decreases with increasing periods of time after ingestion.

Prior to initiating lavage, the patient should be encouraged to drink a glassful of water; dentures and other objects should be removed from the mouth. The lavage tube is gently passed into the stomach, and the stomach contents aspirated prior to the introduction of the lavage fluid or local antidote. Lavaging with about 250 ml of fluid (in adults) should be repeated until the washings are clear. Tap water is commonly used as a lavaging fluid in adults, while in children a normal saline solution or diluted saline solution (one-half dilution) is preferred. In some cases, when the identity of the poison is known, specific lavage fluids are used to inactivate or neutralize the unabsorbed poison (Table 57-1).

Inactivation of poison Antidotes may antagonize poisons by their local or systemic actions.

Local antidotes A local antidote acts by chemically neutralizing poisons remaining in the gastrointestinal tract or physically combining with toxins, by the process of adsorption, thereby preventing or retarding their absorption. Commonly employed local antidotes are given in Table 57-1.

Activated charcoal is a highly effective adsorbent of a large number of poisons. This odorless, tasteless, fine, black powder is quite effective against most organic and inorganic compounds, with the notable exception of cyanide; moreover, it is not very useful in antagonizing the toxic effects of ethanol, methanol, caustic alkalis, and mineral acids. The dose of charcoal used should be at least five times and up to ten times the weight of the ingested poison. It is generally administered as a freshly mixed slurry in water (to the consistancy of thick soup) and should never be swallowed dry.

If both activated charcoal and syrup of ipecac are to be administered to the patient, it is advisable to induce vomiting with ipecac prior to giving charcoal. If charcoal is taken prior to or concurrent with ipecac, it will adsorb the ipecac and thereby block its emetic effects.

The long-advocated "universal antidote," consisting of activated charcoal, tannic acid, and magnesium oxide, is now discredited and should not be used. The last two ingredients lack effectiveness and may even interfere with the beneficial effects of activated charcoal.

Table 57-1 **Locally Acting Antidotes Against Selected Unabsorbed Poisons**

Poison	Antidote	Mechanism of action
Acids, corrosive[a]	Antacid or weak alkali (milk of magnesia).	Neutralization of acid.
Alkalis, caustic (lye)[a]	Weak acid (lemon juice or diluted vinegar).	Neutralization of alkali.
Alkaloids	Potassium permanganate, 1:10,000 (lavage).	Oxidation and inactivation.
Nicotine		
Physostigmine		
Quinine		
Strychnine	———	
Aspirin	Activated charcoal (lavage).	Adsorption, retards absorption.
Arsenic	Protein (milk, egg white).	Adsorption, retards absorption.
Cyanide	Sodium thiosulfate, 5% (lavage).	Precipitation.
Detergents	Soap.	Inactivation.
Fluoride	Calcium (milk, lime water, calcium gluconate or lactate).	Precipitation.
Glutethimide (Doriden)	Castor oil: water, 1:1 (lavage)	Adsorption, retards absorption.
Hydrocarbons[a]	Mineral oil, followed by lavage with sodium bicarbonate, 1-2%.	Slows absorption.
Gasoline		
Kerosene		
Cleaning fluids		
Paint thinner		
Iodine	Starch or flour slurry in water.	Inactivation.
Iron	Sodium bicarbonate, 1% (lavage).	Forms insoluble iron carbonate.
	Deferoxamine, 5-8 g in 50 ml water.	Iron chelation.
Mercury and salts	Sodium formaldehyde sulfoxylate, 5% (lavage) or protein (milk, egg white).	Precipitation.
Methanol	Sodium bicarbonate, 3% (lavage).	Neutralization.
Phenol (carbolic acid)	Vegetable oil (olive or castor) (lavage).	Slows absorption.
Propoxyphene (Darvon)	Activated charcoal in water (lavage).	Adsorption, retards absorption.
Sodium hypochlorite (laundry bleach)	Sodium thiosulfate, 2.5% (lavage).	Inactivation.
Tricyclic anti-depressants	Activated charcoal in water (lavage).	Adsorption, retards absorption.
Unknown	Activated charcoal in water (lavage).	Adsorption, retards adsorption.

[a]Avoid inducing emesis or use of gastric lavage.

Systemic antidotes Compounds in this category act systemically by specifically neutralizing the poison or by antagonizing its effects. This antagonism may be pharmacological (competition for common receptor sites) or physiological (producing an effect that is opposite to that caused by the poison). Examples of specific antidotes to heavy metals and other poisons are given in Tables 57-2 and 57-3, respectively.

Hastening poison elimination Relatively few specific and highly effective systemic antagonists for poisons are currently available. One widely adopted approach in the management of acute poisoning involves enhancement of the urinary elimination of the toxic substance.

Ion trapping You will recall from Chapter 2 that most drugs are chemically

Table 57-2 Antidotes to Heavy Metal Poisons

Generic name (synonym)	Trade name	Useful in poisoning by	Dose	Remarks
Dimercaprol (British Anti-Lewisite)	BAL in oil	Arsenic, gold, mercury; antimony, bismuth, thalium may be useful.	IM: 2.5-5 mg/kg q. 4 h on day 1, thereafter 2.5 mg/kg q. 4-6 h	Potentially dangerous. May cause hypertension, tachycardia, nausea, vomiting, abscesses at injection site; fever in children.
Calcium Disodium Edetate	Calcium Disodium Versenate	Lead.	IV infusion: adults up to 50 mg/kg/day; children up to 33 mg/kg/day in 2 divided doses for 3-5 days. Dilute drug in 250-500 ml.	Adverse effects include fever, malaise, fatigue, thirst, chills.
Penicillamine	Cuprimine	Copper; also lead, gold, mercury.	PO: 1 g (up to 5 g) daily in 4 divided doses.	Primary use for copper removal in treatment of Wilson's disease. Useful for long-term treatment of lead poisoning. Low incidence side effects: skin, blood, kidney disorders.
Deferoxamine Mesylate	Desferal	Iron (should not be used in mild cases).	IV or IM: 500 mg twice at 4-h intervals, then 500 mg q. 4-12 h.	Pain and induration at site of injection. Flushing, gastrointestinal disturbances, muscle spasms, tachycardia, allergic reactions. Contraindicated in severe renal impairment.

Table 57-3   **Systemic Antagonists for Selected Poisons**

Poison	Antidote	Mechanism of action
Amphetamines	Chlorpromazine (25–50 mg, IM), or haloperidol (2.5–5 mg, IM);	Receptor blockade (behavioral effects).
	Propranolol (1–2 mg, IV).	Receptor blockade (peripheral adrenergic effects).
Anticholinergics Antidepressants, tricyclics	Physostigmine (1–4 mg IV).	Receptor blockade.
Anticholinesterases (organophosphates)	Pralidoxime (Protopam) (25–50 mg/kg, IV, repeat in 12 h)	Cholinesterase reactivation.
	Atropine (1–4 mg, IM or IV, repeated at 30-min intervals).	Muscarinic receptor blockade.
Carbon monoxide	Oxygen (inhalation).	Hastens carboxyhemoglobin breakdown.
Cholinergics	Atropine (as above) [NOT Pralidoxime].	Muscarinic receptor blockade.
Cyanide	Amyl nitrate inhalation, sodium nitrite (300–500 mg, IV).	Iron in formed methemoglobin competes with cyanide for cytochromes.
	Sodium thiosulfate (50 ml of 20–50% sol., slow IV).	Inactivates cyanide by forming thiocyanate.
Metals (see Table 57-2)		
Methanol	Ethanol (60 ml initially, then 9 ml hourly for 4 days).	Slows formation of toxic products.
	Sodium bicarbonate (5 mEq/kg, IV).	Corrects acidosis.
Narcotics and derivatives, propoxyphene	Naloxone (0.4 mg, IV), repeat after 5–10 min PRN.	Receptor antagonism.
Strychnine	Diazepam (2–10 mg, IV).	Controls convulsions.

weak acids or weak bases, and that only the nonionized forms of these molecules are capable of crossing such cell membranes as the kidney tubules and being reabsorbed.

The degree of ionization and subsequent excretion of acidic drugs can be markedly enhanced by alkalinizing the urine to pH 8 by administering sodium bicarbonate or lactate or tromethamine (Tham); examples of such acidic drugs include the salicylates and barbiturates (phenobarbital). Conversely, acidifying the urine to pH 4 with ammonium chloride, ascorbic acid, or arginine hydrochloride increases the urinary excretion of such basic drugs as the amphetamines and antihistamines.

Forced diuresis   Administration of large volumes of fluids orally or intravenously causes water diuresis but does not significantly enhance the elimination of the poison. *Osmotic diuresis*, induced by mannitol or urea, is far more effective in removing a toxic substance than water. Still more effective, and widely employed, is the regimen that combines the use of an osmotic diuretic with a chemical that alters the pH of the urine. This method has been demonstrated to reduce barbiturate-induced coma by two-thirds when compared with patients not so treated.

Dialysis   In the dialysis procedure, undesirable compounds in the blood are allowed to diffuse across a semipermeable membrane into a solution of known composition (dialysate). Continuous or regular replacement of the dialysate promotes the most effective diffusion of the poison out of the blood.

Two basic types of dialysis are employed, namely, extracorporeal hemodialysis (the artificial kidney) and peritoneal dialysis. Dialysis procedures are most useful when normal kidney function fails or is insufficient, or when, in the absence of the rapid reduction of body poison levels, the patient will die. Not all drugs and poisons are dialyzable; strongly plasma-protein bound compounds are not efficiently removed by these procedures.

Peritoneal dialysis can be performed in almost any hospital setting and is particularly useful for the treatment of infants and young children. It is simple and does not require elaborate equipment, and hospital personnel need not receive extensive training to safely perform this procedure.

Extracorporeal dialysis is five to ten times more efficient than peritoneal dialysis in removing poisons from the body but requires expensive equipment and highly trained and experienced operators to minimize the adverse reactions that are often associated with this procedure. The use of oil dialysates has been reported to be useful in treating poisonings produced by highly lipid-soluble drugs such as glutethimide (Doriden).

Supportive care Even when specific antidotes or other procedures are available for the treatment of acute poisoning, good supportive nursing care remains essential for the survival and well-being of the patient. Attention should always be focused upon maintaining respiration; managing hypotension, arrhythmias, and other cardiovascular complications; preventing shock; replacing fluid and electrolyte losses; monitoring kidney and liver function; and managing excessive central nervous system stimulation. The position of comatose or stuporous patients should be changed periodically to prevent the development of pneumonitis.

Treatment of Acute Poisoning:
nursing implications

Education

1. Educating the patient, family, and general public about measures needed to prevent accidental poisoning is an extremely important nursing function.
2. Information about poison control centers should be made available to everyone. Instruct the public to post the telephone number of the local poison control center with other emergency numbers. A national network of poison control centers can be contacted at any hour, day or night, for information about potential poisons. The center maintains a computer bank of data about potentially poisonous ingredients of products commonly used in the home.
3. All potentially harmful substances, with the contents clearly labeled, should be stored out of the reach of children.
4. Medications intended for oral use should be kept in a separate area from drugs intended for external use and from poisons.

5. Parents should be discouraged from telling children that medication is candy in order to persuade them to take it.

6. Drugs should never be taken in the dark. Older patients may need reminding to always read the label carefully.

7. Old or unused drugs should be disposed of in the toilet rather than the trash, where children can find them.

8. Caution individuals against transferring drugs or chemicals into other containers, especially those indicating that they contain other substances.

9. Families with young children should be advised not to grow plants that contain potentially harmful substances.

General Nursing Intervention

1. When poisoning is suspected, the physician or poison control center should be contacted immediately to determine the treatment advised or contraindicated.

2. Essential information to be obtained: identification of poison; quantity ingested; time elapsed since ingestion; symptoms the patient is experiencing.

3. Use appropriate measures, such as gastric lavage, induced emesis, and washing eyes or skin, to remove as much poison as possible. Administer antidote if available.

4. When emesis begins, place the face of patient down with head lower than hips to prevent aspiration of vomitus.

5. Provide supportive care to maintain vital functions.

SUPPLEMENTARY READINGS

Arena, J. M., *Poisoning: Toxicology, Symptoms and Treatment* (4th ed.). Springfield, Ill.: Charles C Thomas, Publishers, 1979.

Coleman, A. B., and J. J. Alpert, ed., "Poisoning in Children," *Pediatric Clinics of North America* **17:** 471–758 (1970).

Cooper, P., *Poisoning by Drugs and Chemicals* (3rd ed.). London: Thomas Waide & Sons, 1974.

Doull, J., C. D. Klaasen, and M. O. Amdur, ed., *Casarett and Doull's Toxicology: The Basic Science of Poisons*, 2nd ed. New York: Macmillan, Inc., 1980.

Driesbach, R. H., *Handbook of Poisoning: Diagnosis and Treatment* (9th ed.). Los Altos, Calif.: Lange Medical Publications, 1977.

Gosselin, R. E., H. G. Hodge, R. P. Smith, and M. N. Gleason, *Clinical Toxicology of Commercial Products* (4th ed.). Baltimore: The Williams & Wilkins Company, 1976.

Kaye, S., *Handbook of Emergency Toxicology* (4th ed.). Springfield, Ill.: Charles C Thomas Publishing, 1977.

Loomis, T. A., *Essentials of Toxicology* (3rd ed.). Philadelphia: Lea & Febiger, 1978.

Thienes, C. H., and T. J. Haley, *Clinical Toxicology* (5th ed.). Philadelphia: Lea & Febiger, 1972.

Tong, T. G., "Poisoning and Its Treatment," *Nurse Practitioner* **2**(2): 35–36 (1976), **2**(3): 29–32 (1977).

Index

525